The American Psychiatric Press

Textbook of Geriatric Psychiatry

Second Edition

Edited by

EWALD W. BUSSE, M.D.
AND
DAN G. BLAZER, M.D., PH.D.

The American Psychiatric Press

Textbook of Geriatric Psychiatry

Second Edition

Edited by

EWALD W. BUSSE, M.D.
AND
DAN G. BLAZER, M.D., PH.D.

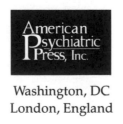

American Psychiatric Press, Inc.

Washington, DC
London, England

Note: The authors have worked to ensure that all information in this book concerning drug dosages, schedules, and routes of administration is accurate as of the time of publication and consistent with standards set by the U.S. Food and Drug Administration and the general medical community. As medical research and practice advance, however, therapeutic standards may change. For this reason and because human and mechanical errors sometimes occur, we recommend that readers follow the advice of a physician who is directly involved in their care or the care of a member of their family.

Books published by the American Psychiatric Press, Inc., represent the views and opinions of the individual authors and do not necessarily represent the policies and opinions of the Press or the American Psychiatric Association.

Copyright © 1996 American Psychiatric Press, Inc.
ALL RIGHTS RESERVED
Manufactured in the United States of America on acid-free paper
99 98 97 96   4 3 2 1
First Edition

American Psychiatric Press, Inc.
1400 K Street, N.W., Washington, DC   20005

Library of Congress Cataloging-in-Publication Data
The American psychiatric press textbook of geriatric psychiatry / [edited by] Ewald W. Busse and Dan G. Blazer. — 2nd ed.
     p.   cm.
   ISBN 0-88048-713-5
   1. Geriatric psychiatry. I. Busse, Ewald W., 1917- . II. Blazer, Dan G. (Dan German) 1944-
    [DNLM: 1. Geriatric Psychiatry. 2. Mental Disorders—in old age.   WT 150 A5124 1995]
RC451.4.A5A518   1995
618.97′689—dc20
DNLM/DLC
for Library of Congress
                                                    95-33558
                                                     CIP

British Library Cataloguing in Publication Data
A CIP record is available from the British Library.

Contents

Contributors ix

Preface xi
Ewald W. Busse, M.D.
Dan G. Blazer, M.D., Ph.D.

The Basic Science of Geriatric Psychiatry

1 The Myth, History, and Science of Aging 3
   Ewald W. Busse, M.D.

2 Physiological and Clinical Considerations of the Geriatric Patient 25
   John W. Rowe, M.D.
   Cathryn A. J. Devons, M.D., M.P.H.

3 Perceptual Changes With Aging 49
   Gail R. Marsh, Ph.D.

4 Neuroanatomy and Neuropathology of Aging 61
   F. Stephen Vogel, M.D.

5 Chemical Messengers 73
   Garth Bissette, Ph.D.

6 Genetics and Geriatric Psychiatry 95
   Ewald W. Busse, M.D.
   Dan G. Blazer, M.D., Ph.D.

7 Psychological Aspects of Normal Aging 105
   Ilene C. Siegler, Ph.D., M.P.H.
   Leonard W. Poon, Ph.D.
   David J. Madden, Ph.D.
   Kathleen A. Welsh, Ph.D.

8 Social and Economic Factors Related to Psychiatric Disorders in Late Life 129
   Linda K. George, Ph.D.

9 Epidemiology of Psychiatric Disorders in Late Life 155
   Dan G. Blazer, M.D., Ph.D.

The Diagnostic Interview in Late Life

10 The Psychiatric Interview of the Geriatric Patient 175
Dan G. Blazer, M.D., Ph.D.

11 Use of the Laboratory in the Diagnostic Workup of Older Adults 191
Dan G. Blazer, M.D., Ph.D.
Ewald W. Busse, M.D.
W. Edward Craighead, Ph.D.
Donald D. Evans, Ph.D.

Psychiatric Disorders in Late Life

12 Cognitive Disorders 213
Elaine R. Peskind, M.D.
Murray A. Raskind, M.D.

13 Mood Disorders 235
Dan G. Blazer, M.D., Ph.D.
Harold G. Koenig, M.D., M.H.Sc.

14 Schizophrenia and Paranoid Disorders 265
Harold G. Koenig, M.D., M.H.Sc.
Caron Christison, M.D.
George Christison, M.D.
Dan G. Blazer, M.D., Ph.D.

15 Anxiety and Panic Disorders 279
Javaid I. Sheikh, M.D.

16 Somatoform and Psychosexual Disorders 291
Ewald W. Busse, M.D.

17 Bereavement and Adjustment Disorders 313
Dolores Gallagher-Thompson, Ph.D.
Larry W. Thompson, Ph.D.

18 Sleep and Chronobiological Disturbances 329
Thomas C. Neylan, M.D.
Mary G. De May, M.D.
Charles F. Reynolds III, M.D.

19 Alcohol and Drug Problems 341
Dan G. Blazer, M.D., Ph.D.

Treatment of Psychiatric Disorders in Late Life

20   Pharmacological Treatment 359
      Jonathan Davidson, M.D.

21   Diet, Nutrition, and Exercise 381
      Robert J. Sullivan Jr., M.D.

22   Psychotherapy 395
      Keith G. Meador, M.D., M.P.H.
      Claudia D. Davis, R.N., M.S.N.

23   Clinical Psychiatry in the Nursing Home 413
      Joel E. Streim, M.D.
      Ira R. Katz, M.D., Ph.D.

24   The Continuum of Care: Movement Toward the Community 433
      George L. Maddox, Ph.D.
      Karen Steinhauser, M.A.
      Elise Bolda, M.S.P.H., Ph.D.

25   The Past and Future of Geriatric Psychiatry 459
      Ewald W. Busse, M.D.
      Dan G. Blazer. M.D., Ph.D.

      Index 475

Contributors

Garth Bissette, Ph.D.
Professor, Department of Psychiatry and Human Behavior, The University of Mississippi Medical Center, Jackson, Mississippi

Dan G. Blazer, M.D., Ph.D.
J. P. Gibbons Professor of Psychiatry and Dean of Medical Education, Duke University School of Medicine, Durham, North Carolina

Elise Bolda, M.S.P.H., Ph.D.
Consultant, Long Term Care Resources Program, Duke University Medical Center, Durham, North Carolina

Ewald W. Busse, M.D.
J. P. Gibbons Professor of Psychiatry Emeritus and Dean Emeritus, Medical and Allied Health Education, Duke University Medical Center, Durham, North Carolina

Caron Christison, M.D.
Assistant Professor of Psychiatry, Loma Linda University, Loma Linda, California

George Christison, M.D.
Assistant Professor of Psychiatry, Loma Linda University, Loma Linda, California

W. Edward Craighead, Ph.D.
Professor, Affective Disorders Program, Department of Psychiatry, and Professor, Department of Psychology, Duke University Medical Center, Durham, North Carolina

Jonathan Davidson, M.D.
Associate Professor, Division of Outpatient Services, Department of Psychiatry, Duke University Medical Center, Durham, North Carolina

Claudia D. Davis, R.N., M.S.N.
Assistant Professor of the Practice of Nursing, Vanderbilt University School of Nursing, Nashville, Tennessee

Mary G. De May, M.D.
Director of Geropsychiatry, California Pacific Medical Center, San Francisco, California

Cathryn A. J. Devons, M.D., M.P.H.
Assistant Professor, Department of Geriatrics and Adult Development, and Assistant Professor, Department of Medicine, The Mount Sinai Medical Center, New York, New York

Donald D. Evans, Ph.D.
Assistant Professor, Division of Medical Psychology, Department of Psychiatry, Duke University Medical Center, Durham, North Carolina

Dolores Gallagher-Thompson, Ph.D.
Co-Director, Older Adult Center, Department of Veterans Affairs Medical Center; Clinical Associate Professor, Department of Psychiatry and Behavioral Sciences, Stanford University School of Medicine, Palo Alto, California

Linda K. George, Ph.D.
Professor, Division of Social and Community Psychiatry, Department of Psychiatry, and Professor, Department of Sociology, Duke University Medical Center, Durham, North Carolina

Ira R. Katz, M.D., Ph.D.
Professor of Psychiatry, Section on Geriatric Psychiatry, University of Pennsylvania, Philadelphia, Pennsylvania

Harold G. Koenig, M.D., M.H.Sc.
Assistant Clinical Professor, Department of Psychiatry, Duke University Medical Center, Durham, North Carolina

David J. Madden, Ph.D.
Associate Research Professor, Division of Medical Psychology, Department of Psychiatry, Duke University Medical Center, Durham, North Carolina

George L. Maddox, Ph.D.
Professor, Department of Sociology, and Program
Director, Long Term Care Resources Program,
Duke University Medical Center,
Durham, North Carolina

Gail R. Marsh, Ph.D.
Associate Professor of Medical Psychology,
Department of Psychiatry; Associate Professor,
Department of Psychology–Experimental; and
Senior Fellow, Center for the Study of Aging and
Human Development, Duke University Medical
Center, Durham, North Carolina

Keith G. Meador, M.D., M.P.H.
Associate Clinical Professor of Psychiatry,
Duke University Medical Center,
Durham, North Carolina

Thomas C. Neylan, M.D.
Assistant Clinical Professor of Psychiatry,
University of California; Psychiatry Service,
Department of Veterans Affairs Medical Center,
San Francisco, California

Elaine R. Peskind, M.D.
Assistant Professor of Psychiatry and Behavioral
Sciences, University of Washington School of
Medicine, Seattle, Washington

Leonard W. Poon, Ph.D.
Director, Gerontology Center, The University of
Georgia, Athens, Georgia

Murray A. Raskind, M.D.
Professor of Psychiatry and Behavioral Sciences,
University of Washington School of Medicine,
Seattle, Washington

Charles F. Reynolds III, M.D.
Professor of Psychiatry and Neurology,
Department of Psychiatry, University of
Pittsburgh School of Medicine,
Pittsburgh, Pennsylvania

John W. Rowe, M.D.
President, The Mount Sinai Medical Center,
New York, New York

Ilene C. Siegler, Ph.D., M.P.H.
Associate Professor, Division of Medical
Psychology, Department of Psychiatry,
Duke University Medical Center,
Durham, North Carolina

Javaid I. Sheikh, M.D.
Associate Professor of Psychiatry and Director,
Geriatric Psychiatry Program, Department of
Psychiatry and Behavioral Sciences,
Stanford University School of Medicine,
Stanford, California

Karen Steinhauser, M.A.
Research Assistant, Department of Sociology,
Duke University Medical Center,
Durham, North Carolina

Joel E. Streim, M.D.
Assistant Professor of Psychiatry, Section of
Geriatric Psychiatry, Department of Psychiatry,
University of Pennsylvania and Philadelphia VA
Medical Center, Philadelphia, Pennsylvania

Robert J. Sullivan Jr., M.D.
Assistant Professor, Department of Medicine,
and Associate Professor, Department of
Community and Family Medicine,
Duke University Medical Center,
Durham, North Carolina

Larry W. Thompson, Ph.D.
Co-Director, Older Adult Center, Department of
Veterans Affairs Medical Center; Professor of
Medicine (Research), Division of Endocrinology,
Gerontology and Metabolism, Stanford University
School of Medicine, Palo Alto, California

F. Stephen Vogel, M.D.
Secretary-Treasurer and Executive Director,
United States and Canadian Academy of
Pathology, Inc., Augusta, Georgia; Professor
Emeritus of Pathology, Duke University Medical
Center, Durham, North Carolina

Kathleen A. Welsh, Ph.D.
Assistant Professor, Division of Medical
Psychology, Department of Psychiatry,
Duke University Medical Center,
Durham, North Carolina

Preface

The first edition of *Geriatric Psychiatry* was published in 1989. The need for a second edition has become obvious as the rapid expansion of scientific knowledge about aging and the diseases of late life has altered the practice of geriatric psychiatry. *The American Psychiatric Press Textbook of Geriatric Psychiatry,* Second Edition, is designed to provide the scholar and the clinician with the scientific facts and the applied skills and knowledge that are so needed in dealing with mental disorders in late life. Consequently, this volume covers not only the wide range of important mental diseases of late life but also the so-called normal age changes that result in biological and behavioral changes in late life.

The chapters are presented in a sequential and integrated fashion, which we hope will enhance the accessibility and usefulness of the information presented. The carefully selected contributors are both basic and clinical investigators and scholars who have demonstrated that they can present very complex material in a manner that is understandable to health professionals as well as other interested and well-informed individuals.

In developing this second edition, we adhered to an eclectic orientation regarding the theory of practice of geriatric psychiatry. Most of the contributors are psychiatrists, but we believed it was appropriate to also include scientists from relevant biomedical and behavioral disciplines. This is particularly true for the chapters that are concerned with the basic sciences, because such knowledge must be incorporated into a comprehensive approach to patient care.

Our experience indicates that the primary target of this text is the psychiatrist who has an interest in and a commitment to geriatrics. This book is of particular value to the candidate seeking certification in geriatrics from the American Board of Psychiatry and Neurology, the American Board of Internal Medicine, and the American Board of Family Practice. All of these examinations place considerable emphasis on geriatric psychiatry and the behavioral aspects of aging.

This second edition includes material prepared during a transition period in the diagnostic nomenclature. Consequently, the diagnostic and statistical information is derived from both DSM-III-R (American Psychiatric Association 1987) and DSM-IV (American Psychiatric Association 1994). Fortunately, this is a minor complication that does not significantly influence the importance of the research and its clinical application.

We wish to express our deepest appreciation for the assistance of our staff, Denise Smith, Jennifer Riley, and Elaine Lamb, for their long hours typing, editing, and organizing the manuscripts.

Ewald W. Busse, M.D.
Dan G. Blazer, M.D., Ph.D.

The Basic Science of
Geriatric Psychiatry

CHAPTER 1

The Myth, History, and Science of Aging

Ewald W. Busse, M.D.

For thousands of years scholars, physicians, theologians, philosophers, and others have written on the subjects of life, aging, and death. Some of their observations and conclusions are casual, a few are frivolous, and some are based on careful study and considered judgment. Some of the older writings are interesting because they provide information regarding social values, the influence of political and economic factors, the level of scientific knowledge, and, in particular, the interpretation of the significance and application of existing knowledge. This summary includes selections from the literature (ancient and past), prose and verse, and myths and events relevant to geriatric psychiatry. Additional examples and details can be found in publications such as those by Gruman (1966), Segerberg (1974), and Cole (1992).

Six percent of the world's population is 65 years of age or older. In the United States in 1990, 31.1 million people (12.5% of the total population) were age 65 or older. Of these, about 18 million were 65–74, 10 million were 75–84, and 3 million were 85 or older. There were 35,808 persons over the age of 100, 80% white and 79% female (Taeuber 1993).

The Prolongation of Youth and Life

Attempts to prolong youth or to restore sexual vigor and physical vitality have been made for many centuries and still occur today. Many such attempts at rejuvenation carry a distinct risk. In fact, Greek mythology teaches that the risk is greater than the gain. The goddess Aurora (also called Eos) with great effort persuaded Zeus to grant her husband Tithonus immortality. Regrettably, she neglected to mention that she also wanted him to remain eternally young. As the years passed, Tithonus became more and more disabled, praying frequently for death. In one account, Tithonus escaped his misery by turning into a cicada. The male of this insect produces a shrill sound similar to the voice of a demented person.

Ancient Greek tales do contain one success story. The sorceress Medea claimed to hold the key that unlocked the door to eternal youth. She mixed a ram's blood, a snake's skin, an owl's flesh, roots, herbs, grass, and other ingredients and then proceeded to fill the veins of King Aeson with this po-

3

tion. The king promptly leaped from his sickbed, bursting with energy and youthful vitality; how long his energetic state lasted is unclear.

Centuries later, a similar injection ended in catastrophe. Pope Innocent VIII (1432–1492) was appropriately named: he requested his physicians to transfuse the blood of young men into his veins. Obviously the blood types were incompatible, for he died almost immediately.

During the 19th century there were a number of famous rejuvenists. Dr. Charles Edouard Brown-Séquard was a distinguished physician who described a syndrome known as the Brown-Séquard syndrome. In 1889 at a scientific meeting in Paris, Brown-Séquard announced that he had discovered a way to make old men young again. He accomplished this by injections of mashed dog testicles. He claimed that he had personally received the injections and that they had improved his potency. Following this announcement, rumors of Brown-Séquard's incredible discovery flowed through Paris and spread around the world. His office was besieged with patients seeking rejuvenation treatment. However, the treatments passed out of favor as adverse reactions developed (Zeman 1967). The Brown-Séquard effort in rejuvenation may seem outrageous, but it does not appear to be so bizarre if one appreciates the status of medical science at that time.

A different approach to rejuvenation—transplanting goat testicles into men—was advocated by John Romulus Brinkley early in the 20th century. He reputedly transplanted the testicles of 6,000 billy goats into the scrota of aging men (Zeman 1967). Brinkley moved to Mexico when he was forced to close his offices in the United States.

Serge Voronoff (1866–1951), a Russian physician in Paris, claimed great success in his efforts to restore youth. Voronoff grafted the testicles of a monkey into an aging man. Elie Metchnikoff (1845–1916), another Russian, had a different approach to the prolongation of life. He advocated removal of the large intestine and ingestion of large amounts of yogurt. Television advertisements shown in the United States for more than two decades suggested that long-lived Cossacks achieved this status by consuming large amounts of yogurt (Zeman 1967).

During the past 30 years, an injection rejuvenating technique has received considerable publicity. The technique was developed by Paul Neihans of Geneva, Switzerland. He injected living cells derived from a lamb embryo into his clients. Considerable success was claimed, and the technique continues to be used; however, there is no doubt that the introduction of a foreign protein into a human body can result in disaster.

Gerocomy

Rejuvenation efforts were abundant in the Near and Far East centuries ago. One that persisted in many societies is "gerocomy," the belief—and the actions derived from the belief—that a man, particularly an older man, absorbs virtue and youth from sexual intimacy with women, especially younger women. The Old Testament indicates that King David believed in and practiced gerocomy. There is clear evidence that the Romans had a similar view. In recent times, gerocomy is believed to have been associated with the downfall of Mahatma Ghandi. In his extensive review of the leader's life, Erik Erikson (1969) noted that notwithstanding Ghandi's expressed preference for celibacy, he was accused of gerocomy, and that this indictment contributed to his political demise.

The Hyperborean Theme

The idea that in remote parts of the world there are people who enjoy remarkably long lives appears in the mythology of cultures throughout the world. The Greek legend of the Hyperboreans held that there was a group of people who lived beyond the north wind in a region of perpetual sunshine. These fortunate people were free from all natural ills. Writing in the first century, Pliny (23–79 A.D.) noted that the Hyperboreans were extremely happy and "aloof from toil and conflict," and that they lived to an extreme old age until, "sated with life and luxury, they leaped into the sea" (Gruman 1966, p. 22).

It is interesting that this idea of people living in remote parts of the world who enjoy a long life persists in the mythology of the centenarians that occurs periodically in news media and scientific literature (see section titled "The Centenarians").

Antediluvian Theme

The idea that people lived much longer in the past has support from the Old Testament. In Genesis are recorded the life spans of 10 patriarchs who lived before the flood. The ages range from 365 years for Enoch to 969 years for Methuselah (Genesis 5:3–32):

Enoch	365 years
Lamech	777 years
Mahalalel	895 years
Enosh	905 years
Kenan	910 years
Seth	912 years
Adam	930 years
Noah	950 years
Jared	962 years
Methuselah	969 years

Because these longevity records appear in the Old Testament, they have posed a problem of interpretation for theologians. Three types of explanation have been put forth: mythical, metaphorical, and literal. The mythical interpretation denies any historical validity. The metaphorical interpretation reasons that each patriarch symbolized a tribe or group that existed for that period of time that carried the name of the founding patriarch. The literal interpretation is that before the Great Flood these patriarchs pursued a moral and proper behavior as well as diet conducive to long life. They were "beloved of God." Not only are such long-lived individuals reported in the Bible, but Greek and Roman historians also refer to a number of persons who attained extreme longevity. Pliny claimed to have identified a number of living individuals whose ages ranged from 150 to 800 years (Gruman 1966).

Other opinions have been expressed regarding the longevity of the patriarchs. The English philosopher and scientist Roger Bacon (c1220–1292) deduced that if, after the fall precipitated by Adam and Eve, human beings were still able to live almost 1,000 years, then the short life span of his own time must be the result not of the will of God but of human ignorance.

The Fountain of Youth

In America the myth of the fountain of youth is well known because it was instrumental in Ponce de Leon's discovery of what is now the state of Florida. The fountain of youth legend is traced by scholars to several possible origins. Two ancient myths involve the Hindu Pool of Youth and the Hebrew River of Immortality. The reading of ancient manuscripts as well as a travel guidebook for Greece prepared by Pausanias apparently played a role in renewing interest in the fountain of youth in the 14th and 15th centuries. In ancient Greek and Roman writings there are two interesting references to fountains with properties that conferred a prolonged life span. Hera, the wife of Zeus, bathed each year in a spring that renewed her maidenhood. In another classical reference, Herodotus (c 484–425 B.C.) recounted a search for a spring and pool whose constant use made people live longer. The water was most unusual; nothing would float on it (neither wood nor anything lighter than wood), but everything sank to the bottom. The water was strangely oily and had a fragrant quality. An Ethiopian king attributed his life of 120 years to using this water (Segerberg 1974).

The Hindu Pool of Youth is linked to the legend of Cyavana, which dates from at least 700 B.C., although the story is probably considerably older than that. Cyavana was an aged and venerable priest who was highly respected by the king. Sukanya, the daughter of the king, was given to Cyavana to be his wife. Throughout some tribulations, the dutiful wife remained loyal to her senile husband. He in turn resolved to correct the situation of their age difference and managed to get to the site of the Pool of Youth. After bathing in it, Cyavana emerged divinely fair, youthful, and wearing brilliant earrings. This Hindu fable was probably transmitted to medieval Europe by either the Arabs or the Nestorian Christians of the Near East (Gruman 1966).

The Myth of Gilgamesh

One of the principal heroic tales of antiquity is the Gilgamesh epic. The Babylonian clay tablets containing the story were discovered among the remains of the library in Nineveh by George Smith of the British Museum. Although the clay tablets were created about 650 B.C., the origin of this story traces back to the Sumerian civilization, or about 3,000 B.C. Translations were difficult but eventually produced the longest and most beautiful Babylonian poem yet discovered in the mounds of the Tigro-Euphrates region, one that ranks among the great literary masterpieces of humankind.

Gilgamesh was a vigorous young king who was exuberant but who also was arrogant and bullied his overburdened subjects. To divert him from his tyrannical behavior, the gods created Enkidu, a man of wild appearance and enormous strength. Gilgamesh and Enkidu engaged in a long, bitter struggle, with neither being able to overcome the other. Recognizing each other's power and skill, they became close friends and decided to travel together to combine their strengths and abilities to seek fame and fortune. These overcompetent superhumans violated divine law by killing sacred animals and by hurling insults at a goddess. The gods decreed the death of Enkidu, who became sick and died. Gilgamesh realized that regardless of his abilities and enormous strength, he too someday would die, and he became obsessed with the desire to obtain the secret of immortal life. He first decided to seek out the prophet Utnapishtim, a Babylonian-type Noah who lived far away. After traveling over land and sea, Gilgamesh finally located Utnapishtim. Utnapishtim told Gilgamesh that to be immortal, he must master sleep by staying awake for 6 days and 7 nights. Gilgamesh was unable to do this. He was then told that there was one last hope, and that was to retrieve from the bottom of the sea a thorny plant that possessed powers of rejuvenation. Gilgamesh succeeded in retrieving the plant from the bottom of the ocean, but on the way home he saw a pool of water and decided to bathe. After bathing, he was unable to resist sleep; while he slept a serpent appeared and ate the precious plant. By eating the plant, the serpent gained the power of shedding its own skin and renewing its life. In addition, the serpent became the symbol of a number of gods of healing.

Alchemy

Alchemy was the medieval chemical science and speculative philosophy; the two objectives of its practice were the transmutation of base metals into gold and the discovery of an elixir of life, which would represent both a universal cure for disease and a means of indefinitely prolonging life. The seeds of alchemy had emerged centuries before. Some can be traced back into Egyptian and Babylonian civilizations. Observation of materials changing provided the basis for alchemical speculation. Alchemists wondered, If a bluish stone treated with fire becomes the red metal (copper), what is the true nature of the substance? Obviously, water is an excellent example because it can evaporate or freeze

into ice or snow. In the 10th century, Ibn-Snia, one of the most famous physicians to emerge between Galen and modern times, worked diligently to find the elixir of life although he rejected the idea that metals could be turned into gold and silver. Alchemy persists today; claims have been reported, such as silver being turned into gold, but none have been proven (Paul 1993).

The twin goals of alchemy filtered into Europe during the twelfth century. In the 13th century, Roger Bacon accepted the tenets of alchemy and promoted his belief that the life span of his day, which usually was not more than 45–50 years, could be tripled with alchemy's help. His reasoning was in part based on the long life spans of Methuselah and Noah: if life spans had once been that long and then had shortened, some reversal must be possible. Bacon became a Franciscan monk in order to pursue a moral and physically clean life. He did recommend the rejuvenating breath of a young virgin, but as a monk he cautioned against any accompanying licentiousness. Bacon reasoned that if disease were contagious, why not vitality? Clearly Bacon's views were related to gerocomy.

The Myth of Cell Immortality

Alexis Carrel (1873–1944) was born and educated in France. Carrel was a very skillful and creative surgeon who encountered frustrations in his career. He left for America in May 1904. At the University of Chicago and later at the Rockefeller Institute, he devoted his work to vascular and cardiac surgery and wound healing. This interest in wound healing led him to an interest in growing tissues outside the body. For his surgical contributions, he won the 1912 Nobel prize for physiology and medicine. He rapidly developed his studies in tissue culture, and on the basis of some of his own apparent successes, he became convinced that some human cells grown in culture were immortal. This claim of possible cell immortality was reported by Carrel and Ebeling beginning in 1912. In spite of numerous objections to his work, Carrel was very persuasive and his belief was widely accepted. In January 1912, Carrel established a series of chick heart fibroblast cultures, one of which was destined to become the immortal cell strain. Both Ebeling and Carrel continued to publish and apparently maintained excellent public relations. Their claimed success of maintaining the cell culture was such that the *New York World Telegram* made periodic inquiry about the health of the cells and reported on their status.

Subsequently it was demonstrated that Carrel and Ebeling had made an error in their methodology that resulted in improper conclusions. The Carrel-Ebeling cell culture was fed an extract taken from chick embryos. This extract actually contained a very few but significant number of new viable cells; hence, the introduction of new cells permitted the culture to survive. It was found that if the extract was carefully prepared, removing all new cells, the cell colony would die.

Although other experiments have suggested that animal and human cells have the capacity to be immortal, it has been demonstrated that all such immortal cell colonies are abnormal in one way or another. At the present time it appears that the only human cells that may be immortal are transformed or abnormal mixoploid cells such as the HeLa cells, which were originally taken from cancerous cervical tissue and grown in culture by George O. Gey in 1950.

Before 1961, the accepted dogma was that cell and tissue cultures were potentially immortal. The death of a cell line was usually attributed to failure to use proper laboratory methods. In 1961, Hayflick and Moorhead first described the finite replicative capacity of cultured normal human fibroblasts and interpreted the phenomenon to be aging at the cellular level. They demonstrated that even when normal human embryonic cells were grown under the most favorable conditions, death was inevitable after about 50 population doublings. Thus, the death of the cell line was an inherent property of the cells themselves.

In 1965, Hayflick reported that culture fibroblasts derived from older human donors divided fewer times than those derived from embryos. Since then, a number of investigators have replicated the work of Hayflick, finding that the number of population doublings of cultured human cells is inversely proportional to donor age. It was subsequently demonstrated that freezing viable normal human cells at subzero temperatures does not alter the memory in the cells for the number of doublings that had previously occurred. These cells have been held for more than 24 years in a frozen state and, when thawed, replicate only the amount of times they would have had they never been frozen.

Gerovital H$_3$

Gerovital H$_3$, an exceedingly controversial compound, has been sold in Europe for many years. It is claimed by its predominantly European advocates to have a variety of curative and restorative powers for disabilities and diseases affecting the elderly, and its reported use by European political and religious leaders is a testament to its popularity. The most active advocate of Gerovital H$_3$ was Professor Anna Aslan of the Geriatric Institute of Bucharest, Romania. Although procaine hydrochloride has been used in Europe as a general tonic for more than 60 years, it was not until 1985, when Professor Aslan began to use it and to proclaim its value, that this particular drug began to receive considerable attention.

Many of Aslan's claims are probably exaggerated, and the resulting questions about the legitimacy of the drug's purported benefits may mask its potential usefulness. Assuming that it does have some pharmaceutical effect, the question is, How is this accomplished? One proposed explanation is that Gerovital H$_3$ is an effective inhibitor of monoamine oxidase. Another possible explanation involves the presence of benzoic acid, which positively influences the availability of needed substances to cells; alternatively, benzoic acid may also enhance the action of the metabolic products, which include para-aminobenzoic acid and at least one other substance that is believed to have favorable effects upon the organism (Busse 1973).

Ostfeld et al. (1977), in a review of 285 articles and books addressing the subject of procaine hydrochloride, concluded that there was no convincing evidence that procaine or Gerovital H$_3$ has any value in the treatment of diseases of older patients, except for a possible antidepressant effect. Thus, it may be that the reported improvements are the result of the relief of complaints associated with depressive conditions.

Limited efforts have been made to produce Gerovital H$_3$ in the United States. A small amount was sold in two western states, but the drug has not been widely marketed in the United States. A major source of Gerovital H$_3$ is the Bahama Islands.

Rejuvenation in the Soviet Union

Zhores Medvedev is a distinguished Russian scientist who has made many contributions to the study of biological aging, including the redundant theory of aging—that the amount of DNA reserve within the genome that can be called upon to maintain vital function plays an important role in determining life span (Busse 1983). Medvedev has published two important books that are relevant to geriatric psychiatry. The first is a historical account of pseudoscience entitled *The Rise and Fall of T. D. Lysenko,* which first appeared in the science underground of the Soviet Union in 1961 and was published in the United States in 1969.

Medvedev's first book vividly recounts how, between 1937 and 1964, Lysenko used a false doctrine and fabricated scientific data to achieve fame and power. Of particular interest to the geriatric psychiatrist is Medvedev's account of a technique of rejuvenation advocated by a disciple of Lysenko's, a woman named O. B. Lepeshinskaya. Around 1949, Lepeshinskaya began to advocate the use of soda baths to prolong life and restore vigor, a practice warmly supported by Lysenko. This approach quickly moved to the drinking of soda water and finally to the introduction of soda into the body by enema. Apparently the latter two techniques were used as alternatives for those who were unable to take frequent soda baths. Lepeshinskaya also claimed that she could make living matter from nonliving material. This account is a vivid example of how vulnerable geriatrics is to the practice of pseudoscience.

The second book, *A Question of Madness,* which Medvedev coauthored with his brother Roy, was published in the United States in 1972. This book is a vivid account of the problems of using psychiatry for incarcerating and harassing political dissenters (Busse 1984).

The Centenarians

Reports of life spans exceeding 100 years have involved three wide-ranging pockets of people. One group, the Viejos, live in Vilcabamba, a small mountain village in Ecuador. The other two pockets are in widely separated regions of Asia—the Hunzukuts of the Karakoram region in Kashmir and the Abkhazians of the Republic of Georgia in the former Soviet Union. Over the past decade, a number of individuals have visited the two groups in Ecuador and Georgia. In February 1978, the National Institute on Aging brought together a number of scientists who had visited Vilcabamba. After three visits to Vilcabamba they concluded that the oldest person in the community was 96 years of age. Similar visits to the Soviet Caucasus and reevaluations found the reports of longevity had been grossly exaggerated (Palmore 1984).

An interesting publication of the Soviet Institute of Gerontology (Chebotarev 1984) reported no individuals who had lived beyond the age of 114. The Soviet scientists concluded that longevity was promoted by physical labor during the course of life, regimens of work alternating with rest, and characteristics of nutrition. The study of Soviet centenarians included data of functional ability. Twenty-five percent of the Soviet centenarians were unable to "self serve," 2% showed psychic disorders, 50% had hearing loss, and 24.3% suffered from impaired vision.

In 1985, of the 28.5 million Americans over the age of 65 years, 32% were between 75 and 84 years old, 10.5% were 85 years and over, and less than 1% had attained the age of 100 years or more.

During the same era, a brief flurry of publicity centered on the "long-lived" Hunzukuts. Hunza is a 2,000-year-old country that has remained virtually isolated from the rest of the world. The statements in the news media claimed that this civilization originated in 330 B.C. when an army division of Alexander the Great of Macedonia broke away, took Persian wives, and purposely lost themselves in the vastness of the Himalayas. These individuals supposedly lived from 120 to 140 years, and men aged 100 years and older fathered children. Hunza women, at age 80, supposedly looked like American women of 40 years. The longevity of Hunzukuts was attributed to a number of factors including exercise, diet, periods of relaxation, and moderation in many things including the consumption of wine. In 1978, a biocalendar health system appeared supposedly based on information attained from the Hunzukuts. In recent years, no additional information has appeared. Consequently, we can only assume that these reports were a fabrication or a distortion of fact.

There is widespread agreement that maximum human life span does not and will not in the foreseeable future exceed 116 years.

Attitudes Toward Aging

Marcus Tullius Cicero, the Roman orator and statesman of the first century (106–43 B.C.), incorporated into his elegant speeches and writings the philosophical views and social values of his time (Gruman 1966). Cicero, at the age of 62, produced an essay on senescence ("de Senectute"; 44 B.C.) in which he suggested that old age was not welcomed equally by different human races. The status the elderly held within a society apparently made a difference. The Spartans capitalized on the experience of older men, and the gerotes, a council of 28 men past 60 years old, controlled the city-state (Thewlis 1924). Cicero argued that successful aging was obtainable if one developed an appropriate attitude and dealt effectively with the four major complaints associated with aging. It is interesting that these same four complaints exist today.

The first complaint was that society excluded the aged from important work of the world. Cicero replied by saying that courageous elders can find a way to make themselves useful in various advisory, intellectual, and administrative functions.

The second charge was that aging undermines physical strength and reduces the individual's value. Cicero answered that bodily decline counts for little compared with the cultivation of mind and character.

The third complaint was that aging prevents or reduces the enjoyment of sensual pleasures, particularly sexual enjoyment. Cicero replied that such a loss has some merit because it allows the aged to concentrate on the promotion of reason and virtue.

The fourth, and final, charge was that old age brings with it increasing anxiety about death. In response to this charge, Cicero followed Plato by saying that death could be considered a blessing, freeing individuals and their immortal souls from their bodily prison on this very imperfect earth. He added that even if one does not believe that the soul is immortal, death remains a virtue, as all things must have limitations and the limitation on the duration of life is not unlike the end of a play in the theater. Cicero concluded by saying that the wise individual is one who submits to the dictates of nature and passes through the vicissitudes of life with a tranquil mind. He implied that the prolongation of life seemed undesirable, particularly if, in old age, one had to go back to being "a crying child in the cradle." Cicero also indicated that he himself had no desire to relive his life or to be summoned back to some starting point.

Maximianus, a Latin poet contemporary with Boethius in the time of the Byzantine emperor Jus-tinian the Great (483–565), wrote six elegies on old age and love that are, according to Lind (1988), "unmatched in ancient or modern poetry" for their explicitly detailed realism and their almost clinical descriptions of the visible and psychological phenomena of aging.

There is nothing prudish about Maximianus' elegies, in which he reflects on the four major loves that occurred during his life. The first was Lycoris, who was either his concubine or a live-in partner and who remained the longest with him but finally left him in their old age. After two subsequent loves, Maximianus met his fourth love, an unnamed Greek performer in Constantinople, with whom he had the most humiliating of all of his sexual experiences—a collapse into impotency.

In his introduction to Maximianus' work, Lind quoted from a number of other medieval poems. The poems contain very negative statements about old age and particularly dwell on how older people become ugly. It is evident that most of the older persons living in medieval times lost their teeth and did not have false teeth. This condition not only interfered with their ability to chew "with toothless gums" but also was a major contributor to their ugliness. It is also very likely that exposure of the face to sun and weather not only increased those skin changes associated with aging, but also increased skin lesions. One poem stated that old men become "so revolting . . . to wife and children and themselves that even fortune hunters pass them by."

Gerontocomia was published in Latin by Gabriele Zerbi in 1482. Zeman (1967) reported finding this fascinating volume and said that Zerbi's work had not previously been quoted by any medical or lay writer since its original publication. Lind (1988, p. 7) attested to the fact that this lengthy manuscript had previously not been translated into English and had been largely overlooked by medical and lay writers. Lind described Gerontocomia as "the first practical manual on the problems of old age." Zerbi dealt with the care of the aged in a rest home, especially selected with regard to climate, exposure, equipment, and staff. He described all of his ideas regarding longevity and maintaining health, advocating exercise, bathing, massage, rest, and diet. He referred to medications that are useful to old people and discussed their ingredients and dosages. One of Zerbi's most fascinating recommendations was the continuing use of human milk for the aged. Zerbi detailed the proper characteristics of the wet nurse and advised that the patient take the milk directly from the nipple. (This custom, which was deeply rooted in antiquity, continues to appear periodically in recent times. In Steinbeck's *Grapes of Wrath,* a dying old man is nursed by a young girl who has just lost her baby.) As to clothing, Zerbi recommended silk over linen. Silk garments are soft and warm, whereas linen is flat textured and therefore cold. He noted that clothes woven with wool and silk keep one moderately warm and dry. Recognizing that death and old age are inevitable, Zerbi stated, "It is impossible therefore to prevent the wasting away of old age, but it is possible to combat and resist it considerably" (Lind 1988, p. 26).

According to Zerbi, there are two kinds of causes of old age: extrinsic and intrinsic. The extrinsic causes are in the realm of the astrologers. The first period of old age is governed by Jupiter, whereas the last stage of old age is governed by Saturn. Zerbi observed that there are very few humans who live beyond 100 years. Those who live that long are said to pass from the leadership of Saturn to that of the moon—which is, in effect, a reversion, since the moon was thought to govern humans at the age of approximately 25 years. Zerbi's comments indicated that because no one can do much about the astrological component, physicians should be more concerned with the intrinsic processes of old age. He further stated that the human body has the beginnings of its generation from "the sperm of both men and women," but apparently the fetus grows as a result of both blood and sperm. Apparently the idea was that when something goes wrong with the composition of the two fluids, problems develop. These problems are claimed to be in the areas of both astrology and medicine; therefore, Zerbi said, "These two masters, the physician and the astrologer, must in particular consult and provide for human nature" (Lind 1988, p. 35).

Luigi Cornaro was born in 1467 in Padua. He was dedicated to maintaining health and prolonging life. At the age of 83 he published one of his most important writings, *Vita Sobria.* In this book he described his regimen of health. He lived to the age of 98 years without any decay in his health or understanding (Gruman 1966).

Sir William Osler, born in Canada in 1849, was considered a superb observer, an excellent teacher, and a scholar who was knowledgeable about medicine, literature, and the humanities (Belkin and Nee-

lon 1992). At the age of 56, he delivered the farewell address to the Johns Hopkins faculty (Berk 1989). In that address, he expressed the belief that with advancing age, professors often lose their usefulness. The address was called "The Fixed Period," a title taken from the name of a novel by Anthony Trollope. The novel describes how a college is created in which men at 60 were retired for a year before being eliminated by chloroform. Osler held the position that productivity in life occurs before the age of 40. This farewell speech resulted in negative reaction both by his colleagues and by the public press. An effort was made to explain it away by characterizing it as an attempt in humor. However, in answer to this storm, Osler said, "The criticisms have not shaken my convictions that the telling work of the world has been done and is done by men under forty years of age. The exceptions which have been given only illustrate the rule. It would also be to the general good if men at sixty were retired from active work. We should miss the energies of some young-old men, but on the whole be of greater service to the sexagenarii themselves."

Osler died in 1919 at age 70. Until approximately a year before his death, he is said to have remained an active teacher, researcher, and statesman. He was buried in Wrens Tower at Oxford.

How It Feels to Grow Old

Walter E. Barton, professor emeritus of psychiatry at Dartmouth Medical School and former president of the American Psychiatric Association, was asked to reflect on how it feels to grow old. His response (1986), at which time he was 80 years old, is a remarkable report and is consistent with general clinical experience in dealing with elderly persons. It is also very similar to reports that have appeared in the literature for many centuries, although the subjects of some of those reports apparently experienced the ravages of aging earlier in life than did Barton. Barton, in his self-observation of aging, commented on visual problems, including glare and the hazards of night driving, the decline in manual dexterity, and the fear of loss of mental acuity. In spite of these and other concerns, Barton observed that "we [Dr. and Mrs. Barton] suffer no depressed mood" and "we have developed the ritual which we observe each Friday when we toast our survival through another week" (Barton 1986, p. 192). In answer to the question, how does it feel to grow old, Barton responded that it felt "disgusting, disagreeable, and terribly terminal." If one is blessed with an intact mind, according to Barton, one can find satisfaction in life and erect defenses against undesirable feelings. However, he did conclude, "The years of the seventies are not so bad, but the eighties, with the rise in chronic illness, are mostly downhill" (p. 192).

A number of psychiatrists have published accounts of how they have observed and reacted to their own aging. The vast majority have said that they feel that their intellect had not deteriorated with aging, but all have emphasized the importance of maintaining activity in a diversity of intellectual and physical activities. They recognize that aging is accompanied by limitations and that it is a difficult process to know when and how to reduce or stop some activities (Busse 1991; Pollock 1992).

Another famous psychiatrist, Francis Braceland—like Barton, a past president of the American Psychiatric Association—said of aging, "When it's quiet I can almost hear brain cells drop out" (Braceland 1978).

The Advantages of Aging

Most people seem to have difficulty thinking of the advantages of aging. Palmore (1979, p. 220) quoted, as an example, this passage from Kanin's *Remembering Mr. Maugham* (1966):

> Somerset Maugham was being honored by the Garrick Club as part of his eightieth birthday celebration. He spoke the customary salutations, paused for a moment and said, "There are many . . . virtues in . . . growing old." He paused, he swallowed, he wet his lips, he looked about. The pause stretched out, he looked dumbstruck. The pause became too long—far too long. He looked down, studying the tabletop. A terrible tremor of nervousness went through the room. Was he ill? Would he ever be able to get on with it? Finally he looked up and said, "I'm just . . . trying . . . to think what they are!

Palmore believed he had documented some major advantages of aging. These include the fact that the aged are the most law abiding of all age groups, except for young children. The aged are much better

citizens and are interested and active in public issues and political affairs. They make an enormous contribution to society by maintaining voluntary participation in community organizations, churches, and recreational groups. Although many are not gainfully employed, they are quite capable of participating in performance tasks. Older workers are stable and dependable and have less absenteeism. Although older persons are equally exposed to crimes of certain types, they are much less likely to be the victims of crime in general than are people in other age groups. Although some of the apparent advantages of aged individuals are under constant pressure, it is obvious that Social Security and other pension systems have improved their economic status, as have lower taxes and other economic benefits such as reduced rates in many hotels, motels, and recreational facilities. Medicare, in spite of its limitations, provides health insurance for many older people who would not otherwise be covered. Undoubtedly there are other advantages. The disadvantages, as is true in all medical publications, appear repeatedly throughout this book.

A Definition of Aging

Aging, in living organisms, usually refers to the adverse effects of the passage of time, although occasionally the term refers to the positive processes of maturation or acquiring a desirable quality. Biological aging is not necessarily confined to the latter years of life; some declines begin with conception. In general, the term does designate those physical changes that develop in adulthood, result in a decline in efficiency of function, and terminate in death. Aging is observed in nearly all animals, but it may not be a universal phenomenon. Hayflick (1994) contended that "there are some animals that do not seem to age at all" (p. 29). Such animals increase in size indefinitely. These nonaging animals include sturgeons, sharks, alligators, and tortoises native to the Galápagos Islands. In flounder, gender makes a difference, as females do not show age changes, whereas the male reaches a fixed size and age. Hayflick stated that "the explanation for this difference is a mystery" (p. 21).

The multiple processes of decline that are associated with growing old can be separated into primary and secondary aging (Busse 1987). *Primary ag-*

ing is held to be intrinsic to the organism, and the decremental factors are determined by inherent or hereditary influences. The rate of aging as a functional decline varies widely between individuals. Further, there are extreme aging variations in systems, organs, and cells. *Secondary aging* refers to the appearance of defects and disabilities that are caused by hostile factors in the environment, including trauma and acquired disease.

This operational separation of primary and secondary aging processes has limitations, because both inherent (hereditary) and acquired decremental age changes are often of multiple etiology. Inherent defects that make the organism vulnerable may not appear unless and until the organism is exposed to hostile precipitating events.

Definitions of aging that have been offered, including those for primary and secondary aging, are not consistently accepted and applied. The aging of living organisms is a universal phenomenon, but the rate of aging can vary between individuals and groups. In humans, aging differences are in part genetically determined but also are substantially influenced by nutrition, lifestyle, and environment (Busse 1987). There are some scientists who define primary aging as first cause and secondary aging as the pathological processes that ensue from the first cause.

Many age changes are relatively benign and allow a person to continue to function, meet personal needs, and maintain a place in society. Age changes are recognized as a decline in efficiency or performance but in the extreme are often labeled a disease. Examples of age changes that can become sufficiently severe to be a disease include a decline in kidney function (creatinine clearance), reduced respiratory performance (forced expiratory volume), an increase in systolic blood pressure (isolated systolic hypertension), and an impaired response to oral glucose tolerance tests (non-insulin-dependent diabetes) (Tobin 1984).

The chronological age of a person is often estimated by changes in appearance and the person's ability to perform tasks associated with activities of daily living and working. As humans age, the skin often becomes wrinkled, dry, and seborrheic, and actinic keratosis appears. Hair becomes gray and thinner; baldness increases. Teeth decay and are lost. In addition, height tends to decrease, as does weight. Chest depth and abdominal depth both increase.

The ear lengthens and the nose broadens. Fat cells invade muscle and muscle strength decreases. Posture and height are affected by musculoskeletal changes. Bone densities, influenced by gender and race, decrease with age; in women especially, the trabecular bones of the hip, wrist, and vertebrae are particularly affected.

The metabolic dimensions that are affected by age include drug absorption, distribution, destruction, excretion, the kinetics of drug binding, and alterations in biological rhythms. Drugs are therefore metabolized in old people differently from the way they are metabolized in younger adults.

Another important age change is the loss of irreplaceable cells, most noticeably in the skeletal muscle tissue, heart, and brain. Striated musculature diminishes by about one-half by approximately 80 years of age. As these muscle cells disappear, they are replaced by fat cells and fibrous connective tissue. Hence, the body achieves increased storage capacities for certain drugs that are stored in fat cells. The loss of brain cells alters important aspects of body metabolism and affects circadian rhythms. The decrease in heart cells results in alterations in certain cardiac functions. Cellular and supportive tissue changes cause pulmonary changes.

In the brain, neurons shrink and are lost, and alterations occur in neuronal synapses and networks. The loss of nerve cells, particularly those in vulnerable areas of the hypothalamus, may contribute to placing the elderly at risk for certain physiological changes and associated mental and emotional aberrations. Aging results in a decline of neurotransmitters such as dopamine, norepinephrine, serotonin, tyrosine hydroxylase, and cholinesterase. The activity of monoamine oxidase increases with age.

Selected Biological Theories of Aging

There are many theories and processes of aging. A satisfactory, unified theory of aging does not exist. In part this is due to the fact that the human body has three major components: cells capable of dividing, cells that cannot undergo mitosis, and interstitial noncellular material. Similar age changes have been identified in one or two of the body components, but rarely are the same changes seen in all three. A number of theories of aging lack adequate scientific proof. For example, at the present time, there is substantial—though not conclusively definitive—evidence that intrinsic cellular or molecular aging changes underlie many of the neuronal or endocrine changes associated with the brain.

Classification of theories. In 1993, the National Institute on Aging published a booklet, "In Search of the Secrets of Aging." It divides the major theories of aging into two categories: program theories and error theories. Program theories hold that aging is the result of sequential switching on and off of certain genes. Defects develop during this switching on and off, and these defects are manifested by senescence. Those who subscribe to error theories maintain that aging is the result of wear and tear processes; these theorists hold that in many mechanisms important parts wear out and cannot be replaced or repaired. Included among the error theories is the "somatic mutation theory," whose proponents maintain that, with increasing age, genetic mutations occur and accumulate, causing cells to deteriorate and malfunction.

In a review of biological theories of aging, Hart and Turturro (1985) categorized theories into cellular, organ, and population based; integrative approaches; and meta-aging. The cellular-based theories are those that emphasize the importance of the inherent limited potential proliferation of cells. These theories are consistent with the fact that animals have decreased cellularity in a number of organs as aging advances. Consequently, aging stem cells exhibit a progressively limited ability to repopulate differentiated daughter cells. The capacity for limited proliferation is linked to some experiments that have demonstrated that the limited proliferation of cells is the result of stochastic changes. Other experiments have been concerned with the somatic-mutation theory of aging and the closely associated "error theory." Finally, cellular aging may be attributed to accumulated effects of damage from the expression of "cell death genes" important to development. This is linked with the observation that during embryogenesis the number of cells retained for further development is reduced by some genetic mechanism. Because cell numbers are reduced in late life, it would be important to understand the underlying mechanism that is needed by the organism early in life but that may be detrimental late in life. In a similar manner, the Hart and Turturro review identifies those theories of aging that are re-

lated to mechanisms of cell death. The final category of aging theories mentioned by Hart and Turturro is meta-aging. This encompasses what the authors refer to as "the theory of the theory of aging." The complexity of such a discussion is obvious, and the development of a unified theory of aging will be extremely difficult because such a theory of biosenescence would have to take into consideration all of the processes an individual undergoes as well as the sequence of environmental interactions that occur within the individual over a lifetime.

Watch-spring theory. One early biological explanation of aging rested on the assumption that a living organism contained a fixed store of energy not unlike that contained within a coiled watch spring. When the spring of the watch was unwound, life ended. This is a type of exhaustion theory.

Another simple theory relates to the accumulation of deleterious material. This particular theory is given some support by the observation that pigments such as lipofuscin accumulate in a number of cells throughout life.

Although these two simple theories may make some contribution to the aging process, there is little evidence that they have any substantial role.

The "aging clock." The hypothalamus is said to be the location of the "aging clock." Age changes within the hypothalamus play a particularly important role in losses of homeostatic mechanisms in the body. Cell loss, an event that is common in late life, occurs within clusters of cells in the hypothalamus. The disappearance of a few critical cells in the hypothalamus may have far-reaching consequences. The remaining aging cells may become less efficient. These changes in the hypothalamus undoubtedly cause important changes within the pituitary that in turn affect other glands and organs within the body. As a consequence, the aging body undergoes many endocrine changes. Alterations within the hypothalamus also affect numerous connections within the brain and play a major role in age changes associated with chemical messengers of the brain.

Stochastic theories. Processes of aging that are associated with random changes such as cell loss or mutation are often termed "stochastic" processes. *Stochastic* implies "a process or a series of events for which the estimate of the probability of certain outcomes approaches the true possibility as the number of events increases" (Busse 1977, p. 16).

The atomic scientist Leo Szilard advanced a stochastic theory based on what he termed "a hit." A hit was not solely the result of radiation, but rather could be considered any event that would alter a chromosome. In addition, Szilard believed that every animal carries a load of what he termed "faults." A fault is a congenital absence or impairment of one of the genes essential to cell function. A cell is capable of operating as long as one of the pair of genes continues to function; however, when both members of a pair of essential genes are incapable of functioning, the cell declines and dies. Therefore, a cell will cease to function effectively if one of the pair carries the fault and the other is the victim of a hit, or if both of the pair are the victims of hits. One reservation about Szilard's theory is that it is applicable only to irreplaceable cells. The second objection to the fault/hit approach is that individuals having pairs of like (homozygous) genes should survive hits much more readily than heterozygous individuals having many dissimilar gene pairs. Yet hybrids, that is, heterozygous individuals with dissimilar genes, live consistently longer than inbreds (homozygous individuals) (Busse 1977).

Holliday (1986) observed that stochastic processes may also be under genetic control, because the frequency of defects in macromolecules or the ability to remove defects is known to be determined by the genotype of the organism.

Deliberate biological programming. The theory of deliberate biological programming has received considerable attention. This theory holds that within a normal cell are stored the memory and the capability of determining the life of a cell. This theory is consistent with the research and conclusions of Hayflick (1965). The memory and capacity to terminate life are found in all normal human diploid cells. In mixoploid or cancer cells this memory or capacity apparently is destroyed, and the cells can duplicate indefinitely.

Cristafalo (1972) reported that the number of doublings is the same for both male and female cells. (Female cells are easily identified by the presence of a bar body, the second sex chromosome.) This observation suggests that the difference in life expectancy between human males and females cannot be attributed to intracellular differences (Weiss 1974).

The free radical theory. A free radical is a chemical molecule or compound that has an odd number of electrons (an unpaired electron) and is highly reactive, in contrast to most chemical compounds, which have an even number of electrons and are stable. Often considered molecular fragments, free radicals are highly reactive and destructive, but they are produced by normal metabolic processes and are ubiquitous in living substances. They can also be produced by ionizing radiation, ozone, and chemical toxins such as insecticides. The oxygen free radical, superoxide (O^{2-}), is an important agent of oxygen toxicity and the aging process. Scavengers of oxygen free radicals exist within cells. Enzymatic defenses involve superoxide dismutase, catalases, and perioxidases. Oxygen free radicals have been linked to DNA damage, the cross-linkage of collagen, and the accumulation of age pigments and cancers (Busse 1983). Nutrient antioxidants include vitamins C and E and beta-carotene (National Institute on Aging 1993a).

Immune system. The immune system performs both surveillance and protective tasks. It is a complex, widespread bodily function that is essential for the preservation of life (Suskind 1980). The destruction of the immune system is well known to people because it is identified with acquired immunodeficiency syndrome (AIDS) (Laurence 1985). Traditionally the immune system has been considered to have two major components. One is the humoral immune response, characterized by the production of antibody molecules that specifically bind the introduced foreign substance. The second is the cellular immune response, by which cells are mobilized that can specifically react with and destroy the invader. Considerable evidence has accumulated that a decrease in the immune competence and alterations in the regulation of the immune system are associated with aging. With increasing age, surveillance is impaired, and there is a decline in the efficiency of the protective mechanism. Furthermore, there is a loss of control so that immune functions become so distorted that they are self-destructive. The impairment of the immune system results in an increased incidence of certain diseases in the aging population. Certain tumors in the aged appear to be related to the failure of the body to recognize and eliminate abnormal cells. Autoantibodies increase with the passage of time, and the presence of autoantibodies identifies subpopulations at risk of early death. The older body has an increased susceptibility to infection, and, in general, effective immunization cannot be induced in late life (Finkelstein 1984).

Cells that cannot divide (i.e., neurons and cardiac muscle cells) may be particularly vulnerable to alterations in the immune system. The loss of nondividing cells in the aging body has been previously mentioned. It may be that this loss is the result of the inability of the immune system to protect these nonreplaceable cells or that the death of the cells may be the result of autoaggressive processes.

Eversion (cross-linkage).   The eversion, or cross-linkage, theory of aging is based on the observation that there are changes in collagen structure associated with aging. Collagen is probably the most important protein in the human body. There are two types of collagen: interstitial and basement membrane. With the passage of time, the ester bonds from within the collagen molecule switch to binding together individual collagen molecules. This aging chain alters the characteristics of connective tissue. Cross-linkage may, in addition, be caused by glycosylation.

Glycosylation (glucose cross-linkage).   Glucose is the body's most abundant sugar and is important to the metabolisms of cells, particularly neurons. Glycosylation is a nonenzymatic reaction between glucose and protein (Cerami et al. 1987). It is known as the browning reaction or the Maillard reaction. Food chemists have known for many years that this process discolors and toughens food. Until diabetes studies, however, it was not understood that glycosylation also takes place within the human body.

Normally, when enzymes attach glucose to proteins within the body, they do so at a specific site on a specific molecule for a specific purpose. In contrast, the nonenzymatic process adds glucose haphazardly to any of several sites along any available peptide chain. The nonenzymatic process apparently increases with aging and culminates with the formation and accumulation of irreversible cross-links between adjacent protein molecules. Cerami et al. (1987) proposed that the nonenzymatic addition of glucose to nucleic acids may gradually damage DNA.

The end products of glycosylation are yellowish-brown and fluorescent and have specific spectro-

graphic properties. Most important for the body is that many of these end products can cross-link with adjacent proteins. The realization that the browning reaction could occur in and potentially damage the body emerged from studies of diabetes. Now it appears that the glucose changes could also play a role in the tissue changes associated with normal aging. Although additional research is needed to understand the importance of glycosylation, it is a promising theory because it appears that treatments could be developed to prevent some of the changes that connect glycosylation with aging.

Genetics of human aging.   Brown and Wisniewski (1983) stated that the genetic nature of the aging process is reflected by the wide range of maximal life spans that animal species may attain. Among mammals, the life span range is from 1 year in the smoky shrew to over 114 years in humans. This wide variation in life spans emphasizes that the aging process is likely to have an underlying basis that is in part encoded in our genes. The genetic basis may involve two types of inherited species-specific differences. The first type relates to development of the organism. This mechanism governs program timings in developmental stages as well as rates of maturation. The second genetic determinant relates to self-maintenance. This mechanism influences the efficiency of enzymatic systems as well as protection and repair of internal and external insults to the machinery. If the DNA process in itself is damaged or declines in efficiency, the functioning capacity of the organism is severely impaired. It is obvious that the numerous biological changes that take place over the life span are very complicated. It is likely that many interacting genes are involved. However, specific genetic defects have been identified that are particularly relevant to certain life-shortening conditions. It is possible that there are other genes that contribute to longer life; however, at this stage of our knowledge, only rarely have specific "longevity" genes been identified that are consistently associated with increased life expectancy. Examples are genes that overproduce superoxide dismutase and catalase; such genes are antioxidants and appear to increase life expectancy (National Institute on Aging 1993b).

McKusick (1982) listed more than 3,000 specific human gene conditions that are known to result in defects within the human organism. These recognized human gene conditions are considered to be genetically autosomal, dominant, or recessive and/or X-linked. It appears that there are rare autosomal-dominant genetic conditions that may increase the average life expectancy. One of these is hypobeta-lipoproteinemia, a condition characterized by abnormally low plasma levels of beta-lipoproteins and associated with decreased susceptibility to atherosclerosis and, presumably, a reduced risk of heart disease.

In Chapter 12, the genetic determinants in dementia are discussed. In brief it is evident that senile dementia of the Alzheimer's type (i.e., at least certain subgroups) does have a genetic component. Creutzfeldt-Jakob's disease appears to be related to two important factors: both a virus and a familial tendency. It may be that heredity produces a susceptibility to infectious viruses. A relatively rare condition, Gerstmann-Sträussler syndrome, is a dementia accompanied by spinocerebellar ataxia that has been shown to have an autosomal dominant inheritance. Interestingly, from a neuropathological viewpoint, this syndrome is associated with neuritic and amyloid plaques, which of course are very common in senile dementia of the Alzheimer's type and are related to congenital defects in chromosome 21 (Barnes 1987).

Martin (1977) reviewed a long list of human genetic conditions to select out those in which physical and physiological changes were usually associated with senescence. He identified the 10 genetic disorders that had the highest number of senescent features and thus that were considered to be associated with the aging process: Down's syndrome, Werner's syndrome, Cockayne's syndrome, progeria, ataxia telangiectasia, Lawrence-Seip syndrome, cervical lipodysplasia, Klinefelter's syndrome, Turner's syndrome, and myotonic dystrophy.

Length of Life: The Sex Differential

In humans and in many other animal species, females outlive males. It is easy to assume that the differences between the two sexes are genetically determined by the presence or absence of the male Y chromosome. It has been suggested that the greater constitutional weakness of males may be due to their having only one X chromosome.

Before 1900, in those nations where data are available, it appears there were slightly more older men than women. After the turn of the century, this situation gradually changed, and by 1940 the situation had reversed itself. Thereafter, the preponderance of older women increased rapidly. In 1985 in the population over 65 years of age, the sex ratio was 147 women for every 100 men; this discrepancy is increasing.

Contrary to the reasonable expectation of the equal balance in males and females at birth, there are in the United States approximately 106–110 white males born for every 100 white females, and approximately 104 black males born for every 100 black females. It has been reported, but not confirmed, that in black populations of several islands in the West Indies, there are fewer males than females at birth (American Association of Retired Persons 1987).

Numerous environmental factors have been investigated to determine their influence on sex ratio at birth. In England and Wales it has been reported that upper socioeconomic groups are likely to have a higher ratio of males to females than do lower socioeconomic groups. During World War II, many European countries observed that the ratio of males to females was higher than during times of peace. It is possible that this was due to the births occurring in younger parents as opposed to older parents during peace time.

At birth, the female in the more developed nations has a life expectancy of 8 or more years beyond that of the male. In 1978, France had the most extreme male/female differences for life expectancy at birth, 8.21 years. Canada was second with a difference of 7.59 years. In 1981, Japan had the best life expectancy at birth: 79.1 years for females and 73.8 years for males, a difference of 5.3 years. In Japan this male/female difference is increasing rather than decreasing—in 1970 there was a difference of 4.4 years and in 1952 a difference of 3.4 years.

Geriatric psychiatry is particularly concerned with the remaining years after the age of 65. In the United States in 1985, a 65-year-old woman could expect to live another 18.6 years, but a man of the same age could anticipate only 14 more years of life (American Association of Retired Persons 1987). This gender imbalance in late life has important social and medical implications. Most older men are married, whereas most older women are widowed or single (divorced or never married). The gender imbalance is enhanced by the practice of men marrying younger females, which expands the pool of older, unmarried women. The recognition of the preponderance of women in modern society undoubtedly affects socioeconomic planning and programs in health care.

Waldron (1986) reviewed the literature as to causes of gender differences in mortality. She noted that in contemporary industrial societies the single most important cause of higher mortality for males has been a greater incidence of cigarette smoking among men. Other gender differences in mortality are related to behaviors that contribute to the males' higher mortality. Such behaviors include heavier alcohol consumption and employment in hazardous occupations. In many nonindustrial societies, where, in many instances, the gender differences in mortality are not as great as in the industrial societies, these factors play a less important role.

In nonindustrial societies, women are more vulnerable to infectious diseases. This may be related to less adequate nutrition and health care for women. Waldron described a wide variety of factors that influence gender differences in mortality. In contrast to men in undeveloped nations, men in the United States tend to have a higher death rate from infectious and parasitic diseases than do women; American men were more vulnerable in 1930 than in 1978. However, one must be cautious in interpreting this information, because, as Waldron pointed out, gender differences do vary somewhat for different types of infections and parasitic diseases.

The genders show differences in their immune capacities; for example, women have higher levels of one of the major classes of immunoglobulins (IgM). In theory this may be attributed to the differences in the sex chromosomes. It appears that the female X chromosome carries one or more genes that influence the production of IgM. The pair of X chromosomes in women could result in higher production of IgM than in the male single X chromosome. It is also true that gender differences may be the result of differences in exposure to infectious disease. Both work and recreational types of exposure may bring men into greater contact with infectious organisms.

Death rates by accidents and other violent causes are much higher for men than for women. Motor vehicle accidents account for a significant

percentage of these differences. Although Waldron did not mention it, the differences caused by motorcycle accidents involving young men is a factor that appears in other U.S. statistics. Men have a much higher death rate than do women from accidental drownings and fatal gun accidents. Suicide is also more prevalent among men, and the incidence increases with age. As noted above, the higher death rate among men may be related to behavioral factors such as heavier alcohol consumption and other types of risk-taking behavior; these behaviors may or may not have a biological component, and cultural influences may also have an effect.

Ischemic heart disease has been consistently higher for men than for women in almost all available international and historical data. However, the magnitude of gender differences for ischemic heart disease has varied considerably in different regions, historical periods, and ethnic groups. The relationship between cigarette smoking and heart disease cannot be ignored. Of interest is the fact that women who smoke do not have the same risk as men. This is attributable to different smoking habits. Not only do men smoke more cigarettes per day, but they inhale more deeply. As to smoking, an often overlooked consideration is that females "may often feel sick as a result of smoking their first cigarette" (Waldron 1986, p. 64) and this may be a deterrent to their developing a smoking habit. Coronary-prone behavior also plays a significant role. There is a greater prevalence of Type A coronary-prone behavior among men than among women. Type A behavior is marked by impatience, competitive drive, and hostility (Busse and Walker 1986).

As to the influence of menopause, there is contradictory evidence regarding the risk of women before or after menopause. There continues to be a debate regarding early onset of menopause. Early onset of natural menopause has been reported to be higher among women who smoke, and this may account in part for the increased risk of myocardial infarction among women with early natural menopause (Waldron 1986).

Mortality due to malignancies is more frequent among males than females over most of the life span. Because of the large variety of cancers, the patterns and causes of gender differences vary for many different types of malignant neoplasms. Furthermore, occupational exposures contribute to the higher cancer rate among men.

Behavioral factors cannot be ignored for either gender. Clearly, the complex interaction of cultural, anatomical, physiological, and behavioral characteristics must be taken into consideration when discussion gender differences in aging, longevity, and mortality.

Waldron (1987) discussed mortality of "older adults"—a category that includes all adults age 40 and over. Ordinarily the years from 40 to 65 would be considered to constitute middle age, with old age beginning at 65. In this older age group, a reversal of certain trends is beginning to show—for example, the gradual decline of ischemic heart disease. Waldron added some additional statistical information regarding the causes of the gender differential in longevity. Of deaths from ischemic heart disease, 50% are attributable to smoking. Ischemic heart disease is the major cause of death linked to atherosclerosis, but atherosclerosis linked to cerebrovascular disease accounts for only 2% of the gender differential in total mortality (National Center for Health Statistics 1984). Waldron concluded that smoking's effects on hormones and on atherosclerosis are responsible for, at most, 25% of the gender differential and total mortality in the United States. She noted that other observations point to behavioral factors as more important causes of gender differences in mortality. Taking high-risk behaviors as a group, behavioral differences appear to be responsible for at least 50% of the gender differential in total mortality in the United States. A question that remains unanswered is, What are the important factors that influence this difference in behavioral risks?

Psychological Theories of Aging

Birren and Renner (1977) expressed the opinion that there was no pressure on the field of psychology to formulate a unified theory of aging or to explain how behavior is organized over time. They did offer a definition of aging for the behavioral sciences that recognizes that there can be incremental functions as well as decremental changes that occur over the adult life span. "Aging refers to the regular changes that occur in mature, genetically representative organisms living under representative environmental conditions" (Birren and Renner 1977, p. 4). Later, Birren and Cunningham (1985) said, "The psychology of aging is concerned with differences in behav-

ior, changes in behavior with age, and patterns of behavior shown by persons of different ages in different periods of time" (p. 18). They also noted that "much of contemporary psychology of aging is a collection of segments of knowledge" (p. 19). Further, this implies that most theories of the psychology of aging are actually microtheories because they do not embrace large amounts of data derived from various domains of behavior.

Baltes and Willis (1977) reached a somewhat similar conclusion: "All existing theories of psychologic aging and development are of the prototheoretical kind and are incomplete" (p. 148). The psychological theories that have appeared are often the extension of personality and developmental theories into middle and late life. Personality theories usually consider the innate human needs and forces that motivate thought and behavior and a modification of these biologically based energies by the experience of living in a physical and social environment.

Baltes recently extended and clarified his concept of the process of the aging mind (Baltes 1993). He emphasizes that it is important to know the full range of human mental performance and potential. Baltes begins with two major aggregations of mental processes: fluid and crystallized intelligence (Hebb 1949). *Fluid intelligence* is described as the mechanics and *crystallized intelligence* as the pragmatics. The fluid mechanisms are considered the basic information processes and are referred to as the hardware. In contrast, the crystallized pragmatics are culturally based and acquired; this is the software of the mind. Baltes is interested in reaching a better understanding of wisdom, as it is often believed to be a characteristic of many elderly persons. Baltes holds that wisdom is the ability to deal with important and difficult matters that are associated with how people conduct their lives and the meaning of life. Wisdom reflects a superior knowledge and includes judgment and sound advice; it is one of the few attributes of late life that is frequently recognized by a large segment of the population.

Schaie (1977–1978) advanced what he called a "stage theory of adult cognitive development" (p. 129). His tentative scheme involved four possible cognitive stages: acquisitive (childhood, adolescence), achieving (young adulthood), responsible and executive (middle age), and reintegrative (old age). Schaie postulated two overlapping cognitive patterns during middle life—a "responsible" component and "executive" abilities—neither of which can be judged by common psychometric testing. He suggested that during the life span there is a transition from "what should I know" through "how should I use what I know" to a "why should I know" phase of life. Schaie has stated the belief that numerous new strategies and techniques will have to be developed in order to fully test a stage theory, and that alterations in the theory will emerge.

Kalish and Knudtson (1976) recommended the extension of the concept (theory) of attachment, common in infant and child psychology, to a lifetime conceptual scheme for understanding the relationships and involvements of older people. They further stated their belief that the concept (theory) of disengagement is not functional and that it should be eliminated. Attachment is a relationship established and maintained by "social bonds" and is distinguished from social contact. Elderly people lose significant early objects of attachment. New attachments are often much weaker, frequently are not mutual, and therefore are vulnerable. Kalish and Knudtson argued that an appreciation and understanding of attachments will provide a better approach to explaining the psychological changes in elderly people. Relevant to the attachment concept is the finding by Lowenthal and Haven (1968) that, more than any other single factor, having a confidant appeared to discriminate between elderly persons who were institutionalized and those who could remain in the community.

There are obvious limitations in the psychological theories of aging; these are quite realistic in view of the complexity of the research. Furthermore, recognizing the complexity of psychological experimentation and theory is essential to an awareness of the considerable psychological investigations that have contributed to a better understanding of human aging. Consequently, the material by Siegler and Poon presented in Chapter 7 ("Psychological Aspects of Normal Aging") is essential to achieving an adequate knowledge of human aging.

Social Theories of Aging

Palmore (1981) proposed five categories of social theories: 1) disengagement, activity, and continuity theories, 2) age stratification, 3) minority group the-

ory, 4) life events and stress theory, and 5) homogeneity versus heterogeneity.

Disengagement theory states that aging invariably causes physical, psychological, and social disengagement (Cumming and Henry 1961). Physical disengagement is attributable to a decline in physical energy, strength, and the slowing of responses. Psychological disengagement refers to the withdrawal of concern from a rather diffuse interest in many people to a focus on those who are directly related to the individual. Some describe this as a shift of attention from the outer world to the inner world of one's own feelings and thoughts. Social disengagement means the reduction of all types of social interaction, including activities such as those related to family, friends, community actions, church participation, and so forth. This theory of disengagement originally held that it was actually good—both for the older person and for society—for the older person to disengage. It was proposed that disengaged older persons tend to be happier and healthier than those who remain active.

Shortly after the appearance of the disengagement theory, the *activity theory* was published (Havighurst 1963). This theory holds that activity positively affects health, happiness, and longevity, and that remaining active is good for both the aging individual and for society.

The *continuity approach* is something of a compromise position between the disengagement and activity theories (Neugarten 1964). Proponents of the continuity approach maintain that older people tend to behave according to a pattern that has been established before late life. At times the person may disengage and other times remain active. It is also apparent that some elderly people will drop one type of activity only to replace it by something that is more suitable to their health status and environment.

Age stratification is really a model of life-span development, but obviously includes late life as a part of the conceptualization. According to Palmore (1981), age stratification conceptualizes society as being composed of different age groups with different roles and different expectations. Each age group must move up through time while responding to changes in environment. Age stratification focuses on distinguishing between age, period, and cohort effects.

The *minority-group theory* relates to differences such as those attributed to race and ethnic groups.

According to this theory, the aged are a minority group and frequently experience the same kind of discrimination that society inflicts upon other minority groups (Busse 1970).

The *theory of life events and stress* holds that those major events usually associated with advancing age are particularly important to health and well-being in late life. A study utilizing this approach must distinguish events that may be welcomed or resisted from those that do not affect all people in a similar manner. Some people resist retirement, whereas others welcome it. Some are unhappy in retirement, and others see it as an opportunity to attain life satisfactions.

Some social theories are related to the age distribution of the population and economic influences. One of these theories holds that the status of the aged is high in static societies and tends to decline with the acceleration of social change (Ogburn and Nimkoff 1940). Another theory is that the status of the aged is inversely related to the proportion of the aged in the population. For the most part, the aged are highly valued in societies in which they are scarce, and their value and status decrease as they become more numerous. The modernization theory of Cowgill and Holmes (1972) suggests that elderly persons are more highly respected in agricultural societies than they are in urbanized societies, and that the status of the aged is inversely proportional to the rate of social change. A more recent study suggests that in some societies in the process of modernization, the status of the aged population goes through phases. During a developmental phase toward modernization, there is an increase in family control of resources, but as modernization continues, the status of elderly people is likely to decline (Gilleard and Gurkan 1987).

Homogeneity and *heterogeneity* are concerned with the issue of whether individuals become more like each other or increasingly different from each other as they age (Maddox and Douglass 1974). One interesting consideration is the possibility that those who survive into late life (i.e., those who are 85 years old and over) have identifiable characteristics that are very similar, whereas these individuals may have been quite different from the other people in the same age group 10–15 years earlier. Another consideration concerns the differences between men and women. Do men and women become increasingly different, or increasingly similar as they age?

All of these theories have been demonstrated to have varying degrees of validity. No satisfactory composite theory of social aging is available that is applicable to all aging people.

Models of Early Aging

The progerias are syndromes that are linked with premature aging. The presence of these disorders does, to a limited extent, provide an opportunity to study accelerated bodily changes that resemble those attributable to aging. Although all of these syndromes are quite rare, two have received particular attention: Hutchinson-Gilford syndrome (Hutchinson 1886; Hastings 1904) and Werner's syndrome.

The early-onset Hutchinson-Gilford syndrome is characterized by dwarfism, physical immaturity, and pseudosenility. Individuals with this syndrome have a peculiar form of hypermetabolism and generally die during their mid-teens of coronary heart disease. Hutchinson-Gilford syndrome affects both sexes and has been described in white, black, and Asian races. The affected individuals look like very old, wizened, small humans with distorted features. This is because their heads are large in comparison to the face, and the ears and nose are small. Scalp hair, eyebrows, and eyelashes are lost. Some of the features that are commonly associated with aging are not increased in Hutchinson-Gilford syndrome. These include tumors, cataracts, and osteoporosis.

The search for the mode of inheritance of Hutchinson-Gilford syndrome continues. The syndrome has been considered to be a rare autosomal recessive condition, but it has been argued that it is more likely a sporadic autosomal dominant mutation because of several observations, including 1) a lower frequency of consanguinity than might be expected, 2) the low frequency of recurrence in families, and 3) a possible parental age effect. The vast majority of cases occur with no siblings affected. For this reason, all of the progerias—and particularly Hutchinson-Gilford syndrome—may be sporadic dominant-type mutations.

Although the life span of fibroblasts of progeria is affected, there have been variations in reports regarding the life spans of individuals with these disorders, making it unclear whether the life span reduction is modest or severe. Furthermore, the suspicion that a basic defect in protein synthesis fidelity is a basic defect in progeria lacks confirmation (Goldstein et al. 1985). Similarly there is confusion regarding the existence or nonexistence of definitive immune abnormalities. As to DNA repair capability, although such a defect is not uncommon, it is not a consistent marker for progeria. One must conclude that the basic metabolic defect is, at this time, unknown.

Werner's syndrome is a later-onset type of progeria. Werner (1904) described, in his doctoral dissertation for graduation from the Ophthalmological Clinic in Kiel, an unusual disorder, under the title "Cataract in Connection with Scleroderma." Werner reported the condition in siblings, two brothers and two sisters between the ages of 36 and 40 years of age. The parents, grandparents, and one sister were healthy.

Because Werner's syndrome differs from normal aging in several respects, Martin (1985) classified this condition as a "segmental progeroid syndrome." The appearance of an individual affected by Werner's syndrome is indeed striking, because the initial impression is that the person is very old. As the disease develops, affected individuals look 20–30 years older than their actual years, and their life span is shortened. Because the disease usually appears before growth is completed, patients with this syndrome frequently have thin limbs and typically are of smaller stature and are less developed than would be expected. Their appearance is striking in that the face develops a tightly drawn, pinched expression. Pseudoexophthalmos, a beak nose, protuberant teeth, and a recessive chin are characteristic features. Cataracts develop early, and in addition to hypogonadism, individuals are likely to have diabetes. Not infrequently, they develop cancer, which contributes to their shortened life expectancy. The connective tissue cells and fibroblasts of these patients have been studied. For instance, Hayflick (1977) mentioned that fibroblast cells derived from such individuals and cultured in vitro undergo significantly fewer doublings than do cell samples from age-matched control subjects.

Progressive mental deterioration is not commonly associated with the progerias, and few postmortem neuropathological studies have been performed on the brains of patients with these syndromes. What we do know at this point is that the usual microscopic changes associated with aging— senile plaques and neurofibrillary tangles—are not characteristic of Werner's syndrome (Ishii et al.

1985). Sumi (1985) reported that Marinesco found small, round eosinophilic inclusions in the nuclei of the neurons in the substantia nigra. According to another review, clinical studies show that approximately 25% of patients with Werner's syndrome have mild neurological defects such as loss of distal deep tendon reflexes, but no systematic psychological or electroencephalogram studies have been reported. It is highly likely, however, that psychological problems are common (Omenn 1977).

Since 1904, at least 250 patients have been reported with similar clinical findings and have been labeled as having "Werner's syndrome." Goto and colleagues (1978) reported on 15 patients with progeria—12 males and 3 females—ranging from 17 to 59 years of age. All patients showed the following signs and symptoms: short stature and light body weight, slender extremities with a stocky trunk, beak-shaped nose, high-pitched and weak voice or hoarseness, juvenile bilateral cataracts, flat feet, and hyperreflexia of the patellar and Achilles tendons. Thirteen of the 15 patients had parents who were consanguineously married, although the article did not contain any further information regarding these consanguineous relationships. It was noted, however, that consanguineous marriages are common in Japan. Goto et al. were able to collect a total of 100 cases in Japan and found that the gender ratio was one to one. They did note that the patients were so similar in their facial characteristics that they could be easily mistaken for identical twins. In an attempt to determine the genetic causation, they found no chromosomal abnormalities.

As to the immunological data, only in one patient did Goto and colleagues find any differences in the titers of IgG, IgA, IgM, and IgE. The only deviation occurred in one patient who had an elevated IgE. They also noted that the ratio of the T-cell subpopulation has been reported to decrease with age; that is, it declines in a normal aging group. However, utilizing the method of Nakai, they found there was a decrease in the T-cell subpopulation among the subjects with Werner's syndrome. Goto and co-workers (1978) did not report the age of death of any of the subjects studied.

Werner's syndrome seems to be somewhat different from Hutchinson-Gilford syndrome in that 10% of Werner's patients develop neoplasms, with a particularly high frequency of sarcomas and meningiomas.

References

American Association of Retired Persons: A Profile of Older Americans, 1986. Washington, DC, American Association of Retired Persons, 1987

Aslan A, Ionescu T, Bordea M, et al: The influence of Gerovital H_3 on the immune cell response in x-rayed Wistar rats. Paper presented at the 13th International Congress of Gerontology, New York, July 12–17, 1985

Baltes PB: The aging mind: potential and limits. Gerontologist 33:580–594, 1993

Baltes PB, Willis SL: Toward psychological theories of aging and development, in Handbook of the Psychology of Aging. Edited by Birren JE, Schaie KW. New York, Van Nostrand Reinhold, 1977, pp 128–147

Barnes DM: Defect in Alzheimer's is on chromosome 21. Science 235:846–847, 1987

Barton WE: How it feels to grow old. Integrative Psychiatry 4:191–192, 1986

Belkin BM, FA Neelon: The art of observation: William Osler and the method of Zadig. Ann Intern Med 116:863–866, 1992

Berk SL: Sir William Osler, ageism, and "the fixed period": a secret revealed. J Am Geriatr Soc 37:263–266, 1989

Birren JE, Cunningham WR: Research on the psychology of aging: principles, concepts, and theory, in Handbook of the Psychology of Aging, 2nd Edition. Edited by Birren JE, Schaie KW. New York, Van Nostrand Reinhold, 1985, pp 5–45

Birren JE, Renner VJ: Research on the psychology of aging, in Handbook of the Psychology of Aging. Edited by Birren JE, Schaie KW. New York, Van Nostrand Reinhold, 1977, pp 3–34

Braceland FJ: Aging ourselves tomorrow, in The 18th Carrier Foundation Symposium. Edited by Garber RS, Sugerman AA. Nutley, NJ, Roche Laboratories, 1978, pp 7–13

Brown TW, Wisniewski HM: Genetics of human aging. Review of Biological Research in Aging 1:81–99, 1983

Busse EW: The aged: a deprived minority. North Carolina Journal of Mental Health 4:3–7, 1970

Busse EW: Longevity and rejuvenators, in Psychiatry Update: Mental Illness in Later Life. Edited by Busse EW, Pfeiffer E. Washington, DC, American Psychiatric Association, 1973

Busse EW: Theories of aging, in Behavior and Adaptation in Late Life, 2nd Edition. Edited by Busse EW, Pfeiffer E. Boston, MA, Little, Brown, 1977, pp 11–32

Busse EW: Biologic and psychosocial bases of behavioral changes in aging, in American Psychiatric Association Annual Review, Vol 2. Washington, DC, American Psychiatric Press, 1983, pp 96–106

Busse EW: The political abuse of psychiatry. Perspectives 4:22–24, 1984

Busse EW: Primary and secondary aging, in The Encyclopedia of Aging. Edited by Maddox GL, Roth G, Atchley R, et al. New York, Springer, 1987, p 534

Busse EW: A gerontologist looks at his own retirement and aging. Generations 15(1), Winter 1991

Busse EW, Maddox GL: Cognitive function and behavior, in The Duke Longitudinal Studies of Normal Aging. Edited by Busse EW, Maddox GL. New York, Springer, 1985, pp 77–96

Busse EW, Walker JI: Heart and neuropsychiatric disorders, in The International Text of Cardiology. Edited by Cheng TO. New York, Pergamon, 1986, pp 976–987

Cerami A, Vlassara H, Brownlee M: Glucose and aging. Sci Am 256:90–96, 1987

Chebotarev DF (ed): Longevity: Medical and Social Aspects. Kiev, USSR, Institute of Gerontology AMS USSR and USSR Gerontological and Geriatric Society, 1984

Cole TR: The Journey of Life. Cambridge, UK, Cambridge University Press, 1992

Cowgill D, Holmes L (eds): Aging and Modernization. New York, Appleton-Century-Crofts, 1972

Cristafalo VS: Animal cell cultures as a model for the study of aging, in Advances in Gerontological Research. Edited by Strehler BL. New York, Academic Press, 1972, pp 68–72

Cumming E, Henry W: Growing Old. New York, Basic Books 1961

Erikson EH: Ghandi's Truth on the Origin of Militant Nonviolence. New York, WW Norton, 1969

Finkelstein MS: Defenses against infection in the elderly: the compromises of aging. Triangle 23:57–64, 1984

Gilleard CJ, Gurkan AA: Socioeconomic development and the status of elderly men in Turkey: a test of modernization theory. J Gerontol 42:353–357, 1987

Goldstein S, Wojtyk RI, Harley CB, et al: Protein synthetic fidelity in aging human fibroblasts, in

Werner's Syndrome and Human Aging (Advances in Experimental Medicine and Biology, Vol 190). Edited by Salk D, Fujiwara Y, Martin GM. New York, Plenum, 1985, pp 495–508

Goto M, Horiuchi Y, Tanimoto K, et al: Werner's syndrome: analysis of 15 cases with a review of the Japanese literature. J Am Geriatr Soc 26:341–347, 1978

Gruman GJ: A History of Ideas About the Prolongation of Life: The Evolution of Prolongevity Hypotheses to 1880. Philadelphia, PA, American Philosophical Society, 1966

Hart RW, Turturro A: Review of recent biological research theories of aging. Review of Biological Research in Aging 2:3–12,3, 1985

Hastings G: Progeria: a form of senilism. Practitioner 73:188–217, 1904

Havighurst R: Successful aging, in Processes of Aging. Edited by Williams R, Tibbitts C, Donahue W. New York, Atherton Press, 1963, pp 81–90

Hayflick L: The limited in vitro lifetime of human diploid cell strains. Exp Cell Res 37:614–616, 1965

Hayflick L: Cellular basis for biological aging, in Handbook of Biology of Aging. Edited by Finch CE, Hayflick L. New York, Van Nostrand Reinhold, 1977, pp 73–86

Hayflick L: How and Why We Age. New York, Ballantine, 1994

Hayflick L, Moorhead PS: The serial cultivation of human diploid cell strains. Exp Cell Res 25:585–621, 1961

Hebb DO: The Organization of Behavior. New York, Wiley, 1949

Holliday R: Testing molecular theories of cellular aging, in Dimensions of Aging. Edited by Bergener M, Ermini M, Stahelin HB. New York, Academic, 1986, pp 21–34

Hutchinson J: Case of congenital absence of hair and mammary glands with atrophic condition of the skin and its appendages. Lancet 1:473–477, 1886

Ishii T, Hosoda Y, Hamada Y, et al: Pathology of the Werner syndrome, in Werner's Syndrome and Human Aging (Advances in Experimental Medicine and Biology, Vol 190). Edited by Salk D, Fujiwara Y, Martin GM. New York, Plenum, 1985, pp 187–214

Kalish RA, Knudtson FW: Attachment versus disengagement: a life-span conceptualization. Human Development 19:171–181, 1976

Kanin G: Remembering Mr. Maugham. New York, Atheneum, 1966

Laurence J: The immune system in AIDS. Sci Am 252:84–93, 1985

Lind LR (trans): Gabriele Zerbi, Gerontocomia: On the Care of the Aged and Maximianus, Elegies on Old Age and Love, translated from the Latin. Philadelphia, PA, American Philosophical Society, 1988

Lowenthal MF, Haven C: Interaction and adaptation: intimacy as a critical variable, in Middle Age and Aging. Edited by Neugarten BL. Chicago, IL, University of Chicago Press, 1968, pp 390–400

McKusick VA: Mendelian Inheritance in Man: Catalogs of Autosomal Dominant, Autosomal Recessive and X-Linked Phenotypes, 6th Edition. Baltimore, MD, Johns Hopkins University Press, 1982

Maddox GL, Douglass EB: Aging and individual differences. J Gerontol 29:555–563, 1974

Martin GM: Genetic syndromes in man with potential relevance to the pathobiology of aging: genetics of aging. Birth Defects 14:5–39, 1977

Martin GM: Genetics and aging: the Werner syndrome as a segmental progeroid syndrome, in Werner's Syndrome and Human Aging (Advances in Experimental Medicine and Biology, Vol 190). Edited by Salk D, Fujiwara Y, Martin GM. New York, Plenum, 1985

National Center for Health Statistics: Monthly Vital Statistics Report 33(9), 1984

Neugarten B: Personality in Middle and Later Life. New York, Atherton Press, 1964

National Institute on Aging: Biochemistry and aging, in In Search of the Secrets of Aging. Washington, DC, National Institute on Aging, May 1993a

National Institute on Aging: The genetic connection, in In Search of the Secrets of Aging. Washington, DC, National Institute on Aging, September 1993b

Ogburn WF, Nimkoff MF: Sociology. Boston, MA, Houghton Mifflin, 1940

Omenn GS: Behavior genetics, in Handbook of the Psychology of Aging. Edited by Birren JE, Schaie KW. New York, Van Nostrand Reinhold, 1977, pp 190–216

Ostfeld A, Smith C, Stotsky B: The systematic use of procaine in the treatment of the elderly. J Am Geriatr Soc 25:1–19, 1977

Palmore E: Advantages of aging. Gerontologist 19:220–223, 1979

Palmore E: Social Patterns in Normal Aging: Findings from the Duke Longitudinal Study. Durham, NC, Duke University Press, 1981

Palmore EB: Longevity in Abkhasia: a reevaluation. Gerontologist 24:95–96, 1984

Paul R: Alchemy altercation at Texas A&M. Science 262:1367, 1993

Schaie KW: Toward a stage theory of adult cognitive development. Journal of Aging and Human Development 8:129–138, 1977–1978

Pollock GH: How Psychiatrists Look at Aging. Madison, CT, International Universities Press, 1992

Segerberg O Jr: The Immortality Factor. New York, EP Dutton, 1974

Sumi SM: Neuropathology of Werner syndrome, in Werner's Syndrome and Human Aging (Advances in Experimental Medicine and Biology, Vol 190). Edited by Salk D, Fujiwara Y, Martin GM. New York, Plenum, 1985, pp 52–61

Suskind GW: Immunological aspects of aging: an overview. Paper presented at the National Institute on Aging Conference on Biological Mechanisms of Aging, Washington, DC, 1980

Taeuber CM: Sixty-Five Plus in America. Malta, United Nations International Institute on Aging, 1993

Thewlis MW: The history of geriatrics, in The Care of the Aged. Edited by Thewlis MW. St. Louis, MO, CV Mosby, 1924

Tobin JD: Physiological indices of aging, in The Baltimore Longitudinal Study of Aging (NIH Publ No 84-2450). Edited by Shock NW. Rockville, MD, National Institutes of Health, 1984, pp 387–395

Waldron I: What do we know about causes of sex differences in mortality: a review of the literature. Population Bulletin of the United Nations 18:59–76, 1986

Waldron I: Causes of the sex differential in longevity. J Am Geriatr Soc 35:365–366, 1987

Weiss AK: Biomedical gerontology: the Hayflick hypothesis. Gerontologist 14:491–493, 1974

Werner O: Uber Katarakt im Verbindung mit Sklerdermie. Doctoral dissertation, Ophthalmological Clinic, Kiel, USSR, 1904

Weisse AB: Osler, aging and the late twentieth century (editorial). Journal of Chronic Diseases 30:473–475, 1977

Zeman FD: Some little-known classics of old-age medicine. JAMA 200:150–152, 1967

CHAPTER 2

Physiological and Clinical Considerations of the Geriatric Patient

John W. Rowe, M.D.
Cathryn A. J. Devons, M.D., M.P.H.

The Physiology of Aging

Over recent decades, increasing interest in aging and the medical problems of older persons has fueled substantial growth in physiological, psychological, and sociological research on aging. Investigators involved in such studies recognize the critical importance of separating pathological from age-related changes. Thus, for physiological studies, careful guidelines are developed to exclude individuals whose results might not represent "normal" aging but would be contaminated with changes related to specific disease processes (Rowe 1985; Shock et al. 1984). Results on the remaining population are felt to represent "normal" aging, with confidence regarding the age specificity of the findings resting more on longitudinal studies of age changes than on cross-sectional comparisons of age differences, which are sensitive to cohort effects. Numerous carefully conducted cross-sectional and longitudi-

nal studies on well-screened, well-characterized populations have demonstrated major effects of age on a number of clinically relevant variables, including hearing, vision, renal function, glucose tolerance, systolic blood pressure, bone density, pulmonary function, immune function, sympathetic nervous system activity, and a variety of cognitive and behavioral measures. Such nonpathological aging effects are important to understand, not only as reflections of the aging process but also—because they serve as a physiological substrate for the influence of age on the presentation of disease—as reflections of response to treatment and the complications that ensue.

The decline in most variables that change with age is linear into the eighth and ninth decades. Although healthy 80-year-olds are more aged than their younger counterparts, having accumulated more of the changes secondary to age, they are not losing function at a more rapid rate.

Although many important physiological variables—including cardiovascular, immune, endocrine, renal, and pulmonary functions—show fairly substantial losses with advancing age, an important characteristic of these data sets is the substantial variability (Rowe 1977, 1985; Shock et al. 1984). The variability often increases with advancing age so that older people become less like each other, not more like each other. In many data sets, one can easily find older persons with minimal or no physiological loss compared with their younger counterparts, whereas the average change in the aged group is a very substantial decrement from the results seen in youth.

Changes in one organ with age are not necessarily predictive of changes in other organs. If an apparently healthy 60-year-old is found on serial prospective measurements to have a cardiac output that is falling at a certain rate, this information is of no value in predicting the rate at which the individual's kidneys, thyroid, sympathetic nervous system, or any other organ is changing with time. This apparent failure of various organs to be synchronized in their age-related changes rules against the presence of a basic biological clock. Currently one cannot construct a variable termed "functional age" that predicts performance on a physiological or psychological test better than does the individual's chronological age.

The variability in human aging from individual to individual is also substantial. In studies of functions that undergo major changes with age, the variance is often large, and one can easily identify apparently healthy 40-year-olds who perform at the same level as the average 80-year-old. Likewise, many 80-year-olds can be found who perform like the average 40-year-old.

Successful and Usual Aging as Subtypes of Normal Aging

The prior focus of research on dichotomizing findings into either disease or "normal" aging categories has important limitations. This approach tends to neglect the substantial heterogeneity among older persons with regard to many physiological and cognitive variables. In addition, it tends to imply that the physiological changes that occur in older individuals in the absence of disease are harmless and do not carry a significant risk. Finally, the identification of certain physiological changes as "normal" suggests that these changes are the natural state of affairs and thus cannot or should not be modified.

The physiological changes that occur with "normal" age, in the absence of disease, are very variable, are in many cases associated with attributable risk for adverse health events, and are potentially modifiable. The contribution of the intrinsic aging process to decrements observed in the aged population may be substantially less than previously recognized, with factors such as personal habits, diet, exercise, nutrition, environmental exposures, and body composition playing more important roles.

Rather than focusing purely on differentiation of the effects of disease versus "normal" aging, investigators conducting gerontological studies should recognize that the "normal" aging group includes two important subsets. One subset is composed of those individuals who demonstrate minimal age-associated losses in a given physiological function (e.g., immune function, bone density, carbohydrate tolerance, renal function, cognitive function). These individuals might be viewed as aging "successfully" with regard to the particular variable under study. Individuals who demonstrate "successful" aging in a constellation of physiological functions, rather than just one, present a state of minimal physiological loss and robust physiological function in advanced age—a pure aging syndrome. This successful aging group represents a small but potentially increasing portion of the overall "normal" aging population, the bulk of which is represented by the second subset under discussion, the group that might be termed the "usual" aging group. For a given physiological variable, individuals in the usual aging group have significant impairments compared with their younger counterparts but do not qualify as having a disease. As noted previously, the physiological losses in the usual aging group are characterized by large interindividual differences, and those individuals with the greatest "age effect" are at increased risk for the emergence of a specific disease or disability.

The pathways of physiological or psychological change that individuals take with advancing age are influenced by the intrinsic aging process and a variety of extrinsic factors, including genetic and environmental influences, personal habits, diet, psychosocial factors, and diseases. We should also be aware that older persons who display "usual aging" for a given function may be able to improve their function and thus potentially reduce their risk of adverse outcomes. Therefore, the focus of study moves gradually from the evaluation of the emergence of diseases in an aging population to elucidation of those factors that regulate the transition of individuals from successful to usual state of aging and vice versa.

With these general considerations in mind, the specific physiological changes associated with aging will be reviewed from two perspectives. First, the types of changes will be discussed because they represent a continuum in the interaction of intrinsic aging and pathology. Second, detailed information will be presented on specific clinically relevant physiological changes in the major organ systems.

The Continuum of Interaction Between Physiology and Pathology in the Elderly

The interaction of age and disease varies from a lack of interaction on one end of the spectrum to the extreme example where the changes that occur with age are often aggravated by extrinsic factors and actually represent disease inasmuch as they have direct, predictable, adverse clinical sequelae. Several specific, clinically relevant points along the continuum can be identified.

Variables That Do Not Change With Age

Perhaps the most important physiological change that occurs with age, from a clinical standpoint, is no change at all. Too frequently clinicians are apt to ascribe a disability or abnormal physical or laboratory finding to "old age," when the actual cause is a specific disease process. An example of this lack of change may be seen in hematocrit. Frequently, elderly individuals will be found to have low hematocrit levels, and the clinician will categorize the patient as having "anemia of old age." The physician may fail to pursue the underlying basis of the anemia, believing that the normal aging process has induced the anemia and that no investigation or treatment is warranted. However, data from several sources, including the Framingham study, indicate that in healthy community-dwelling elderly people there is no change in hematocrit with age (Gordon

and Shurtleff 1973). Thus, a lower hematocrit level in an elderly individual cannot be ascribed to "anemia of old age," but deserves a proper investigation and treatment.

Physiological Changes by Which Specific Diseases Become Less Likely or Severe With Age

Although aging is characteristically considered to be associated with a greater prevalence or severity of disease, it is quite possible that the physiological changes associated with normal aging result in many diseases being less likely or less severe in advanced age. Clearly, some disorders that appear to be based, at least in part, in altered immune system response—such as systemic lupus erythematosus, myasthenia gravis, and multiple sclerosis—are seen much more commonly in younger persons than in older individuals. It is feasible that the changes that occur in the immune system with age might result in a less robust immunological response to the inciting agent or event in these disorders (Gillis et al. 1981). In this regard, recent findings of increased auto-anti-idiotypic antibody production with age suggest a basis for lessened autoimmune disease in elderly persons.

Similarly, some diseases that occur in old age as well as in younger adults clearly run a less virulent natural history in elderly persons. One example may be carcinoma of the breast. Many cancer specialists feel that carcinoma of the breast runs a more virulent and more aggressive course in premenopausal than postmenopausal women. In addition, the likelihood of breast carcinoma responding well to hormonal therapy increases with the number of years after menopause. Thus, elderly individuals with this disease might be expected, on average, to enjoy a more favorable clinical course than their younger counterparts.

Physiological Changes That Alter the Presentation of a Disease

The physiological changes that alter the presentation of a disease are, in general, poorly understood, yet this area has long been recognized as being of major importance to the practice of geriatric medicine. Many diseases that occur in both young and old adults have manifestly different clinical presentations and natural histories in the two age groups. These disorders should not necessarily be looked on as either less or more severe in elderly persons, but just *different*.

One example of a common disorder that presents very differently in the elderly compared with the young is uncontrolled diabetes mellitus. In children and young adults, uncontrolled diabetes is generally manifested by diabetic ketoacidosis, with elevations of blood glucose to levels between 300 and 500 mg/dL and coincident severe metabolic acidosis associated with markedly elevated levels of circulating ketones. Conversely, elderly persons with uncontrolled diabetes will frequently present with hyperosmolar nonketotic coma, altered consciousness, striking elevations of blood glucose (often to levels exceeding 1,000 mg/dL), and a relative or absolute lack of circulating ketones or acidosis.

Impaired Homeostasis in the Elderly: Physiological Changes That Increase the Likelihood or Severity of a Disease

The category of physiological changes that increase the likelihood or severity of a disease encompasses age-related reductions in the function of numerous organs that place the elderly person at special risk for increased morbidity from diseases in those organs.

Cross-sectional and longitudinal studies in carefully screened subjects across the adult age range indicate that increasing age is accompanied by inevitable physiological changes that are separable from the effects of diseases. There is no pleasant plateau of the middle years during which physiological function is stable; instead, there is a progressive, age-related reduction in the function of many organs, including major losses in renal, pulmonary, and immune functions. Simultaneous linear reductions in homeostatic capabilities in several organs result in a geometric reduction in the total homeostatic capacity. When coupled with the functional impairments associated with disease states, this constricted homeostasis is responsible for the markedly increased vulnerability of the elderly to morbidity during acute illness or trauma (such as burns; see Figure 2–1), major surgery, or administration of medications.

Normal aging is associated with a marked reduction in pulmonary function, as reflected in the

forced vital capacity and other measures of lung function. Healthy individuals in the ninth decade of life frequently will have lung function equal to only one-half that of their 30-year-old counterparts. Thus, an acute pulmonary disease, such as bacterial pneumonia, will be more likely to induce a serious clinical manifestation in an elderly person because of the markedly lessened pulmonary functional reserve. Over the past decade, very significant advances have been made in our understanding of the marked reduction in immune competence that occurs with age. Immunosenescence is likely responsible, in some ways, for the increased severity of infections in the elderly population. Thus, an elderly individual with pneumonia may be less likely to contain and control that infection in the respiratory tract than a young individual. Failure of immune function may result in dissemination of that infection to many organs, and a much more serious, if not life-threatening, clinical illness may develop.

An additional example of a mechanism whereby age-related alterations in function increase the prevalence of a disease relates to the development of accidental hypothermia in the frail elderly. This disorder is associated with a high mortality rate and can be seen not only in individuals exposed to unheated rooms in the winter, but also in individuals in adequately heated rooms who appear to spontaneously develop marked lowering of body temperature. This disorder is essentially absent in healthy young individuals and occurs with increasing frequency with advancing old age. Although the mechanisms of accidental hypothermia are poorly

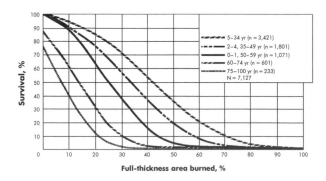

Figure 2–1. Survival of burn patients as a function of the total percentage of body surface burned and age. *Source.* Reproduced with permission from Feller I, Flora JD, Bawol R: "Baseline Results of Therapy for Burned Patients." *JAMA* 236:1945, 1976.

understood, alterations in sympathetic nervous system responsiveness seem likely to be a major contributor.

Physiological Changes That Mimic Specific Diseases

Some changes that occur with aging may be seen to mimic specific clinical entities, thus causing confusion regarding the diagnosis of specific diseases in older persons. Perhaps the best and most widely recognized instance of this is the decrease in carbohydrate economy, reflected in decreased performance on oral or intravenous glucose tolerance tests, that occurs with advancing age in the absence of diabetes mellitus (Davidson 1979). This is discussed in detail later in this chapter (see subsection on carbohydrate metabolism in section "Age-Related Changes in the Major Organ Systems").

Physiological Changes That Have a Direct Clinical Impact

For decades, gerontologists and geriatricians have drawn a clear line between changes that occur with age and those that are associated with specific disease states. We have staunchly defended the view that aging is not a disease but rather a normal process that must be clearly understood to adequately diagnose and treat the increasing burden of illness that will befall a rapidly growing population. Substantial data suggest that this approach is no longer tenable. There is no question that some physiological changes of aging have clearly adverse clinical sequelae. Although a change may represent "normal aging" inasmuch as it is present in the entire population and cannot be avoided, one should not assume that "normal" change is necessarily harmless.

Although one can argue about the specific criteria for the definition of a "disease," one generally acceptable definition would include any process that results in clearly adverse clinical sequelae measured as either morbidity or mortality. Under this definition there are clear changes that occur with advancing age that appear to be normal characteristics of the aging process and that would also qualify as diseases. Of the potentially long list of such processes, three are briefly reviewed.

More than any other biological changes, menopause seems clearly to be accepted as age related.

Although menopause is thus clearly "normal," it has become abundantly clear that this normal change is associated with increased risk for certain diseases such as osteoporosis and atherosclerosis as well as for symptomatic clinical manifestations such as hot flashes, which are associated with sleep disturbances and are so frequent and severe as to be disabling in many individuals (Hannon 1927; McKinlay and Jefferys 1974).

A second change that occurs with normal aging and that has direct adverse clinical consequences is lens opacification, or cataract formation. Posttranslational modifications of central lens proteins with advancing age result in increasing opacity as well as decreasing flexibility of the lens, which is manifested in decreasing capacity to accommodate to near vision (Weale 1963). The reasons for development of cataracts in some individuals and not others are poorly understood. Lens opacification is a common cause of blindness in older Americans. Thus, this normal age-related change, in its most extreme form, would seem to represent a disease.

A third characteristic type of change with advancing age that appears to have direct clinical consequences is arteriosclerosis. This thickening of the walls of major arteries must be distinguished from atherosclerosis, which represents the development of plaques on the vessel intima that encroach on the lumen. Arteriosclerosis appears to be a normal consequence of age-related changes in the extracellular material in arterial walls and is reflected in decreased compliance and increased stiffening of vessels with advancing age (O'Rourke 1970). This is manifested in increased systolic blood pressure, which is discussed in detail later in this chapter (see subsection on aging of the heart in section "Age-Related Physiological Changes in the Major Organ Systems").

Age-Related Physiological Changes in the Major Organ Systems

Endocrine Systems

Gerontological interest in endocrine systems has been based in part on the view that senescence is an incapacity to regulate the internal environment in response to changes in the internal or external milieu. Endocrine systems display a broad spectrum of effects during aging that are of major clinical relevance (Minaker et al. 1984). This rich variety provides the opportunity to increase the understanding of specific common illnesses and evaluate general mechanisms underlying physiological aging.

Evaluation of endocrine systems has generally emphasized anatomical studies and measures of circulating hormone levels under basal conditions and during physiologically relevant stresses. Similar normative changes occur with age in the anatomy of most endocrine glands. Each gland appears to decrease in weight and to develop a patchy, atrophic appearance accompanied by vascular change and fibrosis. Most glands have a tendency to form adenomas.

Basal hormonal levels in animals and humans are generally not influenced by age. Several hormones, however, clearly have reduced serum concentrations of their active form after changes in binding hormones are taken into account. These include renin, aldosterone, and dehydroepiandrosterone. Secretion rates of most hormones decline with advancing age whether lean body mass is adjusted for or not. Substantial declines in the secretion of testosterone, insulin, adrenal androgens, and thyroid hormone are well established. he maintenance of near-normal circulating hormone levels in the face of decreased secretion rates necessarily implies that hormone clearance rates are decreased similarly with age. Although it is not presently known whether the primary defect lies in hormone secretion or in hormone clearance, the implication is clear that the capacity to adjust hormone secretion or to maintain stable levels of plasma hormones is maintained with age. The generation of active metabolites, where examined, suggests there is decreased rate of production of these with advancing age.

Receptor binding appears to show no systematic changes during aging. Although some receptors are clearly decreased, either in affinity or number, the majority are unchanged (Minaker et al. 1984). Postreceptor responses to hormone action appear to decrease with advancing age. This is the case with somatomedins, insulin (particularly with regard to glucose metabolism), catecholamines, and steroid hormones. Elucidation of the mechanisms by which age decreases postreceptor hormone action and the relative contributions to these effects of aging per se and of extrinsic factors represent the next major frontier of gerontological endocrine research. The following section deals with specific changes that occur with age in the physiology of a number of clinically relevant endocrine systems.

Carbohydrate Metabolism

An age-related impairment in the capacity to maintain carbohydrate homeostasis after glucose challenge has been recognized for more than 60 years. Over the past two decades a number of studies have focused attention on elucidation of the underlying mechanisms, and a general consensus is now emerging. Increasing age in individuals without clinical evidence or family history of diabetes is associated with a progressive decline in carbohydrate tolerance, a modest (approximately 1 mg/dL/decade) increase after maturity in fasting blood glucose levels, and a rather striking increase in blood sugar after oral glucose challenge (8–10 mg/dL/decade at 1 hour) (Davidson 1979). Recent studies indicate that at least 22% of Americans aged 65–74 demonstrate impaired carbohydrate tolerance that is not severe enough to warrant a diagnosis of diabetes mellitus (Harris et al. 1987). The increases in postprandial glucose levels seen with aging are also reflected in increased levels of hemoglobin A_{1C}.

Pathogenetic mechanisms postulated to underlie these changes in carbohydrate tolerance include age-related changes in body composition, diet, activity, and insulin secretion and action. In response to oral or intravenous glucose challenges, elderly on high carbohydrate intakes have repeatedly been found to have circulating insulin levels that are equivalent to, or in many cases greater than, levels found in their younger counterparts. This is due in large part to the fact that clearance of insulin is impaired in the elderly. Insulin release is either not influenced or is mildly impaired with age. The major effect of age under these conditions is decrease of the effectiveness of insulin to induce glucose metabolism in peripheral tissues. On diets low in carbohydrate content, older persons demonstrate impaired insulin release as well as insulin resistance.

There is no effect of age on basal hepatic glucose production or the regulation of hepatic glucose production by insulin. There is also no age effect on insulin receptor number or affinity. It appears that the insulin resistance of aging is due to a postreceptor defect in glucose transport into cells.

The carbohydrate intolerance of aging may be an example of "usual" aging rather than "successful" aging and may carry substantial risk. A report from the Honolulu Heart Study evaluated a 12-year risk of stroke in 690 diabetic and 6,908 nondiabetic individuals free of stroke at study entry (Abbott et al. 1987). Diabetes was associated with a clearly increased risk of stroke. In addition, in nondiabetic subjects, the risk of stroke was moderately age-related and was statistically significantly higher for those at the 80th percentile of serum glucose when compared with those at the 20th percentile. Studies focusing on postprandial hyperinsulinemia, a cardinal feature of the insulin resistance of aging, have shown increases in insulin levels to be a significant independent contributor to the incidence of coronary artery disease. In addition to these effects, increases in insulin level are associated with increases in triglyceride level and decreases in high-density lipoprotein cholesterol levels, both of which are known risk factors for heart disease.

Many studies have attempted to identify the relative contributions of aging per se and a number of extrinsic factors to the noted carbohydrate intolerance associated with advanced age. Zavaroni et al. (1986), studying factory workers aged 22–73, evaluated the contributions of obesity, physical activity, family history of diabetes, and the use of diabetogenic drugs to age-related increases in glucose and insulin levels after an oral glucose tolerance test. The initial strong correlations among age, postprandial glucose, and insulin level increases became much weaker when the effects of these other factors were taken into account, so that the correlation between glucose and age was limited to marginal statistical significance, and there was no longer an effect of age on insulin levels. In addition, other studies have shown a significant direct relationship between physical fitness as reflected in maximal oxygen consumption and insulin-stimulated glucose metabolism in nonobese older men. Other studies have shown that the capacity to metabolize glucose is markedly improved in those older persons who are physically trained compared with their less well-trained counterparts.

These findings clearly suggest that much of the observed glucose intolerance and insulin resistance of older people may be caused by factors other than biological aging per se. In addition, the available data suggest that the carbohydrate intolerance of aging may not be "normal" in the sense that it is not harmless. More aggressive approaches to modifying the extrinsic factors associated with impairment of glucose metabolism would be in the best interest of many elderly individuals.

Parathyroid Function

The general consensus derived from a number of careful studies of healthy men and women across the adult age range is that human aging, in the absence of disease, is associated with the development of a very mild form of hyperparathyroidism. There is clear evidence of a gradual and very variable increase in circulating levels of parathyroid hormone with advancing age. As parathyroid hormone is metabolized, fragments accumulate in the blood that are generally excreted by the kidneys. It is not surprising, in view of the marked decrease in glomerular filtration rate (GFR) with age (discussed later in this section), that radioimmunoassays that detect intact hormone, as well as these inactive fragments, indicate an 80% increase in circulating levels of parathyroid hormone between ages 30 and 80 years. However, when assays sensitive only to intact hormone are used, a persistent increase of 30% is still observed over the adult age range. The modest increase in circulating levels of parathyroid hormone is not accompanied by change of total serum calcium, but rather by a slight reduction in ionized calcium that probably represents a stimulus from parathyroid release. This increase in parathyroid hormone is clearly physiologically relevant because it is reflected, in the elderly, in increased levels of urinary cyclic adenosine monophosphate (cAMP).

The major physiological mechanism contributing to a slight decrease in ionized calcium with age and the attendant slight increases in parathyroid hormone level is a well-documented decline in intestinal calcium absorption (Bullamore et al. 1970). This decline is probably due, in turn, to decreases in 1,25-dihydroxy-vitamin D_3 levels, which have been well documented with age and which, in turn, are probably related to decreases in renal mass. Thus it would appear that the primary abnormality with advancing age is a decrease in renal mass.

Although this is very variable, as discussed later in this chapter, in those individuals in which it is physiologically significant, it leads to a progressive cascade of alterations in endocrine and gastrointestinal systems relevant to skeletal integrity that result in the development of mild normocalcemic hyperparathyroidism. It is important to note that the mild hyperparathyroidism of "normal" aging is probably not a major contributing factor to the development of osteoporosis, because individuals with and without hip fracture have been shown to have similar circulating parathyroid hormone levels, with the exception of those few individuals with significant hyperparathyroidism.

Thyroid Function

Normal aging, in the absence of disease, has no major effect on the function of the thyroid gland and no clinically important influence on the results of diagnostic studies (Livingston et al. 1987). Thus, serum levels of thyroxine (T_4), free thyroxine, the 3,5,3'-triiodothyronine (T_3) resin uptake test, and a free T_4 index are not importantly influenced by age. Thyroxine clearance has been shown to decrease with age, but this is coupled with a decrease in the release of T_4, resulting in no major overall change in serum levels. Although minor age-related declines in T_3 have been identified with advancing age, the values remain within the rather broad limits described as "normal" for young populations. It is widely recognized that the most sensitive index of thyroid inadequacy is a modest elevation of circulating thyroid-stimulating hormone (TSH) levels, and thus there has been substantial interest in the impact of age on TSH secretion. A number of studies have shown that TSH is either unchanged or very slightly increased with age but remains within the normal limits. Whereas early studies indicated that the thyrotropin-releasing hormone (TRH) stimulation of TSH was impaired in elderly men but not in elderly women, more recent evidence suggests that there is no important influence of age on the TRH stimulation test (Harman et al. 1984). Although thyroid antibodies can be found in higher prevalence in older populations, their presence does not constitute a sensitive or specific screening test for thyroid disease; up to one-third of patients with hypothyroidism have no antithyroid antibodies.

Thyroid gland dysfunction is one of the most common endocrine disorders in the elderly, yet the diagnosis is often difficult to make. Reports of the prevalence of hypothyroidism in the elderly vary widely. In one study by Bahemuka and Hodgkinson (1975), 2.3% of an elderly inpatient group were found to be hypothyroid. The majority of the cases were in women, and a strong association was found with other autoimmune disorders. Patients with hypothyroidism often have nonspecific complaints, such as weakness, memory loss, and constipation. Hypothyroidism can often be accompanied by depressive symptoms. Both the patient and the physician may believe that the symptoms are part of normal aging, and the diagnosis can be missed. The thyroid gland sits lower in the neck in older persons and may even be in the mediastinum, making physical examination more challenging. It is particularly important to watch for the thyroid rising in the neck during examinations.

Because hypothyroidism is so insidious and is relatively common in the elderly, screening is recommended, usually determination of TSH. Savin and colleagues (1985) reported that 14.4% of individuals over 60 years of age have an elevated TSH with a normal T_4, a finding that often represents a prehypothyroid state. Rosenthal et al. (1987) conducted a longitudinal study of elderly persons with an elevated TSH and a normal T_4 and found that those who also had elevated microsomal antibodies were much more likely to go on to develop hypothyroidism.

The elderly represent 10%–30% of all hyperthyroid patients. Symptoms of hyperthyroidism in elderly individuals can be quite different from those seen in younger persons. Patients have been classically described as "apathetic," because of the paucity of symptoms of sympathetic overactivity such as nervousness and tachycardia. Dominant features of presentation of hyperthyroidism in the elderly are likely to be cardiovascular. Angina, atrial fibrillation, and congestive heart failure may be the first signs of hyperthyroidism.

Male Reproductive System

The possible existence of a male climacteric, analogous to the female menopause, has long attracted attention. Early studies suggested a decrease in the level of testosterone and dihydrotestosterone with age. Additional studies on healthy men, who were very carefully screened to exclude those with underlying disease, are mixed, showing either no effect of age on levels of total testosterone, free testosterone, or the major metabolite, dihydrotestosterone, or a modest decline in levels of these hormones (Harman and Nankin 1985; Harman and Tsitouras 1980). Although the majority of current studies show a modest decline in levels, it is clear that this is a variable finding and that many elderly men, even in their 90s, will still have a testosterone level that is not importantly different from that of the average middle-aged man. Normal blood levels reported by some authors may still reflect age-related decreases in secretion of androgens, because androgen clearance falls with advancing age.

Healthy men have shown a modest decrease in luteinizing hormone (LH) levels, a marked increase in follicle-stimulating hormone (FSH) levels, and decreases in LH and FSH response to LH-releasing hormone, suggesting a decrease in pituitary gonadotropin reserve or sensitivity. Prolactin levels are either unchanged or increased slightly with age. In healthy men there appears to be no change in testicular size or in sperm number or morphology.

The Duke Longitudinal Study has shown that 75% of healthy males over the age of 70 have intercourse at least once a month and that 25% of those over the age of 78 are still engaging in regular sexual activity (Pearlman 1972). Martin (1981) found that sexual activity in late life tends to correlate with the degree of sexual activity earlier in life as well as with general health. Sexual response is delayed and greater stimulation is required for a man to obtain an erection, which tends to be less firm in late life. The ejaculatory volume is decreased, and men do not appear to have the need to ejaculate with every episode of intercourse. After ejaculation, there is rapid detumescence of the penis and a rather prolonged refractory period before the man is able to have another erection. There is no correlation between levels of serum testosterone and sexual activity in healthy elderly men.

Female Reproductive System

Menopause is one of the most widely recognized age-related biological changes. Whereas many of the physiological effects of aging discussed in this chapter are modified strongly by extrinsic factors such as lifestyle, diet, and habits, this does not appear to be the case with menopause. The average age of onset of menopause has been remarkably stable at 50–51 years for several centuries and appears unrelated to age of menarche, body composition,

diet, or socioeconomic status. The only possibly important exception is smoking, which appears to hasten menopause. Although widely considered to represent part of the "normal" aging process, menopause clearly should not be considered to be harmless; it is associated with a number of potentially adverse changes, including acceleration of age-related bone loss; increase in the risk of coronary heart disease; changes in the female reproductive and urinary tract, particularly thinning and atrophy of the vagina and urethra; and hot flashes, which occur in approximately 50% of postmenopausal women and can be very disturbing.

The primary physiological change underlying menopause appears to be age-related loss in the number of ova and their associated follicles. The population of ova begins at several million during gestation, falls to 400,000 at menarche, and to less than 100 at menopause. In the years preceding menopause, the reduction in the number of ova is associated with ovarian resistance to FSH stimulation and to reductions in circulating levels of the major estrogen produced by the ovary, 17-beta-estradiol. In the premenopausal period as 17-beta-estradiol levels fall, FSH levels increase, with a variable and less pronounced increase in LH levels as well. After age 45, cycle length declines, with the primary reduction being in the follicular phase, whereas the luteal phase remains stable. As menopause nears, the interval between menses lengthens, and anovulatory cycles begin before the final cessation of bleeding. With the progressive reductions in circulating levels of estradiol, FSH and, to a lesser extent, LH levels rise. Interestingly, administration of gonadotropin-releasing hormone results in even further increases in FSH and LH in postmenopausal women (Carr and MacDonald 1985).

Menopause is a state of relative rather than absolute estrogen deficiency. Postmenopausally, circulating estrogen levels are maintained at a much lower level than before menopause. Castration or adrenalectomy does not further reduce estrogen levels in postmenopausal women; the circulating estrogens—primarily estrone, a physiologically weaker estrogen than estradiol—are produced in extraglandular sites from the metabolism of androstenedione. One of the most important extraglandular sites of estrogen production is adipose tissue, and therefore obese elderly postmenopausal women may have substantial circulating estrone levels.

Osteoporosis

Bone loss occurs in all elderly persons as a result of an imbalance between resorption and formation in bone remodeling. Osteoporosis, the most common metabolic bone disease, occurs when there is loss of bone to such an extent that the skeleton is no longer adequate for mechanical support, and there is an increased susceptibility to fractures, particularly of the vertebral bodies, the distal radius, and the proximal femur. During the course of their lifetimes, women lose about 50% of their cancellous bone and 30% of their cortical bone, and men lose 30% of cancellous bone and 20% of cortical bone (Riggs 1986).

Several studies focusing on osteoporosis prevention have shown that engaging in weight-bearing exercises and increasing dietary calcium and vitamin D intake are useful in increasing bone mass. Women with low bone density can decrease the rate of subsequent bone loss by taking estrogen replacement therapy at the time of menopause. Those patients who have suffered compression fractures as a result of osteoporosis may benefit from additional treatment with new antiresorptive agents such as calcitonin and biphosphonates.

Aging of the Heart

Physiological age-related changes that occur in the heart are of obvious major clinical importance as a substrate for the development of cardiac disease and as a significant predisposing factor in the development of cardiac complications of noncardiac diseases, trauma, or surgery. Perhaps more than most other physiological areas, elucidation of the relative contributions of intrinsic aging per se and those of extrinsic factors has been very difficult in studies of the heart. This is because of the high prevalence of asymptomatic coronary artery disease in the elderly population and the importance of physical fitness in influencing cardiovascular performance. A number of studies have shown that up to 50% of elderly individuals will have severe occlusive disease in at least one coronary artery, although they may not have any symptoms or show any abnormality in a resting electrocardiogram (White et al. 1950). Investigators now use exercise tolerance testing and thallium scanning in an effort to identify and exclude individuals with underlying heart disease from the "normal" aged group. The results of such robust studies show much less decline in cardiac function in old age than did previous studies, which were undoubtedly contaminated by inclusion of individuals with underlying cardiac disease.

The second major factor, physical fitness, is difficult to quantitate in community-dwelling populations. One must be careful not to exclude all individuals except the very fit, because this would yield a superselect group whose results tell us little about normal aging and have little generalizable clinical relevance. One reasonable approach is to study carefully screened men and women across the adult age range, aggressively attempting to exclude those with underlying heart disease and seeking individuals who are not physically trained but who participate fully in the activities of daily living. In the following discussion, the studies cited have generally met these criteria. The literature reviewed deals with the effect of age on cardiac function both under rest and in response to stress in order to provide a broad perspective on the possible clinical implications of the physiological changes in the aging human heart.

Cardiac function at rest. The results of physical examination of the heart are not necessarily altered with age, although nonradiating systolic ejection murmurs, generally attributed to aortic sclerosis, are common in individuals over age 75. The electrocardiogram is also generally not importantly changed with age in the absence of disease.

Studies of carefully screened individuals from across the adult age range fail to identify an effect of advancing age on cardiac output in the sitting position, but show a modest decline in cardiac output in the supine position. This suggests that older persons do not increase their cardiac output in response to the increased preload associated with the supine position as much as their younger counterparts (Rodeheffer et al. 1984).

Important at-rest cardiovascular variables that are not influenced by age include left-ventricular diameter, area, and volume, and ejection fraction. There is a very modest decline in basal heart rate with age, which is compensated for by a slight increase in stroke volume to maintain cardiac output. There is no change in peripheral resistance with age, despite a slight increase in systolic blood pressure—which is discussed at length elsewhere in this chapter (Lakatta 1979).

There is a clear increase in left-ventricular wall thickness with age. This modest cardiac hypertrophy is probably secondary to the increase in systolic blood pressure. Stroke work, the product of stroke volume and systolic blood pressure, thus increases with age. There is no effect of age on myocardial force production or the extent of shortening under basal conditions.

Early diastolic filling falls with advancing age. This is probably due to age-related prolongation of isometric relaxation time and decreases in cardiac compliance, which are secondary to collagen accumulation in the ventricle. Thus, as the ventricle stiffens with age, relaxation is impaired and filling slows. This may become important when cardiac rate is increased and diastole shortens, leading to inadequate filling, pulmonary venous congestion, and dyspnea.

Taken together, these physiological studies suggest that there are no inevitable changes with age in cardiac performance, although some modest modifications primarily relating to decreases in left-ventricular compliance and subsequent impairment of diastolic function are probably secondary to the hypertrophic response to increases in systolic blood pressure.

Cardiac performance under stress. At various levels of exercise, cardiac output rises in older individuals to levels similar to those seen in their younger counterparts. However, maximal heart rate during exercise declines with age, and cardiac output is maintained via an increase in stroke volume and left-ventricular end diastolic volume. Although the left-ventricular ejection fraction declines with age, the absolute amount of blood ejected with each contraction is greater in elderly persons because left-ventricular end diastolic volume is clearly increased, and thus an adequate stroke volume can be maintained at a lower ejection fraction (Lakatta 1979).

These changes in cardiac response to stress appear related to the well-documented age-related blunting of the chronotropic and inotropic response of the senescent myocardium to adrenergic stimulation. Because circulating norepinephrine levels are higher in the elderly, both under basal circumstances and in response to graded exercise, inadequate heart rate response clearly cannot be attributed to catecholamine deficiency. Studies of the physiological mechanisms underlying these findings suggest that they are not related to a decline in adrenergic myocardial receptors but to postreceptor events.

In summary, the senescent human heart is fully capable of maintaining adequate overall function—that is, cardiac output—both under basal circumstances and in response to stress. Specific physiological effects of aging, primarily related to decreased compliance of the left ventricle and impaired diastolic function as well as impaired chronotropic response to stress, lead to specific adaptations. Thus, adequate cardiac output is maintained during exercise via increases in left-ventricular end diastolic volume and stroke volume to compensate for the lack of increase in cardiac output. These physiological changes are important clinically because they may explain the tendency of older individuals to develop pulmonary venous congestion during uncontrolled atrial fibrillation or other forms of supraventricular tachycardia; they may also help to explain the blunted response of the elderly to beta-adrenergic agonist and antagonist stimulation.

Hypertension in the elderly. There have been many recent advances in knowledge about hypertension in the elderly. The commonly held views that hypertension accompanies "normal" aging, that it is harmless, and that antihypertensive therapy is poorly tolerated in older persons have come under attack. The most recent data from clinical trials have given evidence to support the beneficial effects of treatment of hypertension in older persons, and the multitude of new pharmacological agents on the market has made treatment easier than ever before.

There are two types of hypertension seen in older persons. The first, systolic-diastolic hypertension, is defined as a systolic blood pressure greater than 140 mm Hg with a diastolic pressure more than 90–95 mm Hg. The second type is isolated systolic hypertension, which has been found to be of particular importance in the elderly. Isolated systolic hypertension occurs when the systolic blood pressure is greater than 160 mm Hg with a concomitant diastolic blood pressure less than 90 mm Hg.

The Framingham Study is a longitudinal study that was begun in 1948 to explore the epidemiology of cerebrovascular and cardiovascular disease. The

Framingham data demonstrated a disproportionate rise in systolic pressure with age, whereas diastolic pressure appeared to level off at age 55 (Kannel and Gordan 1978). This results in an increased incidence of isolated systolic hypertension associated with aging. Estimates of the prevalence of hypertension among the elderly vary from study to study and are generally thought to be inflated. Figures depend on the age and race of the population studied, blood pressure cutoff values used, and the number of times the blood pressure is measured. Data from the Framingham Study showed a cumulative incidence of isolated systolic hypertension of 418 per 1,000 in men and 533 per 1,000 in women.

There is general agreement that the major pathophysiological factor underlying isolated systolic hypertension is the age-related decrease in arterial compliance (Rowe 1983). Although some systemic changes in circulating catecholamines and the renin-angiotensin system have been shown to occur with age, to date these have not been shown to contribute importantly to the development of isolated systolic hypertension.

The risk of isolated systolic hypertension. The early evidence for an increase in morbidity and mortality associated with isolated systolic hypertension came from several longitudinal studies. Colandrea et al. (1970) reported the findings on 72 elderly patients with isolated systolic hypertension. Over a 4-year follow-up period, 10 hypertensive patients had fatal cardiovascular events compared with one member of the age-, sex-, and diastolic-matched control group. The Chicago Stroke Study (Shekelle et al. 1974) was a 3-year longitudinal study of 2,100 men and women aged 64–74 years. In the group with diastolic blood pressure less than 95 mm Hg and systolic blood pressure greater than 180 mm Hg, the incidence of stroke was 2½ times greater and mortality was 59% higher compared with subjects with normal systolic blood pressure. Data from 30 years of follow-up of the original Framingham Study (Stokes et al. 1989) cohort of 5,070 men and women who were 30–62 years old and free of cardiovascular disease when the study began show that blood pressure is a strong predictor for the development of coronary heart disease and stroke. In another longitudinal study, investigators conducting the Multiple Risk Factor Intervention Trial (MRFIT; Stamler et al. 1989) examined 356,222 men aged 35–57 at entry.

During 6 years of follow-up, more than 2,000 coronary deaths occurred. With this large data set, a clear correlation was found between elevated blood pressure and the risk of coronary heart disease. Elevated systolic blood pressure was even more strongly associated with death from coronary heart disease than was elevated diastolic blood pressure.

The Cardiovascular Health Study (Psaty et al. 1992) provided evidence that isolated systolic hypertension not only is associated with an increased risk of clinically apparent heart disease, but also carries an increased risk of subclinical disease. In a sample of 2,189 community-dwelling persons over age 65 who were not being treated for hypertension and had no known history of clinical coronary heart disease, 195 (9%) had isolated systolic hypertension. Elevation of systolic pressure was associated with electrocardiographic evidence of myocardial infarction, increased left-ventricular mass, diastolic dysfunction, and increased intima-media thickness of the carotid artery.

The benefits of treating hypertension. The original Veterans Administration Cooperative Study proved the benefit of treating mixed systolic and diastolic hypertension. The European Working Party on Hypertension (Amery et al. 1985) was a double-blind, placebo-controlled randomized trial of treatment of 840 persons over age 60 with elevated systolic and diastolic blood pressure. The treatment group received hydrochlorothiazide and triamterene as first-line treatment, and then methyldopa. After 7 years of follow-up, the treatment group had a 38% reduction in cardiac mortality and 32% fewer cerebrovascular events compared with the placebo group. In subgroup analysis, no benefit could be demonstrated for treating hypertension in those over 80 years old.

The Swedish Trial in Old Patients With Hypertension (STOP–Hypertension; Dahlof et al. 1991) was the first study designed specifically to examine the impact of treating systolic and diastolic hypertension in persons 70–84 years old. Patients were treated with hydrochlorothiazide and amiloride as first-line and a beta-blocker as second-line therapy, and were followed longitudinally for up to 65 months. The results demonstrated striking reductions of 45% in cardiovascular morbidity and mortality, 46% in fatal and nonfatal strokes, and 43% in total mortality.

The benefits of treating isolated systolic hypertension. The Systolic Hypertension in the Elderly Project (SHEP Cooperative Research Group 1991) was the first study to clearly show the benefit of lowering systolic blood pressure in the elderly (see Figure 2–2). The SHEP trial was a 5-year, multicenter, double-blind placebo-controlled study designed to assess the ability of antihypertensive drug treatment to reduce the incidence of fatal and nonfatal cardiovascular events and stroke. A total of 447,921 persons over 60 years of age were screened to find 4,736 with isolated systolic hypertension. At the start of the study, the average systolic blood pressure among the participants was 170 mm Hg, with an average diastolic blood pressure of 77 mm Hg. The initial treatment was chlorthalidone (12.5–25 mg); if needed, atenolol (25–50 mg) or reserpine (0.05–0.1 mg) was added. After an average of 4.5 years of follow-up, the treatment group had an average systolic blood pressure of 143 mm Hg, and the placebo group had an average systolic blood pressure of 155 mm Hg. The total incidence of stroke was 5.2 per 100 participants in the treatment group and 8.2 per 100 in the control group, a 36% reduction in stroke incidence. The combined incidence of nonfatal myocardial infarction plus coronary death was 27% lower in the treatment group. The benefit of treatment of isolated systolic hypertension was found for participants of all ages, including those over 80 years old, without regard to race or gender.

These studies demonstrate clearly the beneficial reductions in cerebrovascular and cardiovascular

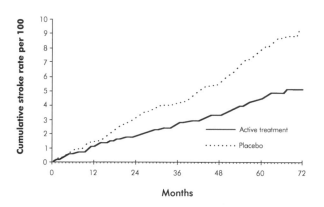

Figure 2–2. Cumulative fatal plus nonfatal stroke rate per 100 participants by treatment group in the Systolic Hypertension in the Elderly Project (SHEP).
Source. SHEP Cooperative Research Group 1991.

disease associated with treating hypertension in elderly persons, particularly those with elevated systolic blood pressure. Treatment should be initiated if the average systolic blood pressure on two visits is greater than 160 mm Hg or diastolic is greater than 90 mm Hg. Evidence from the SHEP trial suggested that treating systolic blood pressure in the 140–160 mm Hg range may be beneficial, but no study has yet been done to confirm this. Low-dose thiazide diuretics are safe and effective in the elderly as first-line therapy.

Renal System

Advancing age is associated with progressive loss of renal mass in humans, with renal weight decreasing from 250–270 g in young adulthood to 180–200 g by the eighth decade. The loss of renal mass is primarily cortical, with relative sparing of the renal medulla. The total number of identifiable glomeruli decreases with age, roughly in accord with the changes in renal weight.

It is generally agreed from histological studies that normal aging, independent of hypertension or renal disease, is associated with variable sclerotic changes in the walls of the larger renal vessels. These sclerotic changes do not encroach on the lumen and are augmented in the presence of hypertension. Radiographic studies in normotensive patients demonstrate an increasing prevalence after the seventh decade of abnormalities similar to those seen in patients with hypertension, including abnormal tapering of interlobar arteries, abnormal arcuate arteries, increased tortuosity of intralobular arteries, and a predilection for age-related vascular abnormalities to occur in the polar region. Smaller vessels appear to be spared, with only 15% of senescent kidneys from nonhypertensive patients displaying arteriolar changes.

Combined microangiographic and histological studies have identified two very distinctive patterns of change in arteriolar-glomerular units with senescence. In one type, hyalinization and collapse of the glomerular tuft is associated with obliteration of the lumen of the preglomerular arteriole, which results in loss of blood flow. This type of change is seen primarily in the cortical area. The second pattern, seen primarily in the juxtamedullary area, is characterized by the development of anatomic continuity between the afferent and efferent arterioles during glomerular sclerosis. The end point is thus loss of the glomerulus and shunting of blood flow from afferent to efferent arterioles.

Renal blood flow.   Renal plasma flow declines progressively from 600 mL/minute in young adulthood to 300 mL/minute by 80 years of age. The primary factor contributing to this decrease appears to be a reduction in the renovascular bed already discussed above. Studies in healthy potential renal donors, ranging in age from 17 to 76 years, indicate that the age-related decrease in flow is not purely a reflection of decreased renal mass, but rather that flow per gram of tissue falls progressively after the fourth decade. There is a highly significant decrease with advancing age in the cortical component of blood flow, with preservation of medullary flow—a finding consistent with the histological studies reviewed above (Hollenberg et al. 1974). These cortical vascular changes probably account for the patchy cortical defects commonly seen on renal scans in healthy older adults. Studies using intravenous administration of vasodilators, including acetylcholine or pyrogen, show similar increases in renal blood flow in all age groups, indicating that the age-related change in renal blood flow is not related to "functional spasm," but appears to be on a fixed or structural basis. Consistent with these findings, vasoconstrictor response to angiotensin is not influenced by age.

Glomerular filtration rate.   The major clinically relevant functional defect arising from the histological and physiological changes with aging in the kidney is a decline in the GFR. Age-adjusted normal standards for creatinine clearance have been established (Rowe et al. 1976). Creatinine clearance is stable until the middle of the fourth decade, when a linear decrease of about 8.0 mL/minute/1.73 m/decade begins. Long-term longitudinal studies indicate substantial variability in the effect of age on creatinine clearance, with as many as one-third of individuals showing no decline in GFR with age. This variability suggests that factors other than aging per se may be responsible for the apparent effect of age on renal function. One important "extrinsic" factor may be blood pressure, because longitudinal studies show that increasing blood pressure levels within the normotensive range are associated with accelerated loss of renal function.

Serum creatinine.   Muscle mass, from which creatinine is derived, falls with age at roughly the same rate as GFR, and so the rather drastic age-related loss of GFR is not reflected in an elevation of serum creatinine. Thus, serum creatinine overestimates GFR in the elderly. A healthy 80-year-old man with a creatinine clearance 32 mL/minute less than his 30-year-old counterpart of the same stature and weight will have the same serum creatinine. Depressions of GFR so severe as to result in elevation of serum creatinine above 1.5 mg/dL are rarely due to normal aging, and so indicate the presence of a disease state.

One must consider not only the effects of age but also those of muscle mass on determining the utility of serum creatinine as an estimate of renal function. Elderly debilitated individuals may have a markedly limited muscle mass and glomerular filtration rates as low as 20–30 mL/minute with serum creatinine levels of less than 2.0 mg/dL. In these cases, renal impairment is often overlooked or, at best, underestimated, and these patients are at risk for the development of iatrogenic complications.

In clinical practice, the doses of many drugs excreted primarily by the kidneys are routinely adjusted to compensate for alterations in renal function. This is particularly true of digoxin preparations and aminoglycoside antibiotics. Unfortunately, these adjustments are usually based on serum creatinine values, with the resultant predictable overdose in elderly patients. Dose adjustment should ideally be based on creatinine clearances, even if a timed urine specimen of only a couple of hours is available. If no timed urine specimen can be obtained and only serum creatinine is available, the influence of age must be considered. This can be accomplished by use of the following formula (Cockcroft and Gault 1976):

Creatinine clearance (mL/minute) =

$$\frac{(140 - \text{age}) \times \text{weight (kg)}}{72 \times \text{serum creatinine (mg/dL)}}$$

(15% less in females).

Pulmonary System

A central theme of this discussion regarding the physiological changes with age has been the importance of extrinsic factors, including personal habits, diet, and so forth, as modifiers of the aging process in the absence of disease. Just as increasing levels of blood pressure in the normotensive range influence renal function and physical fitness affects cardiovascular capacity, cigarette smoking and exposure to hazardous environmental conditions clearly accelerate the progressive changes that occur in pulmonary function in the absence of disease. In this section we discuss the changes that occur in the lung in the absence of obvious extrinsic factors such as cigarette smoking or evidence of pulmonary disease. We focus on four major areas: pulmonary mechanics, gas exchange, control of respiration, and pulmonary defense mechanisms.

Pulmonary mechanics. Changes with age in the compliance of both the lung and the chest wall account for many of the observed alterations in pulmonary volumes with age. Under normal conditions, the natural tendency of the chest wall to expand is matched by the natural tendency of the lung to collapse so that, under static conditions, lung volume is constant. With advancing age the chest wall becomes stiffer, developing a greater tendency to expand. Simultaneously, the lung becomes stiffer and thus has less of a tendency to collapse. These changes, taken together, explain the finding that functional residual capacity—the volume at which the tendency of the lung to collapse inward is balanced by the tendency of the chest wall to expand outward—increases progressively with advancing age. This increase in functional residual capacity is accompanied by a decrease in vital capacity—or the amount of air exhaled following a maximal inhalation—and an increase in residual volume. Total lung capacity either remains constant or declines very slightly with age (Weiss 1980).

Numerous studies have shown that the major flow rates used in clinical measurements of pulmonary function (i.e., the forced vital capacity and the forced expiratory volume in 1 second) decline with age. These changes are very variable, however, and many individuals demonstrate very minor declines.

Gas exchange. The primary determinant of gas exchange is the match of the distribution of blood flow and ventilation in the lung. The decreases in compliance with aging result in closure of airways in the lower portions of the lungs during much of the respiratory cycle and a mismatch of ventilation

and perfusion. These changes, along with increases in physiological dead space, result in progressive declines in arterial oxygen concentration after adulthood. Normal arterial PO_2 for the aged can be estimated by the following formula:

$$PO_2 = 100 - 0.34 \times age.$$

Despite the decline in PO_2 with age, there is no change with age in arterial CO_2 content or pH.

Control of respiration. Advancing age is associated with a progressive blunting of both the central and the peripheral components of the system that controls respiration. It is unknown whether this decreased respiratory drive is the result of reduced responsiveness to decreases in PO_2 or increases in PCO_2, or whether it is caused by reduced output from the central respiratory center. Ventilatory drive, as measured by the ventilatory response to hypoxia and hypercapnia, is blunted with normal aging. The magnitude of this effect is slight, however, and it generally does not have clinical significance (Kronenberg and Drage 1973).

Pulmonary defense mechanisms. Pulmonary defense mechanisms play a critical role in the prevention of respiratory tract infections. Recognition of the important increase in the prevalence and severity of pneumonia in the elderly has led to substantial study of the influence of normal aging on pulmonary defense mechanisms. In addition to the substantive age-related alterations in systemic immune function—particularly cell-mediated immunity—age-related impairments have been identified in local nonimmune defense mechanisms, including the cough reflex, as well as in laryngeal reflexes and in the rate at which mucus is transported by cilia up the trachea so that it can be expectorated. These changes, when combined with systemic immune changes, place the elderly at enhanced risk for respiratory infection. However, it must be emphasized, as with many other variables, that physiological changes with age are very variable and that many healthy older persons have respiratory tract defense mechanisms that are within the normal range for younger adult populations.

In summary, there are very substantial reductions in respiratory function with advancing age.

Decreases in defense mechanisms make respiratory infection more likely. Decreases in the compliance of the lung and chest wall lead to alterations in gas exchange, which provide older individuals with decreased respiratory reserve. This decreased reserve often becomes critically important in the presence of respiratory infection. In this regard, it is of particular interest to note that longitudinal studies indicate that forced vital capacity is a statistically significant predictor of future mortality in community-based population studies. As such, this measure of respiratory function may begin to approach a useful "biomarker of aging" that provides an index, other than birth date, of the rate of physiological change in at least one clinically important organ system.

Gastrointestinal System

Esophagus.   Esophageal function is not importantly influenced by normal aging in the absence of disease. Although a modest decrease has been found in the amplitude of peristalsis in the esophagus, and older persons are more likely to have other nonspecific motility disturbances, these changes are not generally of clinical relevance. To date, there have been no clear physiological changes identified as underlying the clearly increased prevalence of hiatus hernia with advancing age.

Stomach and duodenum.   The impaired acid-secreting capacity of the aged stomach is well documented. With advancing age, maximal stimulated gastric acid decreases 10 mEq/hour/decade in men and slightly less in women. The term *gastric atrophy* is generally reserved for individuals with very low or no acid secretion, whereas *atrophic gastritis* refers to the range of decreased acid production values seen in older persons. An indirect index of gastric acid secretion may be found in the ratio of circulatory pepsinogen I (PI) (which is secreted by mucous and chief cells in the gastric fundus) to pepsinogen II (PII) (secreted by cells in the gastric fundus, cardia, and antrum). When a PI/PII ratio less than 2.9 is considered to be indicative of gastric atrophy, the prevalence of this disorder increases from 24% between the ages of 60 and 69 years to 37% over age 80 years (Krasinski et al. 1986). Impaired gastric acid production has several clinically relevant consequences, including decreased gastric emptying, lowered intrinsic factor levels, enhanced propensity for bacte-

rial overgrowth, and elevated proximal intestinal pH, which influences nutrient and drug absorption. Long-term studies show that atrophic gastritis tends to persist and that superficial gastritis progresses slowly to atrophic gastritis.

Other studies of gastric physiology with advancing age show minor changes. There are no major effects of age on gastric motility, emptying, or the absorption of simple sugars.

Small intestine.   As gastric acid secretion decreases with age, the sterility of the gastrointestinal tract is threatened. Elderly individuals have higher counts of coliform bacteria in the small intestine than their younger counterparts. Blood supply to the intestine is not altered with age.

Absorption of nutrients to the small intestine is, in general, well preserved in the elderly. Although occasional deficits do exist, such as in fat absorption, these are minor and have limited, if any, clinical significance.

With regard to vitamins and minerals, there is, as mentioned previously, a progressive reduction in absorption of calcium with advancing age. This is most likely related to decreases in circulating levels of 1,25-dihydroxy-vitamin D_3, rather than structural or primary physiological changes in the intestine. There is a slight decline in the circulating levels of B_{12} with age, which may be related to B_{12} malabsorption secondary to bacterial overgrowth, but the declines are generally not significant enough to result in clinical evidence of B_{12} deficiency. Absorption of folic acid is adequate in most elderly persons. This may be due to the fact that the tendency toward decreased absorption induced by higher intestinal pH is compensated for by folate production from increased bacterial flora (Russell et al. 1986). Vitamin A absorption increases with age, most likely secondary to age-related declines in the unstirred water layer barrier and increases in pH, thus placing elderly persons who ingest large doses of vitamin A supplements at risk for vitamin A toxicity.

Liver, biliary tract, and pancreas.   There are no changes with age in the size or weight of the liver. Standard liver function tests, which have widespread clinical application, are not influenced by age; nor is the bromosulfophthalein retention test. There are, however, important age-related declines in hepatic blood flow and oxidizing systems. The primary clinical impact of these changes is pharmacological because they impair the metabolism and increase the half-life of many agents that are modified primarily via hepatic mechanisms. These pharmacological changes are discussed in detail in Chapter 20. Exocrine pancreatic function is not importantly influenced by age.

Colon.　The high prevalence of constipation or other symptoms of colonic dysfunction has led to the widespread belief that there are major changes with age in the physiology of the colon. On the other hand, a number of studies have shown that the physiology of the large bowel is intact with age in the absence of disease. The reflex responsible for defecation is intact with aging. It has become clear that age-related impairments in large bowel function, which have become so common as to be considered a part of normal aging, are not related to inevitable physiological changes with age as much as they are to insufficient dietary fiber, medication use, inadequate food intake, laxative abuse, and inadequate exercise in the elderly.

Thermoregulation

Advancing age is associated with progressive restriction in the capacity to regulate body temperature. Although older people are able to maintain their body temperature within narrow normal limits under ordinary conditions, they are much more likely to exhibit altered thermal regulation under stress. In most older people with altered temperature regulation, the physiological changes with age are aggravated by concomitant disease states or the administration of medications that impair thermoregulatory function.

Hypothermia.　Older persons are at especially high risk for accidental hypothermia, which occurs when the body's core temperature is unintentionally reduced below 35°C (95°F). Typically the older person with hypothermia is not a victim of exposure to severely cold weather. More commonly seen is a frail, multiply impaired person who may have fallen asleep next to an air conditioner or developed sepsis with paradoxical hypothermia. The physiological changes that occur with aging that predispose the elderly to accidental hypothermia include decreases in temperature sensitivity, body mass, shiv-

ering, and response to catecholamines. Additional important risk factors seen in the elderly include diseases such as diabetes, malnutrition, hypothyroidism, stroke, Parkinson's disease, reduced physical activity, consumption of alcohol, and the administration of medication such as tranquilizers, sedatives, and antidepressants. The greatest impediments to recognition of accidental hypothermia are lack of consideration of the diagnosis and failure to use low-reading thermometers. Patients with hypothermia are often lethargic, dysarthric, and ataxic. The abdomen is cool to the touch, and shivering is often absent. Sinus bradycardia, arrhythmias, and congestive heart failure can be potentially life-threatening complications. The treatment of choice is slow warming with close attention to heart rate, blood pressure, and blood glucose.

Hyperthermia.　Hyperthermia is also an important threat to the elderly person's health: two-thirds of all victims of heat stroke are over 60 years old. Typically, hyperthermia in the elderly is not the result of exertion in extreme heat. It is more likely the consequence of a frail person's failing to recognize a gradual increase in ambient and body temperature. In addition to impaired temperature sensitivity, older people have a delayed and less robust sweating response to thermal stimuli as well as delayed vasodilation that interferes with heat loss. As in accidental hypothermia, use of tranquilizers and other psychoactive medications may impair thermoregulation and increase the risk of heat stroke in the elderly. Immediate, aggressive treatment should be instituted to bring the body temperature down.

Afebrile infection.　Many healthy elderly persons are capable of developing a fever in the presence of significant infections, although the excursion of the temperature curve is less dramatic than in similarly infected younger people. In addition, a significant subset of older persons do not experience a fever in the presence of quite severe infections, especially bacteremia and pneumonia. In these cases, the patients are often very old and have other conditions that interfere with fever development such as hypothyroidism, renal failure, malignancy, or have been administered salicylates or steroids. Although the precise mechanism of the failure of some elderly to mount a fever has yet to be completely elucidated, there is evidence to suggest there is a reduced production of interleukin-1 associated with aging. It is therefore prudent not to rely too heavily on the presence of fever as an index of infection, especially in frail very old patients.

Illness Behavior in the Elderly

Underreporting of Illness

An important factor underlying functional impairment in the elderly is the failure of many persons to seek assistance. Studies in several countries with various health care systems indicate that symptoms of serious and treatable diseases often go unreported (Anderson 1966; Rowe 1977). Health problems reported by frail elderly persons are thus frequently only the tip of the iceberg of treatable illness.

This apparently self-destructive behavior springs from the notion on the part of older individuals that advanced age is necessarily accompanied by illness and functional decline and that many symptoms are thus to be expected rather than treated. Other contributing factors include cognitive impairment, fear of the nature of the underlying illness, and concern about the costs and other negative aspects of hospitalization, diagnostic evaluation, or unpleasant treatment.

As Besdine (1982) has pointed out, nonreporting of symptoms of underlying disease in elderly persons is an especially dangerous phenomenon when coupled with the passive American organizational structure of health care delivery, which lacks prevention-oriented or early detection efforts. He noted that aged persons, burdened by society's and their own ageist views of functional loss with aging, cannot be relied on to initiate appropriate health care for themselves, especially early in the course of an illness.

Multiple Diseases

The coexistence of several diseases has a profoundly negative influence on health and functional independence in the elderly. The number of pathological conditions in a person is strongly related to age. Elderly individuals who live in the community have 3.5 important disabilities per person (Anderson 1966), and the hospitalized elderly have evidence of 6 pathological conditions per person (Wilson et al. 1962). The entire array of diseases present in an in-

dividual patient must be considered as treatment plans are developed.

Atypical or Altered Presentation of Disease in the Elderly

A fundamental principle of geriatric medicine is that many diseases are manifested by signs or symptoms in the elderly that differ from those in their younger counterparts. These alterations can take two major forms. First, specific characteristic symptoms of a disease in middle age may be replaced by other symptoms in old age. For instance, in acute myocardial infarction, some studies have suggested that elderly persons are less likely than younger adults to present with chest pain (Pathy 1967). On the other hand, acute myocardial infarction is not "silent" in older persons; instead, they have a variety of other acute signs and symptoms, including syncope, and the sudden onset of left-ventricular failure (Besdine 1980). The second difference is that elderly persons may present with nonspecific signs and symptoms (Besdine 1980), such as confusion, weakness, weight loss, or "failure to thrive," instead of specific symptoms indicating the organ or organ system affected.

Importance of Functional Change With Advancing Age

Function, the ability to manage daily routines, is of major concern to the elderly person. The emphasis in the provision of health care to the elderly should be on maintaining functional capability. Most older persons living in the community are cognitively intact and fully independent in their activities of daily living. Unfortunately, major activity limitations due to chronic conditions become increasingly common with aging. Major functional impairment is seen in only 5% of those aged 65–74, whereas by age 85 this rises to 35%–40%. Even if one maintains functional independence into old age, the risk of becoming frail for a long period is still high. For independent persons between the ages of 65 and 70 years, "active life expectancy," that portion of the remaining years characterized by independence, represents about 60%, a portion that falls to 40% by age 85.

Evaluation of the elderly patient should focus on what the patient can do, relative to what he or she should be able or wishes to do, and on identification of recent functional deficits that may be reversible. Although a complete and precise diagnosis is essential, the functional impact of each diagnosis should be evaluated. Specific diagnoses often have little relation to functional status, and the length of the diagnosis list provides little insight into the specific needs and capabilities of a given elderly person. A long list of diagnoses may give a physician the false impression that a patient is impaired and frail when this may not be the case at all. Thus, diagnoses themselves are often a weak criterion for assessing the health status and needs of an elderly individual.

Approach to Comprehensive Functional Assessment of the Elderly

Functional assessment is most useful when a standard systematic approach is used. The Subcommittee on Aging of the American College of Physicians developed a useful, simple approach to routinely screen the functional status of older persons (Lachs et al. 1990). The approach focuses on specific target areas that represent a common source of functional disability but are often missed when conventional history and physical examination techniques are used. These areas are discussed below.

Sensory impairments become increasingly common with aging and can be devastating for the older person. Poor vision can contribute to isolation and increase the risk of falls. Visual loss, particularly from cataracts, can be prevented by screening and appropriate referrals. Hearing loss is also associated with isolation, worsening confusion, and depression. Hearing aids can substantially improve the quality of an elderly person's life.

Activities of daily living scales are useful in determining the elderly person's ability to function independently. Some of these include the ability to bathe, dress, toilet, transfer, and groom oneself independently. Activities of daily living instruments are used to evaluate measures such as ability to use the telephone, shop, cook, handle finances, and use transportation independently.

Falls and impaired mobility are common in the elderly and can be screened for simply by observing a patient rise from a chair, walk, and sit down again. Patients' homes should be examined for obstacles such as loose rugs whenever possible, and environ-

mental adaptations (such as bath bars) should be fitted as needed. Physical therapy and appropriate use of canes and walkers can prevent injuries.

Urinary incontinence is a common problem for the elderly, which many older persons may be reluctant to discuss. Unless the physician queries the patient about involuntary loss of urine, an existing problem may remain undetected. There are many reversible causes of incontinence such as infections, fecal impactions, medical conditions such as diabetes mellitus, and medications such as diuretics, sedatives, and anticholinergics. Urological consultation can be helpful in treating mechanical causes of incontinence.

Nutritional deficiency in the elderly can be multifactorial and can reflect factors such as illness, depression, or the inability to shop or cook. Monitoring weight at each visit is an appropriate screening tool.

Cognitive impairment is a common problem in the elderly that can be missed unless specifically tested for. Reliable, easily administered, brief tests of mental status, such as the Mini-Mental State Examination (Folstein et al. 1975), provide valuable data regarding the mental status of elderly persons whose apparently slight cognitive impairment may be incorrectly labeled as "normal" for their age (Kane and Kane 1981). If mental status is found to be impaired, reversible causes such as medications, thyroid disease, B_{12} or folate deficiency, or depression should be sought and treated.

Old age can be a time of many *losses* for older persons—loss of spouse, friends, job, and health. Depression is common in the elderly; it can be devastating for many patients and can have serious consequences. Simply asking patients if they ever feel sad or depressed can open a conversation. Mood assessment scales such as the one designed by Yesavage and Brink (1983) are useful questionnaires for further investigation.

Another important dimension of functional assessment is evaluation of the patient's *social and economic status*. The health care of elderly persons, perhaps more than any other group, is influenced by the social support system available to them. The network of current and informal supports, such as family or friends, has an important role in modulating the clinical impact of underlying disease and is often the major determinant in decisions to institutionalize elderly people. For every impaired elderly person in a nursing home, there are approximately two equally impaired elderly people living in the community, who often remain there by virtue of the critical role of informal support systems, which provide approximately 80% of their long-term care.

Health Promotion and Disease Prevention in the Elderly

Not many years ago, it would have seemed paradoxical to discuss health promotion and disease prevention in the elderly. Recently, however, this has become an important theme in geriatrics in view of both the remarkable increases in longevity and the awareness that the physiological and pathophysiological changes associates with advancing age may be much more reversible than was previously appreciated.

Primary prevention consists of identifying and reversing risk factors that may predispose an elderly person without disease to developing disease in the future. This includes the judicious use of the major vaccines which all elderly persons should receive: tetanus-diphtheria toxoid, influenza virus vaccine, and pneumococcal vaccine. One should not assume that risk factors are necessarily cumulative in their impact or that little is to be gained by altering long-term habits. This plasticity of aging organ systems is reflected in findings that moderate exercise (30 minutes three times weekly) retards age-related loss of bone mineral content in elderly women, including individuals in their ninth decade of life living in long-term care facilities. Similarly, even though elderly smokers have a much higher risk of cardiac mortality than nonsmokers, quitting smoking in late life is associated with a rapid and sustained reduction in mortality from coronary disease.

Secondary prevention consists of early detection of disease before symptoms are evident. Cancer is the second leading cause of death in the elderly, and 50% of all cancers occur in the elderly (Boring et al. 1991). Early detection of diseases such as cancer through screening is clearly an attractive proposition. It is not possible, nor would it necessarily be desirable, to screen for all cancers. Therefore several criteria exist for what makes a disease amenable to screening: the disease should be prevalent, it should have an impact on quality of life, and there should exist a treatment that will prolong life if instituted in

the asymptomatic period of an illness. Tests should be sensitive, specific, acceptable to the patient, and available at a reasonable cost.

There are several recommended strategies for cancer screening in the elderly. The American Cancer Society (1980) suggests screening for breast cancer with monthly self-examination, and yearly physical examination and mammography. Cervical cancer should be screened for annually with Papanicolaou smears until three or more are negative after age 65. Colon cancer screening is advocated with yearly digital rectal examinations, testing for fecal occult blood, and sigmoidoscopy every 3–5 years. Annual physical examination of the skin and oral cavity and palpation of the prostate should be conducted.

Another aspect of secondary prevention in the care of the elderly is recognition that physiological or pathological changes so common in advancing age as to be considered part of "normal aging" should not be considered to be without risk and are better considered reflections of "usual" aging. Thus, although systolic blood pressure increases with advancing age, it is also clear that this rise is associated with an increased risk of stroke and coronary heart disease. Elevations in blood sugar represent another potentially harmful aging change that is usually considered harmless.

Figure 2–3 displays the risk associated with usual aging. The curve farthest to the right, labeled "Death," displays the current age-specific mortality experience in the United States. This rather rectangular curve is typical for developed nations. The next curve, labeled "Disability," depicts the proportion of the population, at any age, who are without disability. With advancing age, the proportion of disabled individuals in the population increases rather dramatically. The next curve, labeled "Disease," represents a theoretical estimate of the increasing emergence with advancing age of specific disease processes such as cardiac disease, dementia, osteoporosis, and hypertension.

As can be seen, at any given age the proportion of individuals who are still living can be divided into those who have not yet developed disease, those who are diseased but have not yet developed disability from their disease, and those who have developed disability from their disease. The major aim of early health promotion efforts targeting pathological aging is to compress the emergence of dis-

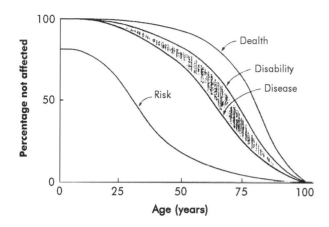

Figure 2–3. The relation of age to survival, disability, disease, and risk of disease in the U.S. population.
Source. Adapted from World Health Organization: "The Uses of Epidemiology in the Study of the Elderly" (Technical Report Series 706). Geneva, Switzerland, World Health Organization, 1980. Used with permission.

ease. Tertiary prevention efforts seek to identify existing disease at a point when rehabilitative intervention can still lessen disability. Thus, the goal of prevention in older adults is to shift the disease and disability curves to the right so that they approximate the mortality curve.

The final curve on Figure 2–3, labeled "Risk," provides a theoretical estimate of the proportion of the nondiseased population, at any age, who have developed physiological age-related changes that carry considerable risk and who thus might be considered to be experiencing what we have termed "usual" aging. The population below the disease curve then can be broken into a population further below the risk curve (those who are aging "successfully") and a larger population of individuals who lie between the risk and disease curves, who might be said to demonstrate usual aging. The goal of geriatric health-promotion efforts aimed at successful aging would be to shift this risk curve to the right. The strategies likely to be effective in facilitating the transition from usual to successful aging include social, behavioral, biomedical, and pharmacological interventions.

In this chapter we have attempted to present a broad review of current knowledge regarding the physiological changes associated with aging and the principles governing thorough evaluation of elderly patients. Although these factors are critical to proper care of all elderly patients, they may play especially important and often neglected roles in those individuals for whom old age is complicated by psychiatric illness. The emerging database on the general physiology of aging provides a proper backdrop for detailed discussion of age-related and disease-related alterations in the central nervous system.

References

Abbott RD, Donahue RP, MacMahon SW, et al: Diabetes and the risk of stroke: the Honolulu heart program. JAMA 257:949–952, 1987

American Cancer Society: Guidelines for the cancer-related checkup. Cancer 30:194, 1980

Amery A, Brixko P, Clement D, et al: Mortality and morbidity results from the European working party on high blood pressure in the elderly trial. Lancet 1:1349–1354, 1985

Anderson WF: The prevention of illness in the elderly: the Rutherglen experiment in medicine in old age: proceedings of a conference held at the Royal College of Physicians. London, Pitman Medical, 1966

Bahemuka M, Hodkinson HM: Screening for hypothyroidism in elderly inpatients. BMJ 2:601–603, 1975

Besdine RW: Geriatric medicine: an overview, in Annual Review of Gerontology and Geriatrics. Edited by Eisdorfer C. New York, Springer, 1980, pp 135–153

Besdine RW: The data base of geriatric medicine, in Health and Disease in Old Age. Edited by Rowe JW, Besdine RW. Boston, MA, Little, Brown, 1982, pp 1–14

Boring CC, Squires TS, Tong T: Cancer statistics, 1991. CA Cancer J Clin 41:19–36, 1991

Bullamore JR, Wilkinson R, Gallagher JC, et al: Effect of age on calcium absorption. Lancet 2:535–537, 1970

Carr BR, MacDonald PC: The menopause and beyond, in Principles of Geriatric Medicine. Edited by Andrus R, Bierman EL, Hazzard WR. New York, McGraw-Hill, 1985, pp 325–336

Cockcroft DW, Gault MH: Prediction of creatinine clearance from serum creatinine. Nephron 16:31–41, 1976

Colandrea MA, Freedman GD, Nichaman MZ, et al: Systolic hypertension in the elderly: an epidemiologic assessment. Circulation 41:239–245, 1970

Dahlof B, Lindholm LH, Hanson L, et al: Morbidity and mortality in the Swedish Trial in Old Patients With Hypertension (STOP–Hypertension). Lancet 338:1281–1285, 1991

Davidson MB: The effect of aging on carbohydrate metabolism: a review of the English literature and a practical approach to the diagnosis of diabetes mellitus in the elderly. Metabolism 28:1095–1101, 1979

Feller I, Flora JD, Bawol R: Baseline results of therapy for burned patients. JAMA 236:1943–1947, 1976

Folstein MF, Folstein SE, McHugh PR: Mini-Mental State: a practical method for grading the cognitive state of patients for the clinician. J Psychiatr Res 12:189–198, 1975

Gillis S, Kozak R, Durante M, et al: Immunological studies of aging: decreased production of and response to T cell growth factor by lymphocytes from aged humans. J Clin Invest 67:937–942, 1981

Gordon T, Shurtleff D: Means at each examination and inter-examination variation of specific characteristics: Framingham study—exams 1–10, in The Framingham Study: An Epidemiological Investigation of Cardiovascular Disease. Edited by Kannel WB. Washington, DC, National Institutes of Health, 1973, pp 1–53

Hannon JH: The Flushings of the Menopause. London, Balliere, Tindall & Cox, 1927

Harman SM, Nankin HR: Alterations in reproductive and sexual function: male, in Principles of Geriatric Medicine. Edited by Andrus R, Bierman EL, Hazzard WR. New York, McGraw-Hill, 1985, pp 337–353

Harman SM, Tsitouras PD: Reproductive hormones in aging men, I: measurement of sex steroids, basal luteinizing hormone, and Leydig cell response to human chorionic gonadotropin. J Clin Endocrinol Metab 51:35–40, 1980

Harman SM, Wehmann RE, Blackman MR: Pituitary-thyroid hormone economy in healthy aging men: basal indices of thyroid function and responses to constant infusions of thyrotropin-releasing hormone. J Clin Endocrinol Metab 58:320–326, 1984

Harris MI, Hadden WC, Knowler WC, et al: Prevalence of diabetes and impaired glucose tolerance and plasma glucose levels in the U.S. population aged 20–74 years. Diabetes 36:523–534, 1987

Hollenberg NK, Adams DF, Solomon HS, et al: Senescence and the renal vasculature of normal man. Circ Res 34:309–316, 1974

Kane RA, Kane RL: Assessing the Elderly: A Practical Guide to Measurement. Lexington, MA, Lexington Books, 1981

Kannel WB, Gordan T: Evaluation of cardiovascular risk in the elderly: the Framingham study. Bull NY Acad Med 54:573–591, 1978

Krasinski SD, Russell RM, Samloff IM, et al: Fundic atrophic gastritis in an elderly population: effect on hemoglobin and several serum nutritional indicators. J Am Geriatr Soc 34:800–806, 1986

Kronenberg RC, Drage CW: Attenuation of the ventilatory and heart rate responses to hypoxia and hypercapnea with aging in normal men. J Clin Invest 52:1812–1819, 1973

Lachs MS, Feinstein AR, Cooney LM, et al: A simple procedure for general screening for functional disability in elderly patients. Ann Intern Med 112:699–706, 1990

Lakatta EG: Alterations in the cardiovascular system that occur in advanced age. Fed Proc 38:163–167, 1979

Livingston EH, Hershman JM, Sawin CT, et al: Prevalence of thyroid disease and abnormal thyroid tests in older hospitalized and ambulatory persons. J Am Geriatr Soc 35:109–114, 1987

McKinlay S, Jefferys M: The menopause syndrome. British Journal of Preventive and Social Medicine 28:108–115, 1974

Martin CE: Factor affecting sexual functioning in 60- to 79-year-old married males. Arch Sex Behav 10:399–420, 1981

Minaker KL, Meneilly GS, Rowe JW: Endocrinology of aging, in Handbook of the Biology of Aging. Edited by Finch C, Schneider EL. New York, Van Nostrand Reinhold, 1984, pp 433–456

O'Rourke MF: Arterial hemodynamics in hypertension. Circ Res 27 (suppl 2):123–124, 1970

Pathy MS: Clinical presentation of myocardial infarction in the elderly. Br Heart J 29:190–199, 1967

Pearlman CK: Frequency of intercourse in males at different ages. Medical Aspects of Human Sexuality 6:92, 1972

Psaty BM, Furberg CD, Kuller LH, et al: Isolated systolic hypertension and subclinical cardiovascular disease in the elderly: initial findings from the cardiovascular health study. JAMA 268:1287–1291, 1992

Riggs BL, Melton LJ III: Involutional osteoporosis. N Engl J Med 314:1676–1686, 1986

Rodeheffer RJ, Gerstenblith G, Becker LC, et al: Exercise cardiac output is maintained with advancing age in healthy human subjects: cardiac dilatation and increased stroke volume compensate for a diminished heart rate. Circulation 69:203–213, 1984

Rosenthal MJ, Hunt WC, Garry PJ, et al: Thyroid failure in the elderly: microsomal antibodies as a discriminant for therapy. JAMA 258:209–213, 1987

Rowe JW: Clinical research in aging: strategies and directions. N Engl J Med 297:1332–1336, 1977

Rowe JW: Systolic hypertension in the elderly (editorial). N Engl J Med 309:1246–1247, 1983

Rowe JW: Health care of the elderly. N Engl J Med 312:827–835, 1985

Rowe JW, Andres R, Tobin JD, et al: The effect of age on creatinine clearance in men: a cross-sectional and longitudinal study. J Gerontol 31:155–163, 1976

Russell RM, Krasinski SD, Samloff IM, et al: Folic acid malabsorption in atrophic gastritis: possible compensation by bacterial folate synthesis. Gastroenterology 91:1476–1482, 1986

Savin CT, Castelli WP, Hershman JM, et al: The aging thyroid: thyroid deficiency in the Framingham study. Arch Intern Med 145:1386–1388, 1985

Shekelle RB, Ostfeld AM, Klawans HL Jr: Hypertension and risk of stroke in an elderly population. Stroke 5:71–75, 1974

SHEP Cooperative Research Group: Prevention of stroke by antihypertensive drug treatment in older persons with isolated systolic hypertension: final results of the Systolic Hypertension in the Elderly Program (SHEP). JAMA 265:3255–3266, 1991

Shock NW, Greulich RC, Anores RA, et al: Normal Human Aging: The Baltimore Longitudinal Study of Aging. Washington, DC, U.S. Department of Health and Human Services, 1984

Stamler J, Neaton JD, Wentworth DN: Blood pressure (systolic and diastolic) and risk of fatal coronary disease. Hypertension 13 (suppl):I2–I12, 1989

Stokes J, Kannel WB, Wolf PA, et al: Blood pressure as a risk factor for cardiovascular disease: the Framingham study—30 years of follow-up. Hypertension 13 (suppl):I13–I18, 1989

Weale RA: The Aging Eye. New York, Harper & Row, 1963

Weiss ST: Pulmonary system, in Health and Disease in Old Age. Edited by Rowe JW, Besdine RL. Boston, MA, Little, Brown, 1980, pp 369–379

White NK, Edwards JE, Dry TJ: Relationship of the degree of coronary atherosclerosis with age in men. Circulation 1 (pt 2):645–654, 1950

Wilson LA, Lawson IR, Brass W: Multiple disorders in the elderly: a clinical and statistical study. Lancet 2:841–843, 1962

World Health Organization: The uses of epidemiology in the study of the elderly (Technical Report Series 706). Geneva, Switzerland, World Health Organization, 1980

Yesavage J, Brink TL: Development and validation of a geriatric depression scale: a preliminary report. J Psychiatr Res 17:37–49, 1983

Zavaroni I, Dall'Aglio E, Bruschi F, et al: Effect of age and environmental factors on glucose tolerance and insulin secretion in a worker population. J Am Geriatr Soc 34:271–275, 1986

CHAPTER 3

Perceptual Changes With Aging

Gail R. Marsh, Ph.D.

Alterations in the anatomy and physiology of sensory systems occur with aging. Some of these changes have been identified and can be correlated with the changes in perception that have also been reported in elderly persons. However, with the multiple feedforward and feedback systems that characterize all of our sensory systems, it is not always possible to know how specific perceptual changes are related to the underlying changes in the anatomy and physiology. The emphasis here will be to describe the changes in perception, relating them to aging changes in anatomy and physiology when possible.

Much of what we feel, taste, see, hear, and smell is altered and is somewhat controlled by the context in which the stimuli occur. These "automatic" aspects of our sensory systems are influenced by age, both by alterations in the sensory systems and by the increasing loss of specific sensory input that strips each sensory system of its basic sensory input. In some cases, "noise"—that is, extraneous, self-generated sensory input—is added to the system as well. Recent sophisticated advances in experimental procedures have made it possible to take such effects into account and permit us to better understand some of the causes behind perceptual alterations that occur with age.

Vision

Four major alterations occur in the eye and visual system with age: 1) flattening of the corneal surface, which reduces refractive power; 2) alterations in the crystalline lens, making it scatter light and absorb some of the shorter wavelengths; 3) loss of the ability of the lens to accommodate changes in visual focus; and 4) loss of the retinal elements and neuronal processing systems required to process and interpret the images that reach the retina. With advanced age, the most common visual problems include cataracts, glaucoma, and macular degeneration. In the following sections of this discussion of vision I discuss how perception is changed along the usual dimensions measured in vision and briefly explore the currently known correlational changes in anatomy and physiology.

Acuity

The ability to perceive a clear image by resolving small spatial details when looking squarely at an object, whether it be near to the observer or far distant, is evaluated by measuring the observer's acuity. Acuity for distant objects (often tested by the Snellen chart) is termed *far vision*. Acuity for stimuli close to the observer, or *near vision*, begins to noticeably decrease for most persons between the ages of 40 and 55. This is due largely to the fact that the crystalline lens, which continuously grows, becomes too large and begins to prevent accommodation to near objects—it can no longer be sufficiently brought back toward a spherical shape.

However, even far vision shows decrements in acuity past age 40. This loss of visual acuity may not be as noticeable to the observer because we rarely call upon our far vision to provide information in the same manner as we challenge our visual system at close range—as with fine print. The decrease in far acuity with age seems to be approximately linear, and has been reported by a number of researchers in studies using large populations (Pitts 1982). In one study (Gittings and Fozard 1986), the investigators followed subjects longitudinally for about 15 years and found that far acuity dropped steadily throughout adult life but the decrement did not become noticeable until about age 65. Gittings and Fozard also found decreases in near vision acuity, which dropped off steeply at about age 40–45 and leveled off between 55 and 60. The acuity measurement likely would have gone lower if the measuring scale could have gone lower. In measures of corrected near vision, the drop was not as steep, but persisted in much the same manner as that for far vision.

The physical change that would likely explain the changes in near vision acuity in the early years as demonstrated in these longitudinal studies is the decreasing control of the crystalline lens. Because no accommodation by the lens was necessary in the tests of far vision, the explanation for loss of acuity in far vision is more likely to comprise difficulties in delivering a clear image to the retina and alterations in the neural systems interpreting the image. Losses of retinal receptors (Marshall et al. 1980) and a decreased number of neuronal fibers leaving the retina (Dolman et al. 1980) occur with age. Also, by age 60, the loss of neurons in the macular area in the primary visual cortex is about 25%, and by age 80 this loss is very substantial—about 50% (Devaney and Johnson 1980). The neurons in the visual cortex that represent the macular area are the most important for the majority of our modern-day visual activity, and it is specifically that portion of the retina that is involved in Snellen chart measurements of acuity.

Several other, more peripheral, factors also degrade the image on the retina and affect far vision acuity tests. One of these factors is glare. Glare is nothing more than stray light reaching the retina. This stray light is generated by random deflection of light away from the focused image in the crystalline lens and in the vitreous humor. This stray light on the retina is "noise" added to the image that reduces the ability of the visual system to generate a clear perception of the stimulus. Loss of retinal elements due to injury or lack of sufficient blood supply also becomes a factor in old age. There can be significant loss of cones between the ages of 40 and 60, and after age 70 there may be increasing deterioration in blood supply. With sclerosing of blood vessels and deterioration of the pigmented epithelium (which supports the retinal elements), there can be increased entry of new blood vessels, which tend to be leaky. This can lead to patchy deterioration of the retina in the area where leakage occurs.

Another major problem that occurs with aging is a reduction in the amount of illumination reaching the retina. In the younger, healthy adult, the iris retracts to admit more light when the available light in the environment is lowered. However, with increasing age, the iris reacts with less vigor as illumination is lowered, and therefore less light reaches the retina. In well-lit environments, there is little difference between young and old, but in increasingly subdued lighting, elderly persons are at an increasing disadvantage because the iris fails to continue drawing open once twilight levels are reached. Weale (1961) showed that under bright twilight conditions, only about one-third of the available illumination reached the retina of a 70-year-old as compared with a younger adult; in making this calculation, Weale took into account all of the factors noted above.

Given the above information, it would not be surprising to find that older persons have more difficulty performing adequately on visual tasks under conditions of low illumination. Indeed, Sivak and Olson (1982) found that, compared with younger adults, older adults had to have the distance to road signs reduced by about one-third before they could read the signs. Added to these difficulties in seeing at night on the highway are those associated with glare and recovery from glare (essentially the same as a photopic recovery curve). Glare, of course, can occur in the daytime, as when driving into the sun, but is perhaps most often encountered in nighttime driving as the result of confronting oncoming head-lights. Glare affects all drivers, but seems to have increasing effects in persons over age 45 (Wolf 1960). The amount of time needed to recover from glare nearly doubles between ages 25 and 75. Many older persons are aware of their difficulties driving at night and voluntarily abstain. However, it should be noted that none of the currently used, standard meth-ods of measuring the visual acuity of drivers can identify these nighttime perceptual difficulties.

Contrast Sensitivity

Measurements of acuity continue to dominate the clinical assessment of vision because such measure-ments take good account of a critical aspect of vision with relatively straightforward testing. However, another method of assessing vision, *contrast sensitiv-ity testing,* has become popular in research on vision. Acuity testing strongly emphasizes the ability of the visual system to resolve fine details at the center of the visual field when presented with targets that have high contrast to their background. Acuity test-ing leaves unmeasured aspects of peripheral vision, as well as the ability to see gradual changes in visual texture and larger objects in the visual field. With the use of contrast sensitivity measurement tools, it is possible to assess these other aspects of vision as well as visual acuity.

The stimulus used in testing contrast sensitivity is a *sine-wave grating.* Put simply, a sine-wave grating is a set of vertical, alternating light and dark areas, much like a series of light and dark stripes, except that instead of sharp changes, the light and dark areas change gradually, governed by the sine wave function. The speed with which they change is termed *spatial frequency,* and the amount of change between light and dark is the *contrast.* Typically, a series of such gratings—progressing from low spa-tial frequencies to high—are presented, with each frequency started as a white field; the extent of con-trast is slowly enhanced until the observer can first detect the grating.

Low-frequency gratings are equally well detec-ted by both old and young adults. However, for in-termediate- and high-spatial-frequency gratings, adults age 70 and older have significantly poorer sensitivity compared with younger persons (Kline

et al. 1983; Owsley et al. 1983). The losses at high spatial frequencies predict the losses found with the Snellen chart, which depends only on high-contrast, high-frequency targets. However, intermediate-fre-quency loss implies losses for tasks such as seeing road signs or other medium-visual-angle targets. That such losses are indeed present was supported by the findings of Owsley and Sloan (1987), who found that older persons were less able to detect or identify faces at low contrast. Again, such losses seem to be tied to losses in the nervous system, and appear to be not due to difficulties in the crystalline lens or other media of the eye; experiments with young adults forced to work with distortions of the visual image meant to mimic such aging changes did not show the losses seen in older adults (Owsley et al. 1983).

Depth Perception

The amount of disparity in degrees of visual angle between the images of the left and right eye can be increased until the observer detects the sensation of depth. In adults between 30 and 40 years old, about 100 degrees of disparity is required, but this gradu-ally increases to about 200 degrees by age 60, and to 300 degrees by age 80 (Greene and Madden 1987). Depth perception can be severely impaired in per-sons with a cataract in one eye (Schor and Heck-mann 1989), which is likely due to the loss of ability to compare the two visual fields at the required level of detail.

Peripheral Vision

Wolf (1967) and Burg (1968) established that the ex-tent of the visual field remains fairly constant until age 55. At that point, they noted the start of some shrinkage of the width of the peripheral field, espe-cially in the temporal field. Peripheral vision was shown to drop to about two-thirds that of the young adult By about age 75, and to about half that of the young adult by age 90. In more recent studies, in-vestigators testing for subjects' ability to localize tar-gets within the 30 degrees of central vision while being distracted by other targets in the peripheral areas of vision have found significant reductions in ability with age (Ball et al. 1988; Sekuler and Ball 1986). Target localization test results are clearly more predictive of performance on tasks such as driving and are likely more predictive of the kinds of deficits that older adults will show under most life circumstances than are the purely static tests for visual field limits. The use of these tests has underscored the complex nature of perception—that is, of sensory perception as a blending of the individual's reception of sensory stimuli and his or her cognitive processing of those stimuli.

Loss of peripheral vision typically does not elicit the same kind of complaints that are usually associated with loss of function in the foveal area. This may be due to the fact that some of the functions of the peripheral areas are more automatic and are therefore less available to conscious awareness. For instance, detection of motion in the periphery usually elicits an automatic saccadic eye movement to bring the eliciting stimulus onto the fovea for further examination. When such motion is simply not seen, no eye movement is generated, but the person would notice no loss of function.

Temporal Factors

The aging visual system holds an image longer than does the visual system of the young adult. This is most easily seen in the threshold for *flicker fusion.* This test involves a light flickering at a rate that increases until the observer reports perceiving a continuous light—that is, flicker fusion. This flicker fusion threshold is lower in older persons, and although this finding is partially due to a lower amount of light reaching the retina, thresholds remain significantly different when corrections are made for this factor, especially after age 60 (McFarland et al. 1958; Wolf and Shraffa 1964). The lower flicker fusion threshold among older persons implies the existence of a change in the central nervous system, a hypothesis that is also supported by the fact that the photoreceptors can follow the flicker to much higher frequencies than the flicker thresholds at any age.

Another method of showing that aging increases the retention of a visual stimulus was demonstrated by Kline et al. (1982). These investigators presented older and younger subjects with sequential flashes of red and green light (which blend into yellow) and demonstrated that, in older adults, the red and green lights could be shown at much longer separations and still be perceived as a yellow blend instead of two separate flashes of red and green. Eriksen and colleagues (1970) demonstrated a similar integration of two light flashes to achieve a perception of greater brightness. In these experiments, the perception of brightness was shown to occur over a longer separation of flashes among the older adults who participated in the experiments as compared with the younger subjects.

Backward masking is another way of showing how long an individual takes to analyze a stimulus in the early stages of processing in the visual system. The masking is achieved by following a target stimulus with another stimulus that either has more visual features or is a more intense image than the first, so that the second acts as a masking stimulus. Such masking may be achieved by delivering both stimuli to the same eye or by delivering the target stimulus to one eye and the masking stimulus to the other. Masking is much more easily achieved in older persons, and at longer time intervals between the target and masking stimulus (Walsh 1976).

Dynamic Visual Acuity

Dynamic visual acuity is the ability to identify a finely detailed target in motion. Burg (1966) found that this measure of acuity dropped off more rapidly with age than did static acuity. Henderson and Burg (1974) found that poor scores on this measure correlated with increased numbers of traffic accidents, a finding that did not hold when static acuity scores were considered. The natural conclusion is that eye movement under the control of the slow pursuit tracking system must deteriorate in elderly persons. This is confirmed by findings from more recent studies. Long and Crambert (1990) noted that dynamic acuity, tested across age groups, worsens as the speed of the target is increased. They also determined that static and dynamic acuity are not correlated, and that if the moving targets are presented transiently so that no eye movement can be initiated while the target is present (and with retinal illuminance equated between groups), there is no difference between young and old subjects.

In addition to experiencing difficulty in identifying moving targets, elderly persons are less able to detect motion in a target. Testing with both simple stimuli—such as lines and dots (Whitaker and Elliott 1989)—and more complicated stimuli—such as drifting or oscillating sine-wave gratings (Buckingham et al. 1987)—has produced essentially the same conclusion: slight decrements occur in detection of motion during middle age, but a much more substantial decline occurs after age 60.

Kline and Schieber (1985) proposed that one convenient way of thinking about the changes in vision with aging is to think of a sustained transient shift. This theory was based on the concept that the visual system has two different modes (or channels) that emerge from two different types of neurons found in different sites on the retina. The sustained channel is based largely in the fovea, holds a sustained response to stimuli, is capable of high spatial resolution, and can integrate input over a long time period. The transient channel is peripherally located, responds chiefly to moving or flashing stimuli, has poor spatial resolution, and functions to draw our attention to moving stimuli—usually with an automatic eye movement. Kline and Schieber hypothesized that the transient system deteriorates faster with aging than does the sustained system, thus creating many of the aging alterations noted above.

Color Distortion

The ability to distinguish hues diminishes with age, especially after age 70 (Dalderup and Fredericks 1969). The difficulty in distinguishing hues is greater with shorter wavelengths (the blue-green end of the spectrum) than with the longer wavelengths (the red end of the spectrum). This effect has been shown to be enhanced in the elderly (Knoblauch et al. 1987), often being ascribed to the filtering effect of the crystalline lens that grows increasingly yellow with age (Weale 1986). However, even early evidence showed that this does not entirely explain color distortion in older persons, because elderly observers who had undergone surgical removal of the lens had the same difficulties with distinguishing colors at the blue end of the spectrum as did elderly subjects with intact lenses (Lakowski 1962). More recent studies have confirmed that the loss of sensitivity in perceiving blue-green colors is dependent on alterations in photoreceptors and the central nervous system (Owsley and Sloane 1990).

Aging and Visual Pathology

In the aged eye there is greater risk of breakage of the small blood vessels due to deterioration of the vascular walls. Such leakage of blood both occludes

the photoreceptors and initiates breakdown of the vitreous humor during the clearing of the vascular leak. This leads to the formation of pockets of fluid next to the retina, which, of course, do not support the retina, allowing it to sag forward and leading to further deterioration due to tearing and bleeding. Such vascular pathology leads to loss of perception initially due to the development of small vacuoles in the visual field; these vacuoles usually increase in number with age, and some become larger. This problem is exacerbated by hypertension and by diabetes. Deterioration of the pigmented epithelium, a very active tissue that supports the rods and cones, tends to occur more in macular areas. Further, epithelial deterioration is self-perpetuating, because this deterioration tends to initiate invasion of the retina by blood vessels from the choroid, which are fragile and are very likely to break or leak.

Loss of retinal elements in the peripheral field is better tolerated than the loss of retinal elements in the macular area for two reasons. First, the input to retinal ganglion cells in the peripheral field comes from many rods, whereas input to ganglion cells in the macula comes from cones on—or very close to—a one-to-one ratio. Second, it is likely that more of the peripheral area of the eye is given over to more automatic functions that are not consciously registered, unlike what occurs in the macular area. However, even in the macular region, an area that is destroyed will be perceptually filled in by the visual system unless the person is using his or her vision in such a manner—as in reading—that the lack of input from a specific area is often forced to conscious attention.

Diabetes represents a risk factor for visual loss because the condition is associated with the formation of new—and fragile—blood vessels in the eye that have a tendency to break or leak. Glaucoma, a disease characterized by increased intraocular pressure, tends to destroy peripheral vision first and thus is often not noticed until macular functions are invaded. Glaucoma causes direct and irreversible neural damage due to pressure on the optic nerve at the point where it exits the eye.

All of these pathologies—macular degeneration, diabetes, and glaucoma, as well as vascular and other pathologies secondary to physical alteration—tend toward low incidence before the age of 60; the incidence begins to increase rapidly after age 70.

Audition

Difficulties with hearing are often encountered with increasing age. About 25% of individuals over the age of 65 report some difficulty with their hearing, with the difficulty becoming more intense and more common among those in older age groups. Mild to moderate hearing loss seems not to produce psychological difficulties, but persons with losses of more than 40 decibels in the frequencies needed for understanding speech are at greater risk of emotional difficulties and significant reductions in life satisfaction (Gilhome-Herbst 1983). Unfortunately, many older persons with significant hearing loss deny their difficulty and do not accept appropriate therapy. Also, many elderly individuals do not participate in appropriate therapeutic programs because of limited professional and public awareness of the existence of such programs (Shadden and Raiford 1984).

Auditory Threshold

The most notable change in hearing with advancing age is a loss of sensitivity to sound, especially in the higher frequencies. The range for human hearing is roughly 20–20,000 Hz, but the most widely used clinical hearing test assesses audition in the range of 250–8,000 Hz. As a result, statistics for large populations of older persons are not usually available except for this more restricted range.

The ability to perceive sound within the range of 50–1,000 Hz remains relatively unchanged until advanced old age. However, above 1,000 Hz there is a distinct decrement in sensitivity beginning at about 45 years of age that worsens with higher frequency and advancing age (Lebo and Reddell 1972; Spoor 1967). In all cases, men show this effect to a greater degree than women. Longitudinal studies have demonstrated about the same kinds of changes that are seen in cross-sectional studies (Brandt and Fozard 1990; Moller 1981).

The decrease in an individual's ability to perceive sound is mostly the result of the growing insensitivity of the cochlea to input, which, in turn, is due to four major physiological changes: 1) loss of elasticity of the basilar membrane, 2) loss of sensory receptors on the basilar membrane, 3) loss of neurons (eighth nerve), and 4) atrophy of the stria vas-

cularis. The stiffening of the basilar membrane restricts the amplitude of membrane response and, because the membrane cannot bend as sharply as before, the input is spread out over many sensory receptors instead of stimulating only those at the precise frequency of input. This, in addition to the growing lack of receptors and neurons, results in a less precise initial signal for the auditory system. The atrophy of the stria vascularis decreases the ability of the cochlea to generate a response at any frequency (Schuknecht 1974). Unfortunately, this also precipitates a phenomenon known as *loudness recruitment*—at levels of input that are just above conversational levels, sound quickly passes through a comfortable hearing range and becomes painfully loud.

The most widely discussed model for loss of hearing sensitivity with aging is exposure to noise, especially loud noise for prolonged periods; the supposition by some is that such exposure can lead to a loss of receptors. However, this model has only moderate support and is contradicted by data gathered from persons living in quiet environments (Hinchcliffe 1959). The authors of the most frequently cited study in which a population living in a quiet environment was compared with a populating living in a noisy environment strongly suggest an alternative interpretation: a significant genetic and dietary difference leading to quite different health profiles between the two populations (Rosen et al. 1964). Medications have only been sparsely examined as possible mediators or causal agents in hearing deficits. It has been established that a propensity for noise-induced damage can be increased by some drugs such as kanamycin (Prazma 1981). In addition, some drugs—the most popular being aspirin—have been reported to temporarily enhance the ability of noise to degrade perception (McFadden and Plattsmier 1983).

Speech Perception

With aging, the ability to perceive speech declines faster than would be predicted from the results of pure-tone sensitivity tests. However, these declines in speech perception are relatively minor under quiet listening conditions. Much larger deficits are encountered when the listener must work under more difficult listening conditions, such as with background noise or when distortions exist in the presented signal. Speech is a complex signal that involves many frequencies, but in the presence of sufficient cues that provide a linguistic context, it has enough redundancy to enable complex analysis by the central nervous system to recover misperceived words. Thus, age differences were significantly reduced in one experiment when linguistic cues were given to help subjects perceive words presented against a "cocktail party" background (Dubno et al. 1984). However, under cocktail-party background noise conditions, stereo sound cues can help younger individuals to localize a point in space to which to listen as an aid to perceiving target words, but older individuals are not helped by these same stereo sound cues (Warren et al. 1978).

Altering speech by interrupting it briefly every 62.5 milliseconds (8 Hz) produces a linear decline in speech perception from 100% perception in 20-year-olds to only 30% in 80-year-olds (Bergman et al. 1976). This effect seems to be due to central nervous system losses, because increasing the ratio of speech-filled time to silent time improved perception for the young but did not aid the older listeners (Bergman 1980).

Gustation

Taste perception is divided into four aspects—salty, sweet, sour, and bitter. These aspects are generally studied independently because there is no general model for how humans blend them when tasting a substance. In addition, humans almost always use the sense of smell together with the four aspects of taste, but here we will address taste separately from smell.

The intensity of the taste stimulus is thought to be dependent on the number of taste receptors stimulated (Arvidson and Freiberg 1980; Smith 1971), and before about 1970, investigators studying receptor number and location reported large losses in these receptors over the adult years. However, more recent studies (Arvidson 1979; Miller 1988) have demonstrated a large variability between individuals that cannot be accounted for by the variable of age. Thus, other factors—health, hormones, genetic variability, or mouth hygiene, for example—may be more important than age in determining taste receptor density and pattern. Changes in the amount and makeup of saliva—increasing viscosity and a

change in pH—take place with aging. All of these can function to make tasted substances less accessible or excitable to the receptor. Also, the presence of dentures can alter the access of tasted substances to parts of the oral cavity as well as altering the mouth environment in other ways.

Threshold measures of the four aspects of taste have usually been reported to deteriorate with age, but the most recently available evidence suggests that age losses reported in earlier studies may have been exaggerated. In more recent studies (Weiffenbach et al. 1982), which involved elderly persons living in communities rather than nursing home populations, investigators reported only mild changes associated with age, and when loss of taste perception was identified in an individual subject, the loss was often in only one of the four taste aspects. This loss of a single dimension of taste, of course, might distort the individual's general perception of taste, but this has not been specifically addressed in the research literature. If there is a difference of some magnitude in taste perception to be found, it is likely to be attributable to two factors other than advancing age: a history of tobacco smoking or medication use.

When testing at suprathreshold levels, especially levels well above threshold, there is no difference between young and old persons in their perception of intensity of the tasted substance (Bartoshuk et al. 1986). Just above the taste detection threshold there seems to be what looks like a mild lingering taste in the mouth that masks tasted substances for the elderly. This may be due to problems with oral hygiene, periodontal disease, or effects of dentures. Typically denture use and other possible interfering factors, such as periodontal disease, have not been controlled in taste studies.

Olfaction

The sense of smell has consistently been reported to decline with age; investigators generally agree that the likely cause is an increasing loss of receptors in the nasal epithelium in older persons, although a cause for this deterioration other than infection or inflammation has not been specified. The earliest studies of olfaction involved the use of odorants that were noxious or that were used to protect the public (such as the odorant added to the residential supply of natural gas). Investigators in more recent studies have used a more comprehensive range of stimuli and more extensive psychophysical methods.

Using a total of 18 odorants, Venstrom and Amoore (1968) found that for almost all the odorants, elderly subjects were substantially less able to detect the stimuli until concentrations of the odorants reached much higher levels than those required for detection by younger adults. When stimuli are presented at clearly suprathreshold levels, elderly subjects show some flattening in their intensity response curve compared with young adults (Stevens and Cain 1987). This effect is not evidenced in taste studies, which have found relatively little difference between younger and older subjects. The ability to identify—that is, to name—odorants at suprathreshold levels has also been shown to strongly decline among persons over age 60 (Doty et al. 1984; Wysocki and Gilbert 1989). These experiments were done using very large populations; the data derived from these studies are not confounded by such variables as the general poor health of test subjects, nor are the conclusions suspect because of population biases (for example, reliance on nursing home populations). Currently, no theory has been proposed that can model how perception of specific classes of odorants should or will decline with age (Murphy 1986).

Identification of foods and their enjoyment decreases with age, and the hedonic tone of food description is much more negative among elderly persons than among younger people (Schiffman 1977). As can be seen from the above discussion, much of the difficulty with food enjoyment and identification comes from losses in the sense of smell rather than from losses in taste perception. Thus, enhancement of food odors can significantly enhance the acceptance of foods by elderly individuals (Schiffman and Warwick 1988).

Somesthesis

The ability to detect touch on the skin decreases with age. A fairly good correlation exists between the loss of sensitivity in nonhairy skin with aging and the loss of Meissner's corpuscles (Kenshalo 1986). However, it is reasonable to assume that there must be some loss of free nerve endings as well, because the cornea also shows decreased sensitivity with aging,

and free nerve endings are the sole source of innervation of the cornea (Millodot 1977). The skin also becomes less deformable with aging, preventing adequate stimulation of all of the receptors in the skin. The loss of specialized nerve endings and the less elastic skin could also lead to poorer detection of a two-point threshold (i.e., the ability to discriminate whether one or two points is being touched on the skin), which has also been reported for the elderly (Axelrod and Cohen 1961; Stevens 1992). The age loss for two-point discrimination showed the greatest decline on the finger, and far less on the arm. In the elderly, the loss was enhanced by the loss of finger warmth and could be partly reversed by warming.

Loss of sensitivity to vibratory stimulation is mostly seen at higher frequencies of stimulation—above about 50–80 Hz (Verrillo 1980). These higher frequencies are thought to be selectively stimulating to the Pacinian corpuscles on ligaments and tendons, thus indicating aging losses in that system. A similar loss is not seen at the lower frequencies of stimulation; frequencies below 50 Hz tend to stimulate only the soft tissues—skin and muscle. However, Kenshalo (1986) did note a decrement in response in the feet of elderly persons to both high- and low-frequency stimulation as compared with younger individuals. A similar decrement was not seen in the hands. The greater loss in the lower extremities of elderly persons had been reported before; however, in this case it was thought to reflect a general aging effect rather than an injury or neuropathy, since it was seen in most subjects and all subjects had been screened for neuropathies.

Pain is a sensation that must be measured on at least two dimensions: sensory and affective. Unfortunately, no methods are currently available that can clearly distinguish between the various interpretations of results as being due to changes in response bias, to affective labeling, and/or to altered sensitivity levels. Most studies have involved the use of radiant heat as the source of painful stimuli and have yielded reports of some decrease in sensitivity to pain with age. However, some investigators have reported the results of studies that showed no difference between young and old subjects (Kenshalo 1986). Discrepancies have also been shown in the results of studies using other sources of pain (e.g., electrical tooth pulp stimulation). In studies of suprathreshold sensitivity to pain, investigators have reported some indication of an *intensity recruitment* effect in elderly persons (Harkins et al. 1986). Intensity recruitment is a phenomenon similar to loudness recruitment (described above in the Audition section). Intensity recruitment in pain studies is defined as a sudden upswing in intensity after a more linear pattern of response increments at lower stimulation levels. Harkins and colleagues interpreted the results as being of sensory, rather than affective, origin.

Conclusions

Sensory changes are to be expected with increasing age and usually can be accommodated as a normal part of aging. The pathologies of the senses can exacerbate these changes manyfold and can sometimes be mistaken for normal aging unless carefully examined. Treatments for many of the pathologies have been or are being developed. Too often the treatments are not widely used because they are not widely discussed among professionals or the general public. Better communication regarding such clinical advances will be a welcome bridge over the current information gap.

The practical aspects of some of the sensory declines associated with age have not always been addressed in the past, although they have received more attention recently. For example, the effects of sensory and cognitive changes on the ability to drive a motor vehicle received special attention in a recent review (Barr 1991). That review also included special attention to what may also be a necessary adjunct to tests of sensory function: an assessment of the extent to which subjects may be suffering from cognitive decline that affects the efficiency with which sensory signals can be processed. In future studies, investigators may be able to address how cognitive and sensory areas may overlap in important ways, and also how sensory changes can be dealt with to improve life quality and satisfaction.

References

Arvidson K: Location and variation in number of taste buds in human fungiform papillae. J Dent Res 87:435–442, 1979

Arvidson K, Freiberg U: Human taste: response and taste bud number in fungiform papillae. Science 209:807–808, 1980

Axelrod S, Cohen LD: Senescence and embedded-figure performance in vision and touch. Percept Mot Skills 12:283–288, 1961

Ball K, Beard BL, Roenker DL, et al: Age and visual search: expanding the useful field of view. J Opt Soc Am [A] 5:2210–2219, 1988

Barr RA: Recent changes in driving among older adults. Hum Factors 33:597–600, 1991

Bartoshuk LM, Rifkin B, Marks LE, Bars P: Taste and aging. J Gerontol 41:51–57, 1986

Bergman M: Aging and the Perception of Speech. Baltimore, MD, University Park Press, 1980

Bergman M, Blumenfeld VG, Cascardo D, et al: Age-related decrement in hearing for speech: sampling and longitudinal studies. J Gerontol 31:533–538, 1976

Brandt LJ, Fozard JL: Age changes in pure-tone hearing thresholds in a longitudinal study of normal human aging. J Acoust Soc Am 88:813–820, 1990

Buckingham T, Whitaker D, Banford D: Movement in decline? Oscillatory movement displacement thresholds increase with age. Ophthalmic Physiol Opt 7:411–413, 1987

Burg A: Visual acuity as measured by dynamic and static tests: a comparative evaluation. J Appl Psychol 50:460–466, 1966

Burg A: Lateral visual field as related to age and sex. J Appl Psychol 52:10–15, 1968

Dalderup LM, Fredericks MLC: Color sensitivity in old age. J Am Geriatr Soc 17:388–390, 1969

Devaney KO, Johnson HA: Neuron loss in the aging visual cortex of man. J Gerontol 35:836–841, 1980

Dolman CL, McCormick AQ, Drance SM: Aging of the optic nerve. Arch Ophthalmol 98:2053–2058, 1980

Doty RL, Shaman P, Appelbaum SL, et al: Smell identification ability: changes with age. Science 226:1441–1443, 1984

Dubno JR, Dirks DD, Morgan DE: Effects of age and mild hearing loss on speech recognition in noise. J Acoust Soc Am 76:87–96, 1984

Eriksen CW, Hamlin PM, Breitmeyer BG: Temporal factors in perception as related to aging. Perception and Psychophysics 7:354–356, 1970

Gilhome-Herbst K: Psychological consequences of disorders of hearing in the elderly, in Hearing and Balance in the Elderly. Edited by Hinchcliffe R. London, Churchill Livingstone, 1983, pp 174–200

Gittings NS, Fozard JL: Age-related changes in visual acuity. Exp Gerontol 21:423–433, 1986

Greene HA, Madden DJ: Adult age differences in visual acuity, stereopsis, and contrast sensitivity. American Journal of Optometry and Physiological Optics 64:749–753, 1987

Harkins SW, Price DD, Martelli M: Effects of age on pain perception: thermonociception. J Gerontol 41:58–63, 1986

Henderson RL, Burg A: Vision and audition in driving (report TML-5297). Washington, DC, U.S. Department of Transportation, 1974

Hinchcliffe R: The threshold of hearing as a function of age. Acoustica 9:303–308, 1959

Kenshalo DR: Somesthetic sensitivity in young and elderly humans. J Gerontol 41:732–742, 1986

Kline DW, Schieber F: Vision and aging, in Handbook of the Psychology of Aging, 2nd Edition. Edited by Birren JE, Schaie KW. New York, Van Nostrand Reinhold, 1985, pp 296–331

Kline DW, Ikeda D, Schieber F: Age and temporal resolution in color vision: when do red and green make yellow? J Gerontol 37:705–709, 1982

Kline DW, Schieber F, Abusaura LC, et al: Age and the visual channels: contrast sensitivity and response speed. J Gerontol 38:211–216, 1983

Knoblauch K, Saunders F, Kusuda M, et al: Age and illuminance effects in Farnsworth-Munsell 100-hue test. Applied Optics 26:1441–1448, 1987

Lakowski R: Is the deterioration of colour discrimination with age due to lens or retinal changes? Farbe 11:69–86, 1962

Lebo CP, Reddell RC: The presbycusis component in occupational noise–induced hearing loss. Laryngoscope 82:1399–1409, 1972

Long GM, Crambert RF: The nature and basis of age-related changes in dynamic visual acuity. Psychol Aging 5:138–143, 1990

Marshall J, Grindle J, Ansel PL, et al: Convolution in human rods: an aging process. Br J Ophthalmol 63:181–187, 1980

McFadden D, Plattsmier HS: Aspirin can potentiate the temporary hearing loss induced by noise. Hear Res 9:295–316, 1983

McFarland RA, Warren B, Karis C: Alterations in critical flicker frequency as a function of age and light:dark ratio. J Exp Psychol 56:529–538, 1958

Miller IJ Jr: Human taste-bud density across adult age groups. J Gerontol 43:B26–B30, 1988

Millodot M: The influence of age on the sensitivity of the cornea. Invest Ophthalmol Vis Sci 16:240–242, 1977

Moller MB: Hearing in 70- to 75-year-old people: Results from a cross-sectional and longitudinal population study. Am J Otolaryngol 2:22–29, 1981

Murphy C: Taste and smell in the elderly, in Clinical Measures of Taste and Smell. Edited by Meiselman HL, Rivlin RS. New York, Macmillan, 1986, pp 343–371

Owsley C, Sloan ME: Contrast sensitivity, acuity, and the perception of real-world targets. Br J Ophthalmol 71:791–796, 1987

Owsley C, Sloane ME: Vision and aging, in Handbook of Neuropsychology, Vol 4. Edited by Boller F, Grafman J. Amsterdam, Elsevier, 1990, pp 229–249

Owsley C, Sekuler R, Siemsen D: Contrast sensitivity throughout adulthood. Vision Res 23:689–699, 1983

Pitts DG: The effects of aging on selected visual functions: dark adaptation, visual acuity, stereopsis, and brightness contrast, in Aging and Human Visual Function. Edited by Sekular R, Kline D, Dismukes K. New York, Alan R. Liss, 1982, pp 131–159

Prazma J: Otoxicity of aminoglycoside antibiotics, in Pharmacology of Hearing. Edited by Brown RD, Daigneault EA. New York, Wiley, 1981, pp 131–159

Rosen S, Plester D, El-Mofty A, et al: Relation of hearing loss to cardiovascular disease. Transactions of the American Academy of Ophthalmology and Otology 68:433–444, 1964

Schiffman S: Food recognition by the elderly. J Gerontol 32:586–592, 1977

Schiffman S, Warwick ZS: Flavor enhancement of foods for the elderly can reverse anorexia. Neurobiol Aging 9:24–26, 1988

Schor D, Heckmann T: Interocular differences in contrast and spatial frequency: effects on stereopsis and fusion. Vision Res 29:837–847, 1989

Schuknecht H: Pathology of the Ear. Cambridge, MA, Harvard University Press, 1974

Sekuler R, Ball K: Visual localization: age and practice. J Opt Soc Am [A] 3:864–867, 1986

Shadden BB, Raiford CA: Factors influencing service utilization by older individuals. J Commun Disord 17:209–224, 1984

Sivak M, Olson PL: Nighttime legibility of traffic signs: conditions eliminating the effects of driver age and disability glare. Accident Analysis and Prevention 14:87–93, 1982

Smith DV: Taste intensity as a function of areas and concentration: differentiation between compounds. J Exp Psychol 87:163–171, 1971

Spoor A: Presbycusis values in relationship to noise-induced hearing loss. International Audiology 6: 48–57, 1967

Stevens JC: Aging and spatial acuity of touch. J Gerontol 47:P35–P40, 1992

Stevens JC, Cain WS: Old-age deficits in the sense of smell as gauged by thresholds, magnitude matching, and odor identification. Psychol Aging 2:36–42, 1987

Venstrom D, Amoore JE: Olfactory threshold in relation to age, sex, or smoking. Journal of Food Science 33:290–298, 1968

Verrillo RT: Age-related changes in the sensitivity to vibration. J Gerontol 35:185–193, 1980

Walsh DA: Age differences in central perceptual processing: a dichoptic backward-masking investigation. J Gerontol 31:178–185, 1976

Warren LR, Wagener JW, Herman GE: Binaural analysis in the aging auditory system. J Gerontol 33:731–736, 1978

Weale RA: Retinal illumination and age. Transactions of the Illuminating Engineering Society 26:95–100, 1961

Weale RA: Aging and vision. Vision Res 26:1507–1512, 1986

Weiffenbach JM, Baum BJ, Burghauser R: Taste thresholds: quality-specific variation with human aging. J Gerontol 37:372–377, 1982

Whitaker D, Elliott D: Toward establishing a clinical displacement threshold technique to evaluate visual function behind cataract. Clinical Vision Science 4:61–69, 1989

Wolf E: Glare and age. Arch Ophthalmol 64:502–514, 1960

Wolf E: Studies on the shrinkage of the visual field with age. Highway Research Record 167:1–7, 1967

Wolf E, Shraffa AM: Relationship between critical flicker frequency and age in flicker perimetry. Arch Ophthalmol 72:832–843, 1964

Wysocki CJ, Gilbert AN: National Geographic Smell Survey: effects of age are heterogeneous, in Nutrition and the Chemical Senses in Aging: Recent Advances and Current Research Needs. Ann N Y Acad Sci 561:12–28, 1989

CHAPTER 4

Neuroanatomy and Neuropathology of Aging

F. Stephen Vogel, M.D.

As the animal kingdom evolved phylogenetically, structural characteristics of the nervous system were shared and modified progressively over countless millennia. Late in this course of events, the human brain acquired the facility for cognition. Unfortunately, this acquired attribute is labile. It is transient in each individual brain and its loss is indicative of senescence.

Clearly, cognition necessitates highly specialized anatomic and molecular properties. In this chapter I focus initially on these structural attributes and then use them as an informational base to assess the pathogenesis of the intellectual decline that accompanies chronological age.

Neuroanatomic Considerations

The adult human brain weighs approximately 1,350 g. This weight represents glia (astrocytes, oligodendroglia, and ependyma), myelin, blood vessels, and an astronomical number of neurons. The latter has been estimated conservatively at 20 billion. It is an important concept that each neuron is

essentially an individual unit of structure whose function is integrated into a consortium, a network of allied nerve cells. The functional capacity of a neuron becomes immutable with anatomic development and cell maturation; but clearly, embryonic neuroblasts have the latitude to evolve functions in accord with the needs of the host when these needs are expressed early in embryonic development. Thus, a single cerebral hemisphere assumes bilateral motor and sensory functions in the presence of the congenital abnormality of hemiatrophy of the brain.

The structural character of a neuron is established during embryonic and early postnatal development. Both nerve cells and glia originate from the germinal mantle, a marginal zone in the immediate subependymal area that is densely populated with primitive neuroectodermal cells. Here—and only here, with the rarest exception—do neurons undergo mitotic division, an event of the first trimester of embryonic development. The progeny of these divided neurons migrate outwardly into the cerebral cortex, being assisted directionally in their migration by slender glial filaments that serve as "guide wires" that stretch from the germinal mantle to the cortex. Having gained a permanent cortical position, the neurons differentiate and relinquish their capacity for replication. This imposed inability to divide is not without compensation. Only by giving up the ability to replicate do neurons attain stability of structure, an attribute that is a prerequisite to cognition. Anatomic stability permits the accumulation of information in the present, allows its recall from the past, and facilitates the formulation of concepts for the future. Unalterably, it also defines an inescapability of aging, because metabolic errors and metabolic deficiencies now become accumulative. Metabolic defects cannot be eliminated by cell division, in a manner that characterizes somatic cells. In summary, the structural stability of the human nervous system is simultaneously the prerequisite to cognition and the attribute that is cardinal to aging.

Each nerve cell is bounded totally by a three-layered plasma membrane (*unit membrane*) that is regionally specialized in structure to form axons, dendrites, and synapses. As with all cells, the plasma membrane of nerve cells controls the flow of metabolites between the neuron and its environs, namely the vasculature and the neuropil. Selected areas of the plasma membrane serve as sites of electrical activity, notably at synapses, where the transfer of signals from neuron to neuron is facilitated. The neuronal nucleus is situated in the perikaryon, that is, the cell body or *soma*. The nucleus generally varies proportionally in size to that of the nerve cell, ranging from 5 mm to 100 mm. Analogously with all other cells, its DNA regulates protein synthesis. However, in neurons, the production of protein must sustain not only the soma but also the dendrites and axons. The vulnerability imposed by this physical relationship is underscored in the "dying-back phenomenon," a characteristic of amyotrophic lateral sclerosis. Herein the distal segments of motor axons are the initial site of structural degeneration, presumably as a manifestation of a metabolic inadequacy within the perikaryon.

The perikaryon contains the ribosomes that synthesize proteins. Ribosomes are either free lying, being single or clustered as polyribosomes, or attached to the endoplasmic reticulum, a structural relationship referred to as *Nissl substance.* A neuron may show chromatolysis, characterized structurally as a swelling of the cytoplasmic compartment, a frag-

mentation of Nissl substance, and a displacement of the nucleus to the plasma membrane. These morphological alterations signify cell injury and are accompanied by functional compromises.

Mitochondria are largely restricted to the perikaryon. As in most cells, the mitochondria of the nervous system function as a source of energy through glycolysis, a chain reaction that uses glucose to produce adenosine triphosphate, with its high-energy bonds. However, nerve cells are distinctive in their obligate need for glucose and also in their inability to store glycogen. These characteristics increase their dependence on circulatory glucose and oxygen for uninterrupted aerobic metabolism. Thus, hypoxia and hypoglycemia promptly initiate such pathological entities as insular sclerosis, laminar necrosis, and a loss of Purkinje cells, among others. Lysosomes also frequent the perikaryon and serve as reservoirs of hydrolytic enzymes. Disturbances in their numbers and presumably in their functional capacities to perform autophagocytosis cause them to become engorged with lipoprotein waste material. These *lipofuscin granules* are evidence of metabolic wear and tear. They accumulate with age, but not in a uniform or time-predictable pattern. The motor neurons of the spinal anterior horns are particularly vulnerable. Their rate of accumulation is accelerated by metabolic insults, such as hypoxia. The lengthy distance between the perikaryon and the synapse has necessitated a specialization of lysosomes. Nerve transmission across the synapse initiates the production of vesicles; these are modified lysosomes that conduct autophagic activities as pinocytotic or exocytotic vesicles.

Microtubules, neurofilaments, and microfilaments are specialized structures in neurons. Microtubules measure 20–30 nm; neurofilaments, 10 nm; and microfilaments, 5 nm. Microtubules are long, unbranched cylinders. They are formed principally of the protein tubulin. In nerve cells, microtubules reside predominately in the perikaryon, where they may appear individually or in small clusters. They are present in lesser numbers in axons. Compounds such as colchicine bind with microtubules and impair their functional participation in axoplasmic transport. Neurofilaments are unique to nerve cells. They are abundant in large axons, where they outnumber the microtubules. In small axons and dendrites, microtubules predominate. The ratio of neurofilaments to microtubules is altered moderately as a corollary of age. However, in patients with Alzheimer's disease it is modified to an extreme as the result of neurofibrillary tangle formation.

Microfilaments are abundant in growing nerve processes. They are also present in neuroglia. Compounds such as cytochalasin B greatly interfere with the role of microfilaments in cell motility and presumably also in neuronal axoplasmic transport.

The *synapse* (a term derived from the Greek, meaning to connect or to join) is a locus of specialized anatomy that permits the directional flow of "information" from neuron to neuron. Its directionality is best appreciated in the constancy of the circuitry that defines flow from sensory to motor neurons, and never in the reverse. A synapse is an approximation of the membranes of two neurons, always physically separated by a space approximately 20 nm in width. The contact between an axon to a cell body is termed an axosomatic synapse; between an axon and a dendrite, an axodendritic synapse; between two axons, an axoaxonic synapse; and between two dendrites, a dendrodendritic synapse. At such sites of juxtaposition, neurons release substances that diffuse through the intracellular clefts and serve as neurotransmitters or neuromodulators. The movement of neurotransmitters, ions, or metabolites from one neuron into the synaptic cleft may initiate or modify a function of several contiguous cells, even glia. In addition, the anatomic proximity of juxtaposed membranes permits direct electrical interaction between contiguous nerve cells. The polarity of a synapse is defined by structure; thus the presynaptic terminal is distinguished by the presence of synaptic vesicles, whereas the postsynaptic processes are marked anatomically by an increased density of the plasma membrane. Functional specialization of synapses is reflected in their shape and size, and also in the number and configuration of synaptic vesicles. For example, small vesicles (20–40 nm in diameter), by their size, indicate a content of acetylcholine and characterize the synapse as cholinergic, and medium-sized vesicles (50–90 nm) denote the presence of monoamine transmitters. Large vesicles (120–150 nm) characterize neurosecretory cells, such as those of the hypothalamus, which supply polypeptide hormones to the pituitary. The security of information about the more precisely characterized neurotransmitters, such as acetylcholine, gamma-aminobutyric acid, and do-

pamine, has lent false assurance to our fragmentary knowledge about the numerous, and still putative, neuroactive polypeptides such as somatostatin, vasopressin, endorphins, and the like. The limited knowledge concerning the normal functional roles of these compounds imparts considerable uncertainty to hypotheses that suggest their specific roles in the causation of disease processes such as Alzheimer's disease. Thus, a diminished concentration of acetylcholine in the terminal state of Alzheimer's disease necessitates a clear distinction between causation and an epiphenomenon before its significance assumes meaning.

In this brief discussion I have focused on the individual neuron and the structural characteristics that evolve through cell differentiation. To a degree, I have also reviewed the process of maturation, that is, the evolution of the topography of the nervous system. Ancillary events such as myelinization should not go unnoticed; however, the integrity of myelin seems not to be cardinal to the phenomenon of aging. Its loss seemingly is not a primary event in the aged human nervous system, and therefore my principal concern will remain with the functional unit, the neuron.

The embryonic events of angiogenesis are also important to the functionality of neural tissues. Abnormal angiogenesis may be responsible for congenital malformations of the nervous system. More important, the continued patency of the cerebral blood vessels is clearly cardinal to aging, for it is frequently compromised by atherosclerosis and by hypertensive fibromuscular hyperplasia.

It should be noted that the complex events of embryonic development are accompanied by programmed neuronal cell death, termed *apoptosis*. The word *programmed* warrants underscoring because it reflects the purposeful transiency of biological units within an organism. Thus, defective and superfluous neurons are lost even during this early interval of life. The analogy could be drawn to the "thinning" of a corn field during its most active growth phase. At the point of completed neuronal division, is it then appropriate to characterize the human nervous system as a "sculptured" entity, cast in stone and irreversibly devoid of development or repair, subject only to "aging," to disease, and to degeneration? Ostensibly, this concept has validity, for neurons cannot replicate, oligodendroglial cells cannot remyelinate, and cerebral blood vessels are limited in their capacity for structural repair. But even in the human nervous system there is a reparative process termed *plasticity* that suggests that mature neurons have at least a limited capacity to form axonal sprouts and perhaps new synapses. Optimistically, it has been suggested that the formation of new synaptic circuitry confers an added ability to learn, an acquired capability to remember new facts, and a facility to develop new skills. As indicated above, during embryonic development, the migration of neurons, and particularly the development of dendritic processes and the formation of synapses, are dictated largely by the functional needs of the host. Whether plasticity serves a purposeful need in the adult human nervous system as a reaction to tissue injury or as a response to a neurological deficit, however, remains beyond current knowledge.

It has been demonstrated that neural tissue can be grafted into an alien nervous system. However, again, the capability of these cells to perform useful repair of neurological deficits remains uncertain. In this regard, information cannot be transposed directly from laboratory animals to man. The "grafting" into the human brain of embryonic or adult cells selected because of their capability to elaborate substrate (such as dopamine) merely supplies this compound regionally and makes it available to metabolically compromised cells. As is true with exogenously administered L-dopa, this substrate temporarily restores a degree of functionality to the substantia nigra but does not correct the progressive metabolic defect that ultimately leads to neuronal cell death. At this point, substitution therapy ceases.

What, then, is unique about the human nervous system that enables it to fulfill the functionality of cognition? One can note quantitative differences in the relative mass of the neocortex in humans versus that in lower animals, but these quantitative variables are minor when compared with the grandeur of intellectual function in humans as contrasted with its absence—or at least near absence—in lower animals. One is obliged, however, to admit that our own intellectual capacities do not provide us with meaningful insight into the origin or the modus operandi of cognition. Being required to acknowledge this major deficit in knowledge, we presume to ask, Why does age, or the passage of time, quantitatively modify the cognitive capacities of the human nervous system?

Pathology of Organic Mental Disorders

Unfortunately, the concept of aging and dementia have been inseparably allied. Thus, the inescapable passage of calendar years has encouraged an acceptance of an age-related cognitive decline. In this context, dementia is viewed as an unavoidable corollary of "old age." For example, in 1906, Alois Alzheimer described the occurrence of neuritic plaques, excessive intraneuronal filaments, and granulovacuolar degeneration in the severely atrophic brain of a 51-year-old woman whose illness was dominated by dementia. Although identical morphological alterations had been previously observed—generally in lesser degrees—in individuals of greater chronological age, Alzheimer insisted that this disorder was distinctive because of its relationship to an early decade of life. The entity was termed "presenile dementia" to distinguish it from a disorder that occurred with identical morphology after the age of 65, a disease referred to as "senile dementia." Unfortunately, the rarity of postmortem examinations on patients in mental institutions delayed the realization that neuritic plaques, neurofibrillary tangles, and granulovacuolar degeneration are seemingly the morphological expression of a single disease process, irrespective of age. Thus, the terms "presenile" and "senile dementia" have been set aside for the unified designation *Alzheimer's disease*. Clearly, disease states (notably, Alzheimer's disease, cerebrovascular disease, and Pick's disease) occur with increased incidence in the human nervous system with advanced chronological age. For this reason it is important to examine these entities while seeking ancillary information to the question, Do anatomic and functional alterations occur in the brain as a result of age alone, apart from a disease process?

A list of known causations of dementia would also include Creutzfeldt-Jakob's disease. However, the transmissibility of Creutzfeldt-Jakob's disease to laboratory animals—and also its unfortunate transmission from human to human by corneal transplantation, by pituitary growth extracts, and by contaminated surgical instruments—clearly characterizes it as an infectious process. This characterization removes Creutzfeldt-Jakob's disease from the "degenerative" or "aging" category and thus from our immediate consideration.

Alzheimer's Disease

Neurons and neuritic processes are lost during the course of Alzheimer's disease. Gyri narrow, sulci widen, and cortical atrophy becomes apparent both by computerized tomography and at postmortem examination. The atrophic brain of Alzheimer's disease is generally diminished in weight by approximately 200 g. Importantly, however, the histological features of Alzheimer's disease can be present in a nervous system unaltered in weight or gross appearance (Terry et al. 1991). When atrophy is present, and it usually is, typically it is bilateral and symmetrical, and its distribution is predominately frontal and temporal (Hooper and Vogel 1975; Terry et al. 1981). The degree of atrophy in the parietal and occipital lobes is regularly minimal. The cerebellum is uninvolved, and this importantly distinguishes the clinical attributes of Alzheimer's disease from those of Creutzfeldt-Jakob's disease. The meninges are not thickened; this feature separates Alzheimer's disease from general paresis or dementia paralytica, with which it shares the characteristics of bilaterality and symmetrical frontal lobe atrophy (Khachaturian 1985; Probst et al. 1991a) (Figure 4–1).

Three morphological alterations serve to individualize Alzheimer's disease: neuritic plaque formation, neurofibrillary degeneration, and granulovacuolar alteration (Gibson 1985). In view of the chronicity of the disease process, it is remarkable that astrocytes generally remain so quiescent throughout the entire course of this prolonged disease process. The minimal extent of astrogliosis distinguishes Alzheimer's disease from Pick's disease and from Creutzfeldt-Jakob's disease; in both of the latter diseases, astrocytic proliferation adds firmness to the cortical tissues and provides a diagnostic criterion during histological examination. Notwithstanding the occasional coexistence of congophilic angiopathy, the cerebral blood vessels ostensibly respond neither in structure nor in patency to the presence of Alzheimer's disease. Interestingly, there is no quantitative variance in the formation of senile plaques or neurofibrillary tangles at the margin of a cortical infarct that might incidentally be present in the cerebrum of an individual patient.

As mentioned above, the cardinal lesions of Alzheimer's disease are the neuritic or Alzheimer plaque, the neurofibrillary tangle, and granulovacuolar degeneration. The latter two are intra-neuronal processes, whereas the neuritic plaque is a focal, roughly spheroid area of transformation in the neuropil. Although senile plaques and neurofibrillary tangles are individual and totally distinct in morphology, they conform closely in their geographic distributions. Generally, both predominate in the frontal and temporal cortices and are particularly prominent in the hippocampus. Neurofibrillary degeneration per se is not restricted to patients with Alzheimer's disease but may be observed, for example, in the pigmented neurons of the substantia nigra in patients with postencephalitic parkinsonism.

The senile, or neuritic, plaque is a focal, rather discrete area of abnormality, globoid in shape, several hundred microns in diameter, and regularly situated in the gray matter. Magnification by electron microscopy discloses the initial alteration to be characterized by segmental enlargement, or aneurysmal dilatation, of each neuritic process that traverses the domain of the plaque. These segmentally enlarged, sausage-shaped neurites become engorged with degenerated mitochondria and

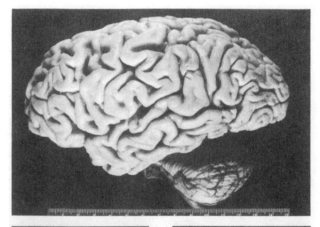

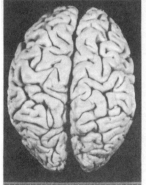
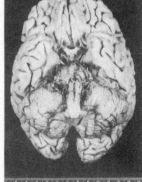

Figure 4–1. Alzheimer's disease. At autopsy, the brain of a 72-year-old man with a 5-year history of dementia weighed 1,225 g and showed moderate cortical atrophy most marked in the frontal and temporal lobes.

lysosomes, presumably because of stagnation of axoplasmic flow. The globoid lesion curiously remains individual. It attains, and retains, uniformity in size without further enlargement. It may cluster with other plaques, but avoids coalescence. The early lesions have a faint argentophilia and thus appear as fine delicate areas of argentophilic, filamentous material. As the senile plaque ages, it acquires density. This composition results from a deposition of native compounds such as acid mucopolysaccharides and glycoproteins and, importantly, from the addition of alien substances, notably amyloid. As a result of these accumulations, plaques become stainable by a variety of agents such as Congo red and Alcian blue, among others (Figures 4–2 and 4–3).

The senile plaque, as an architectural creation, is totally alien to the cellular and molecular composition of the brain. However, this is not the case with neurofibrillary tangle formation, an entity that borrows its structural blueprint, as well as its molecular composition, from the 10-nm neurofilaments that are normally present within neurons and that are sparsely distributed in the perikaryon and axon for the purpose of propelling axoplasmic flow. The filaments that constitute the fibrillary tangle deviate significantly from normal, both in number and in their paired, intertwined, helical structure. There remains a degree of order, however, for each individual filament retains an approximate diameter of 10 nm; moreover, the circumferential twist of the two filaments occurs at predictable intervals of 80 nm. Unfortunately, there is a void of knowledge

concerning the nature of the stimulus and the molecular events that initiate and conduct the excessive production of neurofilaments and also cause them to wed into helical formations. Although the nature of this stimulus is obscured, the stimulus itself seemingly is not restricted to Alzheimer's disease. As has been mentioned, neurofibrillary tangles develop in the pigmented neurons of the substantia nigra in patients with postencephalitic parkinsonism as well as in the cerebral neurons of pugilists (Wisniewski et al. 1979).

The helical configuration is unique to the neurons of the human central nervous system and is not a borrowed characteristic from members of the lower animal kingdom. Neurons of elderly monkeys and dogs accumulate excessive filaments, but these threads do not become paired or helical in configuration. The phenomenon of helical formation is not necessarily related to overproduction. In progressive supranuclear palsy (Steele-Richardson-Olszewski syndrome), the intraneuronal filaments attain quantitative excess without helical formation (Tellez-Nagel and Wisniewski 1973). Neurons altered by neurofibrillary degeneration are generally numerous in the entorrhinal cortex, among the pyramidal cells of the hippocampus, and in the amygdala. They are also readily evident in the cortex of the frontal and temporal lobes and are generally less numerous in the parietal and occipital areas, with only an occasional example in the brain stem. It is of interest that the neurons that normally accumulate lipofuscin pigment are not appreciably disposed to de-

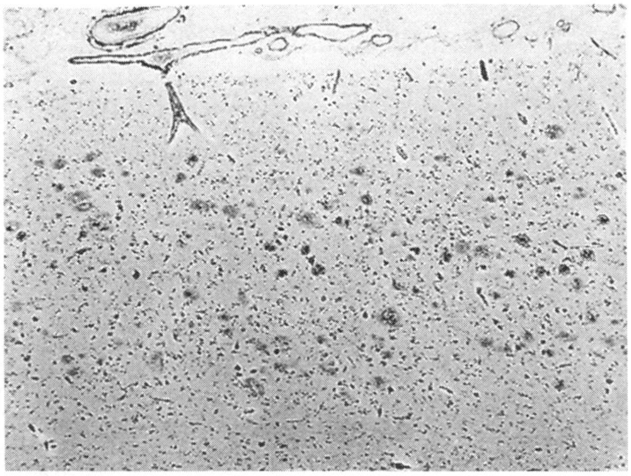

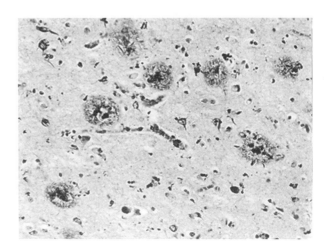

Figure 4–2. Alzheimer's disease. The entorrhinal cortex of the brain in Figure 4–1 contains numerous neuritic plaques. King stain, 52×.

Figure 4–3. Alzheimer's disease. The neuritic plaques are remarkably discrete, spherical, and of uniform size. Their dense core is amyloid. King stain, 250×.

velop neurofibrillary tangle formation, even though lipofuscin, termed "wear-and-tear pigment," is viewed as an expression of "aging." It is also of interest that neurons involved by granulovacuolar degeneration, generally the pyramidal cells of the hippocampus, eschew neurofibrillary degeneration, although contiguous neurons may be severely altered by the accumulation of neurofilaments (Figures 4–4 and 4–5).

Granulovacuolar degeneration is the least conspicuous item in the triad of cytological transformations in Alzheimer's disease (Woodard 1962). Involved neurons portray a fine vacuolization of the cytoplasm, and each vacuole harbors one or several hyperchromatic granules. The significance of granulovacuolar degeneration escapes current understanding, but it is specific to Alzheimer's disease, and it is not coexistent in the same neuron with the formation of lipofuscin pigment or neurofibrillary degeneration.

A number of hypotheses have been formulated concerning the pathogenesis of Alzheimer's disease. All but the most recent have lost degrees of credibility, and the very recent are too current to have withstood vigorous scientific scrutiny. With the advent of electron microscopy, magnification of early plaques disclosed the neuritic processes—the axons and dendrites—to be aneurysmally dilated and to be engorged with particulate cytoplasmic debris. This morphology was interpreted as being indicative of diminished integrity of the plasma membrane, possibly the result of impaired peroxidation. The administration of vitamin E provided no evidence of therapeutic benefit. Shortly thereafter, aluminum intoxication was implicated (Crapper et al. 1976, 1980; Perl and Brody 1980). However, skepticism about the possible role of aluminum intoxication persisted because quantitative tissue assays marginally exceeded the level of instrumental precision, were equivocally elevated in all cases, and were not elevated in youthful patients with Down's syndrome before the inception of plaque formation. Furthermore, environmental exposure to aluminum among bauxite workers was not associated with an increase in Alzheimer's disease. The deposition of aluminum in neural tissue is now generally viewed as an epiphenomenon of chelation. Attention was then directed toward Meynert's nucleus, and, by analogy to parkinsonism, this nucleus was envisioned as the counterpart of the substantia nigra,

wherein the deficiency of transmitter substance concerned cholinergic compounds rather than those of the dopaminergic system (Braak and Braak 1991; Coyle et al. 1983; Davies and Maloney 1976; Johnston et al. 1979; Rogers et al. 1985; Whitehouse et al. 1982). More currently, the role of beta-amyloid deposition has come under active investigation. That beta-amyloid is deposited in the neuritic plaques and very often in cerebral blood vessels (this latter process known as congophilic angiopathy) is unquestioned (Citron et al. 1992; Glenner and Wong 1984; Haass et al. 1992; Hendriks et al. 1992; Probst et al. 1991b; Quon et al. 1991; Rumble et al. 1989; Sandhu et al. 1991; Wasco et al. 1992; Wirak at al.

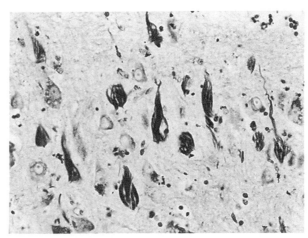

Figure 4–4. Alzheimer's disease. The pyramidal cell layer of the hippocampal cortex of the brain in Figure 4–1 shows numerous neurons with advanced neurofibrillary degeneration. King stain, 325×.

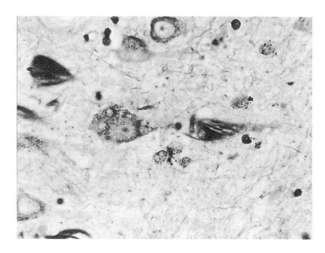

Figure 4–5. Alzheimer's disease. Neurofibrillary degeneration spares neurons with granulovacuolar degeneration. King stain, 680×.

1992). However, beta-amyloid's pathogenic relationship to Alzheimer's disease is brought into question by its absence, as evidenced by electron microscopy, in early-evolving plaques (Wisniewski et al. 1989). A serendipitous observation is currently receiving attention in the public press (Strittmatter et al. 1993). Such findings suggest that individuals born with a disproportionately high concentration of a hematogenous blood protein, apolipoprotein E_4, bear an increased risk for the development of Alzheimer's disease. The predominant member of this family of blood proteins is apolipoprotein E_3 (or apo-E_3), a normal transporter of cholesterol in transcellular traffic. Ostensibly, apo-E_3 also fulfills a normal physiological role through its binding properties with tau, a microtubular protein of neurons, thereby imparting a stability of structure. It is further suggested that the E_4 molecule inadequately fulfills this latter function, and thus the gene defect that causes an overproduction of apo-E_4 above that of E_3 creates structural instability in neuronal microtubules; this instability, in turn, is expressed morphologically as neurofibrillary degeneration. Unfortunately, there are only incomplete models of Alzheimer's disease among laboratory animals (Martin et al. 1991). However, efforts are being made to develop this important source of information in transgenic animals (Quon et al. 1991). The regular and precocious occurrence of Alzheimer's disease in individuals with Down's syndrome remains an unfortunate but valuable source of information against which the validity of current and subsequent theories must ring true (Burger and Vogel 1973; Masters et al. 1985).

Pick's Disease

Classically, the term Pick's disease, or *lobar sclerosis*, signifies asymmetric involvement of a single lobe, notably the frontal or temporal lobe. Atrophy may attain extreme proportions. Occasionally, a case of Pick's disease may show more generalized involvement and may be bilateral and symmetrical. Alternatively, constituent areas of the basal ganglia may be markedly involved. Histologically, the involved cortex is severely depleted of neurons and heavily populated with an overgrowth of astrocytes. The hallmark of this disease is evidenced in the residual neurons, many of which are "ballooned" and within some of which are one or several faint eosinophilic,

argentophilic inclusions, termed *Pick's bodies*. Pick's bodies are formed of densely aggregated neurofilaments (Muñoz-Garcia and Ludwin 1984) (Figures 4–6, 4–7, and 4–8).

Thus, the excessive production of neurofilaments characterizes many disease states—notably Pick's disease, by the formation of Pick's bodies; Alzheimer's disease, with the expression of neurofibrillary degeneration; parkinsonism, by the formation of Lewy bodies; and progressive supranuclear palsy. Is the excessive production of neurofilaments a manifestation of age? I would think not, but instead would attribute excessive production of neurofilaments to a specific metabolic disturbance rather than to a universal event of aging. Even the brains of centenarians do not always reflect quantitative alterations in neurofibrillary production, and when present—as in Alzheimer's disease or Pick's dis-

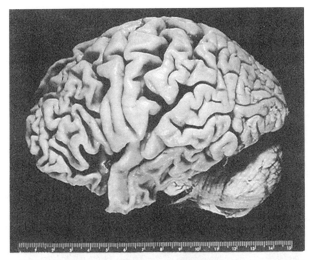

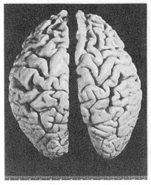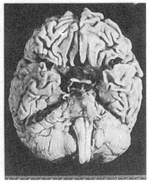

Figure 4–6. Pick's disease. At autopsy, the brain of a 73-year-old man who was institutionalized for 5 years with dementia weighed 1,075 g. There is severe cortical atrophy in the frontal and temporal lobes.

ease—the alterations are typically restricted to selected regions or nuclear systems. In summary, both Pick's disease and Alzheimer's disease are more reasonably termed "disease states" rather than aging phenomena.

Multi-Infarct Dementia

The stenosis or occlusion of small vessels leads to small infarcts, termed *lacunae*. When the clinical state emphasizes dementia, the term *multi-infarct dementia* is then appropriate. Approximately 15% of individuals institutionalized because of severe dementia will be found at postmortem examination to have multiple small cerebral infarcts (Tomlinson et al. 1968, 1970). These lacunae individually measure less than 1 cm across and, although they are randomly distributed, are usually most numerous in the basal ganglia, the thalamus, and the corona radiata. A loss of cognition generally denotes a global insult to cerebral function. In cases of multi-infarct dementia, the impairment in integrated neuronal activity probably reflects an interference in the associated pathways in the white matter. The term *Binswanger's disease* has been applied to the morphological constellation of cerebral arteriosclerosis, multiple microinfarcts, and a diffuse pallor of myelin (Figure 4–9).

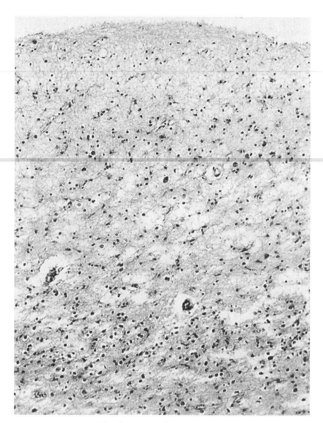

Figure 4–7. Pick's disease. The entorrhinal cortex is almost totally depopulated of neurons and shows marked fibrillary astrogliosis. Luxol fast blue, 100×.

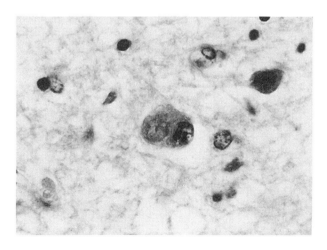

Figure 4–8. Pick's disease. A residual neuron is ballooned; the nucleus is displaced eccentrically and the cytoplasm contains a Pick body. Luxol fast blue, 1,000×.

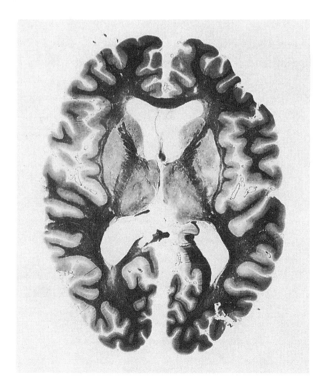

Figure 4–9. Multi-infarct dementia. A whole mount of a horizontal section shows rarefaction and multiple lacunae, particularly in the right basal ganglia and thalamus. Luxol fast blue.

The Brain and Time

The focus in this section is on that nebulous entity, the aged brain untouched by disease. It is self-evident that with the passage of time the accumulation of intraneuronal metabolic errors diminishes the ability of neurons to function and, at some interval thereafter, to survive. These events pertain to each nerve cell individually, for each is a structural unit and each is incapable of replication. As evidenced by the rate of neuronal depopulation, the end point of lethal metabolic errors is attained at an earlier chronological age in cortical neurons than in those of the brain stem or spinal cord.

It is also clear that the biological or metabolic requirements of individual neurons are further challenged by systemic events and exogenous toxins. Unquestionably, the depopulation of neurons is accelerated by impaired circulation. Substrates such as oxygen and glucose are diminished, and cellular toxic waste materials, such as lactic acid, tend to accumulate, and neurons are functionally impaired and structurally lost.

As mentioned at the beginning of this chapter, the very essence of cognition necessitates stability of structure, but biological systems (whether they are bacteria, amoebae, or hepatic cells) perpetuate biological activity only through a capacity for replication. Thus, stability and longevity are incongruous attributers. Cognition cannot be otherwise than transient in the presence of time (Terry 1991; Terry et al. 1981).

References

Braak H, Braak E: Alzheimer's disease affects limbic nuclei of the thalamus. Acta Neuropathol 81:261–268, 1991

Burger PC, Vogel FS: The development of the pathologic changes of Alzheimer's disease and senile dementia in patients with Down's syndrome. Am J Pathol 73:457–476, 1973

Citron M, Olterscorf T, Haass C, et al: Mutation of the beta-amyloid precursor protein in familial Alzheimer's disease increases beta-protein production. Nature 360:672–674, 1992

Coyle JT, Price DL, Des Long MR: Alzheimer's disease: a disorder of cortical cholinergic innervation. Science 219:1184–1190, 1983

Crapper DR, Krishman SS, Quitkat S: Aluminum neurofibrillary degeneration and Alzheimer's disease. Brain 99:67–80, 1976

Crapper DR, Quitkat S, Krishman SS, et al: Intranuclear aluminum content in Alzheimer's disease, dialysis encephalopathy and experimental aluminum encephalopathy. Acta Neuropathol 50:19–24, 1980

Davies P, Maloney AJ: Selective loss of central cholinergic neurons in Alzheimer's disease (letter). Lancet 2:1403, 1976

Gibson PH: Relationship between numbers of cortical argentophilic and congophilic senile plaques in the brain of elderly people with and without senile dementia of the Alzheimer type. Gerontology 31:321–324, 1985

Glenner GG, Wong CW: Alzheimer's disease: initial report of the purification and characterization of a novel cerebrovascular amyloid protein. Biochem Biophys Res Commun 120:885–890, 1984

Haass C, Koo EH, Mellon A, et al: Targeting of cell-surface beta-amyloid precursor protein to lysosomes: alternative processing into amyloid-bearing fragments. Nature 357:500–503, 1992

Hendriks L, van Duijn CM, Cras P, et al: Presenile dementia and cerebral haemorrhage linked to a mutation at codon 692 of the beta-amyloid precursor protein gene. Nature Genetics 1:218–221, 1992

Hooper MW, Vogel FS: The limbic system in Alzheimer's disease: a neuropathologic investigation. Am J Pathol 85:1–13, 1975

Johnston MV, McKinney M, Coyle JT: Evidence for a cholinergic projection to neocortex from neurons in basal forebrain. Proc Natl Acad Sci USA 76:5392–5396, 1979

Khachaturian ZS: Diagnosis of Alzheimer's disease. Arch Neurol 42:1097–1105, 1985

Martin LJ, Sisodia SS, Koo EH, et al: Amyloid precursor protein in aged nonhuman primates. Proc Natl Acad Sci USA 88:1461–1465, 1991

Masters CL, Simms G, Weinman NA, et al: Amyloid plaque core protein in Alzheimer's disease and Down syndrome. Proc Natl Acad Sci USA 82:4245–4249, 1985

Muñoz-Garcia D, Ludwin SK: Classic and generalized variants of Pick's disease: a clinicopathological, ultrastructural, and immunocytochemical comparative study. Ann Neurol 16:467–480, 1984

Perl DP, Brody AR: Alzheimer's disease: x-ray spectrometric evidence of aluminum accumulation in neurofibrillary tangle-bearing neurons. Science 208:297–298, 1980

Probst A, Langui D, Ulrich J: Alzheimer's disease: a description of the structural lesions. Brain Pathology 1:229–239, 1991a

Probst A, Langui D, Ipsen S, et al: Deposition of B/A4 protein along neuronal plasma membranes in diffuse senile plaques. Acta Neuropathol 83:21–29, 1991b

Quon D, Wang Y, Catalano R, et al: Formation of beta-amyloid protein deposits in brains of transgenic mice. Nature 352:239–241, 1991

Rogers JD, Brogan D, Mirra SS: The nucleus basalis of Meynert in neurological disease: a quantitative morphological study. Ann Neurol 17:163–170, 1985

Rumble B, Retallack R, Hilbich C, et al: Amyloid A_4 protein and its precursor in Down's syndrome and Alzheimer's disease. N Engl J Med 320:1446–1452, 1989

Sandhu FA, Salim M, Zain SB: Expression of the human beta-amyloid protein of Alzheimer's disease specifically in the brains of transgenic mice. J Biol Chem 266:21331–21334, 1991

Strittmatter WJ, Saunders AM, Schmechel D, et al: Apolipoprotein E: high-avidity binding to beta-amyloid and increased frequency of type 4 allele in late-onset familial Alzheimer's disease. Proc Natl Acad Sci USA 90:1977–1981, 1993

Tellez-Nagel I, Wisniewski HM: Ultrastructure of neurofibrillary tangles in Steele-Richardson-Olszewski syndrome. Arch Neurol 29:324–327, 1973

Terry RD, Masliah E, Salmon DP, et al: Physical basis of cognitive alterations in Alzheimer's disease: synapse loss is the major correlate of cognitive impairment. Ann Neurol 30:572–580, 1991

Terry RD, Peck A, De Teresa R, et al: Some morphometric aspects of the brain in senile dementia of the Alzheimer type. Ann Neurol 10:184–192, 1981

Tomlinson BE, Blessed G, Roth M: Observations on the brains of non-demented old people. J Neurol Sci 7:331–356, 1968

Tomlinson BE, Blessed G, Roth M: Observations on the brains of demented old people. J Neurol Sci 11:205–242, 1970

Wasco W, Bupp K, Magendantz M, et al: Identification of a mouse brain cDNA that encodes a protein related to the Alzheimer's disease–associated amyloid-beta protein precursor. Proc Natl Acad Sci USA 89:10758–10762, 1992

Whitehouse PJ, Price DL, Struble RG, et al: Alzheimer's disease and senile dementia: loss of neurons in the basal forebrain. Science 215:1237–1239, 1982

Wirak DO, Bayney R, Ramabhadran TV, et al: Deposits of amyloid beta protein in the central nervous system of transgenic mice. Science 255:1443–1445, 1992

Wisniewski K, Jervis GA, Moretz RC, et al: Alzheimer neurofibrillary tangles in diseases other than senile and presenile dementia. Ann Neurol 5:288–294, 1979

Wisniewski HM, Wegiel J, Wang KC, et al: Ultrastructural studies of the cells forming amyloid fibers in classical plaques. Canadian Journal of Neurological Sciences 16:535–542, 1989

Woodard JS: Clinicopathologic significance of granulovacuolar degeneration in Alzheimer's disease. J Neuropathol Exp Neurol 21:85–91, 1962

CHAPTER 5

Chemical Messengers

Garth Bissette, Ph.D.

The concept of biochemical substances controlling the communication between nerve cells (or neurons) can be traced to the latter part of the 19th century when the famous argument between the classical anatomists Ramón y Cajal and Camillo Golgi was finally resolved in Cajal's favor. Cajal and Sherrington had described very small gaps between the processes of adjacent nerve cells, which they termed "synapses" after the Greek word meaning "to touch." Based on his technique of silver staining, Golgi had held that the nerve cells actually connected into a neural network.

We now know that Golgi could claim partial victory in that such networks have been shown to exist in certain invertebrates; however, the vast majority of species that have been examined do, in fact, have synaptic clefts between neurons that are in communication with each other. These areas are composed of specialized membrane thickenings across which biochemicals are released from the presynaptic neuron into the intracellular space. These substances then diffuse across this gap to their corresponding receptor sites on adjacent postsynaptic neurons or glial cells or to presynaptic autoreceptors. These receptors are also specialized areas of the cell membrane where proteins that span the receptive cell's membrane are able to recognize and bind their specific biochemical molecules (or *ligands*). The usual result of this binding is a conformational change in the receptor protein that can open a channel through the membrane that is selective for a particular ionic element, such as calcium, potassium, or sodium. Alternatively, the binding of the ligand to the receptor can initiate a cascade of changes upon molecules that are associated with the receptor, so-called second-messenger species such as adenosine or guanosine triphosphate (ATP or GTP) or inosine 3'-triphosphate (IP3) and diacylglycerol (DAG). These, in turn, alter other membrane and intracellular proteins by a series of biochemical reactions, often involving the addition or deletion of a phosphate group on the target molecule. It is now well established that many different receptors may bind the same type of neurotransmitter molecule with very different postsynaptic effects. These events usually have one of two effects on the receiving neuron: a decrease in its firing rate, termed *inhibition,* or an increase in its activity, termed *excitation.* The actual biomolecules that are released across the synapse and bind to a receptor that then produces a discrete physiological change are termed *chemical neurotransmitters,* and they come in a wide assortment of classes and molecular individuality within these classes. (Refer to Figure 5–1.)

The first substance identified as a chemical neurotransmitter was acetylcholine in the 1920s. Otto Loewi and Sir Henry Dale independently demonstrated that this substance was secreted from the endings of nerve cells of the peripheral nervous system when their fibers were stimulated and that it had predictable and reproducible effects on heart rate and blood pressure. The subsequent identification in the 1940s of epinephrine and norepinephrine in the peripheral nervous system set the stage for work that would eventually allow development of techniques for staining specific components of the synthetic and degradative biochemical pathways in the central nervous system (CNS). Between 1950 and 1970, these and related procedures led to the identification of what are now considered to be the "classical" CNS neurotransmitters: acetylcholine; the so-called biogenic amines, which include the catecholamines norepinephrine, epinephrine, and dopamine; and the indolamine serotonin (5-hydroxytryptamine). This work also led to the recognition that the amino acid gamma-aminobutyric acid (GABA) was an inhibitory neurotransmitter. These classical neurotransmitters are derived from amino acid precursors by sequential biochemical steps that are under the control of specific enzymes. The presence of these enzymes indicates that the neuron is capable of producing the particular neurotransmitter under investigation, and their presence, when coupled with selective staining procedures, allows mapping of the location of the nerve cells that are producing the neurotransmitter. It was this technique that allowed the first practical application of this developing knowledge to the treatment of a neurodegenerative disease. The identification of the dopamine cells of the substantia nigra as the primary target of the degenerative process in Parkinson's disease led to an effective therapy that is still used today, although the cause of the neuronal degeneration and a cure have not yet been discovered. This success reinforced the interest in discovering neurochemical pathologies in other neurodegenerative diseases, such as Alzheimer's disease and Huntington's chorea, as well as offering hope for effective therapies in mental illness based on rational drug design.

Since the 1970s, a plethora of newly discovered transmitter substances have been reported. The dis-

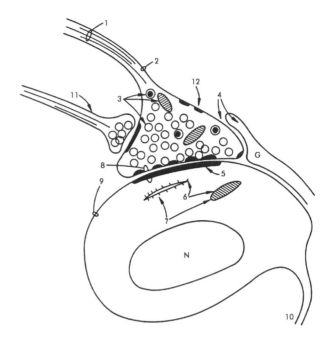

Figure 5–1. Twelve steps in the synaptic transmission process in an idealized synaptic connection: **1.** Transport down the axon. **2.** Electrically excitable membrane of the axon. **3.** The organelles and enzymes present in the nerve terminal for synthesizing, storing, and releasing the transmitter, as well as for the process of active reuptake. **4.** Enzymes present in the extracellular space and within the glia for catabolizing excess transmitter release from nerve terminals. **5.** The postsynaptic receptor that triggers the response of the postsynaptic cell to the transmitter. **6.** The organelles within the postsynaptic cells that respond to the receptor trigger. **7.** Inter-action between genetic expression of the postsynaptic nerve cell and its influences on the cytoplasmic organelles that respond to transmitter action. **8.** The possible "plastic" steps modifiable by events at the specialized synaptic contact zone. **9.** The electrical portion of the nerve cell membrane that, in response to the various transmitters, is able to integrate the postsynaptic potentials and produce an action potential. **10.** Continuation of the information transmission by which the postsynaptic cell sends an action potential down its axon. **11.** Release of transmitter, subjected to modification by a presynaptic (axoaxonic) synapse; in some cases an analogous control can be achieved between dendritic elements. **12.** Release of the transmitter from a nerve terminal or secreting dendritic site may be further subject to modulation through autoreceptors that respond to the transmitter that the same secreting structure has released. G = glia; N = nucleus. *Source.* Reproduced with permission from Cooper JR, Bloom FE, Roth RH (eds): *The Biochemical Basis of Neuropharmacology.* New York, Oxford University Press, 1991, p. 44.

covery of the excitatory amino acids glutamate and aspartate, as well as the identification of other inhibitory amino acids—including glycine, serine, and several others—greatly expanded the list in this class of neurotransmitter substances. The nucleotides adenosine and guanosine have now been shown to be neurotransmitters as well as components of the genetic code and, when phosphorylated, second messengers. Chains of from 3 to over 40 amino acids, termed *neuropeptides,* have been shown to act as messenger molecules and represent a new class of neurotransmitters whose final tally may include more than 200 distinct species. Only recently, the neuronal production and neurotransmitter status of the diffusible gas nitric oxide has been recognized.

To qualify as a neurotransmitter, most of the criteria discussed below must be met, although in many cases, technical problems or insufficient resources for the appropriate research have prevented the accumulation of sufficient evidence for all of the criteria to be met. First, the substance must be found within neurons in a subcellular compartment (usually synaptic vesicles) that allows its release into the synaptic cleft. Second, the biochemical machinery necessary to produce the substance must be localized within the same neuron. Third, the substance must be released from the neuron by physiological mechanisms. Fourth, synthetic forms of the molecule must evoke the same response as does the endogenous candidate when applied directly to the receptive neurons. Fifth, specific receptors linked to a physiological response must be present on the cells in communication with the neuron containing the neurotransmitter candidate. Sixth, mechanisms must be present to end the effect of the secreted putative neurotransmitter. (These mechanisms usually involve degradation of the neurotransmitter in the synaptic cleft by specific degradative enzymes or reuptake by the presynaptic neuron.) Seventh, and finally, it must be possible to block the action of the neurotransmitter substance by pharmacological agents that prevent binding to or activation of the receptor for the neurotransmitter.

In the review that follows I focus on the neurotransmitters that have fulfilled all or almost all of these criteria. To allow adequate discussion of these neurotransmitters in the allotted space, however, it is necessary to omit from consideration many other interesting substances that have thus far been shown to meet only one or more of these criteria but that may eventually achieve the status of true neurotransmitters. For a more comprehensive review of the various neurotransmitters and their associated biochemistry, I encourage readers to refer to the excellent sixth edition of *Biochemical Basis of Neuropharmacology* (Cooper et al. 1991).

Acetylcholine

Acetylcholine (ACh) was the first biochemical recognized as a neurotransmitter substance. It produces initiation of skeletal muscle contraction and mediates parasympathetic effects and preganglionic autonomic neurotransmission in the peripheral nervous system. It is a simple molecule, constructed by joining an acetyl group from the donor molecule, acetylcoenzyme A (acetyl-CoA), with a molecule of choline derived from a variety of metabolic sources. The enzyme that couples these two molecules into one molecule of acetylcholine is termed choline acetyltransferase (CAT), and its presence in neurons indicates that the neuron uses ACh as a neurotransmitter. The rate of acetylcholine synthesis is directly coupled to the firing rate of the cholinergic neuron. However, it is not the rate of CAT activity that controls the amount of ACh synthesis when demand increases. Rather, it is the rate at which choline can be transported across the neuronal cell membrane from its extraneuronal pool that mediates availability of choline to CAT for synthesis. This transport process is performed by the high-affinity choline transporter that resides in the cell membrane of cholinergic neurons. The high-affinity characterization is to distinguish this mechanism from the alternative low-affinity choline transport mechanism that virtually all cells have to maintain membrane integrity through synthesis of choline-containing phospholipids. The high-affinity transporter molecule has not yet been cloned (Knipper et al. 1991), but it requires energy from neuronal metabolism to function. Because this activity quickly degrades at death, few studies of the high-affinity transporter in humans have been attempted. Research using laboratory animals has demonstrated that at death, the concentration of choline in brain tissue increases severalfold. This is thought to be due to the rapid hydrolysis of ACh by its degradative enzyme, acetylcholinesterase (AChE). One molecule of AChE can hydrolyze 5,000 molecules of ACh per second, and blockade of AChE is the mechanism of action of many insecticides and of nerve gases developed for use in war. This enzyme is found on the surface of cell membranes and in soluble form in the extracellular fluid, but is not confined to cholinergic cells. Because it is present in large quantities in tissues such as the electric organ of freshwater electric eels, it was purified to homogeneity earlier than any other enzyme related to chemical neurotransmission in the brain; this allowed immunohistochemical mapping of its distribution in the brain relatively early in the history of this research. More recent work using the specific cholinergic marker CAT has confirmed that much of the previous AChE mapping evidence does truly delineate the major CNS cholinergic pathways. Many brain regions, such as the striatum, contain short interneurons that use ACh as a neurotransmitter; however, the long projection neurons that contain ACh are found in only a few discrete regions: the dorsal tegmental nuclei of the midbrain, where both descending projections to the brain stem and ascending projections to the limbic forebrain arise, and the magnocellular neurons of the septum and diagonal band/nucleus basalis region. The septal neurons give rise to cholinergic projections to the hippocampus, and the basal nucleus projects topographically to the entire cortex. (See Figure 5–2.)

It is the cholinergic neurons in this latter region that have been shown to be one of the major targets of degeneration in Alzheimer's disease; the dementia associated with Alzheimer's disease has been postulated to result from the decreased synaptic availability of ACh in these cortical projections from the nucleus basalis. The nucleus basalis ACh neurons are often found to contain the neuropeptide galanin (GAL), and the GAL terminals that innervate the ACh neurons in this region become hypertrophied in persons with Alzheimer's disease. In an attempt to achieve a therapeutic effect in these patients similar to that which has been successful in patients with Parkinson's disease, some investigators have tried using precursor enrichment in the form of dietary choline. Disappointingly few practical benefits have been derived in terms of decreasing the dementia already present or in slowing its inexorable progress. Recently, a drug that blocks AChE, tacrine hydrochloride (tetrahydroaminoacridine, or THA), has been approved by the U.S. Food

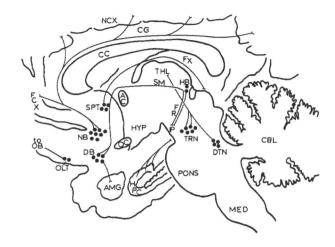

Figure 5–2. Cholinergic systems. Parasagittal view of a schematized primate brain showing the distribution of cholinergic cell bodies (*solid circles*) and their projections. Note that although some of these systems have also been confirmed in the human brain, most of our current knowledge of cholinergic systems stems from studies in the rodent brain. AC = anterior commisure; AMG = amygdala; CBL = cerebellum; CC = corpus callosum; CG = cingulate gyrus; DB = diagonal band; DTN = dorsal tegmental nucleus; FCX = frontal cortex; FR = fimbria; FX = fornix; HB = habenula; HPC = hippocampus; HYP = hypothalamus; MED = medulla; NB = nucleus basalis; NCX = neocortex; OB = olfactory bulb; OLT = olfactory tubercle; P = pineal; PONS = pons; SM = stria terminalis; SPT = septum; THL = thalamus; TRN = thalamic red nucleus.
Source. Reproduced with permission from Watson SJ, Khachaturian H, Lewis ME, et al: "Chemical Neuroanatomy as a Basis for Biological Psychiatry," in *American Handbook of Psychiatry.* Edited by Berger PA, Brodie HKH. New York, Basic Books, 1986, p. 17.

and Drug Administration for use in treating patients with Alzheimer's disease. However, not all patients respond, and those who do have not experienced the relief of symptoms that would be expected of a truly effective therapy (Lamy 1994).

Recent research at the Joseph and Kathleen Bryan Alzheimer Disease Research Center at Duke University Medical Center has been directed at understanding why such therapies have been so limited in benefit, as these strategies are conceivably addressing the reduced synaptic availability of ACh in Alzheimer's disease. Using a rapid autopsy protocol that enables access to postmortem tissue within 2 hours of death, this group of researchers were able to measure the activity and amount of high-affinity choline uptake (HACU) transporter while it remained biochemically viable. The amount of HACU transporter is regulated by its synthesis relative to its degradation, although its activity is believed to be regulated by the firing rate of the neuron that uses it. Large increases (100%) in the activity and the number of HACU transporter sites were observed in cortical tissue from patients with Alzheimer's disease compared with control subjects without dementia and those with dementia from a cause other than Alzheimer's disease (Slotkin et al. 1990, 1994). Thus, in individuals with Alzheimer's disease compared with control subjects, the mechanism for delivery of choline to the surviving cholinergic neurons appears to be upregulated, and the precursor replacement therapy should effectively raise intraneuronal choline levels. Whether this large increase in HACU activity is related to increased neuronal firing rates or represents a pathological increase remains unknown; however, it seems that attempts to increase the synthesis of ACh in patients with this disease are unlikely to succeed in the face of this already maximally accelerated uptake.

The flexibility of the choline moiety in the ACh molecule allows this neurotransmitter to interact at very different binding sites; this is represented physiologically by the presence of two general classes of receptors for ACh: nicotinic and muscarinic receptors. Named for the respective pharmacological agents that specifically stimulate these receptors, these two classes represent both ligand-gated, ionic channel (nicotinic) type I receptors and second-messenger–linked membrane protein (muscarinic) type II receptors. Type I receptors usually have four membrane-spanning segments and mediate fast (millisecond) responses, whereas type II receptors have seven membrane-spanning domains and in most cases are linked to second messengers. The nicotinic receptors are present at the site of innervation of skeletal muscle, as well as in discrete regions of the CNS, including limbic areas thought to mediate emotion and reward. Muscarinic receptors are the predominant ACh receptors in the CNS and act either directly on ion channels for potassium, calcium, or chloride or through second messengers linked to the receptors by G proteins (phosphorylated guanine compounds used as an energy source). The effector systems activated by G proteins either can open or close channels or can stimulate or inhibit other components of the signal

transduction cascade (such as adenylate or guanylate cyclase, phospholipases, and phosphodiesterases). The tools of molecular biology have been used to identify four molecularly distinct forms of the nicotinic receptor and five forms of the muscarinic receptor. Previously, only a few of these receptor subtypes had been characterized pharmacologically, and thus the existence of different molecular phenotypes does not guarantee differences in ligand-binding affinity. It is a well-recognized neurobiological principle that, as endogenous ligand availability is altered over a long enough period of time, the corresponding receptor population will usually attempt to compensate for a reduced signal, often by increasing the number of receptors or—more rarely—by increasing the affinity for the ligand. Because some reports have indicated that certain of these subtypes of muscarinic M_2 ACh receptor populations may be decreased in patients with Alzheimer's disease, efforts are now under way to develop specific agonists for muscarinic and nicotinic receptor subtypes that can be administered peripherally. Although such goals are laudable, the excitement generated by their eventual achievement must be tempered with the realization that unless the cause of the degeneration can be identified and its progress halted, little more than temporary respite can be offered by such pharmacotherapies.

Specific alterations in various aspects of ACh neuronal systems in the aging brains of humans and laboratory animals have been recently reported. The concentration of CAT in the occipital, but not the cingulate, cortex of aged macaque monkeys was found to be decreased compared with that in younger control animals, as were the occipital concentrations of neuropeptide Y, somatostatin, serotonin, and norepinephrine (Beal et al. 1991). Other investigators have reported deficits in the number of cholinergic neurons and in ACh synthesis and release in aged humans, as well as deficits in muscarinic receptor numbers and plasticity in aged humans and laboratory animals (Muller et al. 1991). Release of ACh from brain tissue obtained at surgery from nondemented patients has been demonstrated to decline with the age of the patient (Feuerstein et al. 1992), and brain slices from a strain of senescence-accelerated mice were found to have decreased ACh release compared with controls from a strain of normally aging mice (Zhao et al. 1992). Meyer and colleagues (1994) have reported deficits in the release of ACh from aged (24-month-old) rat brains as compared with tissue from 2-month-old controls, a finding that is similar to deficits seen after membrane peroxidation damage. Decreases in both nicotinic (Schroder et al. 1991) and muscarinic M_2 (Nordberg et al. 1992) receptors in the cortex of patients with Alzheimer's disease have been reported, whereas M_2 ACh receptors in the thalamus were increased (Nordberg et al. 1992). The decrease in muscarinic ACh receptors in aged rat brains is not accompanied by reductions in muscarinic ACh-receptor messenger ribonucleic acid (mRNA), and therefore receptor synthesis is not the target mechanism for these age-related changes (Blake et al. 1991). In another study involving aged rat brains versus brains from younger controls, investigators noted a doubling of muscarinic ACh receptors on astrocytes along with a decrease in neuronal ACh receptors (Van Der Zee et al. 1993). These reports demonstrate that overall cholinergic function declines during normal aging and that its regulation is severely adversely affected at all levels in brain regions affected in Alzheimer's disease. However, the assumption that all or most of the age-related changes in learning and memory are due to cholinergic deficiency should not be made without consideration of the many other neurotransmitter systems that are altered in aging (see Decker and McGaugh 1991 and Palmer and De-Kosky 1993 for review).

Gamma-Aminobutyric Acid

The amino acids are part of the general metabolic pool, and this fact has hindered recognition of their role in synaptic transmission. It also poses problems in attempts to separate the metabolic components from the neurotransmitter component in assays using cellular homogenates. The amino acids are also components of larger neurotransmitter molecules, the neuropeptides and endocrine hormones, the cleavage of which also ultimately produces free amino acids. Several amino acids are now known to fulfill most of the criteria for neurotransmitter molecules, and they can be classified as producing predominantly excitatory or inhibitory effects on their postsynaptic target neurons.

The principal inhibitory neurotransmitter in mammalian brains is the amino acid GABA. Found almost exclusively in the CNS, GABA is produced

through the decarboxylation of glutamic acid by the enzyme glutamic acid decarboxylase (GAD), which is the rate-limiting step in GABA formation. The GABA signal is terminated by transamination to yield glutamate and succinic semialdehyde. The enzyme responsible for this step is GABA-transaminase, which is usually found in association with succinic semialdehyde dehydrogenase, the enzyme that metabolizes the by-product of GABA transamination. These degradative enzymes are found in many tissues, but GABA and GAD are almost exclusively confined to the CNS. A reuptake mechanism to retrieve synaptic GABA for reuse by the presynaptic neuron is mediated by the GABA-transporter protein, which requires sodium for activity (Lam et al. 1993). Relatively high (micromolar) concentrations of GABA are found in certain areas of the brain, such as the hypothalamus and striatum. Neurons containing GAD are usually local circuit interneurons, but some projection neurons—such as the globus pallidus to substantia nigra projection—also use this inhibitory neurotransmitter (see Figure 5–3). Other neurotransmitters colocalized within certain GABA-ergic neurons are ACh, serotonin, dopamine, glycine, histamine, neuropeptide Y, vasoactive intestinal peptide, substance P, and somatostatin. The inhibitory effect of GABA is mediated by two distinct receptor subtypes: GABA-A and GABA-B. GABA-A receptors produce inhibition by hyperpolarization of the postsynaptic neuron through an increase in the permeability of chloride ion channels, whereas GABA-B receptors are linked to second messengers and act by decreasing calcium or increasing potassium ion channel conductance. Similar to the nicotinic ACh receptors, GABA-A receptors are composed of five subunits, whereas GABA-B receptors more closely resemble the muscarinic ACh receptor with its second-messenger linkage. The benzodiazepine anxiolytic drugs, the barbiturates, and ethanol all interact with the GABA-A receptor, and this interaction is the physiological basis for the pharmacological ability of these substances to potentiate each other's effects when they are administered concomitantly. Many anticonvulsant drugs act by stimulating GABA receptors, and blockade of GABA or glycine receptors initiates convulsions.

Age-related changes in GABA neuronal systems have been reported in laboratory animals and in human brain tissue. Changes in GABA content and rate

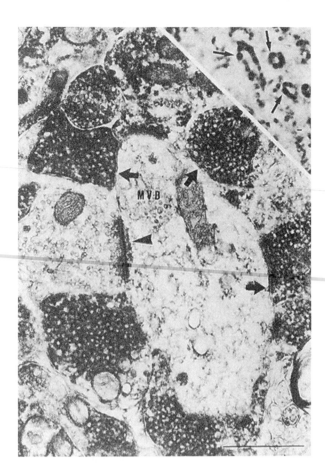

Figure 5–3. Terminals containing glutamic acid decarboxylase (GAD) in the substantia nigra from specimens incubated in anti-GAD serum. *Insert:* Semithin (1 μm) section of the pars reticulata with obliquely and transversely sectioned dendrites that are encircled by punctate structures containing GAD-positive reaction product (→). Scale bar = 1 μm. The accompanying electron micrograph shows an obliquely sectioned dendrite in the substantia nigra, surrounded by many axon terminals filled with GAD-positive reaction product that are equivalent to the puncta seen in the insert. Some of the terminals form symmetrical synapses (←), whereas the unstained terminal contains round synaptic vesicles and forms an asymmetrical synapse (➤) with this dendritic shaft, multivesicular body (MVB). Scale bar = 1 μm. *Source.* Reproduced with permission from Ribak CE, Vaughn JE, Saito K, et al: "Immunocytochemical Localization of Glutamate Decarboxylase in Rat Substantia Nigra." *Brain Res* 116:288, 1977.

of synthesis seem to show regional and strain specificity. Some researchers who have studied aged (24-month-old) Wistar rats have described no change in GABA content in the striatum or cerebral cortex, with decreased rates of GABA synthesis in the cortex but not the striatum (Carfagna and Moretti 1990).

Others have reported striatal elevations of GABA in aged (20-month-old) Fischer 344 rats (Donzanti and Ung 1990). The number and density of GABA neurons in the amygdala (Lolova and Davidoff 1991) and cerebellar (Lolova and Davidoff 1990) regions of aged (26-month-old) Wistar rats were reported to be decreased compared with the number and density of such neurons in 3-month-old rats. The GABA-A receptors in the hippocampus of aged (24-month-old) Wistar rats have been reported to be present in normal numbers and to demonstrate normal pharmacological functions (Ruano et al. 1993), whereas aged (24-month-old) Fischer 344 rats have been shown to have decreased binding of pharmacological agents selective for the GABA-A receptor in cerebral cortex and cerebellum, which was apparently associated with a 70% decrease in mRNA for the GABA-A receptor in the cortex but not in the cerebellum (Mhatre and Ticku 1992). Recent surveys of inhibitory amino acid concentrations in 52 discrete regions of aged human brain tissue have emphasized the heterogeneity of regional changes, and investigators found fewer changes than have been reported for aged rats (Banay-Schwartz et al. 1993). The picture emerging from this research indicates that although it is clear that GABA systems are altered during the aging process, great care must be taken in extrapolating results from one or two brain regions or one species to other areas and species.

Dopamine

Dopamine (DA) is one of three catecholamine neurotransmitters, the others being norepinephrine (NE) and epinephrine (EPI). The catecholamines share a similar molecular structure based on the amino acid tyrosine, with additions or deletions of certain biochemical side groups that distinguish one from the others. DA is formed by the decarboxylation of a previously hydroxylated tyrosine moiety under the control of the enzymes tyrosine hydroxylase and dopa decarboxylase. Upon release into the synapse, DA is recaptured by a specific DA transporter protein (see Hitri et al. 1994 for review) in the presynaptic membrane; unbound DA is metabolized by the enzymes monoamine oxidase (MAO) and catechol-*O*-methyl transferase (COMT) to the metabolic products homovanillic acid (HVA) and dihydroxyphenylacetic acid (DOPAC). In contrast to

ACh synthesis, DA synthesis is rate limiting at the tyrosine hydroxylase step, and the activity of this enzyme is stimulus regulated. DA is heterogeneously distributed in the CNS, with most of the neurotransmitter found in projection neurons of the hypothalamus and midbrain. The DA neurons of the substantia nigra and the ventral tegmental areas of the midbrain project topographically to the striatum and limbic forebrain regions, where they appear to mediate voluntary movement and emotional aspects of pleasure and reward, respectively. DA-containing neurons have been observed to include other neurotransmitters, such as the neuropeptides met-enkephalin, cholecystokinin, and neurotensin (Figure 5–4).

DA receptors are pharmacologically divided into two classes, the D_1 and D_2 receptor subtypes; molecular techniques have also permitted identification of D_3, D_4, and D_5 forms of the D_1 and D_2 basic classes, as well as the existence of a long and a short form of the D_2 receptor. The D_1 receptor is predominately postsynaptic and usually is found to stimulate adenylate cyclase activity and phosphoinositide turnover. The D_2 receptor is found at both postsynaptic sites and on the axons, dendrites, and soma of presynaptic, DA-producing neurons (autoreceptors). The D_2 receptor usually is found to inhibit

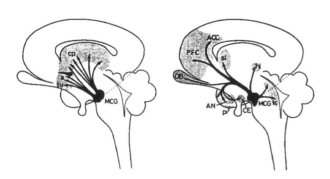

Figure 5–4. Dopamine neurons and their pathways in the human brain. a = nucleus accumbens; ACC = anterior cingulate cortex; AN = amygdaloid nuclei; CE = entorrhinal cortex; cp = nucleus caudatus-putamen; hl = lateral habenular nucleus; lc = locus coeruleus; MCG = mesencephalic dopamine cell groups; OB = olfactory bulb; PFC = prefrontal cortex; pi = piriform cortex; sl = lateral septal nucleus; tu = olfactory tubercle. *Source.* Reproduced with permission from Lindvall O, Bjorklund A: "Neuroanatomical Localization of Dopamine in the Brain and Spinal Cord," in *Handbook of Schizophrenia,* Vol 2. Edited by Henn FA, DeLisi LE. Amsterdam, Elsevier, 1987, p. 63.

adenylate cyclase activity, but it can also exert effects through inhibition of calcium channel passage and potassium conductance, as well as through phosphoinositide turnover changes. Autoreceptors can exert effects on DA release, synthesis, and storage through distinct mechanisms, allowing highly integrated regulation of DA synaptic availability. Drugs that alter DA synaptic availability either can exert effects directly at the receptor or can alter reuptake, synthesis, or degradation. The stimulant drugs cocaine, amphetamine, and methylphenidate inhibit reuptake of DA in the synaptic cleft by the DA transporter, whereas the classical antipsychotic drugs block D_2 dopamine receptors by binding to the DA recognition site. In patients with Parkinson's disease, the degeneration of the DA neurons of the substantia nigra produces tremor and bradykinesia, and these symptoms are temporarily reversed by precursor enrichment in the form of L-dopa administration. The remaining DA neurons increase their rate of DA synthesis to compensate for the reduced synaptic availability at the terminal sites of innervation, and increased amounts of precursor aid this process. However, as the remaining DA neurons degenerate, the synthetic acceleration of these neurons eventually fails to compensate for the reduced synaptic availability, and treatment becomes ineffective. In patients with schizophrenia, the blockade of D_2 dopamine receptors by antipsychotic drugs provides significant relief from the intrusive thoughts and auditory hallucinations that often accompany this disease. The long-term use of these drugs presents the risk of eventual development of tardive dyskinesia and its associated movement disorder. Thus, although these DA system–directed treatments are undeniably effective in treating certain symptoms in patients with these diseases, they do not cure the disease, they are associated with significant limitations, and the risk of side effects complicates their chronic use.

Research involving possible dopaminergic effects on age-related changes has focused on various parts of the brain, but changes have been found mainly in the striatum. Several research teams have observed decreases in DA receptors in the striatum of aging human patients through the use of imaging techniques and D_2 dopamine receptor ligands that cross the blood-brain barrier (Antonini et al. 1993; Iyo and Yamasaki 1993; Rinne et al. 1993), whereas postmortem tissue studies in normal human brain tissue have shown an age-related decrease in DA content relative to HVA metabolite concentrations in this region (Kish et al. 1992). A precipitous decline in the content of the DA transporter protein mRNA in the substantia nigra of human brain tissue was observed in postmortem samples from subjects over the age of 57 years (Bannon et al. 1992). Studies of aged laboratory animals have confirmed and extended these findings of DA pathology in aging humans; reports have been published describing decreased striatal D_2 receptors, DA content, and tyrosine hydroxylase activity in aged (24-month-old) rats (Fernandez-Ruiz et al. 1992) and decreased DA release from the striatum measured in vivo in aged (24- and 30-month-old) Fischer 344 rats (Friedemann and Gerhardt 1992). In contrast, hippocampal DA content and turnover, as well as tyrosine hydroxylase activity, were shown to be unchanged in aged (26-month-old) rats (Venero et al. 1993). Several groups have reported age-related decreases in D_2 receptor mRNA in the striatum of aged (24-month-old) rats compared with younger control animals (Mesco et al. 1991; Merchant et al. 1993), but another team did not find such changes in D_2 receptor mRNA in 18-month-old rats (Sakata et al. 1992). In contrast to the findings reported from work with human brain tissue, DA transporter density has not been shown to decrease with age in Fischer 344 rats up to 24 months of age (Inglefield and Richfield 1992); however, this rat strain does show reduced DA-induced stimulation of all the inositol phosphate isoforms in the striatum, hippocampus, and cerebral cortex of aged rats compared with younger controls (Undie and Friedman 1992). Thus, strain and species differences are apparent in the research literature on DA and aging , although there is generally agreement as to striatal DA-mechanism pathology in aging.

Serotonin

Serotonin, or 5-hydroxytryptamine (5-HT), is an indolamine that is produced by enzymatic alteration of the amino acid tryptophan; it was named for its potent effects on the smooth muscle of blood vessels. Because only a small percentage of the total 5-HT in the body is contained in the CNS, the neurotransmitter status of this molecule was not established until many years after its discovery. The rate-limiting step in the synthesis of 5-HT is the hydroxylation of neuronally available tryptophan by tryptophan hydroxylase, which is subsequently decarboxylated by 5-hydroxytryptophan decarboxylase to yield the functional neurotransmitter molecule. MAO removes an amino group, and further oxidation yields the principal 5-HT metabolite 5-hydroxyindoleacetic acid (5-HIAA).

Serotonin in the synaptic cleft can be recaptured by the presynaptic neuron via the specific 5-HT transporter protein. This transporter protein, cloned relatively recently (Blakely and Berson 1991), is the target of a wide variety of drugs that are useful in reducing the symptoms of major depressive disorder, although this therapeutic result is achieved only after 2–3 weeks of treatment; a similar response can also be elicited, over the same time frame, by drugs that block the NE transporter. Three classes of 5-HT receptors in the CNS have been characterized pharmacologically: $5-HT_1$, $5-HT_2$, and $5-HT_3$. Use of molecular techniques has also allowed identification of subtypes of some of these receptors. The category of $5-HT_1$ receptors now includes $5-HT_{1A}$, $5-HT_{1B}$, $5-HT_{1C}$, and $5-HT_{1D}$ subtypes; the $5-HT_2$ receptors include $5-HT_{2A}$ and $5-HT_{2B}$ subtypes. At last count, 13 molecular subtypes of 5-HT receptors had been identified (Teitler and Herrick-Davis 1994). These subtypes all appear to be linked to second messengers via G proteins, yet the actual second messenger and the effect—stimulatory or inhibitory—of the receptor on these second messengers can be quite different for the various subtypes of 5-HT receptors. The similarity in the shape of the 5-HT molecule and the chemical shape of various psychoactive drugs has promulgated much research into the mechanisms of the effects of these compounds. The hallucinogenic drugs lysergic acid diethylamide (LSD), mescaline, and psilocin all have profound effects on the activity of 5-HT–containing neuronal systems. Whether these effects are due to an agonist or antagonist effect at various 5-HT receptor sites is an issue that has not yet been resolved; however, the current data indicate that a decrease in median raphe 5-HT neuronal firing rates correlates with the effects of these drugs. The distribution of 5-HT neurons in the CNS resembles that of the catecholamines, with the major concentrations of neuronal cell bodies in the midbrain dorsal raphe nucleus and smaller cell groups in the median raphe of the brain stem. The projections from the dorsal raphe course through the median forebrain bundle in the lateral hypothalamus to innervate the entire cortex and limbic systems, and may mediate certain emotional states (see Figure 5–5).

Aging-related changes in 5-HT neuronal systems have been reported in both human and laboratory animal subjects, including the decreased numbers of 5-HT$_2$ receptors with increasing age shown in postmortem samples of human frontal cortex (Arranz et al. 1993) and as visualized by positron-emission tomography in living patients (Iyo and Yamasaki 1993). Nonhuman primates were reported to have decreased concentrations of 5-HT and several other neurotransmitter candidates in occipital cortex, but not cingulate cortex, when rhesus macaques aged 30 or more years were compared with 4- to 6-year-old animals (Beal et al. 1991). Hip-

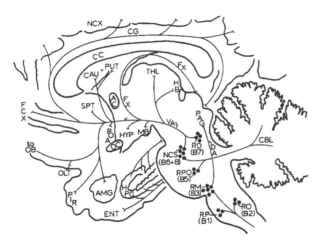

Figure 5–5. Serotonergic systems. This schematic parasagittal view of a primate brain depicts the serotonin cell groups *(solid circles)* and their major projections. These groups were designated B$_1$ through B$_9$ by Dahlstrom and Fuxe (1964). AC = anterior commisure; AMG = amygdala; CAU = caudate nucleus; CBL = cerebellum; CC = corpus callosum; CG = cingulate gyrus; DA = dorsal ascending pathway; ENT = entorrhinal cortex; FCX = frontal cortex; FX = fornix; HB = habenula; HPC = hippocampus; HYP = hypothalamus; MB = mammillary bodies; NCS = nucleus centralis superior; NCX = neocortex; OB = olfactory bulb; OC = optic chiasm; OLT = olfactory tubercle; PAG = periaqueductal gray; PIR = piriform cortex; POA = preoptic anterior hypothalamus; PUT = putamen; RD = raphe dorsalis; RM = raphe magnus; RO = raphe obscurus; RP = raphe pallidus; RPO = raphe pontis; SPT = septum; THL = thalamus; VA = ventral ascending pathway.
Source. Reproduced with permission from Nieuwenhuys R, Voogd J, van Huijzen C: *The Human Central Nervous System.* New York, Springer-Verlag, 1981, p. 230.

pocampal 5-HT synthesis and turnover are reported to be increased with age in rats; this is in contrast to the lack of demonstrated age-related changes in catecholamine turnover and tyrosine hydroxylase activity (Venero et al. 1993), although a decreased number of 5-HT–containing neuronal fiber networks and an increase in swollen and folded 5-HT fibers were observed in several subcortical forebrain and hypothalamic nuclei of 28-month-old rats compared with 3-month-old control rats (Davidoff and Lolova 1991). Reduced numbers of 5-HT neurons in the dorsal raphe nucleus of aged rats were also reported (Lolova and Davidoff 1992). Concentrations of 5-HT were reduced and 5-HT turnover was apparently increased in aged rats relative to younger controls, whereas 5-HT$_{1B}$ and 5-HT$_2$ receptors were decreased in density in the hypothalamus, striatum, hippocampus, and cerebral cortex (Gozlan et al. 1990). Increased concentrations of the 5-HT metabolite kynurenine have been observed in cerebrospinal fluid (CSF) in 28- to 32-month-old Wistar rats compared with 4- to 6-month-old controls (Wada et al. 1994). Release of 5-HT by the specific 5-HT reuptake inhibitor and releasing agent fenfluramine is reported to be less effective in inducing increased exploratory activity in old (22-month-old) Fischer 344 rats compared with 4-month-old controls (Handa et al. 1993). This concatenation of results suggest that specific 5-HT neuronal systems are affected by aging, but the regions involved are often affected to different extents and possibly by different mechanisms.

Norepinephrine

The catecholamine NE was first shown to be a neurotransmitter in the peripheral nervous system and was later demonstrated to be a component of the CNS. The development of staining techniques for visualization of the catecholamines in tissue sections greatly facilitated research into NE's neurotransmitter role in both the CNS and the peripheral nervous system. As the neurotransmitter of postganglionic sympathetic peripheral nerves, NE's effects on a variety of organ systems are well known, although its role in the CNS is not as well delineated. Like DA, NE is synthesized by sequential modifications of a tyrosine amino acid substrate. DA is further hydroxylated by dopamine-β-hydroxylase to yield NE after modifications of tyrosine induced by tyrosine hydroxylase and dopa decarboxylase. After release into the synapse, NE is metabolized by MAO and COMT to form the major degradative product 3-methoxy-4-hydroxyphenylglycol (MHPG). Similar to what happens with 5-HT and DA, released NE is also recaptured by the presynaptic neuron via a NE transporter protein. This protein has now been cloned, and its sequence has been found to be highly homologous with that of the GABA transporter protein (Melikian et al. 1994). (Refer to Figure 5–6.)

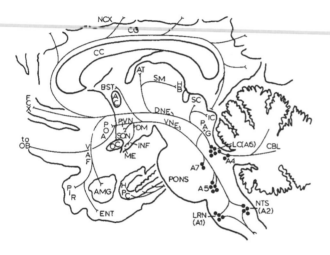

Figure 5–6. Noradrenergic systems. This schematized parasagittal view of a primate brain shows the location of major norepinephrine-producing cell bodies *(solid circles)* and their major projections. These cell groups were designated A$_1$ through A$_7$ by Dahlstrom and Fuxe (1964). AC = anterior commisure; AMG = amygdala; AT = anterior thalamus; BST = bed nucleus of the stria terminalis; CBL = cerebellum; CC = corpus callosum; CG = cingulate gyrus; DB = diagonal band; DM = dorsomedial hypothalamus; DNE = dorsal noradrenergic efferents; ENT = entorrhinal cortex; FCX = frontal cortex; HB = habenula; HPC = hippocampus; IC = inferior colliculus; INF = infindibulum; LC = locus coeruleus; LRN = lateral reticular nucleus; ME = median eminence; NCX = neocortex; NTS = nucleus tractus solitarius; OB = olfactory bulb; OC = optic chiasm; PAG = periaqueductal gray; PIR = piriform cortex; POA = preoptic anterior hypothalamus; PONS = pons; PVN = paraventricular nucleus of the hypothalamus; SC = superior colliculus; SM = stria medullaris; SCN = suprachiasmatic nucleus; VAF = ventral ascending fibers; VNE = ventral noradrenergic efferents.
Source. Reproduced with permission from Nieuwenhuys R, Voogd J, van Huijzen C: *The Human Central Nervous System.* New York, Springer-Verlag, 1981, p. 228.

Blockade of the NE transporter protein for 2–3 weeks by specific NE uptake inhibitor drugs results in amelioration of depressive symptoms in patients with major depressive disorder. However, because this therapeutic effect is also elicited by specific 5-HT transporter inhibitors, it is probably mediated by some adaptive regulatory response to the sequelae of transporter inhibition rather than by the inhibition itself. The receptor subtypes that mediate the actions of NE at the postsynaptic site were originally divided into two classes—alpha and beta adrenoreceptors—based on location and pharmacology, with further subdivision into alpha 1 and 2 and beta 1 and 2. Use of molecular techniques has permitted expansion of this classification to seven specific subtypes to accommodate the very different effects on second-messenger systems mediated by these G protein–linked, seven-membrane domain receptors. The NE neurons in the CNS reside predominantly in two distinct midbrain regions: the locus coeruleus and the dorsal tegmental nucleus. The locus coeruleus provides the major NE projection to the forebrain and the hypothalamus, where NE mediates a variety of behavioral and endocrine effects associated with responses to physiological challenges; this region often shows degeneration of NE-containing neurons in patients with Alzheimer's disease. The neuropeptides GAL and neuropeptide Y have been identified within NE neurons, but the significance of this colocalization is not yet known. An intimate relationship between the NE and the corticotropin-releasing factor (CRF) neuronal systems exists; CRF is released from nerve terminals in the locus coeruleus to elicit increases in NE neuronal firing rates in the locus coeruleus. Through NE projections to the hypothalamus, this noradrenergic activity in the locus coeruleus subsequently induces CRF mRNA production in the paraventricular nucleus of the hypothalamus, where CRF is available for transport to the median eminence and eventual release to the pituitary. Thus, the neurotransmitter that plays such an essential role in the sympathetic nervous system's response to stress is apparently well placed to mediate the CNS responses to stressful stimuli in addition. Anxiolytic drugs, such as the benzodiazepines, reduce the firing rate of NE locus coeruleus neurons, a fact that further strengthens the hypothesis that this circuit mediates arousal states in mammals.

Evidence for NE alterations in aged humans and laboratory animals generally supports the view that humans do not exhibit beta-adrenergic receptor changes in the brain with age, whereas most brain regions of aged rats do show decreased numbers of the NE receptors (see Scarpace et al. 1991 for review). In rats, this finding may be due to increased concentrations of NE in the cerebral cortex of aged versus younger animals (Godefroy et al. 1991), although decreased NE concentrations in the hypothalamus and midbrain nuclei have also been reported (Ida et al. 1982). The ability of $alpha_1$ NE receptor agonists to stimulate phosphoinositide second-messenger hydrolysis was shown to be decreased in the thalamus and cerebral cortex of aged (28-month-old) Fischer 344 rats relative to younger controls (Burnett et al. 1990), although Harik and co-workers (1991) reported no decrease in the numbers of these receptors in aged rats of this strain, and the ability of stress to decrease frontal cortex concentrations of NE also was shown to be attenuated in aged (22-month-old) rats of this strain relative to 7-month-old controls (Lorens et al. 1990). These findings indicate that NE systems do exhibit age-related changes, but the distribution and complexity of these changes are not as great as those reported for some of the other classical neurotransmitters.

Glutamic Acid

Glutamic acid (GLU), or glutamate, is the prototypical excitatory amino acid neurotransmitter, although the evidence for its role in vertebrate neurotransmission has accumulated relatively slowly as a result of the many roles that glutamate plays in cellular metabolism. Because glutamate is both the precursor for GABA and a transmitter itself, its presence in nerve endings cannot reveal whether GLU is being used as a transmitter, and the additional presence of the glutamate transporter protein (Kanner et al. 1993; Kawakami et al. 1994) does not disclose how a neuron is using GLU. The additional problem of lack of regional specificity in neuronal excitation after application of the excitatory amino acids has been interpreted as being attributable to the fact that almost all neurons have receptors for the excitatory amino acids. The ability of these excitatory amino acid transmitters (including aspartate) to excite virtually all neurons to which they are applied has been

exploited through the use of excitotoxic analogs of GLU: kainic acid, quisqualic acid, and ibotenic acid. These agents apparently stimulate the neurons to which they are applied until those neurons die of exhaustion, thus allowing the formation of a relatively discrete, localized lesion of cell bodies without an interruption of neighboring axons or adjacent terminals.

The best evidence for a neurotransmitter role of GLU is derived from the various receptor subtypes that recognize this agent. Originally classified on the basis of whether the receptor would or would not bind the N-methyl-D-aspartate (NMDA) analog, these GLU receptors have now been divided into five distinct groups. The NMDA receptor recognizes aspartate as well as GLU and contains at least four other functional subcomponents, making it similar to the benzodiazepine/GABA receptor complex. The NMDA receptor forms a membrane channel that is permeable to sodium and calcium ions when opened and that contains a modulatory site that recognizes glycine. The hallucinogenic drug phencyclidine (PCP, or "angel dust") and the investigative drug MK801 bind to the NMDA receptor complex and prevent ion passage through the channel. The kainate GLU receptor subtype (which preferentially binds kainic acid) and the quisqualate-preferring AMPA-receptor subtype (which is named for its ability to specifically bind 3-hydroxy-5-methyl-ioxyazole-4-propionic acid, or AMPA) are both ligand-gated ion channels that pass sodium and potassium ions when open. The fourth GLU receptor subtype is also an ion channel receptor and is named AP-4, after its specificity for the compound 1-2-amino-4-phosphonobutyrate. The fifth GLU receptor subtype, the metabotropic, or APCD, receptor (named for its specificity in binding trans-1-aminocyclopentane-1-3-dicarboxylic acid), is linked to the IP3/DAG second-messenger signal transduction pathway, and thus represents a membrane receptor more like the muscarinic ACh receptor than the nicotinic (channel) receptor. The neurons containing these various GLU receptor subtypes are distributed among several brain regions and are particularly enriched in the hippocampus, where they form long projection neurons among the different hippocampal subfields. The pathological involvement of GLU neurons in the devastating sequelae of cerebral infarction (stroke) and in epileptic foci, as well as in learning and memory disorders—and the potential for specific manipulation of the various receptor subtypes—makes this ubiquitous neurotransmitter system an attractive target for a wide variety of pharmacological agents.

Both human and laboratory animal data detailing alterations in GLU-containing neuronal systems in aging processes have been reported. Binding of the NMDA receptor antagonist MK801 in postmortem human frontal cortex has been shown to decline with age due to decreased numbers of these GLU receptor subtypes (Piggot et al. 1992); however, no such changes with age were seen on examination of tissue from the hippocampus or entorrhinal cortex (Court et al. 1993). Concentrations of GLU in human putamen specimens did not change with age (Kornhuber et al. 1993); however, elevations in the GLU concentration of the anterior striatum of aged (20-month-old) Fischer 344 rats compared with 6-month-old controls was reported (Najlerahim et al. 1990), as were age-related elevations in lateral striatum GLU concentrations of this particular rat strain (Donzanti et al. 1993). In several studies, investigators have demonstrated age-related changes in rodent GLU receptor subtypes, including a finding of a 30% decrease in telencephalic AMPA binding by both radioligand binding and immunoreactivity measures in 24-month-old mice compared with 3-month-old control animals (Bahr et al. 1992) and a 35% decrease in NMDA receptor density in the forebrains of 20-month-old mice compared with 3-month-old controls (Cohen and Muller 1992). Two different strains of aged (30-month-old) mice have been shown to have decreased binding of NMDA, kainate, and AMPA receptor subtypes in the parietal cortex and hippocampus compared with 3-month-old controls (Magnusson and Cotman 1993). A senescence-accelerated strain of mice exhibited higher GLU concentrations in the hippocampus and cerebral cortex than did a normally aging strain; when the strains were compared at 3 and 14 months of age, the researchers found decreased NMDA receptor binding in the cerebral cortex of the old mice in the age-accelerated strain (Kitamura et al. 1992). The NMDA receptors that bound radiolabeled GLU in the hippocampus and cerebral cortex exhibited decreased densities in aged (29-month-old) rats relative to 3- or 7-month-old rats when MK801 was used as the displacing ligand (Tamaru et al. 1991), but showed decreases in NMDA receptors in the caudate/putamen and nucleus accumbens septi—not

the cerebral cortex—of aged rats when 3-((+)-2-carboxypiperazin-4-yl)propyl-l-phosphonic acid was used as the radiolabeled ligand (Miyoshi et al. 1991). The electrically stimulated release of GLU from the medial prefrontal cortex in aged (27- to 30-month-old) rats was attenuated compared with that in younger (3- to 4-month-old) rats (Cobo et al. 1993), although GLU concentrations were reported to be unchanged in this and three other cortical regions in aged (24- to 26-month-old) rats relative to 3- to 4-month-old controls (Cobo et al. 1992). There is little doubt that GLU systems are altered in normal aging and in persons with Alzheimer's disease (Francis et al. 1993), as these human and animal data indicate. What remains to be seen is whether these changes result from primary alterations in other neurotransmitter systems or occur independently, and if GLU changes might contribute to the further loss of other neurotransmitters during the aging process.

Histamine

Because histamine is found in mast cells of the reticular activating system, and because it is difficult to separate the histamine component from the CNS tissue component, researchers experienced great difficulty in establishing the role of histamine in CNS neurotransmission. It is now confirmed that histamine is formed in specific neurons by decarboxylation from the amino acid histidine. Both dopa decarboxylase and a specific histidine decarboxylase can accomplish this step. Although histamine can be oxidized or methylated, the predominant inactivation step in the mammalian brain is methylation by histamine methyltransferase. Using antibodies to histidine decarboxylase, researchers have mapped the distribution of histamine-containing neurons and have identified two distinct cell groups. The major group is found in the mammillary body region of the posterior hypothalamus; the other group is found in the mesencephalic reticular formation. These two regions send projections to the cortex and limbic system through fiber bundles in the lateral hypothalamus (median forebrain bundle).

Three forms of histamine receptors can be distinguished pharmacologically: H_1, H_2, and H_3. The H_1 receptor seems to mediate excitatory effects of histamine, whereas H_2 is inhibitory and linked to adenylate cyclase as a second messenger. The H_3 receptor may be an autoreceptor for histamine presynaptic neurons, and their activation inhibits histamine synthesis and release. There have been surprisingly few reports of age-associated changes in histamine neuronal systems in either humans or laboratory animals.

Neuroactive Peptides (Neuropeptides)

Neuropeptides comprise one of the most recently discovered classes of neurotransmitter substances. They were originally purified to obtain just a few milligrams from hundreds of thousands of sheep and pig hypothalami, the section of the brain in which several neuropeptides that function as regulators of pituitary hormones are found in relatively large concentrations (see Bissette and Nemeroff [in press] for a review of peptide biology). Whereas the amino acid neurotransmitters such as GABA and GLU are found in micromolar concentrations in enriched brain regions, and the biogenic amines (DA, NE, 5-HT) and ACh are found in nanomolar concentrations in their neuronal terminal regions, the neuropeptides are found in picomolar and femtomolar concentrations per gram of brain tissue.

Ranging in size from 2 to more than 40 amino acids in length, these small proteins are constructed according to the same transcription/translation mechanism that provides the synthetic and degradative enzymes that are responsible for metabolism of the classical neurotransmitters. The DNA strand encoding the neuropeptide precursor—a larger protein termed a *prohormone*—is transcribed into mRNA sequences within the cell nucleus. The resulting prohormone mRNA sequence is translated into a protein at the ribosome and packaged into vesicles at the Golgi apparatus. The vesicles are transported to the nerve terminal presynaptic region; during this procedure, the active peptide is cleaved from the prohormone sequence at pairs of dibasic residues by specific cleavage enzymes. The active neuropeptide is then released into the synaptic cleft by vesicular fusion with the nerve terminal membrane and crosses the extracellular space in the synaptic cleft to bind to the appropriate receptors. Because only a few of the amino acids in any peptide make up the recognition site at the receptor-binding site, it is pos-

sible for fragments of the active peptide to retain all or some of the activity of the intact active form. It is also possible for peptides with similar sequences, or with sequences that fit the active site of a particular receptor, to exhibit cross-reactivity at a receptor. Similarly, the degradative peptidase enzymes that remove the active peptide from the synapse are designed to cleave the peptide bond at certain amino acids or at one end of the peptide chain, and thus may degrade more than one neuropeptide substrate. In addition, several copies of the active peptide may be contained in the prohormone sequence, allowing quick amplification of the neuropeptide signal on demand.

The various neuropeptides known to reside in the CNS are grouped into families according to sequence similarities, receptor activity, and similarity of physiological effects. These include the tachykinins (substance P, kassinin, eledoisin, bradykinin), which mediate blood pressure responses; the endogenous opioids (endorphins, enkephalins, and dynorphin), which produce analgesia in neuronal systems associated with pain sensation; the posterior pituitary hormones vasopressin and oxytocin, which are involved in maintenance of water balance and milk production, respectively; the glucagon-related peptides (vasoactive intestinal peptide, peptide histidine leucine, and peptide histidine methionine); and the pancreatic polypeptide-related peptides (neuropeptide Y, peptide YY, avian pancreatic polypeptide, and human pancreatic polypeptide). Many of these related neuropeptides are derived from different regions of the same prohormone precursor protein.

Other interesting neuropeptides are apparently unrelated to larger families, as is the case for neurotensin and neuromedin N. These two neuropeptides are encoded in the same prohormone, and their respective coding sequences are separated by a single pair of dibasic amino acids. Neurotensin produces hypothermia, potentiates the effects of barbiturates, and induces analgesia after direct CNS delivery. This fascinating neuropeptide also blocks the effects of DA in various brain regions. Synthesis of neurotensin is induced by antipsychotic drug administration in laboratory animals. Because group mean neurotensin CSF concentrations are often decreased in schizophrenic patients relative to nonpsychiatrically ill control subjects, the hypothesis that neurotensin may act as an endogenous neuroleptic or antipsychotic agent has been proposed. (For a comprehensive review of the neurobiology of neurotensin, see Kitabgi and Nemeroff 1992.) The current list of CNS neuropeptides approaches 100 distinct entities; three representative neuropeptides will be discussed here: thyrotropin-releasing hormone, corticotropin-releasing factor, and somatostatin.

Thyrotropin-Releasing Hormone

The first hypothalamic releasing factor to be purified was thyrotropin-releasing hormone (TRH). The isolation of TRH was the result of an intense competition between two research teams, whose leaders eventually shared the Nobel Prize in medicine for this effort (for a review of TRH neurobiology, see Metcalf and Jackson 1989). The release of thyrotropin (thyroid-stimulating hormone, or TSH) from the anterior pituitary is induced by the release of a TRH molecule from nerve terminals in the median eminence into the pituitary portal system; the TRH molecule eventually binds to a TRH receptor on thyrotrophs of the pituitary.

The TRH molecule is composed of three amino acids (pGLU-HIS-PRO-NH_2), which are joined between the amide terminus of one amino acid and the carboxyl terminus of the next amino acid in a "peptide" bond. The TRH molecule is further modified by a cyclized amino terminus (pGLU) and an amidated carboxyl terminus (NH_2) to protect it from degradation by the specific peptidase enzymes that degrade the neuropeptides into constituent amino acids. The TRH molecule is small enough to cross the blood-brain barrier after peripheral administration, which is not the case for larger neuropeptides and biomolecules, although the half-life of TRH in serum is only a couple of minutes.

The major metabolite of TRH is a cyclized HIS-PRO dipeptide that exhibits biological activity of its own within the brain (Banks et al. 1993). The TRH receptor is membrane bound and is primarily associated with the IP3/DAG second-messenger signal transduction system; synthesis of TRH receptor mRNA is regulated by local concentrations of TRH. Neurons containing TRH are found in highest concentrations in the hypothalamus, but TRH is also found in neurons of the anterior preoptic hypothalamus and septal nuclei. Thyrotropin-releasing hormone is found within 5-HT neurons of the

medullary raphe nuclei, and TRH nerve terminals impinge on the 5-HT neurons of the dorsal raphe midbrain nuclei that project to the entire cortex. The ability of TRH to reverse the sedative effects of barbiturates and ethanol is thought to reside in the septal region, whereas TRH applied to thermosensitive neurons of the preoptic anterior hypothalamus increases the firing rate of cold-sensitive neurons and decreases the firing rate of warm-sensitive neurons. In laboratory animals, it has been demonstrated that thyrotropin-releasing hormone is released from the hypothalamus after exposure to cold, following hemorrhage, or in association with restraint. Patients with major depressive disorder often exhibit reduced activity (blunting) of TRH pituitary receptors, and an increased incidence of antithyroid antibodies has been identified in the blood of such patients; groups of depressed patients have shown increased mean TRH concentrations in CSF compared with psychiatrically healthy control subjects (Banki et al. 1988). These findings suggest that hypersecretion of TRH may be associated with depressive disorder (Bissette 1991b).

Age-related changes in the hypothalamic-pituitary-thyroid axis have been observed in aged (22- to 24-month-old) Wistar rats relative to 3- to 5-month-old controls. Older rats had less TRH in the median eminence, with normal levels of TRH receptors in the mediobasal hypothalamus and higher numbers in the anterior pituitary than did the younger rats (Donda et al. 1989). The increase in TRH receptors in the older rats was associated with an apparent increase in accumulation of TRH in the pituitary, and with normal TSH blood levels and release of TSH from the pituitary. Thus, the endocrine activity of TRH systems appears to be affected by age, although there is little evidence for such changes in extraendocrine TRH systems.

Corticotropin-Releasing Factor

CRF was finally isolated and purified by Vale and colleagues (1981) in the early 1980s, after being intensively sought by various research teams for more than 20 years. The CRF molecule is 41 amino acids in length, and the sequence of CRF in rats and humans has been shown to be identical (for a review of CRF neurobiology, see DeSouza and Nemeroff 1990). CRF-binding protein, a specific carrier protein present in blood and brain, somewhat sequesters bound CRF from the action of peptidases and prevents access to the CRF receptor in the bound configuration. The release of CRF from the median eminence—where processes from cell bodies in the paraventricular nucleus of the hypothalamus terminate—into the pituitary portal system evokes the release of several related peptides derived from the prohormone precursor protein pro-opiomelanocortin (POMC), including beta-endorphin and adrenocorticotropic hormone (ACTH). The CRF receptor active site is directed toward the carboxyl terminus of CRF; the receptor is linked to the adenyl cyclase second-messenger signal transduction system and stimulates the action of this enzyme when the receptor is activated. Outside the hypothalamus, CRF neurons project from the central nucleus of the amygdala to limbic and brain stem nuclei, and CRF is found in interneurons of the cortex and hippocampus. This distribution underscores CRF's putative role in mediating the higher CNS responses to stress and adumbrates a role for CRF in emotional responses to adverse stimuli (see Bissette 1989 and 1991a for reviews). The release of hypothalamic CRF is induced by a variety of stressful stimuli in laboratory animals (Chappell et al. 1986), and exogenous CRF administered directly into the CNS of laboratory animals has been shown to elicit fearful and anxious behaviors.

Patients with major depressive disorder often exhibit a blunted ACTH response after challenge with exogenous CRF; show early escape from the inhibition of ACTH and cortisol secretion after administration of the synthetic glucocorticoid dexamethasone; have higher group mean concentrations of CRF in cerebrospinal fluid than do nonpsychiatrically ill control subjects (Banki et al. 1987; Nemeroff et al. 1984); and have reduced numbers of CRF receptors in the frontal cortex, as demonstrated by Nemeroff and co-workers on postmortem examination of brain tissue of depressed patients who committed suicide (Nemeroff et al. 1988). These findings are consistent with the interpretation of a dysregulated hypersecretion of CRF in patients with affective disorders. In patients with Alzheimer's disease, CRF interneurons in the cortex are targets of degeneration (Bissette et al. 1985); hypothalamic and nucleus basalis CRF neurons are apparently less affected. The corresponding CRF receptor population in the cortex of patients with Alzheimer's disease demonstrates proportional in-

creases (upregulation) in the number of CRF receptors per region without changes in receptor affinity (see Nemeroff et al. 1989 for a review of neuropeptide alterations in patients with Alzheimer's disease). Thus, a clinical need exists for both antagonists (to block the apparent CRF increases in synaptic availability in major depressive disorder) and agonists (to ameliorate the deficit in CRF synaptic availability in Alzheimer's disease) at the CRF receptor. (Refer to Figure 5–7.)

Evidence for decreased resiliency with increasing age in almost all levels of the hypothalamic-pituitary-adrenal axis response to stress exists in both laboratory animal studies and human studies (see Seeman and Robbins 1994 for a review of the human data and Sadow and Rubin 1992 for a review of the animal data). This decreased resiliency appar-

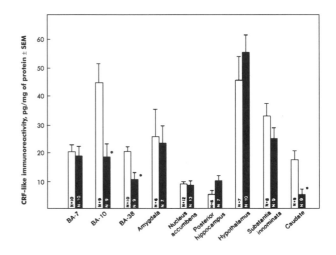

Figure 5–7. Regional brain concentration of corticotropin-releasing factor–like immunoreactivity (CRF-LI) in patients with senile dementia of the Alzheimer's type and in control subjects. Graphs represent concentrations of CRF-LI in brain regions from patients dying of senile dementia of the Alzheimer's type (*solid bars*) and control subjects (*open bars*). Number of samples from each brain region is shown inside respective bars. Concentration of CRF-LI is shown as mean ± SEM and is reported as picograms per milligram (pg/mg) of protein. Statistical significance was sought by Student's *t* test and is represented by an asterisk, which indicates $P < .01$. BA = Brodmann's area; SEM = standard error of the mean. *Source.* Reproduced with permission from Bissette G, Reynolds GP, Kilts CD, et al: "Corticotropin-Releasing Factor–Like Immunoreactivity in Senile Dementia of the Alzheimer Type: Reduced Cortical and Striatal Concentrations." *JAMA* 254:3068, 1985.

ently results in increased hypothalamic concentrations of CRF in aged (25-month-old) Sprague-Dawley rats compared with 3-month-old controls (Scaccianoce et al. 1990). Decreased concentrations of CRF in the frontal cortex of aged (26-month-old) Wistar rats relative to 18-month-old mature control rats—with no age-related change in hypothalamic CRF—has also been reported (Kowalski et al. 1992), indicating that strain differences may be present in these findings.

Somatostatin

Somatostatin (somatotropin release-inhibiting factor, or SRIF) was isolated by Brazeau and colleagues (1973) soon after TRH was isolated. Somatostatin was originally described as consisting of 14 amino acid molecules with a disulfide bridge between the two cysteine residues in the naturally occurring form (see Reichlin 1987 for a review). It was later shown that a larger, 28-amino acid form of SRIF was also produced when the SRIF prohormone was cleaved, and that the distribution of these two forms of somatostatin (SRIF-14 and SRIF-28) was different in various brain regions. The larger version, SRIF-28, is the predominant form in the endocrine axes (where SRIF inhibits the release of growth hormone, TSH, and ACTH as part of a dual control mechanism that regulates anterior pituitary hormone secretion) and in the gut (where SRIF inhibits the release of many digestive hormones). The smaller version, SRIF-14, although originally isolated from the hypothalamus, is the principal form of SRIF in the extrahypothalamic regions of the CNS, where SRIF functions as an inhibitory transmitter; in addition, it is often found to be localized in neurons containing the inhibitory amino acid GABA.

Interneurons throughout the cerebral cortex contain SRIF, and scattered SRIF neurons are also seen in the amygdala, hippocampus, and limbic forebrain regions. The receptors for SRIF are selective in their preference for either form of the SRIF molecule. Using molecular techniques, investigators have recently described five SRIF receptor subtypes. Octreotide, a SRIF receptor agonist, is used to control secretion of gut hormones from tumors that produce excess hormone; however, no centrally acting SRIF receptor agonists or antagonists are approved for clinical use. As SRIF is reduced in concentration in the CSF of patients with a wide variety of diseases that affect cognitive function—including Alzheimer's disease, Parkinson's disease with dementia, Huntington's chorea, multiple sclerosis, major depressive disorder, schizophrenia—and during states of delirium, a receptor agonist directed at CNS receptors for SRIF may be useful in reversing some symptoms of dementia (see Bissette and Myers 1992 for review). However, unlike what happens with CRF receptors, the degeneration of SRIF cortical interneurons in patients with Alzheimer's disease is not accompanied by upregulation of SRIF receptor number or affinity.

Somatostatin concentrations decreased in the striatum and increased in the hippocampus in 14-month-old Wistar rats compared with 3-month-old rats, but did not change further in this or other regions in rats 14–26 months of age (Kowalski et al. 1992). Thus, the available evidence indicates more pathological involvement of SRIF neuronal systems in diseases such as Alzheimer's disease rather than widespread changes in SRIF systems as a consequence of aging alone.

Conclusions

Additional chemical messengers undoubtedly will be discovered in the future as the laborious and tedious biochemical methods of protein purification are replaced by the elegant techniques of molecular biology, and as it becomes increasingly possible to ideally amplify a molecule and determine its structure. However, as discussed in this chapter, this is just the starting point for demonstrating neurotransmitter status. The successful wedding of the classical biochemical, physiological, and behavioral techniques to the exquisitely precise manipulations of molecular genetics promises to reveal ever-increasing complexity and interdependence among the various transmitter molecules and the neuronal systems that use them. Already drugs are being developed not on the basis serendipitously discovered activity but according to a design intended to create a specific interaction with one or more receptor subtypes in the CNS. The results of using these rationally designed drugs to treat patients with diseases with known pathological mechanisms will soon be known. However, the potential bonanza that drives the pharmaceutical industry in this area are the exciting possibilities inherent in being able to specifically affect the precise pathological target in diseases for which no effective treatment currently exists. It must be emphasized, however, that without funding for research to find the specific pathological targets and to sponsor the development of valid laboratory animal models to test nascent therapies, such a dream will remain unrealized for many more years. Unfortunately, given the attendant suffering and death that accompany severe illness, current priorities for biomedical research funding do not justify an optimistic outlook for the near future.

References

Antonini A, Leenders KL, Reist H, et al: Effect of age on D_2 dopamine receptors in normal human brain measured by positron emission tomography and ^{11}C-raclopride. Arch Neurol 50:474–480, 1993

Arranz B, Eriksson A, Mellerup E, et al: Effect of aging in human cortical pre- and postsynaptic serotonin binding sites. Brain Res 620:163–166, 1993

Bahr BA, Godshall AC, Hall RA, et al: Mouse telencephalon exhibits an age-related decrease in glutamate (AMPA) receptors but no change in nerve terminal markers. Brain Res 589:320–326, 1992

Banay-Schwartz M, Palkovits M, Lajtha A: Heterogeneous distribution of functionally important amino acids in brain areas of adult and aging humans. Neurochem Res 18:417–423, 1993

Banki CM, Bissette G, Arato M, et al: Cerebrospinal fluid corticotropin-releasing factor–like immunoreactivity in depression and schizophrenia. Am J Psychiatry 144:873–877, 1987

Banki CM, Bissette G, Arato M, et al: Elevation of immunoreactive CSF TRH in depressed patients. Am J Psychiatry 145:1526–1531, 1988

Banks WA, Kastin AJ, Akerstrom V, et al: Radioactively iodinated cyclo(His-Pro) crosses the blood-brain barrier and reverses ethanol-induced narcosis. Am J Physiol 164:E723–E729, 1993

Bannon MF, Poosch MS, Xia Y, et al: Dopamine transporter mRNA content in human substantia nigra decreases precipitously with age. Proc Natl Acad Sci USA 89:7095–7099, 1992

Beal MF, Walker LC, Storey E, et al: Neurotransmitters in neocortex of aged rhesus monkeys. Neurobiol Aging 12:407–412, 1991

Bissette G: CNS CRF in stress: radioimmunoassay studies, in Corticotropin-Releasing Factor: Basic and Clinical Studies of a Neuropeptide. Edited by DeSouza EB, Nemeroff CB. Boca Raton, FL, CRC Press, 1989, pp 21–28

Bissette G: Neuropeptides involved in stress and their distribution in the mammalian central nervous system, in Stress, Neuropeptides and Systemic Disease. Edited by Kaufman PG, McCubbin JA, Nemeroff CB. San Diego, CA, Academic Press, 1991a, pp 55–72

Bissette G: The role of thyrotropin-releasing hormone in depression. Biol Psychiatry 2:556–558, 1991b

Bissette G, Myers B: Mini review: somatostatin in Alzheimer's disease and depression. Life Sci 51:1389–1410, 1992

Bissette G, Nemeroff CB: Neuropeptides: biology and regulation, in Comprehensive Textbook of Psychiatry, 6th Edition. Edited by Kaplan HJ, Sadock BJ. Baltimore, MD, Williams & Wilkins (in press)

Bissette G, Reynolds GP, Kilts CD, et al: Corticotropin-releasing factor–like immunoreactivity in senile dementia of the Alzheimer type: reduced cortical and striatal concentrations. JAMA 254: 3067–3069, 1985

Blake MJ, Appel NM, Joseph JA, et al: Muscarinic acetylcholine receptor subtype mRNA expression and ligand binding in the aged rat forebrain. Neurobiol Aging 12:193–199, 1991

Blakely RD, Berson HE: Cloning and expression of a functional serotonin transporter from rat brain. Nature 354:66–70, 1991

Brazeau P, Vale W, Burgus R, et al: Hypothalamic peptide that inhibits the secretion of immunoreactive pituitary growth hormone. Science 179: 77–79, 1973

Burnett DM, Bowyer JF, Masserano JM, et al: Effect of aging on alpha$_1$-adrenergic stimulation of phosphoinositide hydrolysis in various regions of rat brain. J Pharmacol Exp Ther 255:1265–1270, 1990

Carfagna N, Moretti A: GABA content and synthesis in the aging rat brain. Exp Gerontol 25:545–552, 1990

Chappell PB, Smith MA, Kilts CD, et al: Alterations in corticotropin-releasing factor–like immunoreactivity in discrete rat brain regions after acute and chronic stress. J Neurosci 6:2908–2914, 1986

Cobo M, Exposito I, Porras A, et al: Release of amino acid neurotransmitters in different cortical areas of conscious adult and aged rats. Neurobiol Aging 13:705–709, 1992

Cobo M, Exposito I, Mora F: Aging, prefrontal cortex, and amino acid neurotransmitters: differential effects produced by electrical stimulation. Neurobiol Aging 14:187–190, 1993

Cohen SA, Muller WE: Age-related alterations of NMDA-receptor properties in the mouse forebrain: partial restoration by chronic phosphatidylserine treatment. Brain Res 584:174–180, 1992

Cooper JR, Bloom FE, Roth RH, eds: The Biochemical Basis of Neuropharmacology. New York, Oxford University Press, 1991

Court JA, Perry EK, Johnson M, et al: Regional patterns of cholinergic and glutamate activity in the developing and aging human brain. Brain Res Dev Brain Res 74:73–82, 1993

Dahlstrom A, Fuxe K: Evidence for the existence of monoamine-containing neurons in the central nervous system. Acta Physiological Scandinavica 62:1–55, 1964

Davidoff MS, Lolova IS: Age-related changes in serotonin-immunoreactivity in the telencephalon and diencephalon of rats. J Hirnforsch 32:745–753, 1991

Decker MW, McGaugh JL: The role of interactions between the cholinergic system and other neuromodulatory systems in learning and memory. Synapse 7:151–168, 1991

De Souza EB, Nemeroff CB: Corticotropin-Releasing Factor: Basic and Clinical Studies of a Neuropeptide. Boca Raton, FL, CRC Press, 1990

Donda A, Reymond MJ, Lemarchan-Beraud T: Influence of age on the control of thyrotropin secretion by thyrotropin-releasing hormone in the male rat. Neuroendocrinology 49:389–394, 1989

Donzanti BA, Ung AK: Alterations in neurotransmitter amino acid content in the aging rat striatum are subregion dependent. Neurobiol Aging 11:159–162, 1990

Donzanti BA, Hite JF, Yamamota BK: Extracellular glutamate levels increase with age in the lateral striatum: potential involvement of presynaptic D_2 receptors. Synapse 13:376–382, 1993

Fernandez-Ruiz J, De Miguel R, Hernandez ML, et al: Comparisons between brain dopaminergic neurons of juvenile and aged rats: sex-related differences. Mech Ageing Dev 63:45–55, 1992

Feuerstein TJ, Lehmann J, Sauermann W, et al: The autoinhibitory feedback control of acetylcholine release in human neocortex tissue. Brain Res 572:64–71, 1992

Francis PT, Webster M-T, Chessell IP, et al: Neurotransmitters and second messengers in aging and Alzheimer's disease. Ann N Y Acad Sci 695:19–26, 1993

Friedemann MN, Gerhardt GA: Regional effects of aging on dopaminergic function in the Fischer 344 rat. Neurobiol Aging 13:325–332, 1992

Godefroy F, Bassant MH, Lamour Y, et al: Effect of aging on dopamine metabolism in the rat cerebral cortex: a regional analysis. J Neural Transm Gen Sect 83:13–24, 1991

Gozlan H, Daval G, Verge D, et al: Aging associated changes in serotoninergic and dopaminergic pre- and postsynaptic neurochemical markers in the rat brain. Neurobiol Aging 11:437–449, 1990

Handa RJ, Cross MK, George M, et al: Neuroendocrine and neurochemical responses to novelty stress in young and old male F344 rats: effects of H-fenfluramine treatment. Pharmacol Biochem Behav 46:101–109, 1993

Harik SI, Sromek SM, Kalaria RN: Alpha- and beta-adrenergic receptors of the rat cerebral cortex and cerebral microvessels in aging, and their response to denervation. Neurobiol Aging 12:567–573, 1991

Hitri A, Hurd YL, Wyatt RJ, et al: Molecular, functional and biochemical characteristics of the dopamine transporter: regional differences and clinical relevance. Clin Neuropharmacol 17:1–22, 1994

Ida Y, Tanaka M, Kohno Y, et al: Effects of age and stress on regional noradrenaline metabolism in the rat brain. Neurobiol Aging 3:233–236, 1982

Inglefield JR, Richfield EK: Preservation of the density of the dopamine uptake complex in aging Fischer 344 rat brain. Neurobiol Aging 13:383–391, 1992

Iyo M, Yamasaki T: The detection of age-related decrease of dopamine D_1, D_2, and serotonin 5-HT_2 receptors in living human brain. Prog Neuropsychopharmacol Biol Psychiatry 17:415–421, 1993

Kanner BI, Danbolt N, Pines G, et al: Structure and function of the sodium and potassium-coupled glutamate transporter from rat brain. Biochem Soc Trans 21:59-61, 1993

Kawakami H, Tanaka K, Nakayama T, et al: Cloning and expression of a human glutamate transporter. Biochem Biophys Res Commun 199:171–176, 1994

Kish SJ, Shannak K, Rajput A, et al: Aging produces a specific pattern of striatal dopamine loss: implications for the etiology of idiopathic Parkinson's disease. J Neurochem 58:642–648, 1992

Kitabgi P, Nemeroff CB (eds): The Neurobiology of Neurotensin (Annals of the New York Academy of Science, Vol 668). New York, New York Academy of Science, 1992

Kitamura Y, Zhao XH, Ohnuki T, et al: Age-related changes in transmitter glutamate and NMDA receptor/channels in the brain of senescence-accelerated mouse. Neurosci Lett 137:169–172, 1992

Knipper M, Kahle C, Breer H: Purification and reconstitution of the high-affinity choline transporter. Biochim Biophys Acta 1065:107–113, 1991

Kornhuber ME, Kornhuber J, Retz W, et al: L-glutamate and L-aspartate concentrations in the developing and aging human putamen tissue. J Neural Transm Gen Sect 93:145–150, 1993

Kowalski C, Micheau J, Corder R, et al: Age-related changes in corticotropin-releasing factor, somatostatin, neuropeptide Y, methionine enkephalin and beta-endorphin in specific rat brain areas. Brain Res 582:38–46, 1992

Lam DM, Fei J, Zhang XY, et al: Molecular cloning and structure of the human (GABATHG) GABA transporter gene. Brain Res Mol Brain Res 19:227–232, 1993

Lamy PP: The role of cholinesterase inhibitors in Alzheimer's disease. CNS Drugs 1:146–165, 1994

Lindvall O, Bjorklund A: Neuroanatomical localization of dopamine in the brain and spinal cord, in Handbook of Schizophrenia, Vol 2: Neurochemistry and Neuropharmacology of Schizophrenia. Edited by Henn FA, DeLisi LE. Amsterdam, Elsevier, 1987, pp 49–99

Lolova I, Davidoff M: Immuno- and histochemical data on changed GABA transmission in aged rat cerebellum. J Hirnforsch 31:423–428, 1990

Lolova I, Davidoff M: Changes in GABA-immunoreactivity and GABA-transaminase activity in rat amygdaloid complex in aging. J Hirnforsch 32:231–238, 1991

Lolova I, Davidoff M: Age-related changes in serotonin-immunoreactive neurons in the rat nucleus raphe dorsalis and nucleus centralis superior: a light microscope study. Mech Ageing Dev 62:279–289, 1992

Lorens SA, Hata N, Handa RJ, et al: Neurochemical, endocrine and immunological responses to stress in young and old Fischer 344 male rats. Neurobiol Aging 11:139–150, 1990

Magnusson KR, Cotman CW: Age-related changes in excitatory amino acid receptors in two mouse strains. Neurobiol Aging 14:197–206, 1993

Melikian HE, McDonald JK, Gu H, et al: Human norepinephrine transporter: biosynthetic studies using a site-directed polyclonal antibody. J Biol Chem 269:12290–12297, 1994

Merchant KM, Dobie DJ, Dorsa DM: Differential loss of dopamine D_2 receptor mRNA isoforms during aging in Fischer 344 rats. Neurosci Lett 154:163–167, 1993

Mesco ER, Joseph JA, Blake MJ, et al: Loss of D_2 receptors during aging is partially due to decreased levels of mRNA. Brain Res 545:355–357, 1991

Metcalf G, Jackson I, eds: Thyrotropin-Releasing Hormone: Biomedical Significance (Annals of the New York Academy of Science, Vol 553). New York, New York Academy of Science, 1989

Meyer EM, Judkins JH, Momol AE, et al: Effects of peroxidation and aging on rat neocortical ACh-release and protein kinase C. Neurobiol Aging 15:63–67, 1994

Mhatre MC, Ticku MK: Aging related alterations in GABA-A receptor subunit mRNA levels in Fischer rats. Brain Res Mol Brain Res 14:71–78, 1992

Miyoshi R, Kito S, Doudou N, et al: Influence of age on N-methyl-D-aspartate antagonist binding sites in the rat brain studied by in vitro autoradiography. Synapse 8:212–217, 1991

Mufson EJ, Cochran E, Benzing W, et al: Galaninergic innervation of the cholinergic vertical limb of the diagonal band (Ch2) and bed nucleus of the stria terminalis in aging, Alzheimer's disease and Down's syndrome. Dementia 4:237–250, 1993

Muller WE, Stoll L, Schubert T, et al: Central cholinergic functioning and aging. Acta Psychiatr Scand Suppl 366:34–39, 1991

Najlerahim A, Francis PT, Bowen DM: Age-related alteration in excitatory amino acid neurotransmission in rat brain. Neurobiol Aging 11:155–158, 1990

Nemeroff CB, Widerlov E, Bissette G, et al: Elevated concentrations of CSF corticotropin-releasing factor–like immunoreactivity in depressed patients. Science 226:1342–1344, 1984

Nemeroff CB, Owens MJ, Bissette G, et al: Reduced corticotropin-releasing factor (CRF) binding sites in the frontal cortex of suicides. Arch Gen Psychiatry 45:577–579, 1988

Nemeroff CB, Kizer JS, Reynolds GP, et al: Neuropeptides in Alzheimer's disease: a postmortem study. Regul Pept 25:123–130, 1989

Nieuwenhuys R, Voogd J, van Huijzen C: The Human Central Nervous System. New York, Springer-Verlag, 1981

Nordberg A, Alavuzoff I, Winblad B: Nicotinic and muscarinic subtypes in the human brain: changes with aging and dementia. J Neurosci Res 31:103–111, 1992

Palmer AM, DeKosky ST: Monoamine neurons in aging and Alzheimer's disease. J Neural Transm Gen Sect 91:135–159, 1993

Piggott MA, Perry EK, Perry RH, et al: [^{3}H]MK-801 binding to the NMDA receptor complex, and its modulation in human frontal cortex during development and aging. Brain Res 588:277–286, 1992

Reichlin S: Somatostatin: Basic and Clinical Status. New York, Plenum, 1987

Ribak CE, Vaughn JE, Saito K, et al: Immunocytochemical localization of glutamate decarboxylase in rat substantia nigra. Brain Res 116:287–298, 1977

Rinne JO, Heitala J, Ruotsalainen U, et al: Decrease in human striatal dopamine D$_2$ receptor density with age: a PET study with [^{11}C]raclopride. J Cereb Blood Flow Metab 13:310–314, 1993

Ruano D, Machado A, Vitorica J: Absence of modifications of the pharmacological properties of the GABA-A receptor complex during aging, as assessed in 3- and 24-month-old rat cerebral cortex. Eur J Pharmacol 246:81–87, 1993

Sadow TF, Rubin RT: Effects of hypothalamic peptides on the aging brain (review). Psychoneuroendocrinology 17:293–314, 1992

Sakata M, Farooqui SM, Prasad C: Post-transcriptional regulation of loss of rat striatal D$_2$ dopamine receptor during aging. Brain Res 575:309–314, 1992

Scaccianoce S, Di Sciullo A, Angelucci L: Age-related changes in hypothalamo-pituitary-adrenocortical axis activity in the rat. Neuroendocrinology 52:150–155, 1990

Scarpace PJ, Tumer N, Mader SL: Beta-adrenergic function in aging: basic mechanisms and clinical implications (review). Drugs and Aging 1:116–129, 1991

Schroder H, Giacobini E, Struble RG, et al: Cellular distribution and expression of cortical acetylcholine receptors in aging and Alzheimer's disease. Ann N Y Acad Sci 640:189–192, 1991

Seeman TE, Robbins RJ: Aging and hypothalamic-pituitary-adrenal response to challenge in humans. Endocr Rev 15:233–260, 1994

Slotkin TA, Seidler FJ, Crain BJ, et al: Regulatory changes in presynaptic cholinergic function assessed in rapid autopsy material from patients with Alzheimer's disease: implications for etiology and therapy. Proc Natl Acad Sci USA 87:2452–2455, 1990

Slotkin TA, Nemeroff CB, Bissette G, et al: Overexpression of the high affinity choline transporter in cortical regions affected by Alzheimer's disease: evidence from rapid autopsy studies. J Clin Invest 94:696–702, 1994

Tamaru M, Yoneda Y, Ogita K, et al: Age-related decreases of the N-methyl-D-aspartate receptor complex in the rat cerebral cortex and hippocampus. Brain Res 542:83–90, 1991

Teitler M, Herrick-Davis K: Multiple serotonin receptor subtypes: molecular cloning and functional expression. Crit Rev Neurobiol 8:175–188, 1994

Undie AS, Friedman E: Aging-induced decrease in dopaminergic-stimulated phosphoinositide metabolism in rat brain. Neurobiol Aging 13:505–511, 1992

Vale W, Spiess J, Rivier C, et al: Characterization of a 41-residue ovine hypothalamic peptide that stimulates secretion of corticotropin and beta-endorphin. Science 213:1394, 1981

Van Der Zee EA, De Jong GI, Strosberg AD, et al: Muscarinic acetylcholine receptor-expression in astrocytes in the cortex of young and aged rats. Glia 8:42–50, 1993

Venero JL, de la Roza C, Machado A, et al: Age-related changes on monoamine turnover in hippocampus of rats. Brain Res 631:89–96, 1993

Wada H, Ito H, Orimo H, et al: Kynurenine specifically increases in the cerebrospinal fluid of the aged rats. Biogenic Amines 10:221–225, 1994

Watson SJ, Khachaturian H, Lewis ME, et al: Chemical neuroanatomy as a basis for biological psychiatry, in American Handbook of Psychiatry. Edited by Berger PA, Brodie HKH. New York, Basic Books, 1986, pp 3–33

Zhao XH, Kitamura Y, Nomura Y, et al: Age-related changes in NMDA-induced [^{3}H]acetylcholine release from brain slices of senescence-accelerated mouse. Int J Dev Neurosci 10:121–129, 1992

CHAPTER 6

Genetics and Geriatric Psychiatry

Ewald W. Busse, M.D.
Dan G. Blazer, M.D., Ph.D.

Remarkable advances in human genetics are affecting the practice of geriatric psychiatry. These advances are highlighted by the explosion of knowledge regarding the molecular genetics of Alzheimer's disease, and are underscored—though in a less dramatic way—by new knowledge concerning many other conditions that affect geriatric patients. Geriatric psychiatrists will be called upon to respond to many questions regarding human genetics as it relates to the pathophysiology of diseases such as Alzheimer's disease, major depression, and late-onset schizophrenic disorders. In this chapter, we review the background of human genetics as it applies to geriatric psychiatry. The history of genetics, the association of genetics and longevity, population genetics, and molecular genetics are explored. Particular emphasis is placed on findings from studies in population and molecular genetics about Alzheimer's disease and the mood disorders.

The Genetic Basis of Aging

The first contributions to genetics derive from studies of plants and animals by plant hybridizers, especially those by the Austrian botanist Gregor Mendel (1822–1884). Although Mendel published his results in 1866, his discoveries remained largely unknown until 1900. The existence of chromosomes and genes was unknown at the time Mendel studied the cross-fertilization of plants, yet three fundamental concepts emerged from his studies that have been confirmed by modern discoveries about cell reproduction. First, each organism is a mosaic of unit characters capable of separate hereditary transmission. Second, a unit character may mask a related unit character completely when the potentials for development of both are present in the same organism. This principle is called *dominance,* and the masked characteristic is referred to as *recessive.* Third, unit characteristics may be segregated during reproduction, regardless of the combinations in which they have been associated.

Sir Francis Galton (1822–1911) studied twins to assess the role of nature (inheritance) and nurture (environment) in the development of various human characteristics. Galton was aware that there were two different types of twins: *monozygotic,* or twins that develop from a single fertilized egg, and *dizygotic,* or twins derived from two eggs fertilized separately. In 1875, he described the life histories of a group of monozygotic twins compared with those of dizygotic pairs. The question Galton posed was, "To what extent does the environment make initially similar twins different over time and make dissimilar twins more alike?" Galton wrote that "there is no escape from the conclusion that nature prevails enormously over nurture" (Galton 1876/1990).

During the middle of the 20th century, significant discoveries in genetics rapidly occurred. In 1944, Avery and colleagues at the Rockefeller Institute discovered that genes (those cellular components responsible for inheritance) were made of deoxyribonucleic acid (DNA). Crick and Watson, in 1953, postulated a structure of DNA, the double helix, and subsequently won the Nobel prize for this discovery (Watson 1968). In 1970, Caspersson and associates discovered that the staining of DNA with fluorescent compounds affected preferentially specific regions of different chromosomes, which made it possible to identify individual chromosomes by fluorescent patterns. The understanding of genetic transmission was closely paralleled by an emerging technology to engineer genetics (Kalin 1985). A technique was developed that permitted the manipulation of bacterial DNA in such a manner that selected regions could be changed while other regions were left intact. This manipulation resulted in the production of recombinant DNA, which has been one of the greatest advances in understanding the human genome in history, and which has opened possibilities for the development of genetic therapies. Through various techniques, genes can now be mapped—in fact, scientists involved in The Human Genome Project are currently in the process of mapping the entire human genome. Through such mapping techniques, remarkable advances in molecular genetics have emerged, including those that we discuss in this chapter.

The Role of the Gene in Longevity

It is a misconception to state that genes alone program the life span; however, it is clear that genes can modulate rates of aging, in part by varying efficiencies of the organism's biological machinery, ranging from metabolism of food to repair of cellular injuries (Martin and Tucker 1994). The conventional wisdom holds that humans have a maximum life expectancy of approximately 120 years, and in fact the fastest-growing segment of the population is that which includes individuals over 85 years old (Curtsinger 1992). It is still unclear to what extent longevity is heritable. The results of twin studies in which monozygotic and dizygotic twins have been compared suggest that the intrapair difference in the age of death is smaller for monozygotic than for dizygotic twins, yet the mean difference in death for both is large—15 years. Therefore, it appears that environmental factors, such as toxins, health habits, and diet, significantly influence longevity (Jarvik et al. 1960). Another approach to assessing the genetic contribution to longevity is to estimate the properties of the human genome that determine genetic variations in human aging. Of the estimated 100,000 informational genes in humans, a reasonable estimate is that perhaps only 70 genes may be characterized as major "aging genes" (Martin 1978; Martin and Tucker 1988).

Longevity Assurance Genes

Some genes are regulatory and some are productive, making proteins that contribute to function and structure. Some genes, not infrequently referred to as "smart genes," can turn off and some can turn on regulatory and productive activities. Faulty regulation can be very destructive to the organism.

Candidate longevity genes perform a number of tasks, including protecting the cells (particularly DNA) from damage, regulating metabolism, maintaining self-proliferation and productivity, and repairing cell damage. Excellent candidates to be named as longevity genes are those that produce scavengers of free radicals and those that can repair damage to cells.

Perhaps the most striking empirical finding regarding longevity is the gender difference in longevity. Although there is no evidence that the maximum life span potential of females is greater than that of males, the average life expectancy of females is significantly greater than that of males. This female advantage is widespread in the animal kingdom and is not limited to humans only (Martin and Tucker 1988). A survival advantage for females has been attributed to the fact that the female sex chromosome is homogametic (two X chromosomes), whereas the male sex chromosome is heterogametic (one X and one Y chromosome). Therefore, the male may be at a disadvantage, for sex-linked recessive alleles are more likely to be expressed (Martin and Tucker 1994). However, the human X female chromosome contains a minimum of 112 genes associated with diseases; the much smaller human male Y chromosome has only one such gene that has been clearly identified (Rennie 1994).

Mitochondrial DNA

Mitochondrial DNA genes exist in all humans, transmitted from mother to all offspring. Human mtDNA is a complex double-stranded circle made up of 16,569 base pairs. It contains only 37 genes, 13 of which encode for polypeptides (Schon and Di Mauro 1994). Mitochondria, cell organelles that are present in virtually all cells with a nucleus (eukaryotic cells), vary in size and number and are the "power source" for the cell. Hence, they are important in many metabolic pathways. Mitochondrial genes are designated as *mtDNA* genes; genes carried in the cell nucleus are *nDNA* genes. The mtDNA is predominantly maternally inherited, with less than 0.1% of these genes contributed by the sperm (Wallace 1992). Hundreds of mitochondria as well as thousands of mitochondrial genes can be found in each cell. Cells can harbor mixtures of mutant and normal mtDNA genes. When a cell divides, both the mutant and the normal mtDNA genes are randomly scattered into daughter cells. Consequently, some cells will have more mutant genes and others will have a higher number of normal mtDNA genes— thus, some cells will function better than others. It is believed that mitochondrial genes are vulnerable to damage by oxygen free radicals (see Chapter 1, "The Free Radical Theory"). Because of their importance in the metabolic process and their vulnerability to damage by oxygen radicals, it is obvious that mtDNA genes could play a major role in aging processes as well as in the genesis of degenerative disorders (Wallace 1992).

To determine the mechanism by which gene action determines longevity, those gene actions that maintain the structural and functional integrity of the mature organism must be investigated (Martin and Tucker 1994). Hayflick and colleagues found that cultures of human fibroblasts undergo a gradual loss of growth potential even in ideal growth environments (Hayflick and Moorhead 1961), and, therefore, it may be that longevity is programmed

into the development of an organism's cells. However, most of the research in this area has focused on gene action that ensures the maintenance of structure and function over time. For example, it has been discovered that genes controlling the production of necessary scavenger enzymes for toxins produced during the normal metabolic cycle may decline in their function with increased age. This fact is illustrated by superoxide, an oxygen free radical produced in the Krebs cycle that can be extremely toxic to tissue. Superoxide is metabolized by the enzyme superoxide dismutase. According to the free radical theory of aging, the activity and efficacy of superoxide dismutase decrease with increased age (Harmon 1971). (See "The Free Radical Theory" in Chapter 1 for a further discussion of this theory of aging.)

Telomeres

A telomere is the terminal region of a chromosome. Although telomeres are composed of DNA, they do not appear to contain genetic information. They are composed of repeating sequences, and the same pattern is repeated until the very end of the chromosome is reached. In cultured normal human cells, the repeated sequence in the telomere is reduced at a fixed rate with each cell division that takes place. Hence, a telomere behaves like an aging clock. Abnormal cells do not undergo telomere shortening, but instead contain telemerase, an enzyme that causes the production of additional telomeres; normal cells lack this enzyme.

One opportunity for investigating longevity and the genetic factors that contribute to longevity is to study the rare but remarkable presenile syndromes. Werner's syndrome (sometimes referred to as "adult progeria" [Salk et al. 1985]), a disorder inherited as an autosomal recessive trait, is attributable to deficiency of a single enzyme. The gene causing Werner's syndrome was recently located on chromosome 8 (Goto et al. 1992). The life expectancy of an individual with Werner's syndrome is significantly shortened: signs of "premature" aging—such as graying of the hair and atrophic changes in the skin—emerge in adolescence. Later, cataracts and other visual problems occur, and diseases associated with older age, such as diabetes and osteoporosis, develop. Death usually occurs during the latter part of the fifth decade, the result of vascular problems or cancer.

Another type of progeria is Hutchinson-Gilford syndrome. This condition is characterized by an earlier onset than Werner's syndrome and is manifested by dwarfism, physical immaturity, and pseudosenility. Affected individuals look like very old, wizened, small humans with distorted features. Their heads are comparatively large, whereas the face, ears, and nose are small. This syndrome has been observed in whites, blacks, and Asians, and is believed to be caused by a defect inherited as an autosomal recessive trait.

A third disorder in which some premature aging is found is Down's syndrome. Individuals with Down's syndrome undergo external signs of premature aging, such as graying of hair, but they also exhibit neuropathological changes remarkably similar to those that occur in patients with Alzheimer's disease, including senile plaques and neurofibrillary tangles. The life expectancy of the patient with Down's syndrome is severely shortened, rarely extending to beyond age 40.

There are many diseases that are associated with shortened life expectancy and that appear to be associated with some genetic predisposition. Most of these diseases, however, require a genetic/environmental interaction for the disease to become manifest. For example, a common and potent environmental carcinogen is aflatoxin, which has been implicated particularly in the development of liver cancer. A genetic mutation has been found to be associated with a familial type of this cancer. Though it is difficult to detect, the mutated gene is found only in tumor cells, not in normal liver cells. Carcinogens such as aflatoxin must be activated by enzymes in the body in order to stimulate the cancer-producing mechanism (the activating forms of these toxins attack DNA, which, in turn, leads to the development of malignancy). Therefore, it is not unreasonable to assume that a genetic predisposition to a shortened life expectancy may be circumvented, at least in part, by reducing exposure to environmental risk factors.

Population Genetics

The study of the genetics of disease can conveniently be divided into population genetics and molecular genetics. Population genetics contributes to our understanding of diseases in late life by establishing genotypic frequencies in the population and exploring the forces that change these frequencies. The samples used in population genetics are twin registries and family studies.

Many twin registries are available throughout the world, and these have proven to be of immense value to scientists in studies of the relative contributions of heredity and environment to the development of disease. Among the best known are the registries from the Nordic countries, especially Sweden, and the National Academy of Sciences twin registry in the United States. Many subjects in these registries are currently among the oldest, and therefore these registries have been especially valuable for studying the diseases of old age. For example, the Swedish twin registry, which provides the best opportunity in the world for exploring differences between twins reared together and twins reared apart, consists of many pairs over the age of 65 who were reared apart. Sweden was an impoverished country during the first two decades of this century. Not infrequently, families to whom twins were born could not support both (or even one) of the twins, and therefore adoption was a common procedure. Meticulous records were kept, and so this most valuable resource is available for investigation of diseases such as Alzheimer's disease and physical abnormalities.

The National Academy of Sciences twin registry was established during World War II by identifying twins enlisted in the armed services. Although it is almost exclusively a registry of male twins, it represents an extremely large reservoir of twins for study. One disadvantage of the National Academy of Sciences registry is that the American twins frequently live at great distances from one another, and there is no large concentration of twins in any given area of the country. (This is not such a problem with the Swedish twin registry, simply because Sweden is a much smaller country.)

Family studies usually begin with a *proband*—that is, a person who has the disease that is under study. The proband frequently is identified through a clinical service (such as a memory disorders clinic) of a hospital or medical center. Family members and the family tree are rostered; interviews as well as biological studies are conducted to determine the frequency and distribution of the disease, or traits related to the disease, within the family. These data are usually presented as a genogram across multiple generations. Such a genogram can assist the investigator in identifying whether a trait is inherited as an autosomal dominant, autosomal recessive, X-linked dominant, or X-linked recessive trait. Unfortunately, most disorders that develop in late life are not inherited via pure Mendelian genetics.

Huntington's disease is the prototypical dementing illness that is inherited as an autosomal dominant trait. The child of an affected parent has a 50% risk of developing the disease. Men and women are equally at risk. Given that the age at onset of the dementia (and accompanying neurological and behavioral problems) is approximately 43 years, the individual carrying the gene is likely to pass through the childbearing years unaffected, for the most part. Within the past several years, the defective gene has been located on chromosome 4p16.3, and several markers for identifying the existence of the defective gene are now available. The defective gene associated with Huntington's disease is an expanded stretch of DNA with a repeating pattern of three nucleotide bases, CAG. The more repeats that occur, the earlier the onset of disease symptoms. However, the number of repeats is unstable from one generation to the next. How this genetic defect results in the disease or how the defective gene may affect neighboring genes is unknown (Gusella and MacDonald 1994). The ability to identify this gene before onset of the disease and during the childbearing years presents an ethical dilemma to both physicians and patient when Huntington's disease is known to be present in the family.

Most psychiatric disorders affecting older adults result from multifactorial inheritance. That is, the inheritance of a trait is governed by many genes. A good example of a multifactorial trait is height, which is distributed in the population according to the normal "bell shaped" curve. The more genes that contribute to a trait (assuming complete penetrance), the more likely it is for that trait to follow a normal distribution in the population. With disorders such as Alzheimer's disease, it is clear that memory difficulties are not distributed normally, but neither do they fall conveniently into normal memory and clear Alzheimer's disease. Therefore, multiple factors undoubtedly contribute to both the inheritance and the expression of the disease, and genetic as well as environmental factors play a role. For this reason, most population genetic investigations involve quantitative genetics. In such studies, examination of the variance in the population of a phenotype, rather than specific genotypes, is the goal of the study.

The overall variance of a characteristic in the population is due to the added effects of genetic variance and environmental variance. Heritability is, therefore, the genetic variance divided by the overall variance within the population. Environmental variance can be divided into both shared and unshared environmental influences—that is, the environmental contribution shared with a relative and those influences independent of relatives. For example, in a study of monozygotic and dizygotic twins, some of whom were reared together, investigators can assume that the difference in the variance of monozygotic twins reared together versus those reared apart is due to shared environment in one group—that is, those reared together. Twins reared apart would have no shared environment. To calculate estimates of the relative contributions of heredity, shared environment, and unshared environment, population geneticists begin with the assumption that monozygotic twins have no hereditary variance, and so whatever differences are found in a characteristic, such as depressive symptoms, are assumed to be due to environmental influences. Dizygotic twins, in contrast, share only one-half of their hereditary contributions to a characteristic. These assumptions are flawed, for even twins reared apart share at least their in utero environment. Also, the genomes of so-called identical twins are not exact carbon copies of each other.

An example of this type of population study was one in which investigators explored the relative contributions of genetic and environmental influences on lipoprotein levels in older twins (Heller et al. 1993). Using the Swedish adoption/twin study of aging, the authors found substantial heritability for serum levels of total cholesterol, high-density lipoprotein cholesterol, apolipoprotein A_1 and B, as well as triglycerides. The researchers found that environmental rearing had a substantial impact on the level of total cholesterol, but affected other lipid measures much less than did the genetic factors, even in these older adults. It did appear, however, that heritability for apolipoprotein B and triglyceride levels decreased with aging.

Most published reports of the heritability of Alzheimer's disease have been from family studies, but twin studies are emerging as an important complement to these early family studies. In 1981, Heston and colleagues studied the relatives of 125 probands who had dementia of the Alzheimer's type, as demonstrated at autopsy. These relatives were more likely to exhibit a history of dementing illness, consistent with genetic transmission. The risk to relatives decreased when the severity of dementing illness decreased, suggesting that a quantitative approach to the study of hereditary/environmental influences in Alzheimer's disease may be appropriate. In addition, when compared with a control group and the general population, the relatives had an increased incidence of Down's syndrome, thyroid problems, and immune system diseases.

A persistent problem in studying the heritability of Alzheimer's disease, however, is that individuals may die before the disease is expressed, and therefore persons carrying the gene to express the illness at a given age are lost from the sample. Statistical procedures have been applied to take this factor into account in studies of heritability. Mohs et al. (1987) investigated the morbid risk of Alzheimer's disease in first-degree relatives of 50 patients who met the criteria for Alzheimer's disease, compared with 45 matched control subjects. Relatives of patients with the disease showed a 46% cumulative incidence of Alzheimer's by the age of 86, four times that found among control subjects. The authors concluded that Alzheimer's disease is commonly distributed as an autosomal dominant disorder, the full expression of which is delayed until oldest-old age, but largely completed by the age of 90.

Breitner et al. (1988) extended these studies and found that early-onset Alzheimer's disease was distinct from late-onset illness, thus postulating different causal mechanisms depending on age at onset. Breitner's group also found that age at onset varies as a familial characteristic, and that only one-third of those individuals who might experience Alzheimer's disease due to heredity will manifest the disorder during their lifetime. Given these findings, these investigators suggested that a dominant gene with a population allele frequency of 0.13 accounted for the expression of Alzheimer's disease.

Breitner and colleagues proceeded from these family studies to twin studies, and to a more quantitative approach to the relative contributions of heredity and environment in Alzheimer's disease (Brandt et al. 1993). They found that the heritability of cognitive status was 30%. Shared environment ac-

counted for an additional 18% of the variance, most of which was related to years of education. Of the cognitive factors studied, the language/attention factor had the highest heritability.

Therefore, the results of population genetic studies of Alzheimer's disease to date suggest autosomal dominant transmission through at least some of the population, although it is highly likely that sporadic cases occur as well. Despite the propensity toward autosomal dominant inheritance, environmental factors do play a role in the expression of the disorder. All of these studies are hindered by the people who would express the disorder but who die before they reach the age at which the disorder would have been expressed.

A number of family studies also have been performed exploring the mood disorders. Mendlewicz et al. (1972) found that among patients with manic-depressive illness, those with an early onset of symptoms were more likely to demonstrate a family history of the disorder. This finding is consistent with a general understanding drawn from family studies of mood disorders (Andreasen et al. 1987). These studies suggest that bipolar illness is more likely to be heritable than unipolar disorders, and that early age at onset is more likely to be associated with a family history than is later age at onset. Stone (1989) performed a retrospective study of patients over age 65 admitted to hospitals because of mania; 26% of these patients had no prior history of mood disorder. Patients with a family history of mood disorder had a significantly earlier age at onset of their illness, again suggesting that the hereditary contribution to a mood disorder is more significant if symptoms first appear in early life rather than in late life. It must be remembered, however, that individuals in late life who manifest a mood disorder may have first experienced a disorder earlier in life that remained clinically unidentified.

Psychiatric symptoms that, alone, do not permit diagnosis of a specific disorder have also been examined in family and twin studies. Jatz et al. (1992) explored symptoms of depression among subjects in the Swedish twin registry. Using the Center for Epidemiologic Studies Depression Scale (CES-D; Radloff 1977), they found that genetic influences explained 16% of the variance in total depression scores and 19% of the variance in the physiologic subscale. Heritability was minimal for the depressed mood and subjective well-being subscales. The influence of family rearing played a substantial role in explaining twin similarity, whereas unique experiences accounted for the greatest proportion of the variance. Heritability of psychomotor retardation was greater for twins 60 years of age and older than for twins under age 60, a finding that contrasts with the results of family studies of mood disorders. These findings substantiate the conclusions from other studies that the etiological factors contributing to mood disorders include biological (heritable) factors, early life experiences (shared environment), and unique experiences (life events that are unshared).

Molecular Genetics

The bridge between population genetics and molecular genetics is the molecular genetic techniques that permit the study of segments of the genome across individuals within a family. There are approximately 200,000 genes in the human genome, and within each gene the base sequence (i.e., the sequence of the four bases of DNA—adenine, thymine, cytosine, and guanine) differs due to random changes or mutations. These changes have been used to produce genetic markers, known as restriction fragment length polymorphisms (RFLPs). These markers of DNA can be used to "detect"—that is, RFLPs mark the genomes of two individuals at sites where the sequence of the bases varies, thereby distinguishing the alleles of the same gene (Whatley and Anderton 1990). Early studies in molecular genetics focused upon the linkage of a gene producing Alzheimer's disease and markers for human leukocyte antigen (HLA). There has been no evidence for linkage of HLA markers with Alzheimer's disease.

Given the histopathological and, indeed, the clinical similarities between patients with Alzheimer's disease and persons in the late stages of Down's syndrome, linkage studies have focused on chromosome 21. Most patients with Down's syndrome develop neuropathological changes that are virtually indistinguishable from those that occur in patients with early-onset (age 35–45) Alzheimer's disease, and an association between Down's syndrome and Alzheimer's disease has been observed in families (Heyman et al. 1983; Oliver and Holland 1985). The cause of Down's syndrome is the production of a third chromosome 21 (trisomy). A triplica-

tion of only a part—namely, this distal part—of the third chromosome may lead to all the pathological features of Down's syndrome. This distal site became an even more attractive candidate for study when it was discovered that the gene coding for the senile plaque amyloid-A4 protein was located on chromosome 21 (Goldgarber et al. 1987). These data suggested, therefore, that the deposition of amyloid-A4 protein in senile plaques was perhaps the cause of Alzheimer's disease. Although more recent evidence has emerged to support this etiological conclusion, it is actually quite unlikely that the amyloid-A4 gene will be established as the cause of Alzheimer's disease. Duplication of the amyloid-A4 gene is not common in Alzheimer's disease (Podlisny et al. 1987) and therefore most cases of Alzheimer's cannot be attributed to this genetic abnormality.

Recent attention has been directed to another protein, apolipoprotein E (apo-E), the gene for which is located on chromosome 19. Apo-E is found in large quantities within the brain. Its synthesis is known to increase when a brain injury occurs, and therefore apo-E is associated with both growth and repair of the nervous system. This protein is localized to the senile plaques (that is, to the amyloid within the senile plaques), to vascular amyloid, and to neurofibrillary tangles, all three of which are found in patients with Alzheimer's disease. In the laboratory, apo-E binds to synthetic beta-amyloid, which is the primary constituent of the senile plaque (Strittmatter et al. 1993b). The appears to be a factor that is associated with late-onset familial Alzheimer's disease, as well as with some sporadic cases (Strittmatter et al. 1993a). In another study, the APOE4 allele was linked with Alzheimer's disease (Corder et al. 1993). In this study, APOE4 appeared to be associated with about half of the cases of Alzheimer's disease.

Some linkage studies focusing on manic-depressive illness have also been performed, but two problems arise concerning their results: first, these studies have not concentrated on elderly subjects; second, their results have been disputed. Egeland et al. (1983) studied an Amish population and found that a strong hereditary component contributed to the frequency of the disease. These researchers also found that manic-depressive illness was linked to a gene located on chromosome 11. This finding has not been verified in other samples.

Genetic Testing and Counseling

Since early 1994, it has been known that all the human chromosomes contain genes that are associated with a variety of diseases. The X sex chromosome contains the maximum number of disease-associated genes (112), whereas only one such gene has been identified on the Y sex chromosome. Chromosome 1 is the leader in the autosome category, with 55 disease-associated genes (Rennie 1994). However, this information must be used with considerable caution, as it appears that only 3% of all human diseases are caused by a single gene. The vast majority of genetic diseases are the result of the interactions of more than one gene. Often the presence of a single defective gene confers merely a predisposition to a disease. Moreover, the expression of a disease in a person who has inherited a single gene for a disease may differ in symptoms and severity from the manifestations of the disease in a person who inherits multiple genes for the disease. Furthermore, as most diseases are multifactorial, it is obvious that genetic testing is associated with serious limitations.

Another important issue that has been raised by the identification of genes associated with specific diseases concerns psychiatrists and patients with psychiatric disorders. Will treatment for psychiatric disorders that may be to any extent attributable to genetic defects be covered by patients' health insurance, or will these disorders be considered "preexisting conditions"? Some illnesses that are currently covered by insurance have only in the last few years been found to be related to genetic factors. These illnesses include diabetes mellitus (the gene for which is located on chromosome 11) and hemophilia (the gene for which is found on the X chromosome). It appears highly likely that many chronic disorders are related to genetic factors, including the autoimmune diseases and the decline in the efficiency of the immune system that are often seen in elderly populations.

Several clinically relevant caveats concerning genetic testing and counseling are appropriate here. First, genetic counseling is a very complicated specialty, and for best results the process requires that the counselor be highly knowledgeable and that the individual being tested be well informed. Second, the privacy of the individual must be given great consideration; unjustified discrimination—from insurance companies or employers, for example—may result from inadvertent disclosure of genetic test results. Third, it is important to remember that knowledge of the presence of a genetic defect is often a considerable source of anxiety for an affected individual, and also for a spouse or partner, siblings, parents, and other interested persons.

In addition to the cautions noted above, it is important to remember that information gained from genetic testing can be used constructively. For example, with some individuals, the technique of preimplantation genetic testing can be used to identify ova or sperm that carry defective genes. The ova and sperm can be fertilized in vitro, and those free of a defect can be implanted in the potential mother. This technique has been successfully used and has resulted in the birth of a daughter known to be free of Tay-Sachs disease (Rennie 1994).

References

Andreasen NC, Rice J, Endicott J, et al: Familial rates of defective disorders: a report from the National Institute of Mental Health Collaborative Study. Arch Gen Psychiatry 44:461–469, 1987

Brandt J, Wealsh KA, Breitner JCS, et al: Hereditary influences on cognitive functioning in older men: a study of 4,000 twin pairs. Arch Neurol 50:599–603, 1993

Breitner JCS, Murphy EC, Silverman JM, et al: Age-dependent expression of familiar risk in Alzheimer's disease. Am J Epidemiol 128:536–548, 1988

Corder EH, Saunders AM, Strittmatter WJ, et al: Gene dose of apolipoprotein E type 4 allele and the risk of Alzheimer's disease in late-onset families. Science 261:921–923, 1993

Curtsinger JW: Demography of genotypes: failure of the limited life-span paradigm in *Drosophilia melanogasler*. Science 258:461–462, 1992

Egeland D, Hofstetter AM: Amish Study I: affective disorders among the Amish, 1976–1980. Am J Psychiatry 140:56–63, 1983

Galton F: Twins and the nature-nurture problem (1876), reviewed in Behavioral Genetics, 2nd Edition. Edited by Plomin RR, DeFries R, McClearin G. New York, WH Freeman, 1990, pp 25–29

Goldgarber D, Lerman MI, McBride OW, et al: Characterization and chromosomal localization of a cDNA encoding brain amyloid of Alzheimer's disease. Science 235:877–880, 1987

Goto M, Rubenstein M, Wever J, et al: Genetic linkage of Werner's syndrome to DNA markers on chromosome 8. Nature 355:735–738, 1992

Gusella JF, MacDonald ME: Huntington's disease and repeating trinucleotides. N Engl J Med 330: 1450–1451, 1994

Hayflick L, Moorhead PS: The serial cultivation of human diploid cell strains. Exp Cell Res 25:585–621, 1961

Harmon DW: The free radical theory. J Gerontol 26: 451–457, 1971

Heller DA, DeFaire U, Pedersen NL, et al: Genetic and environmental influences on serum lipid levels in twins. N Engl J Med 328:1150–1156, 1993

Heston LL, Mastri AR, Anderson E, et al: Dementia of the Alzheimer's type: clinical genetics, natural history, and associated conditions. Arch Gen Psychiatry 38:1085–1090, 1981

Heyman A, Wilkinson WE, Hurwitz BJ, et al: Alzheimer's disease: genetic aspects and associated clinical disorders. Ann Neurol 14:507–515, 1983

Jarvik LF, Falek A, Kallman FJ: Survival trends in a senescent twin population. Am J Hum Genet 12:170–179, 1960

Jatz M, Pedersen NL, Plomin R, et al: Importance of shared genes in shared environments for symptoms of depression in older adults. J Abnorm Psychol 4:701–708, 1992

Kalin N: Ethics and DNA. Vertices (Spring):20–23, 1985

Martin GM: Genetics syndromes in man with potential relevance to the pathology of aging, in Genetic Effects of Aging (Birth Defects: Original Article Series, Vol 14, No. 1). Edited by Bergsma D, Harrison DE. New York, Alan R Liss, 1978, p 5

Martin GM, Tucker MS: Model systems for the genetic analysis of mechanisms of aging. J Gerontol 43:B33, 1988

Martin GM, Tucker MS: Genetics of human disease, longevity, and aging, in Principles of Geriatric Medicine and Gerontology, 3rd Edition. Edited by Hazard WR, Bierman EL, Blass JP, et al. New York, McGraw-Hill, 1994, pp 19–33

Mendlewicz J, Fieve RR, Reiner JD, et al: Manic-depressive illness: a comparative study of patients with and without a family history. Br J Psychiatry 120:523–530, 1972

Mohs RC, Breitner JCS, Silverman JM, et al: Alzheimer's disease: morbid risk among first-degree relatives approximately 50% by 90 years of age. Arch Gen Psychiatry 44:405–408, 1987

Oliver C, Holland AJ: Down's syndrome and Alzheimer's disease: a review. Psychol Med 14:307–322, 1985

Podlisny MB, Lee G, Selkoe DJ: Gene damage of the amyloid precursor protein in Alzheimer's disease. Science 238:666–669, 1987

Radloff LS: The CES-D scale: a self-report depression scale for research in the general population. Applied Psychological Measurement 1:385–401, 1977

Rennie J: Grading the gene tests. Sci Am 270:88–97, 1994

Salk D, Fujiwara Y, Martin GM (eds): Werner's Syndrome and Human Aging (Advances in Experimental Medicine and Biology, Vol 190). New York, Plenum, 1985

Schon EA, DiMauro S: Mitochondrial genome and its mutations. Karger Gazette No. 58, October 1994, pp 2–3

Stone K: Mania in the elderly. Br J Psychiatry 155: 220–224, 1989

Strittmatter WJ, Wisgarber KH, Huang DY, et al: Binding of human apolipoprotein E to synthetic amyloid beta peptide: isoform-specific effects and implications for late-onset Alzheimer's disease. Proc Natl Acad Sci USA 90:8098–8102, 1993a

Strittmatter WJ, Saunders AM, Schmechel D, et al: Apolipoprotein E: high-avidity binding to beta-amyloid and increased frequency of type 4 allele in late-onset familial Alzheimer's disease. Proc Natl Acad Sci USA 90:1977–1981, 1993b

Wallace DC: Mitochondriasis genetics: a paradigm for aging and degenerative diseases. Science 256:628–632, 1992

Watson JD: The Double Helix. New York, Atheneum, 1968

Whatley SA, Anderton BH: The genetics of Alzheimer's disease. International Journal of Geriatric Psychiatry 5:145–159, 1990

CHAPTER 7

Psychological Aspects
of Normal Aging

Ilene C. Siegler, Ph.D., M.P.H.
Leonard W. Poon, Ph.D.
David J. Madden, Ph.D.
Kathleen A. Welsh, Ph.D.

In this chapter we review pertinent findings in five areas concerned with the psychology of aging: 1) experimental and cognitive psychology, 2) neuropsychology, 3) personality and social psychology, 4) health and behavior, and 5) longevity and successful aging. These domains were chosen to reflect the interactive nature of age-related changes and differences in behavior. It is important for clinicians to have a yardstick against which to measure "abnormal" aging. There has been an explosion of interest in the psychology of aging, especially when basic findings are translated for use in the applied and clinical arenas (Poon et al. 1986). When elderly persons only are studied, we have a psychology of the aged rather than of aging. In contrast, the psychology of aging—or the life span view—emphasizes the continuity of patterns of behavior across the life cycle and is consistent with the case history approach in psychiatry. In areas in which cohort variation (social and historical trends) is not important, the best predictors of the behavior of a group of older persons may well be their own behaviors measured at an earlier point in time. To the extent that future generations of elderly persons

Work on this chapter has been supported by a variety of grants for each of the coauthors: Dr. Siegler's work is supported by Grants HL–36587 from the National Heart, Lung and Blood Institute and AG–09276 from the National Institute on Aging; Dr. Poon's work by Grants MH–43435 from the National Institute of Mental Health and AG–09957 from the National Institute on Aging; Dr. Madden's work by Grants AG–02163 and AG–11622 from the National Institute on Aging; and Dr. Welsh's work by Grants AG–05128 and AG–09997 from the National Institute on Aging.

We wish to thank Deborah J. Welke from the Gerontology Center at the University of Georgia and Ron Nelson from the Memory Disorders Clinic at Duke University Medical Center for their assistance in the preparation of this chapter.

are influenced by social change, a psychology of the aged will become increasingly dated; thus, findings on elderly cohorts must be interpreted with attention to the actual time of measurement of the findings reported. However both aspects—psychology of aging and of the aged—have generated important data, and findings in both areas will be reviewed.

In addition to this volume, there are companion handbooks in psychology, adult development, and mental health that would be of interest to readers of this chapter: *Handbook of the Psychology of Aging* (Birren and Schaie 1990), *Handbook for Clinical Memory Assessment of Older Adults* (Poon 1986), *Handbook of Aging and Cognition* (Craik and Salthouse 1992), and *The Handbook of Mental Health and Aging* (Birren et al. 1992). In addition, encyclopedias of aging (Maddox et al. 1987) and adult development (Kastenbaum 1993) are excellent sources of brief essays that review specific topics, and the series *Annual Reviews in Gerontology and Geriatrics* provides current information on a wide range of issues. This chapter builds on previous reviews by Siegler (1980), Siegler and Poon (1989), Poon and Siegler (1991); these publications should be consulted for more detail on the work in psychology of aging published before 1990.

Experimental and Cognitive Psychology

The term *cognition* subsumes the range of human intellectual functioning, including perception, attention, memory, reasoning, decision making, problem solving, and formation of complex structures of knowledge. Investigations of age-related cognitive changes have used both cross-sectional and longitudinal research paradigms and have yielded a complex mosaic of results. Age-related decline can be measured in many cognitive tasks, but areas of preserved functioning are also observed.

When examining the literature comparing cognitive performances among age groups, one should keep in mind that the level of cognition can be affected by a number of individual, environmental, and task characteristics regardless of chronological age (Hultsch and Dixon 1990; Poon 1985). Depending on the task and the situation, some persons tend to excel in certain types of performance and not in others. For example, in some cognitive tasks, some adults with high intelligence and more education

will show minimal decline in their performances with increasing age, whereas adults with lower intelligence and less education show significant decline (Bowles and Poon 1982; Poon and Fozard 1980). For those tasks, intelligence and education rather than chronological age are the important determinants of performance. In some cognitive tasks that are well practiced, the amount of age decline tends to be small or even nonexistent (Salthouse 1982).

Memory Functioning

Although all cognitive processes are intimately interrelated, age-related changes in memory functioning—in both normal and abnormal aging—have received by far the largest share of research effort. (For recent comprehensive reviews, see Craik and Jennings [1992], Hultsch and Dixon [1990], Light [1991; 1992], Poon et al. [1989], and Salthouse [1985a].) The large share of attention on memory performance and aging may be the result of two factors. First, memory decline is one of two major concerns articulated by community-dwelling elderly adults (the other being loss of energy) (Lowenthal et al. 1967). Second, memory dysfunction is a key behavioral benchmark in neuropsychopathology, such as dementia of the Alzheimer type (Kaszniak et al. 1986).

Poon (1985) listed 20 reviews focusing on memory and normal aging that had been published since 1980 and demonstrated the prevalence of the information-processing model in examining age-related differences in memory components, stages, and processes. The information-processing model postulates that information flows from input to output through a series of stages: registration, primary memory, secondary memory, and tertiary memory. Registration is sensory memory, a preattentive and highly unstable system. Primary (short-term) and secondary (long-term) memory (Waugh and Norman 1965) are responsible for the acquisition and retention of new information. Primary memory is conceptualized as a limited-capacity store in which information is still "in mind" as it is being used. If the information is not rehearsed instantaneously so that it can be stored in secondary memory, the information will be lost. Secondary memory is a repository of newly acquired information. Tertiary memory is the repository for well-learned and personal information.

It is important to note that this "linear" model is only one of several theoretical models of memory functioning. Others include, for example, the episodic/semantic memory model (Tulving 1972), the explicit/implicit memory model (Schacter 1987), the level-of-processing model (Craik and Lockhart 1972), and the parallel distributed model (McClelland and Rumelhart 1986). However, the information-processing model has been used extensively in the clinical domain, and the largest amount of data in the study of normal aging and in abnormal memory functioning has been gathered using this model (see Kaszniak et al. 1986 for a review). Findings on age-related differences in memory have been numerous, and only a brief review will be attempted here.

A general theme of memory aging research is that age-related declines tend to increase as the environmental support provided by the task decreases (Craik and Jennings 1992). Memory tasks such as free recall (for example, "Recall the ten words presented earlier") provide little support for the retrieval processes required to perform the task.

Recognition memory measures ("Is *chair* one of the words presented earlier?") provide more support. Age-related declines in memory performance are more evident in recall tasks, which involve self-directed retrieval, than in recognition tasks, although a decline is often observed in recognition as well. Aging is associated with a generalized slowing of virtually all forms of information processing (Cerella 1990; Myerson et al. 1990; Salthouse 1985b), and this slowing affects memory performance as well. Significant age-related slowing is evident in the initial registration of sensory input (Di Lollo et al. 1982), and in the retrieval of information from primary, secondary, and tertiary memory (Anders and Fozard 1973; Madden 1985). The capacity of primary memory (for example, digit span) is relatively constant as a function of age, whereas a significant age-related decline occurs in the capacity of secondary memory (see Tables 7–1 and 7–2). Consequently, aging appears to exert a profound effect in the acquisition and retrieval of new information in secondary memory.

Table 7–1. Cross-sectional experimental evidence for age-related slowing of memory processes

Component affected	Memory store				
	Sensory	Primary	Secondary	Working	Tertiary
Perceptual motor	Positive	Positive	Positive	—	Positive
Decision making	—	Positive	Positive	Positive	Negative

Source. Reprinted with permission from Fozard JL: "The Time for Remembering," in *Aging in the 1980s: Psychological Issues.* Edited by Poon LW. Washington, DC, American Psychological Association, 1980, p. 275.

Table 7–2. Evidence for age-related declines in memory capacity

Type of study and type of evidence	Memory store				
	Sensory	Primary	Secondary	Working	Tertiary
Cross-sectional studies					
Anecdotal	—	Positive	Positive	Positive	Positive
Psychometric	—	Negative	Positive	—	Negative
Experimental	Positive	Negative	Positive	Positive	Negative
Longitudinal studies					
Anecdotal	—	—	—	—	—
Psychometric	—	Negative	Positive	—	Negative
Experimental	—	—	Positive	—	—

Source. Reprinted with permission from Fozard JL: "The Time for Remembering," in *Aging in the 1980s: Psychological Issues.* Edited by Poon LW. Washington, DC, American Psychological Association, 1980, p. 274.

Attention

Age-related changes in attention are important to theories of cognitive aging, because the explanation of so many forms of cognitive performance—ranging from memory (Craik and Lockhart 1972; Hasher and Zacks 1979) to skill acquisition (Shiffrin and Schneider 1977)—involves the concept of attention in some way. As with memory, the investigation of attentional processes has been an active area of cognitive aging research (for reviews, see A. A. Hartley 1992; Madden 1990; Madden and Plude 1993). A fundamental distinction in this research is between selective attention and divided attention. In the former, the relevant and irrelevant sources of information are defined during task performance, allowing attention to be focused selectively on the relevant information. In the latter, multiple sources of information are relevant and must be attended simultaneously. Several investigators have reported that the use of selective attention (such as the use of advance information regarding the location of a target item) is just as efficient in older adults as in young adults (A. A. Hartley et al. 1990; Madden 1983, 1984; Plude and Hoyer 1986). Age-related declines in some forms of selective attention have been reported (Connelly and Hasher 1993; Hasher and Zacks 1988). In contrast, in divided-attention tasks, age-related performance decrements are more consistently evident (Guttentag 1989; McDowd and Craik 1988). An unresolved issue is the information-processing mechanism responsible for age differences in divided-attention performance. The performance differences may represent a slowing of all aspects of task performance (Salthouse et al. 1984), or may be related to a reduction in the availability of cognitive resources, independent of processing speed (Madden 1986a; Tun et al. 1992). Current research using neuroimaging procedures such as positron emission tomography suggests that performance of selective- and divided-attention tasks is mediated by distinct neural systems (Corbetta et al. 1990; La-Berge 1990), and aging may affect these neural systems differentially.

Intellectual Functioning

Research on intellectual functioning has one of the longest and most productive records in the psychology of aging (Schaie 1990; Siegler 1980). Three general patterns of findings can be described. First, the findings on intellectual functioning over the adult life span have been highly consistent. Hertzog and Schaie (1986), for example, reported the results of a new analysis of data from the Seattle Longitudinal Studies in which the data show a high degree of regularity in intellectual functioning across the adult age span. Second, there are two replicated patterns of intellectual performance across the life span. Crystallized abilities or knowledge acquired in the course of the socialization process tend to remain stable over the adult life span. Fluid abilities or abilities involved in the solution of novel problems tend to decline gradually from young to old adulthood (Schaie 1990). For example, McCrae and colleagues (1987) reported consistent declines in divergent thinking (a component of creativity) in cross-sectional, longitudinal, and cross-sequential analyses (a form of time-lag methods). Third, disease and pathology exert profound effects on intellectual functioning. Manton and co-workers (1986) evaluated cognitive and intellectual performance in the Duke Longitudinal Study population. The data indicated clear associations between poorer physical health (from heart disease or dementia) and declining cognitive performance, but not declining mental health, as measured by depression ratings. The findings that relate health factors to measures of intellectual functioning appear to depend upon the sensitivity of the health measures (Anstey et al. 1993).

Investigators holding newer views of intelligence seek to understand the meaning of intelligent behavior across the life cycle by defining prototypes at ages 30, 50, and 70 years (Berg and Sternberg 1992). Although there are global similarities in the prototypes—especially between ages 30 and 70—there are also important differences that emerge when the 30-year-old is compared with the 70-year-old. Cunningham and Haman (1992) provide an excellent, brief review of the work in this area, including the impact of depression (which can be considerable).

Health and Cognitive Functioning

Siegler and colleagues (1980) reviewed the theoretical reasons why physical health changes might account for what has been considered "normal" aging. We now have the results from a series of studies in which such health changes were tested directly.

Hultsch and co-workers (1993) tested a sample

of community-dwelling adults aged 55–86, employing measures of cognitive functioning in eight domains. Of this group, 37% rated their health as excellent, 44% as good, 16% as fair, and 2% as poor. Hultsch et al. reported on the presence and severity of 26 chronic illnesses, illness episodes, and the degree of impairment due to poor health, use of tobacco, drugs, and alcohol, and lifestyle activity patterns. Their findings on self-rated health and cognitive performance support those of Perlmutter and Nyquist (1990), who reported associations of self-rated health with measures of fluid intelligence and memory span. However, these individual differences in self-rated health did not account for most of the observed age differences. Salthouse and colleagues (1990) measured self-rated health, treatment for heart and blood pressure problems, and medication use, and found no evidence that variations in the health measures accounted for the cross-sectional age differences observed in cognitive functioning.

Rodin and McAvay (1992) evaluated changes in self-rated health in a short-term, 3-year longitudinal study of 251 men and women over age 62. Self-rated health tended to be stable: for all pairwise comparisons, 75% of the subjects showed no change, 11% improved, and 14% declined. For those with a negative change in self-rated health, there were baseline differences in new medications and lowered self-efficacy but no changes in illnesses per se. Changes in actual health were strongly related to changes in perceived health, as were psychosocial factors of declines in self-efficacy and increased depressive affect, suggesting that these declines reflect changes in mental health as well as physical health (see also Hooker and Siegler 1992).

Sands and Meredith (1992) evaluated the impact of blood pressure on changes in intellectual functioning and found that about 10% of the decline in performance could be explained by blood pressure changes. These findings essentially replicate those of Elias and co-workers (1990b) from their program of research on the effects of hypertension on cognitive performance. Recent analyses from the Framingham Study (Elias et al. 1993) confirm these findings, and a full discussion of the methodological components of this work can be found in Elias et al. (1995).

Metter and colleagues (1992), given the data from the Baltimore Longitudinal Study of Aging (BLSA), explored the health-cognition relationship based on the following question: When we select 60- and 80-year-old men to be "healthy" by the same criteria, are they the same? These investigators compared healthy (no incidence of heart disease, cancer, stroke) and unhealthy groups of 60-year-olds at age 60 and again at age 80, as well as a new group of healthy 80-year-olds. As expected, those in the healthier group had a significantly better mortality experience. When the healthy 60-year-olds were followed until age 80, only 44% would have qualified as healthy at 80. At age 60, systolic blood pressure and serum cholesterol were associated with good health at age 80. It is important to keep in mind that the burden of illness is not distributed evenly according to social class. House and co-workers (1992) have shown that 75-year-old persons of upper socioeconomic status (SES) have about 1.5 chronic conditions per person, the level that is reached in the lower SES ranges at about age 42–43. Thus, the issue of individual differences in health status are starting to be recognized in the psychology of aging (Siegler 1989, 1990).

Understanding and Remembering Written Information

Earlier studies of verbal memory and aging, using serial or paired-associate learning procedures, revealed substantial age-related deficits (for reviews see Hultsch and Dixon 1990; Poon 1985; Siegler 1980). A number of investigators have asked whether these findings also accurately predict the processing of written or spoken information in everyday life. These questions initiated a number of recent research programs focusing on the investigation of age differences in "discourse," "text," or "prose" processing—the acquisition of written or spoken communications.

The first generation of research on text processing presented contradictory and conflicting findings. Some investigators found clear-cut age deficits (Cohen 1979; Gordon and Clark 1974; Zelinski et al. 1980), although others found no age difference (Harker et al. 1982; Meyer and Rice 1981; Taub 1979). To address these conflicting results, the second generation of research examined in detail the possible contributions of individual differences, the properties of the text to be processed, and the task demand on the observed processing performance (for detailed reviews, see Meyer and Rice 1989; J. T. Hartley 1989). For example, faster presentation rates compromise the comprehension and recall performance of elderly persons more than of young adults (J. T. Hartley 1989). This set of results seems to support the finding of cognitive slowing with increasing age, so that the difficulty of a task would affect the recall performance more in older than in young adults.

The level of education and verbal intelligence could account for some portion of the observed age effects on text recall performance (Meyer and Rice 1989). Age deficits in prose recall were found to be significant for adults with average and low verbal ability. High-verbal old adults (classified as such according to their vocabulary scores on the Wechsler Adult Intelligence Scale—Revised [WAIS-R; Wechsler 1981]) appear to utilize text structure as effectively as young adults (Meyer and Rice 1989) and to take advantage of organized structures to facilitate their processing. On the other hand, low-verbal old adults show less sensitivity to text structures that could assist them in the processing task. The important research objective for everyday appreciation is the identification of factors for subtypes of individuals that could 1) facilitate processing and 2) ensure retention and the long-term maintenance of the facilitated performance.

Madden (1986b) found that recognition memory for words was influenced significantly by both age and verbal ability. Memory performance decreased as a function of increasing age and decreasing WAIS-R vocabulary score. These effects were independent of each other, however, and in fact, the more pronounced age-related decline was found in the subjects with higher verbal ability.

Speech Comprehension

Written material can be scanned and reviewed during processing, but spoken language can only be processed in a serial manner. Older adults have been shown to suffer from deficits in auditory processing (see Olsho et al. 1985 for a review) and speed of processing (Poon 1985); however, older adults do not seem to have disproportionate problems in processing everyday conversations or spoken input from television or radio.

A number of investigators have found clear deficits in the ability of older adults to process spoken language (Cohen 1979; Cohen and Faulkner 1982); for reviews, see Stine et al. (1989) and Tun and Wingfield (1993). One of the major contributors to age-related peripheral hearing decline is presbycusis, which includes loss of sensitivity to higher auditory frequencies, increased tendency to recruitment, and increased probability of phonemic regression or decreased speech intelligibility. An important question for current research programs is how peripheral hearing deficits interact with the available cognitive resources and experiences of older persons. The answer to this question is crucial both for the understanding of speech comprehension performance by older individuals and for the design of methods to compensate for observed deficits.

In an experiment reported by Wingfield et al. (1985), young and elderly subjects processed lists of words varying in linguistic redundancy that were presented at various speeds. Although the performance of all subjects was affected by speech rate and the degree of redundancy, the performance of those in the elderly group was differentially depressed by increasing speech rate and by decreasing linguistic constraints. In other words, the results suggested that the older listeners rely on both the redundancy of language and on linguistic constraints to maintain an acceptable level of performance. Taken together, these preliminary results suggest that older listeners can compensate for peripheral hearing decline and that therapeutic procedures should take into account the individual's cognitive strengths and experiences.

Problem Solving

A series of studies (for example, Denney 1989; J. T. Hartley 1989) was performed in which age-related differences in problem solving were examined with standard psychometric tests and tests imitating problems encountered in everyday situations. Three sets of general observations can be made from these studies. First, tests of performance in everyday problem-solving tasks show that middle-aged adults can, in some situations, perform better than young adults, but performance decline is still evident for the older adults (Denney 1989). Second, traditional laboratory-based problem-solving tasks seem to be predictive of everyday problem-solving performances for older adults. Third, a significant amount of research remains to be done to explore changes of problem-solving styles and strategies in view of declining physical and cognitive abilities of older persons.

Neuropsychology

The psychometric and neuropsychological literature (Albert and Kaplan 1980; Klisz 1978) support the notion of greater decline in the functions of the right hemisphere as compared with those of the left. However, controlled laboratory experiments (such as those conducted by Borod and Goodglass 1980; Nebes et al. 1983; Park et al. 1983) have revealed minimal or no age differences. Thus, the question remains whether there is a differential decline in spatial processing with increasing age. If there is, then a second question must be asked concerning the origin of this decline: Is the observed deficit a result of biologically determined differential decline in the right hemisphere, or is the right-hemisphere decline due to differential disuse of right- compared with left-hemisphere functions over the life span? Although the two questions seem circular, modes of remediation would differ depending on the answers.

From a clinical evaluation perspective, tests of right hemisphere functioning do not always predict everyday spatially related problems. In a study examining the efficiency of shopping routes in supermarkets, Kirasic (1989) reported that, regardless of age group, an individual's psychometric spatial abilities seemed to be poor predictors of shopping efficiency. It would be helpful to pursue how spatial and other cognitive abilities interact in various situational demands to affect successful adaptation among community-dwelling elderly persons.

Research in neuropsychology has also contributed to the understanding of normal aging through broad-based neurobehavioral studies of normal elderly individuals and patients with cognitive syndromes (such as Alzheimer's disease) whose symptoms are often confused with normal aging processes. To separate normal age changes from disease effects, investigators often use longitudinal evaluation to confirm diagnostic placement (Flicker et al. 1993; Katzman et al. 1989) including, when possible, neuropathological verification (Hof et al. 1992; Morris et al. 1991). Researchers in this field also have taken advantage of the advances in neuroimaging to enhance diagnostic accuracy (Rapoport 1991). Excellent reviews of geriatric neuropsychology can be found in Albert and Moss (1988), Huppert (1994), Poon (1986), and Van Gorp and Mahler (1990). Recent updates on structural brain imaging (magnetic resonance imaging, or MRI) and functional brain im-

aging in aging individuals (single photon emission computed tomography, or SPECT, and positron emission tomography, or PET) can be found in Coffey et al. (1992), Hoffman et al. (1989), Parashos and Coffey (1994), and Welsh and Hoffman (in press). Age-related changes in brain morphology are summarized in Chapter 4 of this text and will not be reiterated here.

Most studies involving examination of the cognitive changes associated with aging have focused on one functional domain in isolation—memory, intellect, or attention, for example. Studies focusing on multiple domains simultaneously, as is possible with broad-based neuropsychological designs, have provided some insight into how these different areas of information-processing functions interact and change with aging of the nervous system (Van Gorp and Mahler 1990). In one important early study (Benton et al. 1981), a large sample of normal older adults participated in a battery of neuropsychological tests. The results showed little evidence of generalized decline in cognitive function before age 80. Significant declines were seen in short-term visual memory, serial digit learning, and facial recognition. Subsequent studies have supported the findings that these particular functions (construction, speed of information processing, and nonverbal perceptual processing) are vulnerable to aging (Koss et al. 1991). Similarly, in studies using the Wechsler Adult Intelligence Scales (WAIS, WAIS-R), selective decline in nonverbal performance and relative stability in verbal abilities has been demonstrated with advancing age (Botwinick 1977).

Several interpretations have been proposed regarding the functional and anatomical significance of these findings. One interpretation for the observations concerning the cognitive changes with aging is that age-associated degenerative changes are lateralized to the right hemisphere (Goldstein and Shelly 1981; Klisz 1978; Schaie and Schaie 1977). This hypothesis is based primarily on the observation that right hemisphere brain lesions often produce a discrepancy between verbal and nonverbal performance similar to that seen in aging individuals (Benton 1994; Lezak 1983). Those who argue against this explanation note that neuroanatomical and neuroimaging studies of normal elderly adults fail to show preferential deterioration of right hemisphere structures (Brody 1978; Coffey et al. 1992; Gur et al. 1987; Parashos and Coffey 1994; Welsh and Hoffman, in press). In addition, many investigators have pointed out that the nonverbal subtests of the WAIS/WAIS-R, used as evidence of right hemisphere function, are confounded by their reliance on speed of responding, thereby rendering them less than ideal for comparisons of right- and left-hemisphere integrity (Mittenberg et al. 1989).

An alternative proposal is based on Cattell's construct of "fluid" versus "crystallized" intelligence (Cattell 1963). According to this model, it is hypothesized that fluid intellectual capacities (such as novel, active problem-solving ability) are affected by aging, whereas crystallized intelligence (overlearned, long-held information, usually verbal in nature) is stable across the life span (Horn 1982). Although an intriguing idea, this hypothesis does not appear to be completely adequate when subjected to testing. The results of at least two studies based on factor analysis of a broad-based neuropsychological assessment suggest that other factors, such as speed of information processing, may better account for the age-related changes in performance (Koss et al. 1991; Van Gorp et al. 1990). This "speed of processing" interpretation is consistent with the popular notion elucidated in the cognitive psychology literature (Salthouse 1985b). No hemispheric lateralization is predicted by either the fluid intelligence deficit or the speed of information-processing models. However, the cognitive processes subsumed in each model (such as novel problem solving, attention, and perceptual-motor integration) have all been ascribed in the neuropsychological literature to frontal lobe function (Benton 1994; Lezak 1983).

A current hypothesis, supported by converging lines of evidence from neuropsychology and cognitive psychology, is that normal aging involves specific declines in frontal lobe neocortex and interconnected subcortical brain structures (Albert and Kaplan 1980; Braun and Lalonde 1990; Daigneault et al. 1992; Daigneault and Braun 1993; Mittenberg et al. 1989; Parkin and Walter 1991; Van Gorp and Mahler 1990). In line with this notion, neuropsychological changes reported in frontal lobe damage have been observed in normal aging (Huppert 1994; Van Gorp et al. 1990; Whelihan and Lesher 1985). In contrast, other cognitive changes—such as rapid forgetting—typically associated with Alzheimer's disease and mesial temporal lobe dysfunction (Welsh et al. 1991) are not typical of normal aging (Ivnik et al. 1991; Peterson et al. 1992; Welsh et al. 1994). Brain

imaging studies and neuropathological investigations in normal elderly populations provide additional support for this hypothesis. Whereas generalized brain atrophy and decreases in cerebral blood flow with advanced age have been commonly noted (Parashos and Coffey 1994; Welsh and Hoffman, in press), some investigators report particularly pronounced reductions in frontal lobe blood flow and volume in aged populations (Gur et al. 1987, and Coffey et al. 1992, respectively). Demyelination of subcortical, periventricular brain structures is also common in aging and is associated with signs of frontal lobe deficits on neuropsychological examination (Boone et al. 1992; Coffey et al. 1992; Schmidt et al. 1993). Finally, histopathological studies show selective frontal lobe decline in the aging brain, with the most significant cell loss identified in the superior frontal, precentral, and superior temporal gyri (Creasey and Rapoport 1985; Haug et al. 1983).

Verification of the selective vulnerability of the frontal lobe to aging requires further empirical investigation. Longitudinal studies involving repeat neuroimaging studies (MRI volumetrics) may permit evaluation of structural brain changes associated with aging. Experimental designs that use functional brain imaging (PET or SPECT) under conditions of behavioral activation may also be helpful in sorting out the relative contribution of the various brain areas to the cognitive changes of aging (for review, see Gur et al. 1992; Haxby et al. 1991; Parks et al. 1988).

Applications

The data from research regarding the cognitive psychology of aging help to answer the question of how middle-aged and older adults perform in the workplace and in other situations in which learning of new information is required (Charness and Bosman 1992; Cross 1981; Park 1992; Stagner 1985). As a result of investigation in this area, we no longer ask whether older persons can learn, but instead ponder the question, What is the most effective way to teach older persons the things they want to learn? Willis (1985) reviewed the literature and concluded that older persons' learning capacities are greater and more plastic than had been realized previously, and later extended this discussion to include the competence of the aged, with particular attention to associations between everyday competence (assessed as independence in activities of daily living) and physical as well as mental health (Willis 1991).

Morrell and colleagues (1990) examined how age-related differences in memory could affect the retention of labeling of prescription drugs. Since pictorial input tends to facilitate the organization of information, they evaluated whether verbal, pictorial, or mixed input could facilitate the understanding and recall of information concerning prescriptions. They confirmed the finding that older adults were less able to comprehend prescription information. Younger adults were able to improve their understanding and retention of prescription information when the instructions included a mixed format of written and pictorial information. However, the same type of information was confusing to older adults. Younger adults were also able to remember more prescription information presented in both written and mixed formats. This research demonstrated that there are age-related differences in methods of facilitating the understanding and retention of prescription information. Methods that may work for one age group may not be applicable for another.

Willis and Schaie (1986) evaluated the effects of cognitive training among panel members involved in Schaie's Seattle Longitudinal Study. A group of subjects with a mean age of 72.8 (range 64–95) were classified as "stable" or "decliners" over a 14-year period on measures of inductive reasoning and spatial orientation. Of the 107 subjects, 46.7% were stable, 31% declined on one measure, and 21.8% declined on both measures. A program was devised to provide training on the ability that had declined. Both stable and decliner groups benefited equally and significantly from training. The group of decliners returned to their original levels, and the stable group improved beyond their original levels of performance. These results convincingly indicate that target training on complex tasks can be effective for even very old persons. The implication of these findings is that an older individual past the current retirement age could entertain the option of staying in the work force if he or she wished to do so and could obtain the proper training.

Issues of productivity and age remain important. Sterns and Alexander (1987) presented a comprehensive review of industrial gerontology and pointed out that plant closings, reductions in work

force, and the introduction of new technologies will continue to challenge the role of the older employee in the workplace. The Age Discrimination in Employment Act (ADEA) offers individuals protection from being forced out of the work force prematurely (see Edelman and Siegler 1978 for a history of the act). However, as the preferred retirement age in the United States decreases and longevity increases, it is conceivable that more and more individuals will spend up to 40 years in retirement—say from age 55 to age 95. This may necessitate considerable changes both in the concept of retirement and in its funding.

Personality and Social Psychology

Patterns of Personality Development

The findings of researchers regarding patterns of adult personality development suggest that 1) greater stability in personality across the adult life cycle is seen when it is measured with objective measures of personality (such as self-report paper and pencil) rather than subjective tests (such as ratings from psychiatric interviews); 2) self-esteem is maintained at adult levels in later life; 3) different personality typologies adapt or respond differently to life events; and 4) gender differences are typical. Not all personality patterns are associated with the same consequences. Patterns characterized by better adjustment earlier in life may well lead to more positive outcomes later in life. Although more recent reviews of personality have not led to changes in the conclusions presented above, they do indicate an increased interest in theoretical structures concerning the development and maintenance of personality in middle and later life (Caspi and Bem 1990; Kogan 1990; McCrae and Costa 1990; Whitbourne 1987).

Levinson (1986) views the life cycle as a life structure with alternating periods of building and rebuilding. Roberts and Newton (1987) found that age ranges and themes were similar for women even though the content of the life structure was different. Levinson's system has yet to be applied to the lives of the elderly but should provide a useful paradigm for future research.

Costa et al. (1986), with data from the National Health and Nutrition Examination Survey (NHANES I) Follow-Up Study, reported stability in normal personality, replicating other longitudinal findings

(McCrae and Costa 1984; Costa and McCrae 1986, 1989). They indicated the generalizability of findings that are typically reported on subjects involved in longitudinal studies. Persons who participate in longitudinal studies tend to have better outcomes than those in national samples (Fozard et al. 1990). It is also interesting that in an analysis designed to determine whether the revision of the Minnesota Multiphasic Personality Inventory (MMPI; Hathaway and McKinley 1989) requires different norms for the elderly, an analysis of data from the Normative Aging Study indicated that different norms were not warranted (Butcher et al. 1991).

Frazier and colleagues (1993) recently published a review of the major longitudinal studies of aging with social and psychological content. Field (1991) edited a special issue of the *Journal of Gerontology* focusing on personality, including a useful introductory essay. Field and Millsap (1991) reported on findings from the Berkeley Older Generation Study of 420 men and women first tested in 1928–1929 as young adults, as the parents of children involved in the Berkeley Growth and Guidance Study. Follow-up on the parents has continued for 55 years. Personality characteristics were rated for 21 traits observed during intensive interviews at two times of measurement—1969 and 1988. The ratings were factor-analyzed into five categories: intellect, agreeableness, satisfaction, "energetic," and extraversion. All of the personality components were seen to be stable except for energetic; the changes in mean levels for this component were larger than the correlations would indicate, showing both stability and change in personality functioning, depending on the trait studied.

Schaie and Willis (1991) presented data from the Seattle Longitudinal Study for birth cohorts (1889–1959) who ranged from 22 to 84 years of age at the time of enrollment in the study; the study was conducted over a period of 35 years, with subjects tested in 1956, 1963, 1970, 1977, and 1984. This report updated the previous findings of Schaie and Parham (1976) with personality and psychomotor data derived from the Test of Behavioral Rigidity. Schaie and Willis found significant differences in successive cohorts except on instructional set flexibility, with a modest but statistically significant decline in social responsibility. The findings from this elegant study suggest substantial cohort variation for some personality domains similar to the well-known vari-

ation found for intellectual development: recent generations are more flexible.

Hagberg and colleagues (1991) found evidence of stability in field independence in a longitudinal study of Swedish elderly. In addition, stability of field independence was related to greater survival in the 16-year follow-up period.

In recent years, the results of studies of personality change in later life have become available (Chatterjee et al. 1992; Siegler et al. 1991, 1994; Strauss et al. 1993; R. B. Williams et al. 1995). This set of studies evaluated the impact of Alzheimer's disease on rated personality change. The researchers found consistent increases in the domain of neuroticism, and decreases in the domains of extraversion, openness, and conscientiousness, with stability in agreeableness. These findings are not inconsistent with the patterns defined by Costa and McCrae (1989), as McCrae (1993) maintains that when an individual has a disease in which personality change is a symptom, one would not expect to see stability. The literature on emotion across the life span supports both stability and change in personality (Lawton et al. 1992). Thomae (1992) provides an excellent review of findings on emotion and personality that were derived from the Bonn Longitudinal Study on Aging.

Coping

The literature on coping (for example, Palmore et al. 1979) has often focused on predictable life events, and investigators have generally found that although older persons have fewer stressful life events, 1) their coping capacities are excellent, and 2) their coping capacities differ by gender because the distribution of life events tends to vary by gender (George and Siegler 1982; Siegler and George 1983). Aldwin (1992) looked at stress and coping across the life span and concluded that advanced age is no hindrance to coping behaviors. Kahana's (1992) review of the literature on extreme stress and its implications for adaptation in later life illustrates the impact of such stress on the coping process and the extraordinary resilience of older persons.

Social Interactions and Attributions

Research on the social nature of later life has reemerged with the publication of Carstensen's (1991) view of selectivity theory as a replacement for the disengagement/activity controversy of old. The term *se-*

lectivity refers to the fact that social interactions are chosen for specific reasons and functions in later life. Fredrickson and Carstensen (1990) found that older persons have different preferences for interactions than younger individuals do, leaning toward interactions with more familiar rather than novel persons. However, when younger persons were put into situations invested with a feeling of time limitation (as a way to model aging), they also preferred familiar persons. Rapkin and Fisher (1992a, 1992b) reported the results of their study of goals of older adults and the interactions with levels of life satisfaction. When compared with the findings of Hooker and Siegler (1993), Rapkin and Fisher's results suggest that motivation and goal achievement have different associations in middle and later life.

Information from research on the stress/illness paradigm, life events, and models of coping continues to contribute in significant ways to our understanding of developmental patterns in middle and later life. An excellent review and approach to understanding social factors in health and aging can be found in Felton and Revenson (1990) and in the volume edited by Wykle and colleagues (1992).

Hooker and Kaus (1992) studied health-related possible selves. Respondents were asked to describe their future hoped-for and feared possible selves. Respondents were also measured on their health behaviors and the value they place on health. Health behaviors, rather than health values, were predicted by health-related possible selves. Hoped-for selves were predicted primarily by outcome expectancies; gender was the strongest predictor of feared selves. These findings suggest that older persons are responsive to health promotion messages and will do what they can, while being realistic enough to recognize that, generally, dreaded health events cannot be prevented.

There has been a developing interest in the role of social support as a moderating variable in the lives of middle-aged and older persons. Carstensen (1991) points out that social contact is not the same as social support, and there is evidence that the balance between family and friends as sources of social support may change across the life cycle, with greater continuity for family (Levitt et al. 1993). Studies show a strong relationship between the presence of social support and health, primarily in terms of survival (House et al. 1988). Berkman and colleagues (1993) reviewed the interactions between social support and both cardiovascular disease and mortality. They found that similar patterns of social support existed for men and women, and noted equal consequences for lowered social support for both genders. A number of studies confirmed our expectation that a strong social support system is related positively to physical and mental health and to survival among elderly persons (R. B. Williams et al. 1992). Jackson and Antonucci (1992) provide an excellent discussion of the role of social support in the lives of older persons, and they point out the importance of understanding the mechanisms of social support so that appropriate interventions can be developed.

Health and Behavior

As life expectancy increases, it becomes clear that very different subgroups exist among the elderly (Siegler 1989, 1992). Variations in health, rather than age, may be responsible for a large portion of observed age differences (Siegler and Costa 1985), and these age/health interactions may be mediated by social class (House et al. 1992). Frail, impaired elderly individuals appear to have very little in common with their more robust peers of the same age. Similarly, the data are beginning to show that, even in the middle years, the incidence of premature morbidity and mortality may be reduced by modification of risk factors (Kaplan 1992; Schoenbach 1985). Thus, attention to behavioral factors and their relationship to health is important for practical as well as theoretical reasons (Elias et al. 1990a; Fozard et al. 1990; Siegler 1990). Clipp and co-workers (1992) provide an elegant system for classifying trajectories of physical and emotional health in the Terman gifted sample, which mirrors the understanding that the clinician should have of a particular patient.

Behavioral Medicine

Behavioral medicine is the study of the role that behavioral factors can play in our understanding of the causes and consequences of disease (Rodin 1987). Behavioral medicine, an outgrowth of the tradition in psychosomatic medicine, is particularly useful in the study of aging because so many diseases of the elderly have behavioral components and because elderly persons in general respond to behavioral treatment approaches.

Along these lines, there has been an increase of attention to elderly populations as targets of public health interventions (Phillips and Gaylord 1985). Behavioral factors have been shown to be important predictors of coronary heart disease (CHD) (Friedman and Booth-Kewley 1987; R. B. Williams et al. 1980, 1985), and the application of behavioral strategies has resulted in more successful treatment of patients with arthritis (Verbrugge 1987) and diabetes (Surwit et al. 1982). Little is known about the role of behavioral factors in the etiology of stroke, dementia (Mortimer and Schumann 1981), or cancer (Fox 1978); however, behavioral treatments have proven useful in the management of patients with these conditions (M. M. Baltes 1987). For example, Benfante and colleagues (1991) reported data from the Honolulu Heart Program that indicated smoking continues to be a risk factor for CHD in elderly men. Kaplan (1992) indicates that risk factor modification, even in the later years, improves health and survival. In the New Haven Established Populations for Epidemiologic Studies of the Elderly (EPESE), which began in 1982, investigators explored CHD risk among the elderly (Seeman et al. 1993), using baseline variables to predict CHD outcomes over a 6-year period. The study population comprised a total of 2,812 men and women aged 65 and over. The findings demonstrate important gender differences in risk profiles and reconfirm the continued importance of relative weight, smoking, hypertension medication, and diabetes in determining CHD risk.

There is also evidence that a curvilinear relationship exists between age and "coronary-prone" personality characteristics such as hostility (R. B. Williams 1989); this relationship peaks in adolescence and again in old age (Barefoot et al. 1991, 1993; Siegler 1994; Zonderman et al. 1993). These findings can be compared with those of Lawton and colleagues (1993), who examined the structure of affect and found few differences in hostility between younger (ages 18–30) and middle-aged (ages 31–59) groups, but increases in subjects in later life (age 60 and older). The differences may be due to the age range of the youngest group.

Swan and co-workers (1991) reported on the 27-year follow-up of the Western Collaborative Group Study, the study that indicated that the Type A behavior pattern was an independent risk factor for CHD. These researchers noted that men who were classified as Type A at baseline and the 27-year follow-up evaluation were more likely to be involuntarily retired from work. Although involuntary retirement was associated with poorer mental and physical health, these negative effects could not be attributed to differential distribution of the Type A behavior pattern by type of retirement (i.e., voluntary or involuntary).

Caregiving has been recognized as a normative or expected stress of later life. Vitaliano and colleagues (1994) suggest a model indicating that the stress of caregiving may lead to a heightened incidence of cardiovascular disease in the caregivers, reflecting a breakdown in coping capacity under conditions of unrelenting stress (Vitaliano et al. 1991). Furthermore, Hooker and co-workers (1992) have shown that personality factors in the caregiver are related to coping behaviors and perceptions of stress.

Felton and Revenson (1987) studied middle-aged and older persons with hypertension, rheumatoid arthritis, diabetes, and cancer. Coping was measured by six factor scales analytically derived from the Lazarus Ways of Coping Scale. The resulting interactions of age, coping strategy, and the measure of illness tested underscore the complexity inherent in determining age relationships in this area. Keefe and D. A. Williams (1990) studied coping strategies of patients with chronic pain and found few age differences when the coping task was similar.

Emery et al. (1991) reviewed the effects of physical exercise on personality, mood, cognitive functioning, and behavioral adaptation. Generally, individuals report more positive effects of the exercise intervention than can be shown from the objective data. Although prospective epidemiological studies have shown that physical activity is related to enhanced survival, randomized trials of exercise interventions have yet to show mortality reductions. Thus, although there are many reasons to expect that exercise is beneficial for aging persons, this has not been fully documented.

Longevity and Successful/Unsuccessful Aging

Longevity and successful aging are two distinct constructs, although successful aging is often equated with longevity. An excellent discussion of the psychological understanding of longevity can be found in Woodruff-Pak and Winn (1990).

The bulk of our knowledge about longevity is derived from longitudinal studies with sufficient repeated study durations and sample size to examine the predictive power of specific variables (for example, Thomae 1976) and from studies of the long-lived (e.g., Beard 1991). The attempt to understanding the mechanisms of longevity and successful aging by comparing the long-lived with younger cohorts in cross-sectional studies can be hazardous, because of strong cohort differences in education, health care practices, eating patterns, lifelong experiences, and coping styles (to name just a few of the possible confounding factors).

In the Georgia Centenarian Study, Poon and colleagues (1992a) are investigating cross-sectional differences and longitudinal changes in three panels of community-dwelling and cognitively intact centenarians, octogenarians, and sexagenarians. Included is an examination of influences of and interactions among factors that have been used in studies of successful aging: family longevity, environmental support, individual characteristics, adaptational skills, functional and mental health, nutrition, and life satisfaction (P. B. Baltes and M. M. Baltes 1990). Also included in the Georgia Centenarian Study are activities, personality, coping styles, intelligence, cognition, religiosity, and reminiscence. Although the study is still in its infancy, the researchers have found some interesting characteristics related to the long-lived:

1. Centenarians scored higher in dominance, suspiciousness, and imagination, and lower in active behavioral coping (Martin et al. 1992). Personality factors were found to influence functional abilities and health of centenarians (Martin et al. 1993).
2. Although cognitive resources are lower in the nondemented centenarians than in the younger subjects, the centenarians' problem-solving abilities tend to remain intact. Both functional and mental health are found to influence cognition in the very old, and individuals with higher cognitive functions tend to better sustain their instrumental activities of daily living (Poon et al. 1992b).
3. Religiosity does not seem to change from younger to older cohorts, and religiosity seems to relate strongly to physical but not to mental health (Courtenay et al. 1992).
4. Centenarians tend to eat breakfast more regularly, avoid weight-loss diets and large fluctuations in body weight, and consume slightly more vegetables. On the other hand, centenarians were less likely to consume diets low in fat and to comply with nutritional guidelines designed to reduce the risk of chronic disease (Johnson et al. 1992).
5. Among economic, social, mental health, and cognitive resources, it is evident that economic resources become more important predictors of level of performance of instrumental activities of daily living as individuals age; this has been observed among the octogenarians and is especially true of the centenarians in the study (Poon et al. 1993).

From among the initial findings derived from the Georgia Centenarian Study, one set of questions stands out. As expected, the overall resources tend to be significantly diminished for community-dwelling and cognitively intact centenarians (Martin et al., in press), so why do they tend to perceive themselves to be doing as well as their younger counterparts (Goetting et al., in press)? Are centenarians using special techniques of compensation that they have developed from their lifelong experiences that we should learn if we want to live to be centenarians?

The findings from centenarian studies from Hungary, France, Japan, Sweden, Mexico, and the United States imply that there are different paths to longevity (Poon et al. 1993). For some subtypes or groups of centenarians, strong genetic tendencies or family history of longevity may be most important. For others, the key to longevity may be their ability to efficiently adapt to circumstances throughout their lives, either because of high intelligence and problem-solving abilities or because of adaptive personality types. The debate over nature versus nurture will continue for some time to come.

Although special care must be taken in studying these oldest-old populations, it is generally agreed that such research could result in the discovery of new principles about the aging process or in the validation of the soundness of existing principles. Researchers have only begun to understand the mechanisms underlying longevity and successful adaptation of the oldest-old. Only limited effort has been expended to resolve commonality and differences in these underlying mechanisms across race, gender, ethnic, and cultural domains.

Siegler and O'Keefe (1992) discussed aging and health as part of a policy forum presented by the American Psychological Association. Their review of the role of behavioral factors in health clearly shows—as much of the data presented earlier in this chapter indicate—that for many individuals, old age is really just an extended phase of middle age, with only modest changes in mind and body. Further, adaptation to these changes is well within the range of an individual's capability, and the use of certain behavioral strategies can help to maintain this optimistic pattern of successful aging.

However, there is another side of the story—what might be called "the Grim Side of Gerontology." Cassel and co-workers (1992), in an article entitled "The Price of Success," discussed the implications of the survival of frail elderly persons. For example, there is a cost to society for increased medical care for the frail elderly and for long-term care for persons who depend on others to help them with activities of daily living. The results of research in psychology of aging (for example, see Parmelee et al. 1991) and studies of the frail mentally ill in nursing homes (for example, Strahan and Burns 1991) suggest the tremendous needs of the frail elderly for appropriate care.

Longevity is increasing among both the successfully and the unsuccessfully aging populations, and the definition of "normal" aging—that is, aging without disease—is becoming more difficult to sustain. Clinicians must approach patients with a full knowledge of the variety of medical and psychiatric conditions that can be a part of the normal aging picture, and then set expectations for continued successful or unsuccessful aging for each patient individually.

References

Albert MS, Kaplan E: Organic implications of neuropsychological deficits in the elderly, in New Directions in Memory and Aging: Proceedings of the George Talland Memorial Conference. Edited by Poon LW, Fozard JL, Cermak LS, et al. Hillsdale, NJ, Lawrence Erlbaum, 1980, pp 403–432

Albert MS, Moss M: Geriatric Neuropsychology. New York, Guilford, 1988

Aldwin CM: Aging, coping, and efficacy: theoretical framework for examining coping in life-span developmental context, in Stress and Health Among the Elderly. Edited by Wykle ML, Khana E, Kowal J. New York, Springer, 1992, pp 96–113

Anders TR, Fozard JL: Effects of age upon retrieval from primary and secondary memory. Developmental Psychology 9:411–415, 1973

Anstey K, Stankov L, Lord S: Primary aging, secondary aging, and intelligence. Psychol Aging 8:562–570, 1993

Baltes MM: Behavioral modification, in Encyclopedia of Aging. Edited by Maddox GL. New York, Springer, 1987, pp 56–57

Baltes PB, Baltes MM: Successful Aging: Perspectives From the Behavioral Sciences. New York, Cambridge University Press, 1990

Barefoot JC, Peterson BL, Dahlstrom WG, et al: Hostility patterns and health implications: correlates of Cook-Medley scores in a national survey. Health Psychol 10:18–24, 1991

Barefoot JC, Beckham JC, Haney TL, et al: Age differences in hostility among middle-aged and older adults. Psychol Aging 8:3–9, 1993

Beard BB: Centenarians: The New Generation. Westport, CT, Greenwood Press, 1991

Benfante R, Reed D, Frank J: Does cigarette smoking have an independent effect on coronary heart disease incidence in the elderly? Am J Public Health 81:897–899, 1991

Benton AL: Neuropsychological assessment. Annu Rev Psychol 45:1–23, 1994

Benton AL, Eslinger RJ, Damasio AR: Normative observations on neuropsychological test performances in old age. Journal of Clinical Neuropsychology 3:33–42, 1981

Berg CA, Sternberg RJ: Adults' conceptions of intelligence cross the adult life span. Psychol Aging 7:221–231, 1992

Berkman LF, Vaccarion V, Seeman T: Gender differences in cardiovascular morbidity and mortality: the contribution of social networks and social support. Annals of Behavioral Medicine 15:112–117, 1993

Birren JE, Schaie KW (eds): Handbook of the Psychology of Aging, 3rd Edition. New York, Academic Press, 1990

Birren JE, Sloane RB, Cohen GD (eds): Handbook of Mental Health and Aging. New York, Academic Press, 1992

Boone KB, Miller BL, Lesser IM, et al: Neuropsychological correlates of white-matter lesions in healthy elderly subjects: a threshold effect. Arch Neurol 49:549–554, 1992

Borod JC, Goodglass H: Lateralization of linguistic and melodic processing with age. Neuropsychologia 18:79–83, 1980

Botwinick J: Intellectual abilities, in The Handbook of the Psychology of Aging. Edited by Birren JE, Schaie KW. New York, Van Nostrand Reinhold, 1977, pp 580–605

Bowles NL, Poon LW: An analysis of the effect of aging on recognition memory. J Gerontol 37:212–219, 1982

Braun CMJ, Lalonde R: Les declins des fonctions cognitives chez la personne agée: une perspective neuropsychologique. Canadian Journal of Aging 9:135–158, 1990

Brody H: Cell counts in cerebral cortex and brainstem, in Alzheimer's Disease: Senile Dementia and Related Disorders. Edited by Katzman R, Terry RD, Bick KL. New York, Raven, 1978, pp 345–351

Butcher JN, Aldwin CM, Levenson MR, et al: Personality and aging: a study of the MMPI-2 among older men. Psychol Aging 6:361–370, 1991

Carstensen LL: Selectivity theory: social activity in a life-span context, in Annual Review of Gerontology and Geriatrics, Vol 11. Edited by Schaie KW, Lawton MP. New York, Springer, 1991, pp 195–217

Caspi A, Bem D: Personality continuity and change across the life course, in Handbook of Personality: Theory and Research. Edited by Pervin LA. New York, Guilford, 1990, pp 549–575

Cassel CK, Rudberg MA, Olshansky SJ: The price of success: health care in an aging society. Health Aff (Millwood) (Summer):87–99, 1992

Cattell RB: Theory of fluid and crystallized intelligence: a critical experiment. Journal of Educational Psychology 45:1–22, 1963

Cerella J: Aging and information-processing rate, in Handbook of the Psychology of Aging, 3rd Edition. Edited by Birren JE, Schaie KW. San Diego, Academic Press, 1990, pp 201–221

Charness N, Bosman EA: Human factors and aging, in The Handbook of Aging and Cognition. Edited by Craik FIM, Salthouse TA. Hillsdale, NJ, Lawrence Erlbaum, 1992, pp 495–551

Chatterjee A, Strauss ME, Smyth KA, et al: Personality change in Alzheimer's disease. Arch Neurol 49:486–491, 1992

Clipp EC, Pavalko EK, Elder GH Jr: Trajectories of health: concept and empirical pattern. Behavior, Health, and Aging 2:159–179, 1991–1992

Coffey CE, Wilkinson WE, Parashos IA, et al: Quantitative cerebral anatomy of the aging human brain: a cross-sectional study using magnetic resonance imaging. Neurology 42:527–536, 1992

Cohen G: Language comprehension in old age. Cognitive Psychology 11:412–429, 1979

Cohen G, Faulkner D: Memory for discourse in old age. Discourse Processes 4:253–265, 1982

Connelly SL, Hasher L: Aging and the inhibition of spatial location. J Exp Psychol [Hum Percept] 19:1238–1250, 1993

Corbetta M, Miezin FM, Dobmeyer S, et al: Attentional modulation of neural processing of shape, color, and velocity in humans. Science 248:1556–1559, 1990

Costa PT Jr, McCrae RR: Cross-sectional studies of personality in a national sample, I: development and validation of survey measures. Psychol Aging 1:140–143, 1986

Costa PR Jr, McCrae RR: Personality, continuity and the changes of adult life, in The Adult Years: Continuity and Change. Edited by Storandt MK, VandenBos GR. Washington, DC, American Psychological Association, 1989

Costa PR Jr, McCrae RR, Zonderman AB: Cross-sectional studies of personality in a national sample, II: stability in neuroticism, extraversion, and openness. Psychol Aging 1:144–149, 1986

Courtenay BC, Poon LW, Martin P, et al: Religiosity and adaptation in the oldest-old. Int J Aging Hum Dev 34:47–56, 1992

Craik FIM, Jennings JM: Human memory, in The Handbook of Aging and Cognition. Edited by Craik FIM, Salthouse TA. Hillsdale, NJ, Lawrence Erlbaum, 1992, pp 51–110

Craik FIM, Lockhart RS: Levels of processing: a framework for memory research. Journal of Verbal Learning and Verbal Behavior 11:671, 1972

Craik FIM, Salthouse TA (eds): The Handbook of Aging and Cognition. Hillsdale, NJ, Lawrence Erlbaum, 1992

Creasey H, Rapoport SI: The aging human brain. Ann Neurol 17:2–10, 1985

Cross KP: Adults as Learners. San Francisco, CA, Jossey-Bass, 1981

Cunningham WR, Haman KL: Intellectual functioning in relation to mental health, in Handbook of

Mental Health and Aging, 2nd Edition. Edited by Birren JE, Sloan RB, Cohen GD. New York, Academic Press, 1992, pp 339–354

Daigneault S, Braun CMJ: Working memory and the self-ordered pointing task: further evidence of early prefrontal decline in normal aging. J Clin Exp Neuropsychol 15:881–895, 1993

Daigneault S, Braun CMJ, Whitaker HA: Early effects of normal aging on perseverative and nonperseverative prefrontal measures. Developmental Neuropsychology 8:99–114, 1992

Denney NW: Everyday problem solving: methodological issues, research findings, and a model, in Everyday Cognition in Adulthood and Later Life. Edited by Poon LW, Rubin DC, Wilson BA. New York, Cambridge University Press, 1989, pp 330–351

Di Lollo V, Arnett JL, Kruk RV: Age-related changes in rate of visual information processing. J Exp Psychol [Hum Percept] 8:225-237, 1982

Edelman CD, Siegler IC: Federal Age Discrimination in Employment Law: Slowing Down the Gold Watch. Charlottesville, VA, The Mitchie Company, 1978

Elias MF, Elias JW, Elias PK: Biological health influences on behavior, in Handbook of the Psychology of Aging, 3rd Edition. Edited by Birren JE, Schaie KW. San Diego, CA, Academic Press, 1990a, pp 79–102

Elias MF, Robbins MA, Schultz NR Jr, et al: Is blood pressure an important variable in research on aging and neuropsychological test performance? J Gerontol 45:P128–P135, 1990b

Elias MF, Wolf PA, D'Agostino RB, et al: Untreated blood pressure level is inversely related to cognitive functioning: the Framingham Study. Am J Epidemiol 138:353–364, 1993

Elias MF, Elias PK, Cobb J, et al: Blood pressures affects cognitive functioning: the Framingham Studies revisited, in Quality of Life in Behavioral Medicine Research. Edited by Dimsdale J, Baum A. Hillsdale, NJ, Lawrence Erlbaum, 1995, pp 121–143

Emery CF, Burker EJ, Blumenthal JA: Psychological and physiological effects of exercise among older adults, in Annual Review of Gerontology and Geriatrics, Vol 11. Edited by Schaie KW, Lawton MP. New York, Springer, 1991, pp 218–238

Felton BJ, Revenson TA: Age differences in coping with chronic illness. Psychol Aging 2:164–170, 1987

Felton BJ, Revenson TA: The psychology of health: issues in the field with special focus on the older person, in Aging Curriculum Content for Education in the Social-Behavioral Sciences. Edited by Parham IA, Poon LW, Siegler IC. New York, Springer, 1990, pp 4-1–4-54

Field D: Continuity and change in personality in old age—evidence from five longitudinal studies: introduction to a special issue. J Gerontol 46:P271–P274, 1991

Field D, Millsap RE: Personality in advanced old age: continuity or change? J Gerontol 46:P299–P308, 1991

Flicker C, Ferris SH, Reisbert B: A two-year longitudinal study of cognitive function in normal aging and Alzheimer's disease. J Geriatr Psychiatry Neurol 6:84–96, 1993

Fox BH: Premorbid psychological factors related to cancer incidence. J Behav Med 1:45–133, 1978

Fozard JL: The time for remembering, in Aging in the 1980s: Psychological Issues. Edited by Poon LW. Washington, DC, American Psychological Association, 1980, pp 273–287

Fozard JL, Metter J, Brant LJ: Next steps in describing aging and disease in longitudinal studies. J Gerontol 45:P116–P127, 1990

Frazier L, Hooker K, Siegler IC: Longitudinal studies of aging in social and psychological gerontology. Rev Clin Gerontol 3:415–426, 1993

Frederickson BL, Carstensen LL: Choosing social partners: how old age and anticipated endings make people more selective. Psychol Aging 5:335–347, 1990

Friedman HS, Booth-Kewley S: The "disease-prone personality": a meta-analytic view of the construct. Am Psychol 42:539–555, 1987

George LK, Siegler IC: Stress and coping in later life. Educational Horizons 60:147–196, 1982

Goetting M, Martin P, Poon LW, et al: The economic well-being of centenarians. Journal of Aging (in press)

Goldstein G, Shelly CH: Does the right hemisphere age more rapidly than the left? Journal of Clinical Neuropsychology 3:65–78, 1981

Gordon SK, Clark WC: Application of signal detection theory to prose recall and recognition in elderly and young adults. J Gerontol 29:64–72, 1974

Gur RC, Gur RE, Obrist WD, et al: Age and regional cerebral blood flow at rest and during cognitive activity. Arch Gen Psychiatry 44:617–621, 1987

Gur RC, Erwin RJ, Gur RE: Neurobehavioral probes for physiologic neuroimaging studies. Arch Gen Psychiatry 49:409–414, 1992

Guttentag R: Age differences in dual-task performance: procedures, assumptions, and results. Developmental Review 9:146–170, 1989

Hagberg B, Samuelsson G, Lindberg B, et al: Stability and change of personality in old age and its relation to survival. J Gerontol 46:P285–P291, 1991

Harker JO, Hartley JT, Walsh DA: Understanding discourse—a life-span approach, in Advances in Reading/Language Research, Vol 1. Edited by Hutson BA. Greenwich, CT, JAI Press, 1982, pp 155–202

Hartley AA: Attention, in The Handbook of Aging and Cognition. Edited by Craik FIM, Salthouse TA. Hillsdale, NJ, Lawrence Erlbaum, 1992, pp 3–49

Hartley AA, Kieley JM, Slabach EH: Age differences and similarities in the effects of cues and prompts. J Exp Psychol [Hum Percept] 16:523–537, 1990

Hartley JT: Memory for prose: perspectives on the reader, in Everyday Cognition in Adulthood and Later Life. Edited by Poon LW, Rubin DC, Wilson BA. New York, Cambridge University Press, 1989, pp 135–156

Hasher L, Zacks RT: Automatic and effortful processes in memory. J Exp Psychol [Gen] 108:356–388, 1979

Hasher L, Zacks RT: Working memory, comprehension, and aging: a review and a new review, in The Psychology of Learning and Motivation, Vol 22. Edited by Bower GH. Orlando, FL, Academic Press, 1988, pp 193–225

Hathaway SR, McKinley JC: Minnesota Multiphasic Personality Inventory—2. Minneapolis, MN, University of Minnesota, 1989

Haug H, Barmwater U, Eggers R, et al: Anatomical changes in aging brain: morphometric analysis of the human proscencephalon, in Neuropharmacology (Vol 21: Aging). Edited by Cervos-Navarro J, Sarkander HI. New York, Raven, 1983, pp 1–12

Haxby JV, Grady CL, Ungerleider LG, et al: Mapping the functional neuroanatomy of the intact human brain with brain work imaging. Neuropsychologia 29:539–555, 1991

Hertzog C, Schaie KW: Stability and change in adult intelligence, I: analysis of longitudinal covariance structures. Psychol Aging 1:159–171, 1986

Hof PR, Bierer LM, Perl DP, et al: Evidence for early vulnerability of the medial and inferior aspects of the temporal lobe in an 82-year-old patient with preclinical signs of dementia: regional and laminar distribution of neurofibrillary tangles and senile plaques. Arch Neurol 49:946–953, 1992

Hoffman JM, Guze BH, Baxter LR, et al: [18F]-fluorodeoxyglucose (FDG) and positron emission tomography (PET) in aging and dementia. Eur Neurol 29 (suppl):16–24, 1989

Hooker K, Kaus CR: Possible selves and health behaviors in later life. Journal of Aging and Health 4:390–411, 1992

Hooker K, Siegler IC: Separating apples from oranges in health ratings: perceived health includes psychological well-being. Behavior, Health, and Aging 2:81–92, 1992

Hooker K, Siegler IC: Life goals, satisfaction, and self-rated health: preliminary findings. Exp Aging Res 19:97–110, 1993

Hooker K, Monahan D, Shifren K, et al: Mental and physical health of spouse caregivers: the role of personality. Psychol Aging 7:367–375, 1992

Horn JL: The aging of human abilities, in Handbook of Developmental Psychology. Edited by Wolman BB. Englewood Cliffs, NJ, Prentice-Hall, 1982, pp 847–870

House JS, Landis K, Umberson D: Social relationships and health. Science 241:540–544, 1988S

House JS, Kessler RC, Herzog AR, et al: Social stratification, age, and health, in Aging, Health Behaviors, and Health Outcomes. Edited by Schaie KW, Blazer D, House JS. Hillsdale, NJ, Lawrence Erlbaum, 1992, pp 1–32

Hultsch DF, Dixon RA: Learning and memory in aging, in Handbook of the Psychology of Aging. Edited by Birren JE, Schaie KW. New York, Academic Press, 1990, pp 258–274

Hultsch DF, Hammer M, Small BJ: Age differences in cognitive performance in later life: relationships to self-reported health and activity lifestyle. J Gerontol 48:1–11, 1993

Huppert FA: Memory function in dementia and normal aging: dimension or dichotomy, in Dementia and Normal Aging. Edited by Huppert FA, Brayne C, Connor DO. New York, Cambridge University Press, 1994, pp 291–330

Ivnik RJ, Smith GE, Tangalos EG, et al: Wechsler Memory Scale: IQ-dependent norms for persons ages 65 to 97 years. Psychological Assessment 3:156–161, 1991

Jackson JS, Antonucci TC: Social support processes in health and effective functioning of the elderly, in Stress and Health Among the Elderly. Edited by Wykle ML, Kahana E, Kowal J. New York, Springer, 1992, pp 72–95

Johnson MA, Brown MA, Poon LW, et al: Nutritional patterns of centenarians. Int J Aging Hum Dev 34:57–76, 1992

Kahana B: Late-life adaptation in the aftermath of extreme stress, in Stress and Health Among the Elderly. Edited by Wykle ML, Kahana E, Kowal J. New York, Springer, 1992, pp 151–171

Kaplan GA: Health and aging in the Alameda County Study, in Aging, Health Behaviors, and Health Outcomes. Edited by Schaie KW, Blazer D, House JS. Hillsdale, NJ, Lawrence Erlbaum, 1992, pp 69–88

Kastenbaum R (ed): Encyclopedia of Adult Development. Phoenix, AZ, Oryx Press, 1993

Kaszniak AW, Poon LW, Riege W: Assessing memory deficits: an information-processing approach, in Handbook for Clinical Memory Assessment of Older Adults. Edited by Poon LW. Washington, DC, American Psychological Association, 1986, pp 168–188

Katzman R, Aronson M, Fuld P, et al: Development of dementing illnesses in an 80-year-old volunteer cohort. Ann Neurol 25:317–324, 1989

Keefe FJ, Williams DA: A comparison of coping strategies in chronic pain patients in different age groups. J Gerontol 45:P161–P165, 1990

Kirasic KC: Acquisition and utilization of spatial information by elderly adults: implications for day-to-day situations, in Everyday Cognition in Adulthood and Later Life. Edited by Poon LW, Rubin DC, Wilson BA. New York, Cambridge University Press, 1989, pp 265–283

Klisz D: Neuropsychological evaluation in older persons, in The Clinical Psychology of Aging. Edited by Storandt M, Siegler IC, Elias MF. New York, Plenum, 1978, pp 71–95

Kogan N: Personality and aging, in Handbook of the Psychology of Aging, 3rd Edition. Edited by Birren JE, Schaie KW. New York, Van Nostrand Reinhold, 1990, pp 330–346

Koss E, Haxby JV, DeCarli C, et al: Patterns of performance preservation and loss in healthy aging. Developmental Neuropsychology 7:99–113, 1991

LaBerge D: Thalamic and cortical mechanisms of attention suggested by recent positron-emission tomographic experiments. Journal of Cognitive Neuroscience 2:358–372, 1990

Lawton MP, Kleban MH, Rajagopal D, et al: Dimensions of affective experience in three age groups. Psychol Aging 7:171–184, 1992

Lawton MP, Kleban MH, Rajagopal D, et al: Affect and age: cross-sectional comparisons of structure and prevalence. Psychol Aging 8:165–175, 1993

Levinson DJ: A conception of adult development. Am Psychol 41:3–13, 1986

Levitt MJ, Weber RA, Guacci N: Convoys of social support: an intergenerational analysis. Psychol Aging 8:323–326, 1993

Lezak MD: Neuropsychological Assessment, 2nd Edition. New York, Oxford University Press, 1983

Light LL: Memory and aging: four hypotheses in search of data. Annu Rev Psychol 42:333–376, 1991

Light LL: The organization of memory in old age, in The Handbook of Aging and Cognition. Edited by Craik FIM, Salthouse TA. Hillsdale, NJ, Lawrence Erlbaum, 1992, pp 111–166

Lowenthal MF, Berkman PL, Beuler JA, et al: Aging and Mental Disorder in San Francisco. San Francisco, CA, Jossey-Bass, 1967

Madden DJ: Aging and distraction by highly familiar stimuli during visual search. Developmental Psychology 19:499–507, 1983

Madden DJ: Data-driven and memory-driven selective attention in visual search. J Gerontol 39:72–78, 1984

Madden DJ: Age-related slowing in the retrieval of information from long-term memory. J Gerontol 40:208–210, 1985

Madden DJ: Adult age differences in the attentional capacity demands of visual search. Cognitive Development 1:335–363, 1986a

Madden DJ: Adult age differences in visual word recognition: semantic encoding and episodic retention. Exp Aging Res 12:71–78, 1986b

Madden DJ: Adult age differences in attentional selectivity and capacity. European Journal of Cognitive Psychology 2:229–252, 1990

Madden DJ, Plude DJ: Selective preservation of selective attention, in Adult Information Processing: Limits on Loss. Edited by Cerella J, Rybash J, Hoyer W, et al. San Diego, CA, Academic Press, 1993, pp 273–300

Maddox GL, Atchley RC, Poon LW, et al. (eds): Encyclopedia of Aging. New York, Springer, 1987

Manton KG, Siegler IC, Woodbury MA: Patterns of intellectual development in later life. J Gerontol 41:486–489, 1986

Martin P, Poon LW, Clayton G, et al: Personality, life events and coping in the oldest-old. Int J Aging Hum Dev 34:19–30, 1992

Martin P, Schuette L, Poon LW, et al: Compensating for physical decline: the role of personality. Gerontologist 33:148, 1993

Martin P, Poon LW, Kim E, Johnson MA: Social and psychological resources in the oldest old. Exp Aging Res (in press)

McClelland JL, Rumelhart DE, the PDP Research Group: Parallel Distributed Processing: Explorations in the Microstructure of Cognition (Vol 2 of Psychological and Biological Models series). Cambridge, MA, MIT Press, 1986

McCrae RR: Moderated analyses of longitudinal personality stability. J Pers Soc Psychol 65:577–585, 1993

McCrae RR, Costa PT: Emerging Lives, Enduring Dispositions. Boston, MA, Little, Brown, 1984

McCrae RR, Costa PT: Personality in Adulthood. New York, Guilford, 1990

McCrae RR, Arenberg D, Costa PT Jr: Declines in divergent thinking with age: cross-sectional, longitudinal, and cross-sequential analyses. Psychol Aging 2:130–137, 1987

McDowd JM, Craik FIM: Effects of aging and task difficulty on divided attention performance. J Exp Psychol [Hum Percept] 14:267–280, 1988

Metter EJ, Walega D, Metter EL, et al: How comparable are healthy 60- and 80-year-old men? J Gerontol 47:M73–M78, 1992

Meyer BJF, Rice GE: Information recalled from prose by young, middle, and old adults. Exp Aging Res 7:253–268, 1981

Meyer BJF, Rice GE: Prose processing in adulthood: the text, the learner, and the task, in Everyday Cognition in Adulthood and Later Life. Edited by Poon LW, Rubin DC, Wilson BA. New York, Cambridge University Press, 1989, pp 157–194

Mittenberg W, Seidenberg M, O'Leary DS, et al: Changes in cerebral functioning associated with normal aging. J Clin Exp Neuropsychol 11:918–933, 1989

Morrell RW, Park DC, Poon LW: Effects of labeling techniques on memory and comprehension of prescription information in young and old adults. J Gerontol 45:166–172, 1990

Morris JC, McKeel DW, Storandt M, et al: Very mild Alzheimer's disease: informant-based clinical, psychometric, and pathological distinction from normal aging. Neurology 41:469–478, 1991

Mortimer JA, Schumann LM (eds): The Epidemiology of Dementia. New York, Oxford University Press, 1981

Myerson J, Hale S, Wagstaff D, et al: The information loss model: a mathematical theory of age-related cognitive slowing. Psychol Rev 97:475–487, 1990

Nebes RD, Madden DJ, Berg WD: The effect of age on hemispheric asymmetry in visual and auditory identification. Exp Aging Res 9:87–91, 1983

Olsho LW, Harkins SW, Lenhardt ML: Aging and the auditory system, in Handbook of the Psychology of Aging, 2nd Edition. Edited by Birren JE, Schaie KW. New York, Van Nostrand Reinhold, 1985, pp 332–377

Palmore E, Cleveland WP, Nowlin JB, et al: Stress and adaptation in later life. J Gerontol 34:841–851, 1979

Parashos IA, Coffey CE: Anatomy of the aging brain, in Principles and Practice of Geriatric Psychiatry. Edited by Copeland JRM, Abou-Saleh MT, Blazer DG. New York, Wiley, 1994, pp 35–50

Park DC: Applied cognitive aging research, in The Handbook of Aging and Cognition. Edited by Craik FIM, Salthouse TA. Hillsdale, NJ, Lawrence Erlbaum, 1992, pp 449–494

Park DC, Puglisi JT, Sovacool M: Memory for pictures and spatial location in older adults: evidence for pictorial superiority. J Gerontol 38:582–588, 1983

Parkin AJ, Walter BM: Aging, short-term memory, and frontal dysfunction. Psychobiology 19:175–179, 1991

Parks RW, Loewenstein DA, Chang JY: Brain imaging: positron emission tomography and cognitive functioning, in Cognitive Approaches to Neuropsychology. Edited by Williams JM, Long CJ. New York, Plenum, 1988, pp 189–210

Parmelee PA, Kleban MH, Lawton MP, et al: Depression and cognitive change among institutionalized aged. Psychol Aging 6:504–511, 1991

Perlmutter M, Nyquist L: Relationships between self-reported physical and mental health and intelligence performance across adulthood. J Gerontol 45:P145–P155, 1990

Petersen RC, Smith G, Kokmen E, et al: Memory function in normal aging. Neurology 42:396–401, 1992

Phillips HT, Gaylord SA (eds): Aging and Public Health. New York, Springer, 1985

Plude DJ, Hoyer WJ: Age and the selectivity of visual information processing. Psychol Aging 1:4–10, 1986

Poon LW: Differences in human memory with aging: nature, causes and clinical implications, in Handbook of the Psychology of Aging. Edited by Birren JE, Schaie KW. New York, Van Nostrand Reinhold, 1985, pp 427–462

Poon LW (ed): Handbook for Clinical Memory Assessment of Older Adults. Washington, DC, American Psychological Association, 1986

Poon LW, Fozard JL: Age and word frequency effects in continuous recognition memory. J Gerontol 35:77–86, 1980

Poon LW, Siegler IC: Psychological aspects of normal aging, in Comprehensive Review of Geriatric Psychiatry. Edited by Sadavoy J, Lazarus LW, Jarvik LF. Washington, DC, American Psychiatric Press, 1991, pp 117–145

Poon LW, Gurland BJ, Eisdorfer C, et al: Integration of experimental and clinical precepts in memory assessment: a tribute to George Talland, in Handbook for Clinical Memory Assessment of Older Adults. Edited by Poon LW. Washington, DC, American Psychological Association, 1986, pp 3–10

Poon LW, Rubin DC, Wilson BA (eds): Everyday Cognition in Adulthood and Later Life. New York, Cambridge University Press, 1989

Poon LW, Clayton GM, Martin P, et al: The Georgia Centenarian Study. Int J Aging Hum Dev 34:1–17, 1992a

Poon LW, Martin P, Clayton GM, et al: The influences of cognitive resources on adaptation and old age. Int J Aging Hum Dev 34:31–46, 1992b

Poon LW, Rousseau G, Noble CA, et al: Compensating for instrumental activity of daily living decline in old age: the role of cognitive abilities. Gerontologist 33:48, 1993

Rapkin BD, Fischer K: Personal goals of older adults: issues in assessment and prediction. Psychol Aging 7:127–137, 1992a

Rapkin BD, Fischer K: Framing the construct of life satisfaction in terms of older adults' personal goals. Psychol Aging 7:138–149, 1992b

Rapoport SI: Positron emission tomography in Alzheimer's disease in relation to disease pathogenesis: a critical review. Cerebrovasc Brain Metab Rev 3:297–335, 1991

Roberts P, Newton PM: Levinsonian studies of women's adult development. Psychol Aging 2:154–163, 1987

Rodin J: Behavioral medicine, in Encyclopedia of Aging. Edited by Maddox GL. New York, Springer, 1987, pp 51–58

Rodin J, McAvay G: Determinants of change in perceived health in a longitudinal study of older adults. J Gerontol 47:P373–P384, 1992

Salthouse TA: Adult Cognition: An Experimental Psychology of Human Aging. New York, Springer-Verlag, 1982

Salthouse TA: A Theory of Cognitive Aging. Amsterdam, North-Holland, 1985a

Salthouse TA: Speed of behavior and its implications for cognition, in Handbook of the Psychology of Aging, 2nd Edition. Edited by Birren JE, Schaie KW. New York, Van Nostrand Reinhold, 1985b, pp 400–426

Salthouse TA: Reasoning and spatial abilities, in The Handbook of Aging and Cognition. Edited by Craik FIM, Salthouse TA. Hillsdale, NJ, Lawrence Erlbaum, 1992, pp 167–212

Salthouse TA, Rogan JD, Prill KA: Division of attention: age differences on a visually presented memory task. Memory and Cognition 12:613–620, 1984

Salthouse TA, Kausler WH, Saluts JS: Age, self-assessed health status, and cognition. J Gerontol 45:156–160, 1990

Sands LP, Meredith W: Blood pressure and intellectual functioning in late midlife. J Gerontol 47:P81–P84, 1992

Schacter D: Implicit memory: history and current status. J Exp Psychol [Learn Mem Cogn] 13:501, 1987

Schaie KW: Intellectual development in adulthood, in Handbook of the Psychology of Aging, 3rd Edition. Edited by Birren JE, Schaie KW. New York, Academic Press, 1990, pp 291–309

Schaie KW, Parham IA: Stability of adult personality traits: fact or fable? J Pers Soc Psychol 34:146–158, 1976

Schaie KW, Schaie JP: Clinical assessment and aging, in The Handbook of the Psychology of Aging. Edited by Birren JE, Schaie KW. New York, Van Nostrand Reinhold, 1977, pp 692–723

Schaie KW, Willis SL: Adult personality and psychomotor performance: cross-sectional and longitudinal analyses. J Gerontol 46:P275–P284, 1991

Schmidt R, Fazekas F, Offenbacher H, et al: Neuropsychological correlates of MRI white-matter hyperintensities: a study of 150 normal volunteers. Neurology 43:2490–2494, 1993

Schoenbach VJ: Behavior and life style as determinants of health and well-being in the elderly, in Aging and Public Health. Edited by Phillips HT, Gaylord SA. New York, Springer, 1985, pp 181–216

Seeman T, de Leon CM, Berkman L, et al: Risk factors for coronary heart disease among older men and women: a prospective study of community-dwelling elderly. Am J Epidemiol 138:1037–1049, 1993

Shiffrin RM, Schneider W: Controlled and automatic human information processing, II: perceptual learning, automatic attending, and a general theory. Psychol Rev 84:127–190, 1977

Siegler IC: The psychology of adult development and aging, in Handbook of Geriatric Psychiatry. Edited by Busse EW, Blazer DG. New York, Van Nostrand Reinhold, 1980, pp 169–221

Siegler IC: Developmental health psychology, in The Adult Years: Continuity and Change. Edited by Storandt MK, VandenBos GR. Washington, DC, American Psychological Association, 1989, pp 119–142

Siegler IC: Research paradigms in developmental health psychology—from theory to application: introduction to a special issue. J Gerontol 45:P113–P115, 1990

Siegler IC: Aging and the public health: reflections on Kaplan's report of health and aging in the Alameda County Study, in Aging, Health Behaviors and Health Outcomes. Edited by Schaie KW, House J, Blazer DG. Hillsdale, NJ, Lawrence Erlbaum, 1992, pp 89–95

Siegler IC: Hostility and risk: demographic and lifestyle variables, in Anger, Hostility and the Heart. Edited by Siegman AW, Smith TW. Hillsdale, NJ, Lawrence Erlbaum, 1994, pp 199–214

Siegler IC, Costa PT Jr: Health behavior relationships, in Handbook of the Psychology of Aging, 2nd Edition. Edited by Birren JE, Schaie KW. New York, Van Nostrand Reinhold, 1985, pp 144–166

Siegler IC, George LK: Sex differences in coping and perceptions of life events. Journal of Geriatric Psychiatry, 16:197–209, 1983

Siegler IC, O'Keefe J: Aging and Health: An Overview. Invited Address, Sponsored Legislative Forum at the meetings of the American Psychological Association. Washington, DC, August 1992

Siegler IC, Poon LW: The psychology of aging, in Geriatric Psychiatry. Edited by Busse EW, Blazer DG. Washington, DC, American Psychiatric Press, 1989, pp 163–201

Siegler IC, Nowlin JB, Blumenthal JA: Health and behavior: methodological considerations for adult development and aging, in Aging in the 1980s: Psychological Issues. Edited by Poon LW. Washington, DC, American Psychological Association, 1980, pp 559–612

Siegler IC, Welsh KA, Dawson DV, et al: Perceptions of personality change in patients evaluated for memory disorders. Alzheimer Dis Assoc Disord 5:240–250, 1991

Siegler IC, Dawson DV, Welsh KA: Caregiver ratings of personality change in Alzheimer's disease patients: a replication. Psychol Aging 9:464–466, 1994

Stagner R: Aging and industry, in Handbook of the Psychology of Aging, 2nd Edition. Edited by Birren JE, Schaie KW. New York, Van Nostrand Reinhold, 1985, pp 789–817

Stephens MAP, Kinney JM, Norris VK, et al: Social networks as assets and liabilities in recovering from stroke in geriatric patients. Psychol Aging 2:125–129, 1987

Sterns HL, Alexander RA: Industrial gerontology, in Annual Review of Gerontology and Geriatrics, Vol 7. Edited by Schaie KW, Eisdorfer C. New York, Springer, 1987, pp 243–264

Stine EL, Wingfield A, Poon LW: Speech comprehension and memory through adulthood: the role of time and strategy, in Everyday Cognition in Adulthood and Later Life. Edited by Poon LW, Rubin DC, Wilson BA. New York, Cambridge University Press, 1989, pp 195–221

Strahan G, Burns BJ: Mental illness in nursing homes: United States, 1985. Vital Health Stat [13], No. 105 (PHS 91-1766), 1991

Strauss ME, Pasupathi M, Chatterjee A: Concordance between observers in descriptions of personality change in Alzheimer's disease. Psychol Aging 8:475–480, 1993

Surwit RS, Scovern AW, Feinglos MN: The role of behavior in diabetes care. Diabetes Care 5:337–342, 1982

Swan GE, Dame A, Carmelli D: Involuntary retirement, type A behavior, and current functioning in elderly men: 27-year follow-up of the Western Collaborative Group Study. Psychol Aging 6:384–391, 1991

Taub HA: Comprehension and memory of prose materials by young and old adults. Exp Aging Res 5:3–13, 1979

Thomae H: Patterns of Aging: Findings from the Bonn Longitudinal Study of Aging. Basel, Switzerland, S. Karger, 1976

Thomae H: Emotion and personality, in Handbook of Mental Health and Aging, 2nd Edition. Edited by Birren JE, Sloane RB, Cohen GD. New York, Academic Press, 1992, pp 355–375

Tulving E: Episodic and semantic memory, in Organization of Memory. Edited by Tulving E, Donaldson W. New York, Academic Press, 1972, pp 382–404

Tun PA, Wingfield A: Is speech special? perception and recall of spoken language in complex environments, in Adult Information Processing: Limits on Loss. Edited by Cerella J, Rybash J, Hoyer W, et al. San Diego, CA, Academic Press, 1993, pp 426–457

Tun PA, Wingfield A, Stine EAL, et al: Rapid speech processing and divided attention: processing rate versus processing resources as an explanation of age effects. Psychol Aging 7:546–550, 1992

Van Gorp WG, Mahler M: Subcortical features of normal aging, in Subcortical Dementia. Edited by Cummings JL. New York, Oxford University Press, 1990, pp 231–250

Van Gorp WG, Satz P, Mitrushina M: Neuropsychological processes associated with normal aging. Developmental Neuropsychology 6:279–290, 1990

Verbrugge LM: Sex differences in health, in Encyclopedia of Aging. Edited by Maddox GL, Atchley RC, Poon LW, et al. New York, Springer, 1987, pp 601–604

Vitaliano PP, Russo J, Young HM, et al: Predictors of burden in spouse caregivers of individuals with Alzheimer's disease. Psychol Aging 6:392–402, 1991

Vitaliano PP, Dougherty CM, Siegler IC: Biopsychosocial factors and impaired quality of life as risk factors for and outcomes of CVD in caregivers of people with Alzheimer's disease, in Aging and the Quality of Life. Edited by Abeles RP, Gift HC, Ory MG. New York, Springer, 1994, pp 145–160

Waugh NC, Norman DA: Primary memory. Psychol Rev 72:89–104, 1965

Wechsler D: Wechsler Adult Intelligence Scale—Revised Manual. New York, Psychological Corporation, 1981

Welsh KA, Hoffman JM: Positron emission tomography neuroimaging in dementia, in Handbook of Human Brain Function. Edited by Bigler E. New York, Plenum, in press

Welsh KA, Butters N, Hughes J, et al: Detection of abnormal memory in mild cases of Alzheimer's disease using CERAD neuropsychological measures. Arch Neurol 48:278–281, 1991

Welsh KA, Butters N, Mohs RC, et al: The Consortium to Establish a Registry of Alzheimer's Disease

(CERAD), V: a normative study of the neuropsychological battery. Neurology 44:609–614, 1994

Whelihan WM, Lesher EL: Neuropsychological changes in frontal functions with aging. Developmental Neuropsychology 1:371–380, 1985

Whitbourne SK: Personality development in adulthood and old age: relationships among identity style, health, and well-being, in Annual Review of Gerontology and Geriatrics, Vol 7. Edited by Schaie KW, Lawton MP. New York, Springer, 1987, pp 189–216

Williams RB: The Trusting Heart. New York, Times Books, 1989

Williams RB, Haney TL, Lee KL, et al: Type A behavior, hostility and coronary atherosclerosis. Psychosom Med 42:539–549, 1980

Williams RB, Barefoot JC, Shekelle RB: The health consequences of hostility, in Anger, Hostility and Behavioral Medicine. Edited by Chesney MA, Rosenman RH. New York, Hemisphere/McGraw-Hill, 1985, pp 173–185

Williams RB, Barefoot JC, Califf RM, et al: Prognostic importance of social and economic resources among medically treated patients with angiographically documented coronary artery disease. JAMA 267:520–524, 1992

Williams RB, Briggs R, Coleman P: Carer-rated personality change associated with senile dementia. International Journal of Geriatric Psychiatry 10: 231–236, 1995

Willis SL: Towards an educational psychology of the older adult learner: intellectual and cognitive bases, in Handbook of the Psychology of Aging, 2nd Edition. Edited by Birren JE, Schaie KW. New York, Van Nostrand Reinhold, 1985, pp 818–847

Willis SL: Cognition and everyday competence, in Annual Review of Gerontology and Geriatrics, Vol 11. Edited by Schaie KW, Lawton MP. New York, Springer, 1991, pp 80–109

Willis SL, Schaie KW: Training the elderly on ability factors of spatial orientation and inductive reasoning. Psychol Aging 1:239–247, 1986

Wingfield A, Poon LW, Lombardi L, et al: Speed of processing in normal aging: effects of speech rate, linguistic structure, and processing time. J Gerontol 40:579–585, 1985

Woodruff-Pak DS, Winn M: Longevity, in Aging Curriculum Content for Education in the Social-Behavioral Sciences. Edited by Parham I, Poon L, Siegler I. New York, Springer, 1990, pp 3-1–3-33

Wykle ML, Kahana E, Kowal J (eds): Stress and Health Among the Elderly. New York, Springer, 1992

Zelinski EM, Gilewski MJ, Thompson LW: Do laboratory tests relate to self-assessment of memory ability in the young and old? in New Directions in Memory and Aging: Proceedings of the George Talland Memorial Conference. Edited by Poon LW, Fozard JL, Cermak LS, et al. Hillsdale, NJ, Lawrence Erlbaum, 1980, pp 519–544

Zonderman AB, Siegler IC, Barefoot JC, et al: Age and gender differences in MMPI Content scales. Exp Aging Res 19:241–257, 1993

CHAPTER 8

Social and Economic Factors Related to Psychiatric Disorders in Late Life

Linda K. George, Ph.D

A comprehensive examination of geriatric psychiatry must include the perspectives of multiple disciplines. The authors of previous chapters addressed the physiological, neurological, sensory, and psychological changes that accompany the aging process. In this chapter I examine the social and economic conditions of late life. (For the sake of convenience, henceforth the shorter term *social factors* will be used, although economic factors also are addressed.) Particular attention is paid to the ways that social conditions serve as risk factors for psychiatric disorders, as contingencies that affect the course and outcome of mental illness, and as determinants of mental health service utilization.

An adequate depiction of psychiatric disorders must include a dynamic perspective. The experience of psychiatric disorders varies over time as patients experience onset and remission of symptoms. Help seeking and the course of care also are longitudinal phenomena. The distinctive features of geriatric psychiatry are affected by additional dynamic processes. The aging process itself leads to intraindividual changes that can affect the risk of developing psychiatric disorders and/or the use of mental health services. In addition, the effects of social change—generating cohort differences—also must be examined; it can be documented that over the past decades, social and economic factors have changed substantially across cohorts entering and traversing late life. These cohort differences have important implications for generalizing results across cohorts and for using current knowledge to plan for the future.

Given the importance of age changes versus cohort differences in drawing conclusions about the role of social factors in geriatric psychiatry, these terms merit closer examination. *Age changes* are those changes in organisms that occur simply as a function of age. True age changes will be observed with considerable regularity across time and place because they are developmental. Most biological phenomena (as well as some psychological and so-

This work was supported by grant P50 MH40159 from the National Institute of Mental Health.

cial characteristics) that change with age appear to be driven by this kind of internal, species-specific developmental agenda. Other differences observed across age groups represent the effects of social changes that are external to the individual. The term *cohort* is used to refer to groups of people born at specific times—for example, the 1920 cohort consists of all persons born in 1920. Cohorts that experience different historical and environmental conditions often differ in ways that reflect those external conditions rather than developmental changes. Without longitudinal data from multiple cohorts, it is difficult to empirically distinguish between age changes and cohort differences. Moreover, some phenomena are affected by both age changes and cohort differences (see, for example, George et al. 1981).

Although it is difficult to separate age changes from cohort differences, this distinction is important for three reasons. First, the distinction is critical to attributions of etiology or causality. In their pure forms, age changes reflect developmental phenomena and cohort differences reflect social or environmental conditions. Second, the distinction is relevant to the generalizability of research findings. If a risk factor for psychiatric disorders changes with age, the observed pattern will be broadly applicable across cohorts. If a risk factor differs across age groups because of differences in environmental exposure, the effects of that risk factor (or its distribution in the older population) may be cohort specific. Third, the distinction between age changes and cohort differences is important for the design of interventions. If levels of a risk factor differ substantially across cohorts, interventions can be targeted to the environmental conditions that place certain cohorts at greatest risk. If, instead, a risk factor changes with age, interventions must be targeted toward alteration of a developmental trajectory.

In this chapter, then, I examine two dynamic phenomena simultaneously. First, the processes underlying the occurrence of psychiatric disorders and mental health service utilization is addressed from a social perspective. Second, the degree to which social factors associated with psychiatric disorders and/or mental health service use change with age or differ across cohorts is considered.

This chapter is organized in five sections. The first focuses on social characteristics as risk factors for psychiatric disorders in later life. The social fac-

tors examined include demographic variables (such as race and gender), indicators of social integration (such as social roles and the availability of social support), socioeconomic status, and the experience of acute and chronic stress. The second section examines the degree to which exposure to social risk factors for psychiatric disorders changes with age and varies across cohorts. A central issue here is whether current cohorts of younger and middle-aged adults have experienced or will confront environmental conditions that place them at more or less risk for psychiatric disorders than current cohorts of older adults. The third section focuses on the impact of social factors on the course and outcome of psychiatric disorders in later life. The central question of interest is whether social factors alter the probability or timing of recovery. The fourth section addresses social factors as determinants of mental health service use among older adults. An important distinction is made between help seeking (which reflects the decisions and behaviors of individuals needing mental health services) and provider behavior (that is, how clinicians respond to older persons presenting with psychiatric problems). The final section of the chapter examines the impact of social and economic policies on older adults. These policies and programs have both direct impact—by affecting the likelihood of help seeking for psychiatric problems—and indirect impact—by affecting some social risk factors for mental illness, and thereby influencing the psychiatric status of the older population.

Social Risk Factors for Psychiatric Disorders

Theoretical Model

A consensual model of the precursors of psychiatric disorders has emerged in the literature of the social science, epidemiological, and social psychiatry disciplines. The model remains vague in terms of specific operationalizations and statistical estimation; nonetheless, an overarching theoretical orientation has been forged. Table 8–1 presents the general conceptual model that emerges from previous research. It is a stage model in that each higher stage represents what are hypothesized to be increasingly proximate antecedents of psychiatric disorders.

Table 8–1. Stage model of the social precursors of psychiatric disorders

Stage	Name	Illustrative indicators
I	Demographic variables	Age, sex, race/ethnicity
II	Early events and achievements	Education, childhood traumas
III	Later events and achievements	Occupation, income, marital status, fertility
IV	Social integration	Personal attachments to social structure (e.g., religious participation, community roles), environmental context (e.g., neighborhood stability, economic climate)
V	Vulnerability and protective factors	Social support versus isolation, chronic stressors
VI	Provoking agents and coping efforts	Life events, coping strategies

The first stage consists of demographic variables that are associated with the risk of psychiatric disorders. Virtually all studies of social factors and psychiatric disorders include demographic factors, especially age, race, and gender. The causal mechanisms that underlie these relationships are unclear, however. One suggested explanation is that demographic factors serve as proxies for more mechanistic social factors. For example, the greater prevalence of depressive symptoms reported by women compared with men may be due to gender differences in other risk factors such as marital status, income, and exposure to stress. Alternatively, demographic variables may serve as proxies for biological mechanisms. In this review I emphasize the social meanings of demographic variables. However, possible biological mechanisms should not be overlooked. Indeed, most research emphasizes the multiple types of risk factors that are implicated in the etiology of psychiatric morbidity.

Stages II and III of the model represent events and achievements relevant to mental health outcomes that are distinguished primarily by their timing and recency. Stage II consists of relatively early experiences that are hypothesized to have persistent effects on an individual's vulnerability to psychiatric disorders. Examples of such experiences include childhood traumas (the early death or marital disruption of parents, for example) and educational attainment. Stage III consists of later events and experiences, including family relationships and economic achievements. In most studies, Stage III indicators are based on the current statuses of individuals, reinforcing the temporal distinction between Stages II and III. It should be noted that Stage II risk factors need not be experiences that occurred during childhood or early adulthood; rather,

any experiences that occurred before the time of measurement may be relevant. Again, causal interpretation of relationships between risk factors and psychiatric outcomes is problematic. For example, some investigators view higher levels of education and income primarily as resources that facilitate effective coping; others view them as tapping exposure to environments (e.g., occupational and residential settings) that directly affect psychiatric status. Future research will need to address the specific mechanisms by which these factors affect mental health.

Stage IV consists of risk factors that represent dimensions of social integration. The term *social integration* has been used two ways in previous research. Some investigators define social integration at the individual level, referring to personal attachments to formal aspects of the social structure (religious affiliation and participation in organizations are two examples). Others define social integration at the aggregate level, referring to levels of stability and organization in the broader environments within which individuals function. In this chapter I address social integration at both the individual and the aggregate level, although information is less plentiful for the latter. The rationale for examining social integration as a risk factor for psychiatric disorders rests on the assumptions that lack of social integration is psychologically stressful, impedes effective coping, or both.

Finally, Stages V and VI represent the classes of social risk factors that have received the greatest empirical attention. Vulnerability and protective factors refer to personal assets and liabilities that alter the probabilities of psychiatric problems. Chronic stressors are primary examples of vulnerability factors, and social support is a major illustration of a hypothesized protective factor. Provoking agents and coping efforts are more specific and proximate than vulnerability and protective factors. Life events have been the primary provoking agents examined in previous research and are viewed as sudden sources of stress that may be sufficiently severe to trigger the onset of psychiatric morbidity, especially in the presence of other risk factors. Coping efforts refer to the specific actions taken to confront a particular source of stress. Effective coping may either prevent stresses from generating negative mental health outcomes or minimize their effects. Stages V and VI are distinguished primarily on the basis of specificity and immediacy. For example, although life events and chronic stressors are both important because of the stresses they generate, life events are more discrete and bounded. Similarly, social support is viewed as a generalized resource for defusing stress, whereas coping efforts are specific to particular stressors.

The model in Table 8–1 should be viewed as a heuristic abstraction—as a useful way of summarizing trends in the literature on social risk factors for psychiatric disorders rather than as a model that has achieved consensus among investigators. Undoubtedly, some researchers would classify the social precursors of psychiatric morbidity in somewhat different categories. Moreover, most available studies do not include all the categories of risk factors included in this model. Nonetheless, most studies implicitly or explicitly adopt both the basic categories of risk factors and their ordering. Thus far, the conceptual framework depicted in Table 8–1 has been described in terms of direct effects—that is, the relationships, either bivariate or multivariate, between risk factors and psychiatric outcomes. An additional complexity is the possibility of interactive effects—that the effects of one risk factor are contingent on the presence or level of another risk factor.

In theory, any combination of risk factors may interact to alter the risk of psychiatric disorders. Evidence of such interactions is included in this chapter. I will use one illustration at this point to describe the potential importance of risk-factor interactions. Because of the theoretical and empirical attention it has received, the interaction between life events and social support serves as the illustration. Some investigators propose that life events and social support exert independent effects on mental health outcomes, with life events increasing the risk of psychi-

atric disorders and social support reducing the risk. This is a hypothesis of direct effects. Other investigators suggest that social support buffers the effects of life events on psychiatric outcomes, maintaining that life events increase the risk of psychiatric disorders only (or primarily) among persons who lack adequate social support. This is an interactive hypothesis. Direct versus interactive effects are not mutually exclusive. It is possible, for example, that life events and social support directly affect mental health and that life events are especially damaging in the absence of social support. Thus, examination of the social precursors of psychiatric disorders includes not only consideration of multiple risk factors but also their interrelationships.

One limitation of the model presented in Table 8–1 should be noted. This model is based on research that examines social precursors of *nonorganic* mental disorders. For this reason, and because there are few studies of social risk factors for organic mental illness, this discussion is restricted to exploration of social risk factors for functional psychiatric disorders.

As presented here, there is nothing distinctively age related about the conceptual framework in Table 8–1, and this is a purposeful decision. This general conceptual model can be used to examine age/cohort differences in the relationships between social risk factors and psychiatric disorders, age changes in those relationships, and variability within the older population with regard to those relationships. In this way, the distinctiveness of psychiatric disorders in later life can be empirically revealed.

Methodological Issues

Measuring psychiatric disorders. Psychiatric disorders have been operationalized in a variety of ways. Two dimensions underlie most of this variability: 1) the use of diagnostic versus symptom measures, and 2) the degree to which the measures tap general psychopathology versus specific diagnostic categories. With regard to the first dimension, some instruments are designed to measure psychiatric disorders using formal diagnostic criteria, typically one of the following nosological systems: DSM-III-R (American Psychiatric Association 1987); Feighner diagnostic criteria (Feighner et al. 1972); or Research Diagnostic Criteria (RDC; Spitzer et al. 1978). Other measures are symptom scales in which higher numbers of symptoms are assumed to represent more severe morbidity. Diagnostic and symptom measures can yield different conclusions. For example, several studies suggest that older people report more depressive symptoms, on average, than do middle-aged and younger adults, but that the prevalence of major depression as a diagnosis is lower among older versus younger adults (Blazer et al. 1987a; Henderson et al. 1993).

The second dimension applies primarily to symptom measures. Some scales include symptoms from a spectrum of disorders and generate measures of global psychopathology. Others measure symptoms within a single diagnostic category, such as depression or anxiety. The use of global psychopathology measures is problematic because some risk factors may be important for certain disorders but irrelevant to others. For example, there are substantial gender differences in the prevalence of alcohol abuse/dependence and depression, whereas gender differences are minimal for many other disorders (e.g., Robins et al. 1991).

Differences in measurement strategies, as well as in the specific assessment tools used, complicate cross-study comparisons. When studies reach inconsistent conclusions about the effects of a given risk factor, part of the variability in findings may be due to differences in measurement. On the other hand, when studies reach similar conclusions despite the use of different measurement strategies, confidence in those conclusions is increased.

Sample composition. Sampling variability also accounts for some of the inconsistencies observed across studies. Not surprisingly, samples vary widely in size and composition. Small samples often result in statistical analyses that are "underpowered," and therefore meaningful relationships remain undetected. Compositional differences across samples affect the distributions of both psychiatric disorders and social risk factors. Consequently, sample size and composition must be taken into account when synthesizing research findings across studies.

The age compositions of the samples used in previous research are especially relevant to the discussion in this chapter. Some previous studies of the relationships between social risk factors and psychiatric outcomes relied exclusively on data from older adults. More frequently, however, previous studies used data from samples covering much broader age ranges—typically, all adults age 18 and older. These two types of samples generate different, but valuable, information. Studies based on samples of older adults provide in-depth views of how social factors operate during later life. Investigators who use such designs cannot identify risk factor effects that are specific to old age, however. In contrast, data from age-heterogeneous samples can be used to determine 1) the role of age itself as a risk factor for psychiatric disorders, and 2) whether other risk factors vary in direction or magnitude across age groups.

Complexity of analyses. Differences in the types and complexity of the statistical techniques used across studies also complicate the task of synthesizing findings from previous research. Some studies provide only bivariate estimates of the relationships between risk factors and psychiatric disorders. Although tantalizing, such studies are ultimately unsatisfying because it is not clear whether the observed relationships are meaningful or spurious—that is, whether the relationships will disappear in the face of statistical controls. Investigators increasingly recognize the importance of multivariate analyses in which the relationships between risk factors and psychiatric outcomes are examined with potentially confounding and/or interrelated risk factors statistically controlled. Thus, I have paid primary attention in this chapter to findings from multivariate analyses.

Cross-sectional versus longitudinal studies. As noted previously, the onset and course of psychiatric disorders, as well as related help-seeking behaviors, are dynamic. Although the number and quality of longitudinal studies has increased in recent years, a large proportion of studies of social factors and psychiatric disorders are cross-sectional. Cross-sectional studies can be used to document the existence of hypothesized associations, but they cannot provide evidence of temporal order. Further, cross-sectional data cannot provide information about the lag between exposure to a risk factor and the onset of mental illness. Evidence of temporal order and lagged effects can be obtained only from longitudinal data.

For the purposes of the discussion in this chapter, other kinds of longitudinal data also are needed.

Specifically, information is needed about the extent to which exposure to social risk factors for psychiatric disorders changes with age and varies across cohorts. Fortunately, longitudinal data concerning these changes are quite plentiful. Throughout this chapter I have accorded major attention to results from longitudinal studies.

Evidence Bearing on the Theoretical Model

Evidence bearing on the model presented in Table 8–1 now can be extracted from previous research. Overall, the model receives considerable support, although the amount and quality of evidence varies widely across specific risk factors.

Demographic variables.   Age is related to the risk of psychiatric disorders, but the associations are complex and often inconsistent across studies. By using symptom scales measuring global psychiatric symptoms, a few studies have found higher levels of symptoms among older adults (Warheit et al. 1975), but most have reported the absence of meaningful age differences (Veroff et al. 1981). Evidence is most plentiful with regard to depressive symptoms. In studies based on age-heterogeneous samples, older adults have usually reported levels of depressive symptoms equal to or higher than those reported by younger and middle-aged adults (Blazer et al. 1987a; Mirowsky and Ross 1992). The results of studies of age differences within the older population are inconclusive. Most investigators have reported data showing that depressive symptoms are highest among the oldest old (Blazer et al. 1991; Mitchell et al. 1993), but at least one recent study showed a higher level of symptoms among the younger old (La Gory and Fitzpatrick 1992). In contrast, studies of psychiatric disorders (as opposed to symptom levels) demonstrate a lower prevalence among older versus younger adults for all nonorganic psychiatric disorders (see Robins and Regier 1991 for a review). These age differences are observed for both current and lifetime prevalence. The degree to which these age differences reflect cohort differences remains unclear and represents a priority issue for future research.

Evidence is also mixed concerning gender differences in psychiatric morbidity. Women report higher levels of psychiatric symptoms, especially depressive symptoms, than do men (Blazer et al. 1991; Jones-Webb and Snowden 1993; Kessler 1979). The results of studies based on diagnoses, however, suggest that symptom scales mask considerable variation across specific disorders. Affective and somatic disorders are more prevalent among women, alcohol and substance abuse are more common among men, and schizophrenia and most anxiety disorders are unrelated to gender (Robins et al. 1991). Some evidence suggests that gender differences in depression may narrow substantially in later life. Henderson et al. (1993) found higher rates of depressive symptoms among older women than among older men, but no gender difference in rates of major depressive disorder. Similarly, gender was not a significant predictor of the onset of major depression among older adults in a recent prospective study (George 1992). In a prospective study in Britain, however, Green et al. (1992) found a higher incidence of major depression among older women than among older men.

Evidence concerning the relationship between race/ethnicity and psychiatric morbidity also is mixed. Many studies based on symptom scales and using age-heterogeneous samples have shown higher symptoms among nonwhites, especially African Americans (Kessler and Neighbors 1986; Warheit et al. 1975). Race differences in depressive symptoms among the elderly are less clear cut. For example, La Gory and Fitzpatrick (1992) reported a higher level of depressive symptoms among whites than among African Americans. In contrast, Blazer et al. (1991) report no black-white differences in symptoms. Race differences are rarely observed in studies based on diagnostic measures, with the exception of a higher prevalence of alcohol and drug abuse among nonwhites (Robins et al. 1991). This issue is further complicated by substantial race differences in education and income. Several authors have reported that bivariate relationships between race and psychiatric morbidity disappear when socioeconomic status is statistically controlled (Blazer et al. 1991; Warheit et al. 1975).

Early events and achievements.   There is considerable evidence that early events and achievements have persistent effects on psychiatric status throughout adulthood. Among indicators of socioeconomic status, education is most strongly related to psychiatric morbidity. (An advantage of examining education rather than income is the fact that education is less likely than income to be affected by mental illness; thus, even in cross-sectional studies, causal direction can be assumed with some confidence.) In general, high levels of psychiatric symptoms are strongly related to low levels of education. This pattern is observed in age-heterogeneous samples (Kessler 1979; Veroff et al. 1981; Warheit et al. 1975) and studies of older adults (La Gory and Fitzpatrick 1992; Mitchell et al. 1993). Even when diagnostic measures are used, low education is generally recognized as a risk factor for psychiatric disorder (Holzer et al. 1986; Robins et al. 1991). Limited evidence suggests that the relationship between education and mental illness may be more complex, however. For example, Holzer and colleagues (1986) reported that the relationship between education and major depression is curvilinear, with persons of both very low and very high educational attainment exhibiting a higher prevalence of the disorder.

Although it is commonly assumed that childhood traumas place individuals at increased risk of psychiatric morbidity, it is only recently that this hypothesis has received strong empirical support. There now is evidence that parental divorce/separation, parental problem drinking, childhood physical and/or sexual abuse, and childhood poverty are significant risk factors for a variety of psychiatric disorders during adulthood (Brown and Harris 1978; Greenfield et al. 1993; Kessler and Magee 1993; Landerman et al. 1991; Tweed et al. 1989). Landerman and co-workers (1991) reported that childhood traumas also increase vulnerability to stressful life events during adulthood; this may be one of the mechanisms by which childhood problems exert persistent effects on adult mental health. Although studies to date have focused on age-heterogeneous samples, older adults were included in them. Those data are complemented by findings from clinical studies, some of which have focused specifically on older persons (Kaminsky 1978; McMordie and Blom 1979).

Later events and achievements.   Current and/or recent life conditions also are related to the risk of psychiatric disorder. Income and—to a lesser extent—occupation are related to psychiatric disorder, with low income and low occupational prestige increasing risk (Warheit et al. 1975; Holzer et al. 1986; Robins et al. 1991). These relationships are observed for both symptom scales and diagnostic measures. Although the relationship between income and psychiatric morbidity is strong at the bivariate level, the effects of income are substantially reduced when educational attainment is statistically controlled. Retirement is obviously a common transition of later life—a transition that removes individuals from the occupational structure and results in substantial income loss. Although the research base is small, it does not appear that retirement increases the risk of psychiatric disorders (Atchley 1976; Ekerdt et al. 1983). This conclusion also is compatible with the lower prevalence of psychiatric disorders in later life. Thus, socioeconomic background appears to be a stronger predictor of psychiatric morbidity during late life than do retirement-related changes in economic status.

The relationship between marital status and psychiatric disorders remains ambiguous despite considerable research. In general, marital status appears to be weakly associated with psychiatric morbidity, regardless of whether symptom scales or diagnostic measures are used (Robins et al. 1991). In two recent studies of depression among community-dwelling older adults, the unmarried reported significantly more symptoms of depression than the married (Blazer et al. 1991; Jones-Webb and Snowden 1993). Substantively, however, the differences in symptom levels were quite small. Two additional caveats should be observed. First, undesirable changes in marital status appear to have negative effects on mental health, especially in the few months immediately after marital disruption. However, changes in marital status are typically examined as stressful life events rather than as marital status changes. Second, the protective effects of marriage are confounded with measures of social support. Thus, in multivariate models, the effects of marital status are largely explained by stressful life events and social support.

Evidence linking childbearing to psychiatric disorders is very limited. The few studies available suggest that psychiatric symptoms may be slightly higher among women caring for minor children than among their peers who are not responsible for child care (Kandel et al. 1985; Ross and Huber 1985). However, there is no evidence that childbearing history is related to psychiatric status during later life. Indeed, children are a major source of social support for most older adults.

Social integration.   Although social integration is receiving increased attention, the research base remains small. The available evidence suggests that social integration may protect individuals from psychiatric disorders. At the individual level, participation in religion has received most attention. A growing body of research suggests that church attendance and participation in other religious activities is associated with a decreased risk of psychiatric morbidity, including alcohol abuse (Koenig et al. 1994; Neff and Husaini 1985), depression (Meador et al. 1992; Mitchell et al. 1993), and anxiety disorders (Koenig et al. 1993a, 1993b). Moreover, the studies of anxiety disorders suggest that the effects of religious participation are somewhat stronger for older than for younger adults. Similar, albeit weaker, benefits are reported for participation in voluntary organizations (Grusky et al. 1985; Veroff et al. 1981). Unfortunately, all previous studies in this area were based on cross-sectional data, so causal order remains problematic.

At the aggregate level, most studies have focused on dimensions of the environment such as degree of neighborhood stability; economic conditions, especially levels of unemployment; and neighborhood age or family structure. Overall, research results have been mixed, with some studies showing significant relationships between disruptive environmental conditions and the prevalence of psychiatric disorders and other studies failing to do so (Dooley et al. 1981; Kasl and Harburg 1975). In one recent study of community-dwelling older adults, investigators examined the relationships between selected environmental conditions and depressive symptoms (La Gory and Fitzpatrick 1992). Modest but significant relationships were observed between depression and two environmental parameters: age density of the residential neighborhood and availability of public transportation. Older adults who had fewer age peers in their neighborhoods and/or who lacked access to transportation exhibited higher levels of symptoms. In addition, an interaction was found between environmental variables and functional disability. The effects of disability on depression were stronger for persons who were disadvantaged on one or both of the environmental variables. The environmental variables were examined with other established predictors of depression (such as social support) statistically controlled.

Another indicator of social integration that has received attention in previous research is urban versus rural residence. Studies based on symptom scales have typically shown a higher level of symptoms among urban residents (Brown and Prudo 1981; Comstock and Helsing 1976; Mueller 1981; Schwab et al. 1974). The results of studies based on specific diagnoses suggest a more complex pattern. Using data from urban and rural residents of the southeastern United States, Blazer et al. (1985) found that 1) place of residence was unrelated to prevalence of most disorders, 2) a few disorders, especially major depression, were more prevalent among urban residents, and 3) one disorder, alcohol abuse/dependence, was more prevalent among rural residents. Additional analyses of those data indicated that the urban-rural differences observed were greatest among young adults and were minimal among older persons (Crowell et al. 1986).

Vulnerability and protective factors.   Chronic stress is the vulnerability factor that has been examined most frequently in research to date. Several investigative teams have reported a robust relationship between poverty and depressive symptoms in later life (Krause 1987; La Gory and Fitzpatrick 1992)—an association also observed among all adults (Robins et al. 1991). Chronic illness likewise is a well-documented risk factor for psychiatric disorder in later life, especially for depression (Blazer et al. 1991; Husaini et al. 1991; Moldin et al. 1993). In addition to chronic physical illnesses, an increased risk of depression during late life is associated with other health indicators, including cognitive impairment (Blazer et al. 1987a, 1991), perceived poor health (Blazer et al. 1987a; Henderson et al. 1993), and disability (measured in terms of ADL impairment) (Blazer et al. 1991; Henderson et al. 1993, La Gory and Fitzpatrick 1992; Mitchell et al. 1993). In cross-sectional studies, causal order is problematic for these health measures. Depression may be either a consequence or a cause of disability and perceptions of poor health. Cognitive impairment may be a part of the depressive episode rather than an independent phenomenon. At first glance, it might appear that chronic illness is not subject to these concerns. It is unlikely, for example, that depression can cause diabetes or cardiovascular disease. Although causal direction is less problematic, the etiological role of chronic illnesses in the onset of depression in later life remains unclear. One study has suggested that high rates of comorbid physical and mental illness in later life reflect only the much higher base rates of physical illness among the elderly rather than a causal relationship (George et al. 1988a). In addition, Moldin et al. (1993) report equally high rates of comorbid physical illness and depression among younger and older adults.

An emerging body of research indicates that caregiving for a mentally or physically ill elderly adult represents a chronic stressor that can lead to psychiatric problems. Large numbers of older adults have caregiving responsibilities—usually for spouses, but sometimes for very old parents or siblings. To date, the best research examining the effects of caregiver burden on psychiatric morbidity has focused on family caregivers of demented elderly adults. Recent studies suggest that 30%–50% of caregivers of patients with dementia meet the criteria for a DSM-III diagnosis of major depression (Cohen and Eisdorfer 1989; Tennstedt et al. 1992). Even larger proportions of caregivers suffer high levels of psychiatric symptoms, albeit below the thresholds for diagnosis.

The primary protective factor examined in previous research has been social support. There is consensus that social support is a multidimensional phenomenon. Most investigators recognize at least three major dimensions: 1) social network—the size and structure of the network of people available to provide support, 2) instrumental support—the specific tangible services provided by families and friends, and 3) perceptions of social support—subjective evaluations of satisfaction with the available support. Some investigators examine a fourth dimension: informational support, defined as the extent to which family and friends provide information that can be used when assessing options and confronting stress. The level of interaction with friends and family, as well as the presence or absence of a confidant, also have been addressed as indicators of social support.

There is overwhelming evidence that social support has significant direct effects that protect individuals from psychiatric morbidity. Because of the large body of research supporting this conclusion, I restrict my review here to studies of older adults. It should also be noted that the vast majority of these studies explore the effects of social support on depressive symptoms and disorder. The protective power of social support has been reported in numer-

ous cross-sectional studies and a reassuring number of longitudinal investigations. Available evidence suggests that specific dimensions of social support may be differentially important in protecting against late-life depression. The relationships between social network characteristics and depression have received the least support. Blazer et al. (1991) found that older adults with fewer close relatives reported more depressive symptoms; lack of a confidant also has been related to higher levels of symptoms (Blazer 1983; Murphy 1982). Most studies, however, have failed to show significant relationships between network size or structure and risk of depression (Henderson and Moran 1983; Oxman et al. 1992). Levels of social interaction have consistently distinguished between depressed and nondepressed elders (Arling 1987; Blazer 1983; Essex et al. 1985; Henderson et al. 1986; Smith-Ruiz 1985), but have not been shown to predict the onset of disorder. Some investigators have found that instrumental and informational support decrease the risk of depression, but these effects appear to be highly specific and dependent on the particular stressor under examination (Krause 1986a; Mitchell et al. 1993). There is general consensus that perceptions of social support are most strongly related to depression—and, unlike other dimensions, this conclusion has strong support in both cross-sectional (Blazer et al. 1987a; Dimond et al. 1987; Krause 1986a) and longitudinal studies (George 1992; Holahan and Holahan 1987; Krause et al. 1989; Oxman et al. 1992).

The strong relationships between perceived support and depression have raised interpretive questions. Henderson (1984), for example, worried that the dysphoria associated with depression might "contaminate" perceptions of social support among depressed persons. Several recent studies appear to resolve this concern, however. First, even in longitudinal studies, in which perceptions of social support are measured *before* the onset of depressive disorder, perceived support has had a significant protective effect (George 1992; Krause et al. 1989; Oxman et al. 1992). Second, other longitudinal studies have indicated that although perceived support significantly predicts the onset of depression, baseline levels of depression do not predict subsequent levels of support (Cronkite and Moos 1984; Krause et al. 1989). Thus, the dominant direction of causal influence appears to be from perceived support to depression, rather than the reverse.

Information illuminating the relationships between social support and psychiatric disorders other than depression among older adults is very meager. Several studies involving large proportions of older persons have indicated that the social networks of persons with schizophrenia are unusually small (Cohen and Sokolovsky 1978; Crotty and Kulys 1985; Sokolovsky et al. 1978). Grusky and colleagues (1985) reported that older persons with schizophrenia in the community have even smaller networks than do younger ones. Grusky et al. also found that the composition of the support networks of persons with schizophrenia differed, depending on illness severity. Persons with mild symptoms relied primarily on family members for social support. Individuals with severe symptoms relied primarily on nonfamily for assistance—usually formal service providers. In one study, researchers compared the social networks of older adults with and without late-onset alcohol problems. Dupree et al. (1984) found that those with alcohol problems had much smaller networks than did their peers. All of these studies were based on cross-sectional data; thus, causal order is unclear. Examination of the role of social support in persons with disorders other than depression is a high-priority issue; longitudinal studies would be particularly useful.

Provoking agents and coping efforts.   Life events are the major provoking agents implicated in the onset of psychiatric disorders. Two major strategies have been used to study the effects of life events: 1) studies of aggregated life events (that is, summing the number of events that individuals experience in a given time period); and 2) studies of specific life events (e.g., widowhood or retirement). The results of research based on both strategies suggest that life events—especially those that are perceived as negative—are strongly related to an increased risk of both psychiatric symptoms and specific psychiatric disorders, especially depression, alcohol abuse, and generalized anxiety (Blazer et al. 1987a, 1987b; Cutrona et al. 1986; Dupree et al. 1984; George 1992; Neff and Husaini 1985—Cutrona et al. 1986 and George 1992 are longitudinal studies). These relationships have been observed in both age-heterogeneous samples and samples of older adults. With regard to specific events, bereavement has been shown to be a particularly strong predictor of depression among older adults (Green et al. 1992; Krause 1986b).

Both common sense and social science theory suggest that adequate coping will partially determine whether stress has negative effects on mental health. Scientific efforts to delineate the nature and effects of coping have been fraught with problems; valid methods for assessing coping effectiveness remain unavailable. Studying coping effects is particularly problematic because different stressors elicit, permit, and require different coping strategies. Limited evidence suggests that coping methods alter the probability that stress will have negative effects on mental health; some of that evidence is based on samples of older adults (Felton et al. 1980; Folkman and Lazarus 1980). At this point, investigations of coping appear to be stalled. It is unlikely that further progress will be made unless and until advances in assessing coping effectiveness are realized.

Interactive Effects

Thus far, discussion of evidence bearing on the theoretical model in Table 8–1 has largely been restricted to main effects, both bivariate and multivariate. Three kinds of interactive effects also merit comment: the stress-buffering hypothesis, age-related interactions, and several interactions unrelated to age.

The stress-buffering hypothesis.   A majority of studies support the stress-buffering hypothesis—that is, that stress has stronger negative effects on risk for psychiatric disorder in the absence of social support. This conclusion applies both to studies of age-heterogeneous samples and to research restricted to older adults. Virtually all studies to date have addressed the stress-buffering hypothesis with regard to depressive symptoms and disorders. Several studies, both cross-sectional and longitudinal, have suggested that life events are moderated by the effects of social support (Cutrona et al. 1986; Krause 1986a). Social support also has been shown to buffer the effects of chronic financial strain (Krause 1987) and disability (Arling 1987) during later life. Considerable complexity underlies the moderating effects of social support on stress. For example, Krause (1986a, 1987) showed that stress-buffering effects are observed 1) for some but not all dimensions of social support, 2) for some but not all kinds of specific stressors, and 3) for some but not all dimensions of depressed affect.

Age interactions. Determining whether age interacts with other social precursors of psychiatric disorder is the best strategy for identifying distinctive age differences in the onset of depression. Unfortunately, few investigators have examined age interactions in the risk factors for psychiatric disorders.

One area that has received limited attention is age differences in the effects of specific events on personal well-being. Chiriboga (1982) compared younger and older persons in terms of adjustment to marital separation. His results suggested that marital dissolution has more negative effects for older than for younger adults. Glick and co-workers (1974) performed a longitudinal study of the effects of widowhood. They found that the experiences of younger and older widows differed significantly, although it cannot be concluded that one group fared better, overall, than the other. Younger widows generally exhibited higher levels of psychiatric symptoms than older widows during the first year of bereavement. On the other hand, older widows appeared to confront more difficult and permanent changes in identity because few of them remarried, whereas remarriage was the norm for younger widows.

In perhaps the most comprehensive study to date, George (1992) explored age interactions of the predictors of the onset of major depression in a longitudinal study. Nine social factors were included in the study; six of them exhibited significant interactions with age. Three age groups were examined: young adults (age 18–39), middle-aged adults (age 40–64), and older adults (age 65 and older). The risk of onset of major depression was higher for women, African Americans, and urban residents—but all three of these relationships were significant only among young adults. Lower level of education and the presence of chronic physical illness also increased the risk of depression only among younger adults. An interaction between marital status and age was shown to affect the risk of onset of major depression: being married was a significant protective factor only for the oldest respondents. Three risk factors did not interact with age. With other risk factors statistically controlled, income was unrelated to the risk of depression among all three age groups. In contrast, stressful life events and perceived social support were strongly related to risk of depression among all three age groups. Taken to-

gether, these findings suggest that the effects of social factors on the risk of depression tend to be weaker for older than for younger adults, although the strong effects of stress and social support on persons of all ages should not be overlooked.

Other interactions. Some investigators have tested for gender and race interactions to better understand the role of these factors in psychiatric morbidity in later life. Using data from a sample of older African Americans, Husaini and colleagues (1991) found that several social factors were associated with depression only among women: life events, level of social interaction, and perceived social support. Moldin et al. (1993) found that the effects of chronic physical illness on depression were significantly stronger for older women than for older men. Using data from an age-heterogeneous sample, Jones-Webb and Snowden (1993) found that several risk factors for depression were differentially important for whites and African Americans. Higher socioeconomic status was a significant protective factor only for African Americans; in contrast, younger age increased the risk of depression only among African Americans. Widowhood and unemployment increased the risk of depression only for whites. These findings require replication before firm conclusions can be drawn. It is clear, however, that increased attention should be paid to interactive effects in future research. Interactions provide a rigorous method for identifying the differential importance of social risk factors for specific subgroups of the older population.

Age Changes and Cohort Differences in Social Risk Factors

Thus far, we have considered one set of dynamics affecting psychiatric disorder in later life—the impact of social factors on the risk of mental illness. A second set of dynamics also must be considered: age changes and cohort differences that affect *exposure* to social risk factors for psychiatric morbidity. To the extent that exposure to risk factors varies with age or differs across cohorts, the proportion of the older population at risk of psychiatric disorders also varies. Thus, the six categories of social risk factors will be reexamined, with a focus on age changes and cohort differences that affect their prevalence and distribution during later life.

Demographic variables. Age and gender are largely irrelevant in this context because gender is a fixed characteristic, and age changes are the focus of this discussion. Cohort differences in the age structure of society merit brief note, however. As is well documented, industrialized societies have been aging throughout this century because of increasing life expectancy and declining fertility—and it is predicted that this trend will continue well into the next century (Myers 1990). Consequently, in the future, a larger proportion of the population of mentally ill individuals will consist of older adults. This does not mean that a larger proportion of the older population will experience mental illness—only that the number of mentally ill older adults will increase.

Race/ethnicity is a fixed characteristic. However, there are cohort differences in the ethnic compositions of societies. In the United States, current cohorts of older adults include substantial proportions of immigrants from Europe and Russia. Emigration from these countries declined precipitously after World War II, however, and future cohorts of elderly persons will differ in this regard. Currently there is relatively little legal migration to the United States, with the majority of immigrants coming from Central America, South America, and the Far East. It is not clear how the size and composition of the immigrant population affect the prevalence of psychiatric disorders in later life.

Early events and achievements. Education typically is completed during early adulthood and does not change thereafter. There are substantial cohort differences in average levels of education, however. In comparison with their middle-aged and younger peers, current cohorts of older adults average relatively low levels of education (O'Rand 1990). Given the evidence (noted above) that education is negatively related to the prevalence of psychiatric disorders, higher levels of education may bode well for the mental health of future cohorts.

Childhood traumas become fixed experiences for individuals and do not change over time. Again, however, cohort differences are possible. Although there are few solid data on historical trends, cohort differences in the experience of specific childhood

traumas are likely. Compared with their younger peers, current cohorts of older adults are more likely to have experienced parental death and severe poverty (because of the Great Depression) during childhood (George 1993). Conversely, current cohorts of young adults are substantially more likely to have experienced parental separation or divorce during childhood (Watkins et al. 1987). Children in recent cohorts also have confronted unprecedented rates of parental drug abuse (Robins et al. 1991). The implications of these cohort differences for mental health during later life remain unclear.

Later events and achievements. As with education, occupational attainment and income levels are higher among younger than among older cohorts (Smeeding 1990). In light of the documented mental health benefits of higher socioeconomic status, future cohorts of older adults may be at lower risk of psychiatric disorders than are current cohorts. Family formation factors also differ substantially across cohorts. Compared with current cohorts of older adults, younger adults now are less likely to marry, more likely to marry for the first time at later ages, are more likely to divorce, less likely to have children, and more likely to have fewer children (Watkins et al. 1987). These patterns generate major cohort differences in family size and structure. It is not clear whether or how these family changes will affect psychiatric outcomes during old age.

Social integration. In American society, personal attachments to community structures tend to change with age. Participation in religious, civic, and other organizations peaks during late middle age and declines thereafter as a result of health and mobility problems (Cutler and Hendricks 1990). Consequently, formal social attachments typically decrease, albeit modestly, during later life. Data concerning cohort differences in personal attachments to social structure are rare. Some authors suggest that there has been a trend away from community participation (Bellah et al. 1985). Data supporting that conclusion, however, are scant and of questionable quality. Moreover, even if this trend exists, its meaning is ambiguous. It may be, for example, that recent cohorts invest greater personal commitment in fewer community structures. There are firm data concerning one facet of social integration, however: current cohorts of young and middle-aged adults attend religious services less frequently than have previous cohorts (Roof and McKinney1987).

Conclusions about exposure to social disorganization at the aggregate level are difficult to draw because of the absence of data. Many would argue that increased rates of crime, technological change, and residential mobility signal increasing social disorganization that affects both current cohorts of older adults and the developmental histories of future cohorts of elderly. On the other hand, levels of financial security have increased steadily over this century, resulting in a more materially secure population. Whatever the balance of these trends, substantial numbers of older adults are exposed to sources of social disorganization, including economic dislocations, residential mobility, and even "aging in place" in deteriorating neighborhoods.

Vulnerability and protective factors.   Some chronic stressors are age related. Financial resources decrease and chronic illnesses increase during later life. Cohort differences also may operate. The economic climate of the larger society and the availability of income maintenance policies differ across time and can make financial strain more or less common during later life for specific cohorts. Similarly, medical advances affect both the health status of cohorts before old age and the ability to cure or manage chronic illnesses during later life. Policies that facilitate access to health care also affect the likelihood of impaired physical functioning during later life. The majority of evidence suggests that future cohorts will enter old age with better physical health and greater financial resources than their predecessors. These trends should bode well for decreasing the risk of psychiatric disorders during later life among future cohorts.

Social networks tend both to decrease in size and to change in composition during later life (Antonucci 1990). These changes are largely a function of the death and impairment of age peers. In spite of these changes, the vast majority of older adults are not socially isolated and report adequate levels of emotional and instrumental assistance from family and friends. Cohort differences in the size and structure of support networks are likely. Social trends in family formation strongly suggest that older persons in the future will be less likely to have spouses, children, siblings, and extended kin (Wat-

kins et al. 1987). It is possible, however, that nonfamilial relationships will compensate for these changes.

Provoking agents and coping efforts.   There is considerable evidence that age is related to the occurrence of life events. Compared with their younger peers, older adults average fewer life events overall, but are more likely to experience specific types of life events, especially widowhood, deaths of other family members and friends, and illness onset (Hughes et al. 1988). From a mental health perspective, these patterns have mixed implications. On the one hand, fewer life events should decrease the risk of psychiatric disorders. On the other hand, some events that are more common during later life are strongly related to psychiatric morbidity, especially depression. Neither empirical evidence nor theoretical speculation suggests major cohort differences in the frequency of life events during old age.

Information about the relationship between age and coping efforts is slim and ambiguous. This reflects both the limited research base and the difficulties inherent in studying coping. At this point, there is no evidence of age-related declines or cohort differences in coping effectiveness. These conclusions, however, are based on an absence of data rather than on empirical evidence.

Social Factors That Affect Recovery from Psychiatric Disorders

Given that social factors are substantially implicated in the onset and prevalence of psychiatric disorders during later life, it is plausible to expect that such factors might also influence the course of illness and the timing of recovery. To understand the effects of social factors on recovery, longitudinal data are required, preferably with multiple measurements to provide an accurate picture of the dynamics of recovery and relapse. Fortunately, the number of studies of the course and outcome of psychiatric disorders has increased during the past few years. Limitations continue to characterize this research base, however. One problem is the limited scope of many studies. Many studies exclude older adults and/or social factors. The scope of disorders that have been studied is limited as well. Most studies examine depression, and a few focus on bipolar disorder or alcohol abuse; other disorders have not been studied. Finally, most studies ignore treatment variables, despite the obvious relevance of treatment quality to the likelihood of recovery.

Unipolar Depression and Bipolar Disorder

The results of most studies suggest that 40%–50% of depressed patients will recover from an episode of depression within the 1- to 3-year follow-up interval used in most investigations. Approximately half of the patients who recover will remain free of symptoms or below the diagnostic threshold for a major depressive episode. The remainder of the patients who recover will experience at least one relapse during the follow-up interval; a small proportion will cycle rapidly in and out of depressive episodes. Clearly, there is considerable variability in the prognosis and outcome of depressive disorder, and identification of factors that facilitate or impede recovery is an important research issue.

Whether the likelihood of recovery from a depressive episode is related to age remains unresolved. Several studies that compared older and younger depressed patients showed no age differences in the likelihood of recovery (Andrew et al. 1993; George et al. 1989; Hinrichsen and Hernandez 1993). Other studies have demonstrated that older adults are less likely to recover than middle-aged and younger adults (Cole 1983; Hughes et al. 1992); these differences, although statistically significant, are relatively modest. One author (Cole 1983) suggested that in addition to chronological age, age at onset needs to be explored. He speculated that late-onset depression may carry a better prognosis for recovery than does early-onset disorder.

Gender has been studied as a potential predictor of recovery by multiple investigators. The majority of studies have shown that men are more likely than women to recover from an episode of depression (George et al. 1989; Hughes et al. 1992; Winokur et al. 1993). Again, however, results have been inconsistent. Some investigators have reported that gender is unrelated to recovery (Brugha et al. 1990a; Hinrichsen and Hernandez 1993), and one study showed lower rates of recovery among older men than among older women (Baldwin and Jolley 1986).

Few studies have been performed to examine the role of socioeconomic status (SES) in recovery from depression. In the studies available, education—and, more broadly, SES—did not affect the likelihood of recovery from depression (Andrew et al. 1993; George et al. 1989; Hinrichsen and Hernandez 1993). Despite the consistency of findings across studies, this issue requires additional attention. All of the studies cited here were based on clinical samples. Given that health care settings often serve patient populations that are relatively socially homogeneous, it is not clear that this relationship has received a compelling test.

The role of stress in facilitating or impeding recovery from depression has received considerable attention, although results are, again, not consistent. The effects of life events on the course and outcome of depression have been examined in six previous studies. In three of them, the occurrence of life events was associated with a decreased likelihood of recovery (Brugha et al. 1990a; Holahan and Moos 1991; Murphy 1983). In two of the studies, life events were unrelated to the likelihood of recovery (George et al. 1989; Hinrichsen and Hernandez 1993). Baldwin et al. (1993) suggested that the relationship between life events and recovery from depression may be interactive rather than unidirectional. In their sample, life events reduced the likelihood of recovery among older patients without cerebral disease, but not among those with cerebral disease. Investigators in two studies examined the effects of life events on recovery and relapse among patients with bipolar disorder. Again the results were inconsistent. In one study, the occurrence of events increased the probability of relapse (Hunt et al. 1992); the other study showed no relationship between life events and recovery or relapse (McPherson et al. 1993). McPherson and colleagues (1993) suggested that life events may be important in early episodes of bipolar disease but unimportant in later episodes, by which time the disease is less responsive to external factors. This hypothesis awaits empirical investigation.

Chronic stress has been explored in relation to recovery from depression in a few studies. Chronic physical illness has been examined most frequently. Again, results have been mixed. Hinrichsen and Hernandez (1993) reported no relationship between chronic illness and recovery from depression. In contrast, Baldwin and Jolley (1986) reported that chronic illness lowered the likelihood of recovery in their sample of older adults. Using data from a sample of middle-aged and older patients, Hughes et al. (1993) reported that physical illness reduced recovery from depression among middle-aged subjects, but not among older participants. Using a more comprehensive measure, Vieil and co-workers (1992) studied the relationship between number of chronic stressors and recovery from depression. They found that higher levels of chronic stress were associated with reduced likelihood of recovery.

Social support has been the social factor most frequently studied in relation to recovery from depression during old age. However, the multitude of data available do not translate into clear-cut conclusions. Some of the inconsistent findings undoubtedly reflect differences in sample composition. Additional complexity results from the fact that investigators have examined multiple facets of social support. It is helpful to begin with objective dimensions of social support and to then move to subjective perceptions of support quality.

Results are contradictory with regard to the relationship between size of social network and probability of recovery from a depressive episode. Henderson and Moran (1983) observed no relationship between network size and recovery from depression in their sample of community-dwelling adults. In contrast, in their sample of middle-aged and older depressed patients, George and co-workers (1989) found larger network size to be associated with poorer prognosis. The direction of this relationship is counterintuitive and will be addressed shortly. Presence versus absence of a confidant also is a structural property of the social network. To date, there is no evidence that the presence of a confidant affects the likelihood of recovery from depression (Andrew et al. 1993; Murphy 1983). Marital status is another characteristic of the social network. Three previous studies have scrutinized the relationship between marital status and recovery from depression. In two studies, marital status had no effect on recovery (Andrew et al. 1993; Hinrichsen and Hernandez 1993); in one study, married patients were less likely than unmarried patients to recover from an episode of depression (George et al. 1989). This result also is counterintuitive. We believe that the surprising effects of social network size and marital status on recovery from depression reflect selectivity factors. In the community, undoubtedly a major-

ity of social networks and marital relationships are of high quality; consequently, having larger social networks and being married are likely to have positive effects on mental health. In clinical samples, however, it is likely that patients disproportionately represent individuals whose social networks and marriages are problematic or of poor quality. If the quality of those relationships is poor, it is not surprising that their presence predicts a lower rather than a higher probability of recovery. The importance of exploring the quality of the interpersonal relationships of psychiatric patients has been noted by Pattison et al. (1979) in their discussion of "normal" versus "pathological" relationships. Of course, when measures of quality are introduced, the focus is shifted from objective to subjective facets of social support.

Only one study has addressed the effects of levels of social interaction with network members and receipt of instrumental support on recovery from depression (George et al. 1989). Although both measures were significant in bivariate analyses (with higher levels of interaction promoting recovery and high levels of instrumental assistance impeding recovery), the relationships were reduced to nonsignificance once the patients' perceptions of support were added in multivariate models.

Perceptions of support have received the most attention in previous studies of the course and outcome of depressive disorder. Again, results have been mixed. A few research teams have reported that perceptions of social support are unrelated to recovery (Andrew et al. 1993; Hinrichsen and Hernandez 1993; Hirschfeld et al. 1986). The majority of studies, however, have demonstrated that in prospective designs, perception of high-quality support significantly increases the likelihood of recovery (Blazer et al. 1992; Brugha et al. 1990b; George et al. 1989; Henderson and Moran 1983; Holahan and Moos 1991; Hughes et al. 1993; Vieil et al. 1992). In a similar vein, Pattison et al. (1979) reported that perceived support alleviated the anxiety that accompanied depressive symptoms in their sample but did not affect depressive symptoms per se. Vieil (1990) also found that social support was related to recovery from depression in a complex way: perceptions of poor social support predicted relapses characterized by mood-related symptoms, but not relapses involving primarily vegetative symptoms.

Thus far, this discussion has focused on the direct effects of social factors on the course and outcome of depression. A few investigators also have examined the interactive effects of social factors on recovery. First, the stress-buffering hypothesis, positing that social support is more important among persons experiencing stressful life events than among those without such stress, has been tested in two studies. The findings in one study supported the stress-buffering hypothesis (Holahan and Moos 1991), whereas data from the other study did not (George et al. 1989). Second, social support has been shown to interact with other factors to affect the likelihood of recovery. George et al. (1989) found that perceived social support interacted with both age and gender, such that it was more important for middle-aged than for older adults, and more important for men than for women. The interaction between age and perceived support also has been studied by Hughes et al. (1993).

Recall from the discussion of social factors and the onset of depression that some investigators expressed concern that reports of perceived support by depressed persons may be contaminated by the dysphoria of their illness. This issue also has been raised with regard to the role of perceived support in recovery from depression (Henderson 1984). Results to date have failed to support the contamination hypothesis. First, as noted above, perceived support has been shown to interact significantly in one or more studies with life events, age, and gender. These complex interactions argue against the contamination hypothesis—it would be necessary to explain why the contamination disproportionately affected men, middle-aged adults, and persons who recently experienced stressful life events. Second, in studies in which bivariate correlations were reported, the relationships between perceived support and severity of depressive symptoms were quite modest (typically $r = .2–.3$), suggesting little overlap between the two concepts. Finally, two studies have demonstrated that perceived support is more stable over time than is the presence of depressive symptoms (Blazer et al. 1992; Brugha et al. 1990a), thereby arguing against the position that they reflect the same underlying phenomenon.

Ideally, one would like to know about the relative efficacy of social factors compared with the clinical features of the illness episode in predicting recovery from depression. To date, researchers in two studies have made such "head-to-head" comparisons (Andrew et al. 1993; George et al. 1989). In both studies, social factors were stronger predictors of outcome than were the clinical features of the index episode, although large proportions of variance remained unexplained. Examples of the clinical variables examined include previous episodes and hospitalizations, comorbid substance abuse, comorbid anxiety disorder, severity of symptoms at baseline, and depressive subtype (for example, melancholic versus nonmelancholic).

Although firm conclusions about the relationships between social factors and recovery are generally premature because of inconsistencies across studies, it is clear that social factors are implicated in the course and outcome of depression. Research efforts on these issues is increasing, but considerable additional attention is warranted.

Recovery from Alcohol Abuse/Dependence

Compared with the work that has been done concerning depression, the amount of research on the course and outcome of alcohol abuse and dependence has been very limited. The available evidence suggests, however, that alcoholism is associated with a natural history considerably different from that observed with depression. Using the most extensive longitudinal data available to date, Vaillant (1983) described three major patterns of alcohol-related disorders: 1) a consistent pattern of occasional abuse that does not lead to dependence, 2) an atypical pattern of early and massive alcohol misuse that leads to dependence during early adulthood, and 3) the major pattern, in which "social drinking" on a regular basis leads to persistent heavy drinking and eventual dependence. The population of older alcoholics contains two groups: 1) persons who developed alcoholism earlier in life and who persist in alcohol abuse or dependence during old age, and 2) late-onset alcoholics, for whom problem drinking emerges for the first time during late life (Helzer et al. 1991; Warheit and Auth 1985). Some investigators suggest that late-onset alcoholism is more strongly related to social risk factors than are early-onset alcohol problems (Dupree et al. 1984; Wattis 1983), but evidence for this assertion is scant.

A few researchers have investigated the possible role of social factors in the course of alcoholism, although most studies, unfortunately, are rather dated and/or rely on very small samples. Vaillant (1983) reported that social support and religious participation increased the probability of recovery from acute alcoholism, although these factors explain only a small proportion of the variance in illness duration. Similarly, Helzer et al. (1984) reported that social isolation—primarily, the absence of a spouse or confidant—was a predictor of longer acute episodes of alcoholism and, interestingly, that social isolation was more strongly predictive of recovery for older than for younger persons. Helzer and colleagues also reported that, among older alcoholics, more favorable outcomes were associated with female gender, white race, and higher socioeconomic status. Other studies have supported the conclusion that life events are related to poorer prognosis during later life (Finney et al. 1980; Wells-Parker et al. 1983) and that being married increases the likelihood of recovery, especially among older men (Bailey et al. 1965). Several investigators have also suggested that these social factors are more potent predictors of outcome for late-onset than for early-onset alcoholism (Abrahams and Patterson 1978–1979; Rosin and Glatt 1971; Schuckit et al. 1980).

Help Seeking for Psychiatric Disorders

Social factors have been shown to play a meaningful—albeit not fully understood—role in the onset and course of psychiatric disorders. They also are related both to the likelihood that individuals will seek help for psychiatric problems and to the source from which help is sought.

Mental Health Service Use

The primary theory underpinning research on health service use was developed by Ronald Andersen and colleagues (Andersen 1968; Andersen et al. 1975). This simple yet highly useful theory posited that health service use is a function of three generic classes of antecedents: predisposing variables, enabling factors, and need factors. *Predisposing characteristics* are social and attitudinal variables (such as gender, age, educational level, and attitudes toward physicians) that predispose certain individuals to seek help from medical providers. *Enabling factors* are resources that facilitate health service use

(for example, income level and insurance coverage). *Need factors* are the signs and symptoms of disease and disability that can trigger the decision to seek health care. Andersen developed this theory to identify predictors of differential access to health care. The theory has been used more broadly, however, to examine the major predictors of health service use.

The Andersen model has been used primarily in studies of health service use for physical illnesses, both acute and chronic. However, it also has proven to be useful for understanding the role of social and economic factors in help seeking for psychiatric disorders. Those studies suggest that mental health treatments, especially in the mental health specialty sector, are viewed as more discretionary than are treatments for physical complaints both by the public and by administrators of reimbursement programs (for example, insurance coverage is less likely to exist at all and is more limited for mental health treatments than for services sought for physical illness). As one would hope in a health care system that strives for equity, need factors are the strongest predictors of service use for psychiatric disorders (Kessler et al. 1981; Kulka et al. 1979; Leaf et al. 1985). Nonetheless, predisposing and enabling factors are stronger predictors of service use for psychiatric disorders than they are for physical illnesses. Lower education and income levels, being a member of a racial or ethnic minority, being male, and being old are all associated with lower probability of receiving mental health treatment in the presence of psychiatric disorder (Kessler et al. 1981; Kulka et al. 1979; Leaf et al. 1985).

The relationship between race and utilization of mental health services is especially troubling because race remains a significant predictor of service use after socioeconomic factors are taken into account. Recent research reinforces this fact. Padgett et al. (1994, in press) examined patterns of mental health service use in a well-insured, nonpoor population—federal employees. No racial differences were found for inpatient psychiatric care. However, large differences in outpatient treatment between whites and African Americans were observed for adults of all ages and for the elderly in particular.

Interestingly, research on help seeking by older adults has identified an enabling factor that was omitted from the original Andersen model—that is, social support. Adding social support to the Andersen model requires that we address the interface between formal services provided by physicians and other professional providers and informal services provided by family and friends. Two competing hypotheses have been raised to explain the relationship between formal and informal service use by impaired older adults (Noelker and Bass 1989). The first hypothesis suggests that formal services typically are used as substitutes for informal services. Thus, the *substitution hypothesis* posits that formal services will be used primarily by persons without informal sources of assistance. In contrast, the *supplementation hypothesis* posits that formal services are used most often to supplement the contributions of family and friends. Indeed, the supplementation hypothesis suggests that health professionals and informal providers complement and reinforce one another—for example, by working together to ensure the impaired older adult's maximum compliance with treatment plans. Tests of these competing hypotheses have not been performed with regard to mental health service use. The limited evidence available from research focused on physical illness primarily supports the supplementation hypothesis (Edelman and Hughes 1990; Murdock and Schwartz 1978; Noelker and Bass 1989; Smith 1985; Wan 1987), although some studies support the substitution hypothesis (Krause 1988; Soldo 1985). Given evidence that 1) mental health care is viewed as more discretionary than treatment for physical illness, and 2) the role of social support strongly affects the course and outcome of psychiatric disorders, investigation of these hypotheses in the context of mental health problems is a high-priority issue for future research.

Another issue needs to be addressed with regard to predictors of mental health service use. As applied in previous research, the Andersen model has been used to predict both receipt of any medical care and volume of care received. However, recent evidence suggests that these indicators of service use must be examined separately, using different models. The decision to seek or not seek treatment is largely in the control of the individual; thus, receipt of any care versus no care measures help seeking. In contrast, volume of treatment is largely determined by the physician or service provider. A study by Leaf and colleagues (1985) clearly demonstrated the importance of this distinction. Although need factors were the strongest predictor of any

care, they were not significant predictors of volume of care received. Similarly, women were more likely to seek care for psychiatric problems, but gender was unrelated to volume of care received. Interestingly, only age was a significant predictor of both receipt and volume of care. Both older (age 65 and older) and younger adults (aged 18–24) were less likely to seek mental health treatment than those aged 25–64, and, when treatment was received, the older and younger adults obtained less care.

Although the Andersen model has dominated research on health service use, there are other useful theories. Two major alternatives are the *health belief models* (Kirscht 1974; Rosenstock 1974) and the *congruence theories* (Berkanovic and Telesky 1982). These theories focus on the beliefs, attitudes, and modes of symptom recognition and attribution that underlie decisions to seek medical care. Research based on these alternative theories adds a useful psychological and interpretive dimension to the social determinism of the Andersen model. In general, research based on these models is compatible with findings generated by use of the Andersen model. Of particular interest is the fact that the same subgroups found to be less likely to seek help in research based on the Andersen model (i.e., men, the old, and racial and ethnic minorities) are identified in research based on health belief and/or congruence models to be less likely to recognize symptoms, to make accurate attributions about their cause, and to believe that medical care would be beneficial (see Krause 1990 for a review).

Sector Choice for Treatment of Psychiatric Problems

It is widely recognized that the general medical sector provides the majority of care to persons suffering from psychiatric disorders (Regier et al. 1978; Schurman et al. 1985). There also is considerable concern that mentally ill persons may receive lower quality care when treated in the general medical sector. These concerns are supported by evidence that general medical sector providers often 1) fail to identify psychiatric disorders, 2) fail to treat mental disorders, even when identified, and 3) do not provide the most efficacious treatments to the patients they treat (German et al. 1987; Regier et al. 1978). Inappropriate use of psychotropic drugs is of particular concern, especially for older patients (Blazer 1989;

Vestal 1982). Thus, it is important to understand the determinants of sector choice for treatment of psychiatric disorders.

The majority of older adults seeking outpatient care for mental health problems are diagnosed and treated in the general medical sector. Using data from three community samples, George et al. (1988b) found that older adults were twice as likely to receive mental health treatments from general medical providers than from specialty mental health providers. Leaf et al. (1989) reported similar distributions across general medical and mental health sectors. Using data from the National Ambulatory Medical Care Surveys (NAMCS), Schurman and co-workers (1985) reported that 80% of all older adults with primary or secondary psychiatric diagnoses were treated by primary care physicians. More recent data, from the 1989 and 1990 NAMCS, indicated that both old and young adults are far less likely than the middle aged to receive mental health treatment from psychiatrists (Schappert 1993).

A major reason that the majority of psychiatric disorders are treated in the general medical sector is that primary care physicians typically do not refer patients with psychiatric disorders to mental health professionals. Schurman et al. (1985), for example, reported that primary care physicians refer only 5% of older patients with psychiatric problems to psychiatrists, although the most severely ill are the most likely to be referred. Rates of referral to mental health specialists were lower for older than for young and middle-aged patients. This pattern also has been observed in a health maintenance organization (HMO) setting in which psychiatrists were located in the same building as the primary care physicians (Goldstrom et al. 1987).

As noted above, sector choice is important because there is evidence that general medical providers treat psychiatric disorders differently than do mental health professionals. This issue is especially important because older adults are more likely than their younger peers to obtain mental health treatment in the general medical sector. Both the amount of time spent with patients and the types of treatments used differ between general medical and mental health providers. Schurman et al. (1985) reported that the average outpatient visit for treatment of psychiatric problems was 19.6 minutes for general medical providers compared with 44.3 minutes for mental health providers. The major factor

accounting for this difference is that primary care physicians are unlikely to provide psychotherapy. Psychotherapy is provided in 96% of office visits to mental health professionals, but only in 25% of visits to general medical providers (Schurman et al. 1985). In contrast, general medical providers are far more likely to prescribe psychotropic drugs than are mental health professionals. Schurman et al. reported that 78% of office visits for mental health problems to primary care physicians include the prescription of psychotropic medications, as compared with 25% of visits to mental health providers. Studies restricted to samples of older adults have revealed the same pattern. For example, Burns and Taube (1990) estimated that older adults with psychiatric disorders who are treated in the general medical sector are four times more likely to receive psychotropic drugs than to receive psychotherapy. As Blazer (1989) noted, it is sobering to observe that older adults are the least likely to receive psychiatric care from mental health professionals, but are the most likely to receive psychotropic medications.

In summary, social and economic factors, including age itself, play important roles in determining whether older adults with psychiatric disorders receive treatment and the type of provider from whom treatment is obtained. Evidence indicates that treatment for mental health problems is more strongly affected by social factors than is treatment for physical illness. There also are well-documented reasons for concern about the quality of care received for psychiatric disorders treated in the general medical sector. Moreover, all of these patterns are more frequently evidenced for older adults.

Public Policies and Programs

This chapter would not be complete without consideration of the role of public policies and programs. Public policies and programs are interventions. Not all public policies are intended to affect the risk of psychiatric disorder in later life or help seeking for such problems. Indeed, most policies and programs are intended to achieve very different goals. Nonetheless, because public policies and programs alter distributions of social and economic characteristics of the elderly, they frequently affect—either directly or indirectly—the prevalence and distribution of psychiatric disorders during later life.

In the United States, federal programs for the elderly are concentrated in two areas: income maintenance and health care financing. Social Security retirement benefits are the major income transfers to older Americans, but such income is augmented by other programs such as disability benefits and food stamps. Other policies ensure that older Americans are taxed at lower rates than their younger peers, permitting them to retain larger portions of their incomes. There is substantial heterogeneity in levels of income and assets among older adults. Nonetheless, on the whole, older Americans are less likely than are younger citizens to live in poverty (Smeeding 1990). As noted earlier, socioeconomic status is related both to the risk of psychiatric disorders in later life and to the likelihood that mental health services will be obtained. Thus, federal income maintenance programs undoubtedly affect the prevalence and distribution of psychiatric disorders in later life.

Medicare and Medicaid, the major public health care financing programs in the United States, were designed to serve the elderly and the poor, respectively. Medicare coverage is nearly universal among current cohorts of older adults, and a sizable minority of older Americans are covered by Medicaid. There is indisputable evidence that Medicare and Medicaid have increased accessibility to health services for older adults and the poor. Despite the beneficial effects of Medicare and Medicaid, mental health benefits—especially for Medicare—are much lower than those for physical illnesses. Indeed, even a change in the regulations that govern those programs can alter the availability and quality of health care. Medicare was recently changed to a prospective payment model. Although concerns were raised about the effect of this change on quality of care for psychiatric disorders, one study suggests that quality of care for depressive disorders did not decline after implementation of the prospective payment system, and, in fact, may have improved (Wells et al. 1993). As of this writing, multiple proposals for health care reform are being debated at the federal level. If major changes in public financing of medical care are implemented, they will need to be examined with regard to their implications for treatment of psychiatric disorders in later life.

Space limitations preclude a review of other, less universal policies and programs targeted in whole or in part toward older adults—programs ranging from veterans' benefits to senior centers to subsidized housing. All of these programs, as well as many others, however, have the potential to favorably affect risk factors for psychiatric disorders in later life and/or patterns of help seeking for mental health problems.

One issue emphasized throughout this chapter has been the degree to which risk factors vary across cohorts. Awareness of cohort differences is especially relevant for generalizing over time and anticipating future trends. The public policy arena, however, is one area in which speculation is very difficult because programs are often changed rapidly as a result of shifting political climates and priorities. Anticipation of the future is further complicated by the fact that the psychiatric status of future cohorts will be affected by the policies and programs to which they are exposed during earlier stages of the life course. Thus, we can only note that major policy changes have the potential to generate cohort differences in the prevalence and distribution of psychiatric disorders and in patterns of help seeking for mental health problems during later life.

Summary

Social and economic factors play complex and substantial roles in psychiatric disorders in later life. There is excellent evidence that some factors, such as stress and social support, are strongly related to the risk of psychiatric disorders in later life. For other potential risk factors, the links are less well documented, and additional research is needed. Evidence is accumulating that social factors also are implicated in both the course of and the likelihood of recovery from psychiatric disorders, although additional research is required to resolve the inconsistencies observed in previous studies. Social factors also are strongly related to the likelihood that older adults with psychiatric disorders will seek help for them and to the sources from whom treatment will be obtained. Federal income maintenance and health care financing programs directly affect distributions of social and economic risk factors and thus indirectly affect the prevalence and patterns of help seeking for psychiatric disorders in later life. The greatest and most interesting challenge in this area is monitoring the multiple dynamic processes that intersect and intertwine to affect the risk of experiencing psychiatric disorders, the likelihood of recovering from those illnesses, and the receipt of appropriate treatment for psychiatric disorders in later life.

References

Abrahams R, Patterson P: Psychological distress among community elderly: prevalence, characteristics, and implications for service. Int J Aging Hum Dev 9:1–19, 1978–1979

American Psychiatric Association: Diagnostic and Statistical Manual of Mental Disorders, 3rd Edition, Revised. Washington, DC, American Psychiatric Association, 1987

Andersen R: A Behavioral Model of Families' Use of Health Services. Chicago, IL, University of Chicago Center for Health Administration, 1968

Andersen R, Kravits J, Anderson O: Equity in Health Services. Cambridge, MA, Ballinger, 1975

Andrew B, Hawton K, Fagg J, Westbrook D: Do psychological factors influence outcome in severely depressed female psychiatric inpatients? Br J Psychiatry 163:747–754, 1993

Antonucci TC: Social supports and social relationships, in Handbook of Aging and the Social Sciences, 3rd Edition. Edited by Binstock RH, George LK. San Diego, CA, Academic Press, 1990, pp 205–227

Arling G: Strain, social support, and distress in old age. J Gerontol 42:107–113, 1987

Atchley RC: The Sociology of Retirement. Cambridge, MA, Schenkman, 1976

Bailey M, Haberman P, Alksne H: The epidemiology of alcoholism in an urban residential area. Quarterly Journal of Studies on Alcohol 26:19–40, 1965

Baldwin RC, Jolley DJ: The prognosis of depression in old age. Br J Psychiatry 149:574–583, 1986

Baldwin RC, Benbow SM, Marriott A, et al: Depression in old age—a reconsideration of cerebral disease in relation to outcome. Br J Psychiatry 163:82–90, 1993

Bellah RN, Madsen R, Sullivan WM, et al: Habits of the Heart. Berkeley, CA, University of California Press, 1985

Berkanovic E, Telesky C: Social networks, beliefs, and the decision to seek medical care: an analysis of congruent and incongruent patterns. Med Care 20:1018–1026, 1982

Blazer DG: Impact of late-life depression on the social network. Am J Psychiatry 140:162–166, 1983

Blazer DG: The epidemiology of psychiatric disorders in late life, in Geriatric Psychiatry. Edited by Busse EW, Blazer DG. Washington, DC, American Psychiatric Press, 1989, pp 235–260

Blazer DG, George LK, Landerman R, et al: Psychiatric disorders: a rural/urban comparison. Arch Gen Psychiatry 42:651–656, 1985

Blazer DG, Hughes DC, George LK: The epidemiology of depression in an elderly community population. Gerontologist 27:281–287, 1987a

Blazer DG, Hughes DC, George LK: Stressful life events and the onset of a generalized anxiety syndrome. Am J Psychiatry 144:1178–1183, 1987b

Blazer DG, Burchett B, Service C, et al: The association of age and depression among the elderly: an epidemiologic exploration. J Gerontol 46:M210–M215, 1991

Blazer DG, Hughes DC, George LK: Age and impaired subjective support: predictors of symptoms at one-year follow-up. J Nerv Ment Dis 180: 172–178, 1992

Brown GW, Harris T: Social Origins of Depression: A Study of Psychiatric Disorder in Women. London, Tavistock, 1978

Brown GW, Prudo R: Psychiatric disorder in a rural and an urban population, I: aetiology of depression. Psychol Med 11:581–599, 1981

Brugha TS, Bebbington PE, Sturt E, et al: The relation between life events and social support networks in a clinically depressed cohort. Soc Psychiatry Psychiatr Epidemiol 25:308–312, 1990a

Brugha TS, Bebbington PE, MacCarthy B, et al: Gender, social support, and recovery from depressive disorders: a prospective clinical study. Psychol Med 20:147–156, 1990b

Burns B, Taube C: Mental health services in general medical care and in nursing homes, in Mental Health Policy for Older Americans: Protecting Minds at Risk. Edited by Fogel BS, Furino A, Gottlieb GL. Washington, DC, American Psychiatric Press, 1990, pp 63–84

Chiriboga DA: Adaptation to marital separation in later and earlier life. J Gerontol 37:109–114, 1982

Cohen CI, Sokolovsky J: Schizophrenia and social networks: expatients in the inner city. Schizophr Bull 4:546–560, 1978

Cohen D, Eisdorfer C: Depression in family members caring for a relative with Alzheimer's disease. J Am Geriatr Soc 36:385–389, 1989

Cole MG: Age, age of onset and course of primary depressive illness in the elderly. Can J Psychiatry 28:102–104, 1983

Comstock G, Helsing K: Symptoms of depression in two communities. Psychol Med 6:551–563, 1976

Cronkite RC, Moos RH: The role of predisposing and moderating factors in the stress-illness relationship. J Health Soc Behav 25:372–393, 1984

Crotty P, Kulys R: Social networks: the views of schizophrenic clients and their significant others. Soc Work 27:301–309, 1985

Crowell BA, George LK, Blazer DG, et al: Psychosocial risk factors and urban/rural differences in the prevalence of major depression. Br J Psychiatry 149:307–314, 1986

Cutler SJ, Hendricks J: Leisure and time use across the life course, in Handbook of Aging and the Social Sciences, 3rd Edition. Edited by Binstock RH, George LK. San Diego, CA, Academic Press, 1990, pp 169–185

Cutrona C, Russell D, Rose J: Social support and adaptation to stress by the elderly. Psychol Aging 1:47–54, 1986

Dimond M, Lund DA, Caserta MS: The role of social support in the first two years of bereavement in an elderly sample. Gerontologist 27:599–604, 1987

Dooley D, Catalano R, Jackson R, et al: Economic, life, and symptom changes in a nonmetropolitan community. J Health Soc Behav 22:144–154, 1981

Dupree LW, Broskowski H, Schonfeld L: The gerontology alcohol project: a behavioral treatment program for elderly alcohol abusers. Gerontologist 24:510–516, 1984

Edelman P, Hughes S: The impact of community care on provision of informal care to homebound elderly persons. J Gerontol 45:S74–S84, 1990

Ekerdt DJ, Bosse R, Goldie C: The effects of retirement on somatic complaints. J Psychosom Res 27:61–67, 1983

Essex MJ, Klein MH, Lohr MJ, et al: Intimacy and depression in older women. Psychiatry 48:159–178, 1985

Feighner JP, Robins E, Guze SB, et al: Diagnostic criteria for use in psychiatric research. Arch Gen Psychiatry 26:57–63, 1972

Felton BJ, Brown P, Lehmann S, et al: The coping function of sex-role attitudes during marital disruption. J Health Soc Behav 21:240–247, 1980

Finney J, Moos R, Mewborn CR: Posttreatment experiences and treatment outcome of alcoholic patients six months and two years after hospitalization. J Consult Clin Psychol 48:17–29, 1980

Folkman S, Lazarus RS: An analysis of coping in a middle-aged community sample. J Health Soc Behav 21:219–239, 1980

George LK: Social factors and the onset and outcome of depression, in Aging, Health Behaviors, and Health Outcomes. Edited by Schaie KW, House JS, Blazer DG. Hillsdale, NJ, Lawrence Erlbaum, 1992, pp 137–159

George LK: Sociological perspectives on life transitions. Annu Rev Soc 19:353–373, 1993

George LK, Siegler IC, Okun MA: Separating age, cohort, and time of measurement: analysis of variance or multiple regression. Exp Aging Res 7:297–314, 1981

George LK, Landerman R, Blazer D, et al: Concurrent morbidity between physical and mental illness: an epidemiologic examination, in Mechanisms of Psychological Influences on Physical Health, With Special Attention to the Elderly. Edited by Carstensen LL, Neale J. New York, Plenum, 1988a, pp 9–22

George LK, Blazer DG, Winfield-Laird I, et al: Psychiatric disorders and mental health service use in later life: evidence from the Epidemiologic Catchment Area program, in Epidemiology and Aging. Edited by Brody J, Maddox GL. New York, Springer, 1988b, pp 189–219

George LK, Blazer DG, Hughes DC, et al: Social support and the outcome of major depression. Br J Psychiatry 154:478–485, 1989

German PS, Shapiro S, Skinner EA, et al: Detection and management of mental health problems of older patients by primary care providers. JAMA 257:489–493, 1987

Glick IO, Weiss RD, Parkes CM: The First Year of Bereavement. New York, Wiley, 1974

Goldstrom ID, Burns BJ, Kessker LG, et al: Mental health services use by elderly adults in a primary care setting. J Gerontol 42:147–153, 1987

Green BH, Copeland JRM, Dewey ME, et al: Risk factors for depression in elderly people: a prospective study. Acta Psychiatr Scand 86:213–217, 1992

Greenfied SF, Swartz MS, Landerman R, et al: Long-term psychosocial consequences of childhood exposure to parental problem drinking. Am J Psychiatry 150:608–613, 1993

Grusky O, Tierney K, Manderscheid RW, et al: Social bonding and community adjustment of chronically mentally ill adults. J Health Soc Behav 26:49–63, 1985

Helzer JE, Carey KE, Miller RH: Predictors and correlates of recovery in older versus younger alcoholics, in Nature and Extent of Alcohol Problems Among the Elderly. Edited by Maddox G, Robins LN, Rosenberg N. Rockville, MD, National Institute on Alcohol Abuse and Alcoholism, 1984, pp 83–99

Helzer JE, Burnam A, McEvoy LT: Alcohol abuse and dependence, in Psychiatric Disorders in America. Edited by Robins LN, Regier DA. New York, Free Press, 1991, pp 81–115

Henderson AS: Interpreting the evidence on social support. Soc Psychiatry 19:49–52, 1984

Henderson AS, Moran PAP: Social relationships during the onset and remission of neurotic symptoms: a prospective community study. Br J Psychiatry 143:467–472, 1983

Henderson AS, Grayson DA, Scott R, et al: Social support, dementia, and depression among the elderly in the Hobart community. Psychol Med 16:379–390, 1986

Henderson AS, Jorm AF, MacKinnon A, et al: The prevalence of depressive disorders and the distribution of depressive symptoms in later life: a survey using draft ICD-10 and DSM-III-R. Psychol Med 23:719–729, 1993

Hinrichsen GA, Hernandez NA: Factors associated with recovery from and relapse into major depressive disorder in the elderly. Am J Psychiatry 150:1820–1825, 1993

Hirschfeld RMA, Klerman GL, Andreasen N, et al: Psychosocial predictors of chronicity in depressed patients. Br J Psychiatry 148:648–654, 1986

Holahan CK, Holahan CJ: Self-efficacy, social support, and depression in aging: a longitudinal analysis. J Gerontol 42:65–68, 1987

Holahan CJ, Moos RH: Life stressors, personal and social resources, and depression: a 4-year structural model. J Abnorm Psychol 100:31–38, 1991

Holzer CE, Sheal BM, Swanson JS, et al: The increased risk for specific psychiatric disorders among persons of low socioeconomic status. American Journal of Social Psychiatry 6:259–271, 1986

Hughes DC, Blazer DC, George LK: Age differences in life events: a multivariate controlled analysis. Int J Aging Hum Dev 27:207–220, 1988

Hughes DC, Turnbull JE, Blazer DG: Family history of psychiatric disorder and low self-confidence:

predictors of depressive symptoms at 12-month follow-up. J Affect Disord 25:197–212, 1992

Hughes DC, DeMallie D, Blazer DG: Does age make a difference in the effects of physical health and social support on the outcome of a major depressive episode? Am J Psychiatry 150:728–733, 1993

Hunt N, Bruce-Jones W, Silverstone T: Life events and relapse in bipolar affective disorder. J Affect Disord 25:13–20, 1992

Husaini BA, Moore ST, Castor RS, et al: Social density, stressors, and depression: gender differences among the black elderly. J Gerontol 46:P236–P242, 1991

Jones-Webb RJ, Snowden LR: Symptoms of depression among blacks and whites. Am J Public Health 83:240–244, 1993

Kaminsky M: Pictures from the past: the uses of reminiscence in case work with the elderly. J Gerontol 1:19–31, 1978

Kandel DB, Davies M, Rabers VH: The stressfulness of daily social roles for women: marital, occupational, and household roles. J Health Soc Behav 26:64–78, 1985

Kasl SV, Harburg E: Mental health and the urban environment: some doubts and second thoughts. J Health Soc Behav 16:268–282, 1975

Kessler RC: Stress, social status, and psychological distress. J Health Soc Behav 20:259–272, 1979

Kessler RC, Magee WJ: Childhood adversities and adult depression: basic patterns of association in a US national survey. Psychol Med 23:679–690, 1993

Kessler RC, Neighbors HW: A new perspective on the relationships among race, social class, and psychological distress. J Health Soc Behav 27:107–115, 1986

Kessler RC, Brow RL, Broman CL: Sex differences in psychiatric help-seeking: evidence from four large-scale surveys. J Health Soc Behav 22:49–64, 1981

Kirscht JP: The health belief model and illness behavior. Health Education Monographs 2:387–408, 1974

Koenig HG, Ford SM, George LK, et al: Religion and anxiety disorder: an examination and comparison of associations in young, middle-aged, and elderly adults. Journal of Anxiety Disorders 7:321–342, 1993a

Koenig HG, George LK, Blazer DG, et al: The relationship between religion and anxiety in a sample of community-dwelling older adults. J Geriatr Psychiatry 26:65–93, 1993b

Koenig HG, George LK, Meador KG, et al: The relationship between religion and alcoholism in a sample of community-dwelling adults. Hosp Community Psychiatry 45:225–231, 1994

Krause N: Social support, stress, and well-being among older adults. J Gerontol 41:512–519, 1986a

Krause N: Stress and sex differences in depressive symptoms among older adults. J Gerontol 41:727–731, 1986b

Krause N: Chronic financial strain, locus of control, and depressive symptoms among older adults. Psychol Aging 2:375–382, 1987

Krause N: Stressful life events and physician utilization. J Gerontol 43:S53–S61, 1988

Krause N: Illness behavior in late life, in Handbook of Aging and the Social Sciences, 3rd Edition. Edited by Binstock RH, George LK. San Diego, CA, Academic Press, 1990, pp 228–244

Krause N, Liang J, Yatomi N: Satisfaction with social support and depressive symptoms: a panel analysis. Psychol Aging 4:88–97, 1989

Kulka RA, Veroff J, Douvan E: Social class and the use of professional help for personal problems: 1957 and 1976. J Health Soc Behav 20:2–16, 1979

La Gory M, Fitzpatrick K: The effects of environmental context on elderly depression. Journal of Aging and Health 4:459–479, 1992

Landerman R, George LK, Blazer DG: Adult vulnerability for psychiatric disorders: interactive effects of negative childhood experiences and recent stress. J Nerv Ment Dis 179:656–663, 1991

Leaf PJ, Livingston MM, Tischler GL, et al: Contact with health professionals for treatment of psychiatric and emotional problems. Med Care 23:1322–1337, 1985

Leaf PJ, Bruce ML, Tischler GL, et al: Factors affecting the utilization of specialty and general medical mental health services. Med Care 26:9–26, 1989

McMordie WR, Blom S: Life review therapy: psychotherapy for the elderly. Perspect Psychiatr Care 4:162–166, 1979

McPherson H, Herbison P, Romans S: Life events and relapse in established bipolar affective disorder. Br J Psychiatry 163:381–385, 1993

Meador KG, Koenig HG, Hughes DC, et al: Religious affiliation and major depression. Hosp Community Psychiatry 43:1204–1208, 1992

Mirowsky J, Ross CE: Age and depression. J Health Soc Behav 33:187–205, 1992

Mitchell J, Mathews HF, Yesavage JA: A multidimensional examination of depression among the elderly. Research on Aging 15:198–219, 1993

Moldin SO, Scheftner WA, Rice JP, et al: Association between major depressive disorder and physical illness. Psychol Med 23:755–761, 1993

Mueller D: The current status of urban-rural differences in psychological disorder: an emerging trend for depression. J Nerv Ment Dis 169:18–27, 1981

Murdock SH, Schwartz DF: Family structure and the use of agency services: an examination of patterns among elderly native Americans. Gerontologist 18:475–481, 1978

Murphy E: Social origins of depression in old age. Br J Psychiatry 141:135–142, 1982

Murphy E: The prognosis of depression in old age. Br J Psychiatry 142:111–119, 1983

Myers G: Demography of aging, in Handbook of Aging and the Social Sciences, 3rd Edition. Edited by Binstock RH, George LK. San Diego, CA, Academic Press, 1990, pp 19–44

Neff JA, Husaini BA: Stress-buffer properties of alcohol consumption: the role of urbanicity and religious identification. J Health Soc Behav 26:207–221, 1985

Noelker LS, Bass DM: Home care for elderly persons: linkages between formal and informal caregivers. J Gerontol 44:S63–S70, 1989

O'Rand AM: Stratification and the life course, in Handbook of Aging and the Social Sciences, 3rd Edition. Edited by Binstock RH, George LK. San Diego, CA, Academic Press, 1990, pp 130–150

Oxman TE, Berkman LF, Kasl S, et al: Social support and depressive symptoms in the elderly. Am J Epidemiol 135:356–368, 1992

Padgett DK, Patrick C, Burns BJ, et al: Ethnicity and the use of outpatient mental health services in a national insured population. Am J Public Health 84:222–226, 1994

Padgett DK, Patrick C, Burns BJ, et al: Use of mental health services by black and white elderly, in Handbook on Ethnicity, Aging, and Mental Health. Westport, CT, Greenwood Press, in press

Pattison EM, Lleamas R, Hurd G: Social network mediation of anxiety. Psychiatric Annals 9:56–67, 1979

Regier DA, Goldberg ID, Taube CA: The de facto US mental health services system: a public health perspective. Arch Gen Psychiatry 35:685–693, 1978

Robins LN, Regier DA (eds): Psychiatric Disorders in America. New York, Free Press, 1991

Robins LN, Locke BZ, Regier DA: An overview of psychiatric disorders in America, in Psychiatric Disorders in America. Edited by Robins LN, Regier DA. New York, Free Press, 1991, pp 328–366

Roof WC, McKinney WC: American Mainline Religion. New Brunswick, NJ, Rutgers University Press, 1987

Rosenstock IM: Historical origins of the health belief model, in The Health-Belief Model and Personal Health Behavior. Edited by Becker M. Thorofare, NJ, Slack, 1974, pp 9–27

Rosin A, Glatt M: Alcohol excess in the elderly. Quarterly Journal of Studies on Alcohol 32:53–59, 1971

Ross CE, Huber J: Hardship and depression. J Health Soc Behav 26:312–327, 1985

Schappert SM: Office visits to psychiatrists: United States, 1989–1990. Advancedata 237. Hyattsville, MD, National Center for Health Statistics, 1993

Schuckit MA, Atkinson JH, Miller PL, et al: A three-year follow-up of elderly alcoholics. J Clin Psychiatry 41:412–416, 1980

Schurman RA, Kramer PD, Mitchell JB: The hidden mental health network. Arch Gen Psychiatry 42:89–94, 1985

Schwab J, Warheit G, Holzer C: Mental health: rural-urban comparisons. Mental Health and Society 1:265–274, 1974

Smeeding TM: Economic status of the elderly, in Handbook of Aging and the Social Sciences, 3rd Edition. Edited by Binstock RH, George LK. San Diego, CA, Academic Press, 1990, pp 362–382

Smith K: Sex differences in benzodiazepine use among the elderly: effects of social support. Doctoral dissertation, Duke University, Durham, NC, 1985

Smith-Ruiz D: Relationship between depression, social support, and physical illness among elderly blacks: research notes. J Natl Med Assoc 77:1017–1019, 1985

Sokolovsky J, Cohen C, Berger D, et al: Personal networks of ex–mental patients in a Manhattan SRO hotel. Human Organization 37:5–15, 1978

Soldo B: In-home services for the dependent elderly. Research on Aging 7:281–304, 1985

Spitzer RL, Endicott J, Robins E: Research Diagnostic Criteria (RDC) for a Selected Group of Functional Disorders, 3rd Edition. New York, New York State Psychiatric Institute, 1978

Tennstedt S, Cafferata GL, Sullivan L: Depression among caregivers of impaired elders. Journal of Aging and Health 4:58–76, 1992

Tweed JL, Schoenbach VJ, George LK, et al: The effects of childhood parental death and divorce on six-month history of anxiety disorders. Br J Psychiatry 154:823–828, 1989

Vaillant GE: The Natural History of Alcoholism. Cambridge, MA, Harvard University Press, 1983

Veroff J, Douvan E, Kulka RA: The Inner American. New York, Basic Books, 1981

Vestal RF: Pharmacology and aging. J Am Geriatr Soc 30:191–200, 1982

Vieil HO: Depressed mood and major depressive episodes: differential responsiveness to psychosocial experiences. European Archives of Psychiatry and Neurological Sciences 240:62–65, 1990

Vieil HO, Kuhner C, Brill G, et al: Psychosocial correlates of clinical depression after psychiatric inpatient treatment: methodological issues and baseline differences between recovered and nonrecovered patients. Psychol Med 22:415–427, 1992

Wan TH: Functionally disabled elderly: health status, social support, and use of health services. Research on Aging 9:61–78, 1987

Warheit GL, Auth JB: Epidemiology of alcohol abuse in adulthood, in Psychiatry, Vol 3. Edited by Cavenar JL. Philadelphia, PA, JB Lippincott, 1985, pp 512–537

Warheit GL, Holzer CE, Arey SA: Race and mental illness: an epidemiologic update. J Health Soc Behav 16:243–256, 1975

Watkins SC, Menken JA, Bongaarts J: Demographic foundations of family change. American Sociological Review 52:346–358, 1987

Wattis JP: Alcohol and old people. Br J Psychiatry 143:306–307, 1983

Wells KB, Rogers WH, Davis LM, et al: Quality of care for hospitalized depressed elderly patients before and after implementation of the Medicare Prospective Payment System. Am J Psychiatry 150:1799–1805, 1993

Wells-Parker E, Miles S, Spencer B: Stress experiences and drinking histories of elderly drunken driving offenders. J Stud Alcohol 44:429–437, 1983

Winokur G, Coryell W, Keller M, et al: A prospective follow-up of patients with bipolar and primary unipolar affective disorder. Arch Gen Psychiatry 50:457–465, 1993

CHAPTER 9

Epidemiology of Psychiatric Disorders in Late Life

Dan G. Blazer, M.D., Ph.D.

The epidemiology of psychiatric disorders in late life is the study of the distribution of psychiatric disorders among the elderly and those factors that influence this distribution (MacMahon and Pugh 1970). Roberts (1977) suggested that epidemiology is not only the basic science of preventive and community medicine, but also may serve as the basic science of clinical practice. In this chapter, the goals and findings of psychiatric epidemiologists will be reviewed as they relate to the care of the psychiatrically impaired older adult. In contrast to the substantive sciences, epidemiology is primarily a way of thinking about health and disease beyond the traditional clinical approach (Morris 1975). Platt (1952) described the need for the epidemiological method as follows:

> Wherein then lies the need for training physicians in science . . . ?
>
> First, . . . the training is needed because scientific discipline is the antidote to a surfeit of the art of medicine, which, carried too far, degenerates into medical lifemanship. . . . The clinician who knows only the art . . . may end

by deceiving not only his patients but himself. . . . Self-deception is the sin against which scientific discipline protects. (p. 978)

The evaluation of the impaired older adult is fraught with pitfalls that lead to uncertainty in clinical decision making (Weinstein and Feinberg 1980). Uncertainty can arise from errors in collecting clinical data—for example, the patient may report one complaint but the physician records another. Problems in case identification are especially prevalent in late life, for the older adult may not express those symptoms traditionally associated with psychiatric diagnoses derived from DSM-III-R (American Psychiatric Association 1987). Other data may be ambiguous, for observers may differ in their ability to detect symptoms and signs of a disorder—anxiety, for example. Still further uncertainty may surround the relation between normality and disease. How are clinicians to distinguish the ubiquitous problems of the worried well from serious and treatable psychiatric disorders? Finally, uncertainty about the effects of treatment may derive from a lack of data about the natural history of a disorder.

The beginning of the epidemiological study of psychiatric disorders in the elderly is an understanding of the population at risk—namely, that group of individuals in whom psychiatric disorders may arise. The increasing numbers and percentages of older adults in developed countries compared with younger age groups serves as poignant testimony to the need for increased study of psychiatric disorders and mobilization of services for older adults. A demographic profile and projection of the aging U.S. population is presented in Table 9–1.

Although both the number and the percentage of older adults have increased progressively throughout the 20th century, a dramatic increase will occur in the first half of the 21st century, primarily because of the aging of the "baby boom" generation. Between 1995 and 2030, the number of persons age 65 and older in the United States will double (as it doubled from 1950 to 1985). If the average retirement age remains the same and persons continue the trend to enter the work force in their early 20s, the impact of an aging population upon the economy of the country—not to mention the need for health care—will be dramatic. This can be seen in the profound increase in the age/dependency ratio—that is, the ratio of persons in the work force compared with children or the retired. Flexibility in retirement and other social and economic changes will help modify the impact of this "squaring" of the population pyramid. Nevertheless, this demographic revolution will affect every individual and every institution in our society (Pifer and Bronte 1986).

Although changes in the total number and per-centage distribution of the population across the life span are affected primarily by changes in childbearing patterns, changes in mortality within the aging population have affected the demographics of late life as well. The life expectancies for men and women in 1990 were 71 and 78 years, respectively. Much of the difference between the genders in life expectancy at birth can be accounted for by differences in mortality after the age of 65. For example, on the basis of data available in 1990, a woman who has lived to age 65 can expect to live an additional 19 years, whereas a man can expect to live an additional 15 years. The relative contributions to this difference in longevity of environmental and genetic factors have been debated extensively. Cigarette smoking, more prevalent among men, has contributed to the difference. The more stressful and physically demanding occupations in which men engaged through much of the 20th century may partially explain the difference as well. These potential mortality risks are dynamic across the genders, for more women are entering the workplace at all levels and more women are smoking. Women may have a genetic advantage in life expectancy.

As much as the overall changes in the demographics of the 65+ age group have commanded the attention of health care planners, perhaps an even more dramatic revolution has occurred among the oldest old. Currently, persons 85 years of age and older constitute the most rapidly growing age group in the American population (Rosenwaike 1985). Although this population numbered less than 1 million in 1960, nearly 5 million persons will be 85 years of age and older by 2000, and will represent nearly 15% of the 65+ age group. The oldest old will require increased medical and psychiatric services, for at the age of 85 they enter a time of life characterized by a high prevalence and incidence of dementia and psychiatric symptoms combined with physical illness (such as depression).

What can psychiatric epidemiological studies contribute to mental health services for older adults? Morris (1975) has suggested the following uses of epidemiology:

1. Identify cases (for example, can the symptom pattern of depression in elderly persons be readily identified in community-dwelling as well as clinical [e.g., hospitalized] populations of older adults?)

Table 9–1.   Actual and projected population of older adults (65+) in the United States by year

Year	Population
1900	3,100,000
1920	4,900,000
1940	9,000,000
1960	16,700,000
1980	25,700,000
2000	34,900,000
2020	52,100,000

Source.   Abstracted from Fowles DG: "A Profile of Older Americans: 1990" (DHHS Publication PF3029[1290] D996). Washington, DC, American Association of Retired Persons, Administration on Aging, 1990, pp 1–2.

2. Reveal distribution of psychiatric disorders in the population (for example, what is the prevalence and/or incidence of dementia?)
3. Trace historical trends of mental illness among elderly persons (for example, has the incidence of suicide increased among this population over the past 10 years?)
4. Determine etiology of psychiatric disorders in late life (for example, do social factors contribute more to the etiology of late-life psychiatric disorders than to such disorders in midlife, given lower potential for genetic contributions?)
5. Examine use of psychiatric and other mental health services by elderly persons (for example, do psychiatrically impaired older adults in the community underutilize psychiatric services?)

Each of these functions of epidemiology will be reviewed in this chapter.

Case Identification

Clinicians constantly face the task of distinguishing abnormality from normality. Although most epidemiologists and clinicians agree on the core symptoms of psychiatric disorders throughout the life cycle, the absolute distinction between a case and a noncase—that is, persons requiring psychiatric attention versus those who do not require such care— is not easily established. Many of the symptoms and signs of a psychiatric disorder in late life may be ubiquitous with the aging process, thus blurring the distinction between cases and noncases. Epidemiologists can assist the clinician in identifying meaningful clusters of symptoms and significant degrees of symptom severity. Case identification is also the foundation of descriptive epidemiology: "cases" are the numerator of the equation from which prevalence and incidence estimates are derived in community and clinical samples (the denominator).

What is a case? Copeland (1981) suggests that the question be turned by epidemiologists, with advantage, to "A case for what?" The choice of a construct for a case depends upon the particular scientific or clinical inquiry of the investigator. If, in order to determine the value of a new short-acting sedative–hypnotic agent, the clinician wishes to identify a group of older adults suffering from initial insomnia, the prevalence and severity of a target symptom—initial insomnia—define the case. The sleep difficulty may result from a number of different underlying disorders, but diagnosis would be irrelevant to the purpose of the study. For most clinicians, however, the goal of case identification is to identify subjects experiencing uniform underlying psychopathology (Blazer 1982). According to Goodwin and Guze (1979), diagnosis is prognosis. Diagnostic categories that approximate true disease processes have a number of characteristics, including the following (Weissman and Klerman 1978):

1. A category should be distinguished on the basis of patterns of symptomatology.
2. A category should predict the outcome of a disorder.
3. A category should reflect underlying biological reality, confirmed by family and genetic studies.
4. Laboratory studies should eventually validate a diagnostic category (for example, the use of rapid eye movement latency or the dexamethasone suppression test to delineate melancholic depression).
5. The classification scheme should identify persons who may respond to a specific therapeutic intervention, such as a particular form of psychotherapy or a specific group of medications.

Other authors define a case on the basis of severity of symptoms or the physical, psychological, and social impairment secondary to the symptoms. This approach to case identification is less popular among clinicians, who are more inclined to "treat a disease" than to "improve function." Improved function should derive from remission of the disease. Nevertheless, function has special relevance in the care of older adults. When managing chronic psychiatric disorders, such as primary degenerative dementia of the Alzheimer's type, the improvement or maintenance of physical functioning is a clinician's primary goal. Family members are often more concerned with improved functioning than with alleviation of symptoms. Improved sleep and appetite and a decline in suicidal ideation in a depressed older adult may not translate into a perceived recovery from a depressive episode by the family. Rather, the family may focus on the quality of interpersonal interactions and social functioning.

Regardless of the approach taken to identify cases, most clinicians and clinical investigators want to achieve perfection in the separation of cases from noncases. The epidemiological method depends, for the most part, on a clear distinction between cases and noncases (Kleinbaum et al. 1982), yet most older adults do not ideally fit the psychiatric diagnosis that they receive (Strauss et al. 1979). Regardless of the diagnostic system, unusual or borderline cases that cannot be clearly placed in a single category exist. This has led some investigators to consider the possibility of "fuzzy sets" as a means by which cases can be more realistically distinguished (Clive et al. 1983; Swartz et al. 1986). Not infrequently, older adults manifest more than one disease simultaneously—for example, major depression and primary degenerative dementia. In addition, the prescribed categories of DSM-III-R or DSM-IV (American Psychiatric Association 1994) do not always match the symptoms that can be exhibited by individuals in this population: generalized anxiety, for instance, is not easily disentangled from a major depressive episode in an agitated older adult.

Most natural clustering of older adults into categories is perceptually "fuzzy" (Rosch 1978), for natural processes rarely exhibit necessary and sufficient criteria for sharp distinctions. Boundaries between closely related categories are ill defined. Some of the methods of case identification, such as the symptom checklist and standardized interview approaches that archive symptoms, are adaptive to the development of clusters of both symptoms and subjects with fuzzy boundaries. For example, depressed elderly persons are more likely to express cognitive dysfunction than depressed middle-age persons, yet cognitive dysfunction is part of the depressed syndrome across the life cycle (Blazer et al. 1986). Therefore, psychiatric syndromes—rather than discrete disorders—are more realistic as diagnostic entities in geriatric psychiatry. The most common of these syndromes are memory loss, depression, anxiety, suspicions and agitation, sleep disorders, and hypochondriasis (Blazer 1994).

Regardless of the approach taken to case identification, a diagnosis must be reliable and valid for it to be a useful means of communicating clinical information. To pass the test of reliability, a diagnosis must be consistent and repeatable. Standardized or operational methods for identifying psychiatric symptoms and the availability of specific criteria for psychiatric diagnoses have greatly improved the reliability of case identification by psychiatrists. Reliability, however, does not ensure validity—that is, the test of whether a case identified by a particular method reflects underlying reality. Unlike providers in other medical specialties, clinicians who work with psychiatrically ill patients focus their skills, for the most part, on thoughts, feelings, and actions. No objective standard exists for testing the truth of a particular syndrome identified by symptoms and behavior.

Once the criteria are set for case identification, a number of approaches to identifying cases have been used in psychiatric epidemiological studies of elderly persons. Although each approach contributes to our understanding of psychopathology in late life, each also presents unique problems. Historically, the most frequently used method of case identification in epidemiological surveys has been the chart review method or the establishment of case registries (Farris and Dunham 1939; New York State Department of Mental Hygiene 1960; Pasamanick et al. 1959). In these studies, diagnoses rely on the attending clinician's evaluation of the patient. Variability in criteria used by clinicians, variability in the socioeconomic status of patients, and variability of criteria for disorders across the life cycle may each contribute to a bias in these studies (Clausen and Kohn 1959). Schoenberg et al. (1987) used the chart review method to calculate the incidence of Alzheimer's disease and other disorders characterized by dementia among the population in Rochester, Minnesota. They estimated an average annual incidence of 187.5 new cases per 100,000 population per year.

A second approach to case identification is the use of self-administered symptom scales and personality inventories. Frequently used scales in epidemiological surveys include the Center for Epidemiologic Studies Depression Scale (CES-D), a scale that screens for depressive symptoms (Radloff 1977); the Short Portable Mental Status Questionnaire (SPMSQ; Pfeiffer 1975); and the Mini-Mental State Exam (MMSE; Folstein et al. 1975). The advantage of these scales is that, unlike case registries, they do not subjectively assign patients to a particular diagnostic category; a disadvantage is the lack of diagnostic specificity that can be achieved with their use. For example, the severity of depressive symptoms after the loss of a loved one may be similar to that associated with a major depressive episode with melancholia. A symptom checklist cannot be used to distinguish one from the other, although the diagnosis of, and intervention for, these two disorders would be very different. Blazer et al. (1991) estimated the prevalence of clinically significant depression symptoms among community-dwelling elders in North Carolina to be 9%, although most of these individuals would not be diagnosed with major depression.

In recent years, a commonly used means of case identification in both clinical and community studies has been the standardized interview. The Present State Examination (PSE; Wing et al. 1974), the Schedule for Affective Disorders and Schizophrenia, Lifetime Version (SADS-L; Spitzer and Endicott 1978), and the Diagnostic Interview Schedule (DIS; Robins et al. 1981) are examples of the most frequently used interview schedules. These instruments are generally based on diagnostic systems, such as DSM-III-R, that list specific criteria for a particular diagnostic category. They tend to be reliable and generally are valid. Nevertheless, the standardized interviews are derived from particular diagnostic systems. In addition, there are "trade-offs." The more clinical judgment contributes to the identification of a case, the less reliable cases tend to be (although cases identified by a less structured schedule may reflect clinical judgment better than a highly structured interview that eliminates clinical judgment). For example, the DIS was used in the Epidemiologic Catchment Area (ECA) study (Regier et al. 1988), from which a 1-month national estimate of the prevalence of mood disorders in persons 65 years of age and older was 3.3% (compared with 8.29% for persons 25–44 years old [Regier et al. 1988]).

Finally, one of the more frequently used epidemiological methods in community studies relies on the judgment of a clinician to assess the probability that a psychiatric disorder is present on the basis of data from a survey questionnaire. Clinicians are asked to estimate the chances that a particular individual in the community would be given a psychiatric diagnosis if interviewed clinically. This approach tends to maximize the clinical adjustment in evaluating a forced-response questionnaire. The method suffers, however, because it cannot be used to distinguish among different types of psychiatric impairment and therefore is less clinically relevant. For example, the distinction between major depression and dementia may be blurred, despite the relatively distinct approaches to therapy that are implied in the specific diagnoses. In the Midtown

Manhattan Study (Srole and Fischer 1981), this approach was used in demonstrating that mental health impairment was much more likely to be associated with birth cohort than with age.

Distribution of Psychiatric Disorders

The authors of descriptive studies of the epidemiology of psychiatric impairment have concentrated on either overall mental health functioning or the distribution of specific psychiatric disorders in the population. Reports from these studies usually begin as general observations of the relationship of impairment or specific disorders to such characteristics as age, gender, race, occupation, and social class. These trends provide the template for more in-depth studies of the hereditary, biological, and psychosocial contributors to the etiology of disorders and the epidemiology of mental health care utilization. Frequencies of disorders within the population are usually presented in terms of a proportion: the percentage of persons suffering from a defined impairment or specific disorder within the population. Almost all such studies provide estimates based on community samples of larger populations.

The prevalence of cognitive impairment and dementia in selected community and institutional populations, as determined in selected studies, is presented in Tables 9–2 and 9–3. The prevalence of moderate to severe cognitive impairment usually reported within community populations is approximately 4%–6%, as illustrated by the data presented. Because such studies measure nothing more than cognitive functioning, this prevalence of cognitive impairment must not be assumed to be the prevalence of Alzheimer's disease or actual cerebral impairment. For example, the prevalence of cognitive "impairment" can be biased by the educational level of the population being studied, as well as by other sociocultural factors that may affect performance of cognitive tasks. Most studies of institutional populations show a range of severe cognitive impairment that clusters around 50%. Although the prevalence of dementia in institutional populations is undoubtedly much higher than it is in community-dwelling populations, these prevalence figures must not be misinterpreted as representing the prevalence of dementia in institutions.

Even in community studies performed by clinicians, the prevalence of subtypes of dementia, such as multi-infarct dementia or primary degenerative dementia of senile onset, is not usually reported. Rather, investigators typically report the level of severity of generalized organic brain syndromes (see Table 9–3). Within community populations, these prevalences vary, but most reports hover around 5%. Exceptions have appeared in more recent studies. For example, a two-stage approach to the identification of dementia was reported by Folstein et al. (1985). First, the investigators screened the population using the MMSE. Next, they evaluated in detail those persons who demonstrated impairment on the MMSE. Results from this evaluation were surprising. Although the overall prevalence of dementia was 6.1%, the relative distribution between multi-infarct dementia and Alzheimer's disease (primary degenerative dementia) was different from the 3-to-1 ratio usually reported: 2.8% multi-

Table 9–2.   Prevalence of cognitive impairment in community and institutional populations

Study	Sample	N	Assessment age	Strategy	Prevalence (%)
ECA[1]	1988 U.S. population	5,702	65+	MMSE	4.9
			65–74	MMSE	2.9
			75–84	MMSE	6.8
			85+	MMSE	15.8
EPESE					
New Haven[2]	Community	2,811	65+	SPMSQ (9 items)	5.3
Iowa[2]	Community (entire population of two rural counties)	3,673	65+	SPMSQ (9 items)	1.3
East Boston[2]	Community	3,812	65+	SPMSQ (9 items)	6.0
Durham County[2,3]	Institution	100	65+	SPMSQ	47
Minnesota[4]	Institutionalized Medicaid patients	74	96% were ≥ 65	SPMSQ	59.4
National[5]	Institution	526	x = 83	Chart review	39

Note.   ECA = Epidemiologic Catchment Area; EPESE = Established Populations for Epidemiologic Studies of the Elderly; MMSE = Mini-Mental State Exam (Folstein et al. 1975); MSQ = Mental Status Questionnaire (Kahn et al. 1960); SPMSQ = Short Portable Mental Status Questionnaire (Pfeiffer 1975).
Source.   1. Regier et al. 1988; 2. Huntley et al. 1986; 3. Blazer 1978; 4. Teeter et al. 1976; 5. Burns et al. 1988.

Table 9–3.   Prevalence of dementia in community and institutional populations

Site	Sample	N	Age	Strategy	Prevalence (%)
Europe					
Sweden (Essen-Möller et al. 1956)	Rural community	443	65+	Psychiatric interviews	10.8 mild and 5.0 severe organic brain syndrome
England (Kay et al. 1970)	Community	758	65+	Psychiatric interviews	6.2 severe organic brain syndrome
Netherlands (Heren et al. 1991)	Community	1,259	85+	Standardized interviews	23 dementia (11% with moderate or severe dementia)
United States					
Baltimore (Folstein et al. 1985)	Community	923	65+	Psychiatric interviews and laboratory studies	2.0 Alzheimer's disease; 2.8 multi-infarct dementia; 1.3 mixed or unspecified dementia
Maryland (Rovner et al. 1986)	Institution	50	96% were ≥ 66	Standardized interviews	56 primary degenerative dementia; 22 multi-infarct dementia; 4 Parkinson's dementia
Boston (Evans et al. 1989)	Community	467	65+	Standardized interviews and clinical evaluation	12.3 Alzheimer's disease

infarct dementia versus 2.0% Alzheimer's disease. One explanation for these findings is the relatively high proportion of blacks in the community sample studied (unlike most clinical samples of dementia). In a similar study in Boston (Evans et al. 1989), the prevalence of Alzheimer's disease was estimated at over 12%, with an estimate over 40% for persons 85+ years of age. That the prevalence of Alzheimer's disease is estimated to be twice that of moderate to severe cognitive impairment may at first appear counterintuitive. Nevertheless, a careful diagnostic evaluation may establish Alzheimer's disease even when overall cognitive impairment is not severe.

In Tables 9–4 and 9–5, the prevalence of selected psychiatric symptoms and disorders in community populations is presented. If the entire adult life cycle were included, many of the symptoms reported would find their highest frequencies among elderly persons, especially symptoms of hypochondriasis and sleep difficulties. Most studies of depressive symptoms across the life cycle in the past have documented a higher prevalence in late life (Warheit et al. 1973). A relatively higher frequency of certain symptoms in elderly populations, however, does not necessarily signify an increased frequency of specific psychiatric disorders. The paradox of relatively high reports of depressive symptoms and relatively low reports of the prevalence of major depressive episodes illustrates this point (Blazer 1982). Diagnostic categories, such as those found in DSM-III-R, are clusters of symptoms and signs that derive their validity not from the overall weight of symptomatology but, rather, from regularities in the clustering of history, the persistence of symptoms over time, a predictable outcome, a common pathophysiology, and possibly common biochemical disturbances. As biological markers of psychiatric disorders are identified, laboratory diagnostic techniques will provide information that is complementary to the symptoms reported. As our knowledge progresses in the area of nomenclature, new categories of symptoms may be lumped together to define a particular syndrome. As Morris (1975) noted, each succeeding generation will split and lump groups of symptoms and signs to suit its own purposes, given the current biomedical and clinical understanding of disease entities.

Symptoms, the most objective clinical indicators of psychopathology, may reflect more than one diagnostic entity. On the other hand, symptoms may not be associated with any disorder of interest to the clinician. For example, decreased appetite can result from a number of sources. At a given time, grief reactions, more frequent in late life than at other stages of the life cycle, may be virtually indistinguishable from major depressive episodes if appetite alone is considered. Loss of appetite also accompanies major life adjustments such as a forced change of residence or a decline in economic resources. Most commonly, loss of appetite in late life is a result of poor physical health.

Psychiatric disorders other than depression are also found in a lower prevalence among the elderly than at other stages of the life cycle (Table 9–5). The

Table 9–4. Prevalence of psychiatric symptoms in community populations of older adults

Site	N	Age	Strategy	Disorder	Prevalence (%)
New Haven (Huntley et al. 1986)	2,811	65+	CES-D (≥ 16)	Depression	15
Durham County (Blazer and Houpt 1979)	997	65+	Selected questions	Hypochondriasis	14
San Francisco (Lowenthal and Berkman 1967)	589	60+	Selected questions	Suspiciousness	17
Durham County (Christenson and Blazer 1984)	997	65+	MMPI	Persecutory ideation	4
Iowa (Huntley et al. 1986)	3,217	65+	Selected questions	Trouble falling asleep	14
				Awakes during the night	34
				Sleepy during the day	31
North Carolina (Blazer et al. 1991)	784	65+	DIS	Generalized anxiety	1.9

Note. CES-D = Center for Epidemiologic Studies Depression Scale (Radloff 1977); DIS = Diagnostic Interview Schedule (Robins et al. 1981); MMPI = Minnesota Multiphasic Personality Inventory (Hathaway and McKinley 1970).

Table 9–5.   Prevalence of selected psychiatric disorders in community populations of older adults

Site	N	Age	Strategy	Disorder	Prevalence (%)
ECA (Regier et al. 1988)	5,702	65+	DIS	Major depression	M = 0.4; F = 0.9
				Dysthymia	M = 1.0; F = 2.3
				Alcohol abuse	M = 1.8; F = 0.3
				Schizophrenic/schizo-phreniform disorder	M = 0.1; F = 0.1
England (Kay et al. 1964)	297	65+	Psychiatric interviews	Anxiety and dysthymic disorder	5–10
Liverpool (Copeland 1990)	1,070	65+	Geriatric community	Depressive neurosis	8.5
				Depressive psychosis	3.0

Note.   DIS = Diagnostic Interview Schedule (Robins et al. 1981); ECA = Epidemiologic Catchment Area.

relatively lower prevalence of alcohol abuse among this population has been well documented in the literature, as has been the lower prevalence of schizophrenia and schizophreniform disorders. The virtual absence of these disorders in the ECA data (Regier et al. 1988) may reflect selective mortality. On the other hand, it may also reflect the case-finding techniques used (the investigators did not attempt to assess the homeless). The community data do not include individuals in institutions, and many persons in late life with chronic schizophrenia may be institutionalized. In addition, early-onset schizophrenia may be associated with a "burned-out" symptom picture; this fact, coupled with poor reporting, may mean that an individual's clinical presentation does not meet the criteria for a diagnosis of schizophrenia.

Another question derives from these data: Do unique late-life symptom presentations render the Research Diagnostic Criteria (RDC; Spitzer et al. 1978) and DSM-IV inadequate as a system of nomenclature? DSM-IV provides age-specific categories for children but not for elderly persons. Clinicians who work with older adults, however, have often commented that depression may be masked in late life by symptoms of poor physical health or pseudodementia. Yet there is no compelling evidence for developing a new diagnostic classification specific to older adults. Although DSM-IV may not identify all older persons with significant psychiatric symptoms, those who do qualify for a DSM-IV diagnosis are not unlike persons at other stages of the life cycle (Blazer 1980a; Blazer et al. 1987). The deficiency inherent in DSM-IV is that it poorly differentiates psychiatric symptoms from those that signify the

presence of physical illness and impaired cognition—a situation that may also occur in younger individuals, although it is far more common as a diagnostic problem in late life than in midlife.

The prevalence of psychiatric disorders—other than dementia—in treatment facilities is presented in Table 9–6. As is evident, the prevalence of minor depression and major depression in treatment facilities is much higher than that found in community populations. Many depressed older adults may be selectively admitted to medical inpatient units or to long-term care facilities (because older adults are less likely to use specialty psychiatric care). The lower prevalence of these disorders in the community, therefore, should not lull the clinician into believing that psychiatric problems are of little consequence for older adults.

Historical Studies

Psychiatrists typically follow patients for relatively short periods of time during the course of their illnesses. In addition, they usually interact with each patient within a relatively brief window of historical time. Epidemiological studies add a historical perspective to current cross-sectional findings in population and clinical surveys. Some diseases, such as tuberculosis, are known to wax and wane; new diseases, such as acquired immunodeficiency syndrome (AIDS) dementia, may emerge; and old diseases, such as smallpox, are eradicated or disappear naturally (Morris 1975). Historical studies in psychiatric epidemiology are rare, especially of the elderly. Unlike changes observed with infectious diseases, however, temporal changes that occur with most be-

Table 9–6. Prevalence of selected psychiatric disorders among older adults in selected treatment facilities

Site	N	Age	Strategy	Disorder	Prevalence (%)
Inpatient geriatric evaluation unit (Cheah and Beard 1980)	262	45+ but primarily 55+	Psychiatric interviews	Dysphoria/depression	31.1
Intermediate care facility (Rovner et al. 1986)	50	96% were < 66	Psychiatric interviews	Major depression Paraphrenia	6.0 2.0
Long-term care (Parmelee et al. 1989)	708	65+ 65+	DSM-III-R[1] checklist	Major depression Minor depression	12.4 30.5
Acute-care facility (Koenig et al. 1988)	171	65+	Screening and modified DIS[2]	Major depression Minor depression	11.5 23.0

Note. 1. American Psychiatric Association 1987; 2. Diagnostic Interview Schedule (Robins et al. 1981).

haviors that are of psychiatric interest must be determined over years rather than months; exceptions are the clustering of psychiatric emergencies after the Christmas season and the increase in suicide during the spring season of each year (Hilliard et al. 1981; Lester 1979). Constructs of case identification have changed over the years, and so it is rare to find a study in which similar methods of case identification were applied at two points distant enough in time to establish historical trends. Longitudinal studies are also fraught with methodological problems, especially problems with follow-up.

The study of changes in suicide frequency among older adults during the 20th century illustrates the value of longitudinal studies, despite the methodological problems associated with these designs. Suicide rates in 1980 were positively correlated with age, although the correlation was not as dramatic as it was in the 1970s. As is shown in Figure 9–1, the correlation is almost totally explained by the dramatic increase in frequency of suicide by white men over 60 years old. However, the pattern has changed since 1980, with a 25% increase in suicide among older persons between 1980 and 1985 (Meehan et al. 1991).

The century-long trend for suicide rates increasing with age has flattened. Why has this happened? The suicide rate at any point in time is determined by at least three factors: age, generational or cohort effects, and unique stressors for a particular age group at a particular point in time (that is, period effects). Both age and generational effects were shown to be predictors of suicide in the United States since 1900 in a study by Murphy and Wetzel (1980). The generational effect was illustrated in a

study by Haas and Hendin (1983). Age groups were studied at four points in time from 1908 to 1970. Cohorts entering the 15- to 24-year-old age group showed significantly different suicide rates. The 15- to 24-year-olds in 1908 showed a suicide rate of 13.5/100,000; in contrast, the rate of the same age group in 1923 showed a rate of 6.3/100,000. The 1908 cohort has continued to show higher rates of suicide than the 1923 cohort at every age through life, though both cohorts showed increases in suicide rates with age. In other words, a cohort is presently passing through the 55- through 74-year age window that has always shown lower rates of suicide than the cohort that is currently passing through the 75+-year age window. When examined cross-sectionally, the curve is flattened (Figure 9–1). Younger cohorts (such as the 1946—or baby-boom— cohort) show increased rates of suicide.

In a study of suicides in England and Wales, Murphy and colleagues (1986) were able to demonstrate a marked period effect. In a cohort analysis of recorded suicides from 1921 to 1980, a fall in suicide rates of successively older cohorts was identified. (This finding contrasts with figures in the United States.) Murphy postulated the impact of period events, specifically, World War II and the detoxification of domestic gas. The last hypothesis is especially intriguing. Before the early 1960s, domestic gas in England and Wales contained large amounts of carbon monoxide. One of the more popular means of suicide, particularly among middle-aged and elderly individuals, was putting one's head in a gas oven. As domestic gas was converted to a methane-based product in the 1960s, the rate of gas poisoning in the more elderly groups decreased dramatically. This decrease was not offset by increasing rates of suicide by other means, suggesting that withdrawal of a method of suicide could result in a net saving of life.

It is clear from these historical studies that many factors contribute to changing rates in at least one indicant of psychiatric disorder—that is, suicide. Concomitant changes in other factors are less well understood but may be especially relevant to the study of psychiatric disorders in elderly persons. Klerman et al. (1985) suggest that the relatively low prevalence of depression in the 1980s among late-life cohorts may be the result of a cohort effect. Current cohorts of older adults appear remarkably protected against severe or clinically diagnosed depressive disorders. Younger cohorts, in contrast, have exhibited higher rates of major depression throughout the life cycle. Because there is no reason to expect the rates for younger cohorts to decrease as they enter late life—that is, there is no evidence of a period effect—the prevalence of major depression in late life will probably increase in future years.

An additional historical consideration in the study of psychiatric disorders is the study of incidence and duration of these disorders. Cumulative incidence—the probability of developing a disorder over a specified period of time (usually 1 year)—is less important to the health care provider at a given point in time, but is very relevant to planning for services in the future. The duration of a psychiatric disorder in late life, such as senile dementia, interacts with both incidence and prevalence. For example, the incidence of primary degenerative dementia or senile dementia of the Alzheimer's type appears to have been relatively unchanged over the past 15–20 years (although accurate studies are still lacking). Nevertheless, patients with dementia currently receive better health care and appear to follow the general trend of the aging population—an increased life expectancy. Therefore, in addition to a higher number of cases because there are more older adults at risk, the prevalence of the disorder over time is increasing, leading to a greater burden of dementia within the community (Gruenberg 1978).

Etiological Studies

One of the more important tasks in epidemiology is to identify factors that can either predispose individuals to developing psychiatric disorders or precipitate such disorders (Blazer and Jordan 1985). Both genetic and environmental causative agents can be identified in population studies, yet the significance of this research has only recently achieved some status in psychiatry, and has rarely been applied specifically to geriatric psychiatry.

The contribution of epidemiology to uncovering hereditary trends in mental disorders is best illustrated by the work in senile dementia. Heston et al. (1981) studied the relatives of 125 probands who suffered from dementia of the Alzheimer's type (as identified at autopsy). The risk of dementia in first-degree relatives varied with the age of the person at the onset of dementia. Those persons who were first-degree relatives of someone with Alzheimer's disease were more likely to develop the disease earlier in life, suggesting that the inherited form of Alzheimer's disease is associated with an

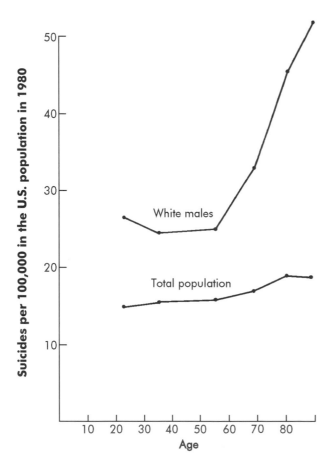

Figure 9–1. U.S. suicide rates in 1980.
Source. Reproduced with permission from Blazer DG, Bachar JR, Manton KG: "Suicide in Late Life: Review and Commentary." *J Am Geriatr Soc* 34:521, 1986.

accelerated onset. In a more recent study by Barclay et al. (1986), a family history for dementia was positive in 35.9% of patients with Alzheimer's disease, compared with 5.6% of individuals who were cognitively intact.

Other investigators have suggested an association between early-onset Alzheimer's disease and Down's syndrome. Heyman et al. (1983) studied 68 patients with Alzheimer's disease who had demonstrated clinical onset before the age of 70. Secondary cases of dementia were found in 17 (25%) of the families, affecting 22 of the probands' siblings and parents. An increased frequency of Down's syndrome was observed among relatives of the probands, a rate of 3.6/1,000, compared with the expected rate of 1.3/1,000. Heston et al. (1981) not only found an excess of Down's syndrome in the families of patients with Alzheimer's disease, but also identified an increased frequency of lymphoma and immune system disorder diatheses among family members, suggesting that immune system disorders and an increased risk for Alzheimer's disease are associated. Another finding that has been shown to be increasingly frequent among patients with Alzheimer's disease is a history of head trauma (Heyman et al. 1983).

Among the more intriguing genetic studies, however, are those of Folstein and Breitner (1981). These investigators suggest that a subtype of Alzheimer's disease may be transmitted as an autosomal dominant trait with complete penetrance (Folstein and Breitner 1981; Chase et al. 1983). In their original investigation, Folstein and Breitner found that the presence of aphasia and apraxia distinguished patients suffering from primary degenerative dementia who had a family history of the disease from those who did not have such a history. In a study of 39 cases of Alzheimer's disease, patients with relatives suffering from the disease were less often able to complete a sentence on the MMSE than those who did not have afflicted relatives ($P < .05$). Among those individuals who were unable to write a sentence, the investigators found a fourfold increased risk of dementia compared with the general population. In a follow-up study, Folstein and colleagues (1985) found that among 54 nursing home patients diagnosed with Alzheimer's disease, 40 were considered aphasic and agraphic and 14 were not. Among the first-degree relatives of the aphasic/agraphic patients with primary degenerative disor-

der, there was a 44% risk of senile dementia by age 90, approaching the 50% rate for a genetic disorder that is autosomal dominant with complete penetrance.

Exposure to physical agents in the environment, such as certain chemicals or the spirochete that causes syphilis, have long been known to be causes of cognitive problems. Exposure to some of these agents may lead to other psychiatric symptoms as well. Two illustrative studies demonstrate the effect of such agents on the brain.

Goodwin et al. (1983) studied 260 noninstitutionalized men and women between the ages of 60 and 94. On clinical examination, these individuals were not found to have serious illnesses or to be clinically malnourished or vitamin deficient. Dietary intake for these subjects was calculated; the nutrients measured included protein, vitamin C, vitamin B_{12}, folic acid, riboflavin, thiamine, niacin, and pyridoxine. Blood samples were obtained to determine the blood levels of these specific nutrients. The investigators discovered a significant relationship between scores on memory tests and blood levels of vitamin C and folic acid in these generally well-functioning older adults. Henderson et al. (1992) found a relationship between Alzheimer's disease and starvation/malnutrition in a case-control study. These results suggest that there may be variables, such as nutrient levels, that provide an opportunity for intervention in the relationship between cognitive functioning and primary (innate) and secondary (environmentally induced) changes with aging. Gerontologists have long sought such intervening variables that may allow clinical intervention to prevent or mitigate deficits that were previously ascribed to primary aging.

Parker and co-workers (1983) investigated the relationship between alcohol use and cognitive functioning. They studied 1,937 employed men and women who were asked about their alcohol consumption during the previous month. In addition, their vocabulary skills and abstraction abilities were examined. Results from the study suggested a linear relationship between the amount of alcohol consumption during the previous month and cognitive impairment. The relationship held both for the men and for those women whose drinking patterns resembled the men's. This model suggests that cognitive performance may be decreased by alcohol consumption before the postintoxication period, and because this relationship is linear, even moderate alcohol intake may lead to impairment in cognitive functioning. The implications of these findings for the elderly are evident.

By far the most frequently investigated environmental factors associated with psychiatric disorders are social factors. The changing roles and circumstances of older adults are considered by many investigators to cause stress for older adults and therefore to contribute to the onset of psychiatric disorders and cognitive difficulties. Blazer (1980b), in a study of 986 community-dwelling older adults, found the crude estimate of relative risk for mental health impairment—given a life event score ≥ 150 on the Schedule of Recent Events (Holmes and Rahe 1967), to be 2.14. A relative risk of 1.73 ($P < .01$) was estimated when a binary regression procedure was used, controlling for physical health, economic status, social support, and age. In a study of individuals 55 years of age and older by Murrell and co-workers (1983), social factors, including widowhood, divorce, separation, and decreased income, were related to depressive symptomatology in the community.

Nevertheless, the study of social factors in relation to psychiatric disorders must not be viewed simplistically. The mitigating effect of social support, the perception of the event (as well as the actual occurrence of the event), the expectancy of the event, and the perceived importance of the event may all contribute to the impact of environmental stress upon the older adult. In a previous study, Blazer (1993) suggested a number of possible hypotheses by which environmental stress and social support may interact with psychiatric disorders:

1. Environmental stressors, including stressful life events, may cause or contribute to the development of a psychiatric disorder. The bulk of the literature on stressful life events as precipitants of depressive disorders is based on this hypothesis.
2. Environmental stressors may decrease physical health status, and the older adult reacts to the decline in physical health by developing a reactive psychiatric disorder (an adjustment disorder with depressed mood, for example).
3. Environmental stressors experienced in the remote past may contribute to physical and psychological changes that predispose the older

adult to develop a psychiatric disorder in late life. Studies of early deprivation (such as the death of a parent in childhood) exemplify this hypothesis.
4. Social isolation may contribute to the onset of a psychiatric disorder. For example, lack of social stimuli may contribute to increased paranoid ideation in an older adult.
5. Environmental stressors may be buffered by the perceived or actual social support. In other words, when actual or perceived social support is decreased, the causal relationship between environmental stress and psychiatric disorder is enhanced.
6. The lack of important specific social relations, such as the absence of a spouse or confidant, may predispose an individual to the development of a psychiatric disorder. Studies of the increased risk for depression in the year after the loss of a spouse or confidant derive not only from the stress of the loss but also from the absence of the relationship in the succeeding year.
7. The absence of a satisfactory social network may lead to decreased frequency of social interaction, which in turn leads to an increased likelihood of developing certain psychiatric disorders. For example, lack of social relations may increase the prevalence of hypochondriacal symptoms and the use of health services (thereby providing an increase in social contact).

Health Service Utilization

Epidemiological studies provide a disturbing profile of the use of mental health services by elderly persons. Although older adults are less likely than those in any other age group to use community-based psychiatric services, they are more likely to use psychotropic medication. In a study of three communities (New Haven, Baltimore, and St. Louis), Shapiro and colleagues (1984) found that 6%–7% of older adults had made a visit to a health care provider for mental health reasons during the 6 months before evaluation. Those in the group aged 65 and older infrequently received care from mental health specialists, even if they were identified in the community as suffering from a DSM-III (American Psychiatric Association 1980) psychiatric disorder or severe cognitive impairment. German et al. (1985) analyzed the data from Baltimore in greater detail. Of those persons under the age of 65, 8.7% had made a visit to a specialty or primary care provider for mental health care during the 6 months before the evaluation. For those aged 65–74, the rate was 4.2%; of those aged 75 and older, only 1.4% received such care. In the 75+ age group, not one person among the 292 individuals interviewed saw a specialty mental health care provider. The investigators concluded that the likeliest source of care for older individuals suffering from emotional or psychiatric problems is their primary care provider, within the context of a visit made for physical medical problems.

In contrast, the use of psychotropic drugs is high among older adults. In a nationwide survey, Mellinger et al. (1978) found that 40% of the men and 44% of the women over age 60 who suffered from psychiatric distress had used a psychotherapeutic drug during the preceding year, and 17% and 20%, respectively, were regular users. A study by Rossiter (1983) from another national survey showed that 23.4% of persons 65 and older were using some central nervous system agent at the time of the survey, a percentage higher than that for any other age group (for example, only 14.4% of the 25- to 54-year-old age group used these agents). The rates may be dropping, however. Hanlon et al. (1992) found that only 12.5% of community-dwelling persons over 65 years of age during 1986 were taking central nervous system drugs. In a review of prescriptions for Medicaid patients residing for at least 1 year in nursing homes in the state of Tennessee, Ray et al. (1980) found that 43% of these individuals had received antipsychotic drugs during the preceding year, and 9% were given such drugs on a chronic basis. These rates may be dropping as well, given the Omnibus Budget Reconciliation Act (OBRA) regulations recently instituted by the federal government.

The value of community surveys does not end with a description of patterns of health services use, however. Such investigations are especially useful for determining the need for services for noninstitutionalized and institutionalized elderly persons. By sampling elderly community-dwelling populations, researchers can collect data on rates of impairment, need for services, perceived needs or demands for services, and the current use of services. This information can be used by government and private agencies to chart effective assessment, treatment, and prevention programs. This development is especially relevant to the care of older adults, as they tend to be isolated, their psychiatric impair-

ment may be masked, and they are less active advocates for their mental health needs than are younger persons.

Such an approach is illustrated by a study done in North Carolina (Blazer 1978). A statewide survey showed that only 8% of the elderly in the community suffering from functional mental impairment were receiving mental health services at the time the survey was conducted. The problem was compounded by the fact that for the elderly, mental health services were not integrated with other available services. The overlap of impairments was documented in this study as well. Blazer and Maddox (1982) reviewed a seven-step model, modified from Wing (1968), to use the data from the 1978 study to develop a new service for older adults. First, a target population was identified through an epidemiological survey of Durham County. Next, the appropriate types of services for this population were determined through a population needs assessment. Because cognitive impairment was highly correlated with impairment in other areas, it was decided that an integrated program of psychotherapy, psychotropic medication management, medical evaluation, and social interaction would be the most appropriate way to develop the necessary services. The third step was to assess the perception of need for services, since this would affect the level of use. Ten percent of the sample expressed some need for counseling, whereas 31% of the cognitively impaired stated that they experienced such a need. Fourth, current use was assessed. Only 10 of the 997 subjects (1%) were receiving any kind of counseling or psychotherapy, although 20% were taking some type of psychotropic medication, almost always prescribed by a primary care physician. The fifth step, closely tied to the fourth, was to assess the impact of other factors on service utilization. One such factor was economic resources. The assumption that those with adequate financial resources would seek private care rather than use a public clinic (as was planned) had to be considered. Because 40% of those who were impaired had inadequate finances, these were identified as persons who would potentially use such a clinic. The sixth step was to address the need for personnel to represent the interdisciplinary requirements described above. It was decided that a part-time staff, including a psychiatrist, a social worker, a physician with experience in geriatric medicine, and a registered nurse with experience in geriatric nursing, as well as a receptionist/secretary, would fulfill these requirements. In addition, it was decided that the staff would make efforts to integrate their services with existing service providers such as primary care physicians and social service agencies. The seventh and final step was to assess the accuracy of these planning efforts after the clinic had been established. Four years after the inception of the clinic, the follow-up assessment revealed that the flow of patients was about as predicted in the planning estimate and that the mix of staff was appropriate to delivering the care conceived initially. Also as anticipated, most of the patients seen were individuals with multiple impairments who could not afford usual medical and psychiatric care.

References

American Psychiatric Association: Diagnostic and Statistical Manual of Mental Disorders, 3rd Edition, Revised. Washington, DC, American Psychiatric Association, 1987

American Psychiatric Association: Diagnostic and Statistical Manual of Mental Disorders, 4th Edition. Washington, DC, American Psychiatric Association, 1994

Barclay LL, Kheyfets S, Zemcov A, et al: Risk factors in Alzheimer's disease, in Alzheimer's Disease and Parkinson's Disease: Strategies for Research and Development. Edited by Fisher A, Hanin I, Lachman C. New York, Plenum, 1986, pp 141–146

Blazer DG: The OARS Durham surveys: description and application, in Multidimensional Functional Assessment: The OARS Methodology—A Manual, 2nd Edition. Durham, NC, Duke University Center for the Study of Aging and Human Development, 1978, pp 75–88

Blazer DG: The diagnosis of depression in the elderly. J Am Geriatr Soc 28:52–58, 1980a

Blazer DG: Life events, mental health functioning and the use of health care services by the elderly. Am J Public Health 70:1174–1179, 1980b

Blazer DG: The epidemiology of late life depression. J Am Geriatr Soc 30:587–592, 1982

Blazer DG: Depression in Late Life, 2nd Edition. St. Louis, MO, CV Mosby, 1993

Blazer DG: Geriatric psychiatry, in The American Psychiatric Press Textbook of Psychiatry, 2nd Edition. Edited by Hales RE, Yudofsky SC, Talbott JA. Washington, DC, American Psychiatric Press, 1994, pp 1405–1421

Blazer DG, Houpt JL: Perception of poor health in the healthy older adult. J Am Geriatr Soc 27:330–334, 1979

Blazer DG, Jordan K: Epidemiology of psychiatric disorders and cognitive problems in the elderly, in Psychiatry, Vol 3. Edited by Michels R, Cavenar JO. Philadelphia, JB Lippincott, 1985, pp 1–12

Blazer DG, Maddox G: Using epidemiology survey data to plan geriatric mental health services. Hosp Community Psychiatry 33:42–45, 1982

Blazer DG, Bachar JR, Manton KG: Suicide in late life: review and commentary. J Am Geriatr Soc 34:519–526, 1986

Blazer DG, Bachar JR, Hughes DC: Major depression with melancholia: a comparison of middle-aged and elderly adults. J Am Geriatr Soc 35:927–932, 1987

Blazer DG, Burchett B, Service C, et al: The association of age and depression among the elderly: an epidemiologic exploration. J Gerontol 46:M210–M215, 1991

Burns BJ, Larson DB, Goldstrom ID, et al: Mental disorder among nursing home patients: preliminary findings from the National Nursing Home Survey Pretest. International Journal of Geriatric Psychiatry 3:27–35, 1988

Chase GA, Folstein MF, Breitner JCS, et al: The use of life tables and survival analyses in testing genetic hypotheses with an application to Alzheimer's disease. Am J Epidemiol 7:590–597, 1983

Cheah KC, Beard OW: Psychiatric findings in the population of a geriatric evaluation unit: implications. J Am Geriatr Soc 28:153–156, 1980

Christenson RM, Blazer DG: Epidemiology of persecutory ideation in an elderly population in the community. Am J Psychiatry 141:1088–1091, 1984

Clausen JA, Kohn ML: Relation of schizophrenia to the social structure of a small city, in Epidemiology of Mental Disorder. Edited by Pasamanick B. Washington, DC, American Association for the Advancement of Science, 1959, pp 69–94

Clive J, Woodbury MA, Siegler IC: Fuzzy and crisp set theoretic-based classification of health and disease: a qualitative and quantitative comparison. J Med Syst 7:317–332, 1983

Copeland JRM: What is a "case"? a case for what?, in What Is a Case? The Problem of Definition in

Psychiatric Community Surveys. Edited by Wing JK, Bebbington P, Robins LN. London, Grant McIntyre, 1981

Essen-Möller E, Larsson H, Uddenberg CE, et al: Individual traits and morbidity in a Swedish rural population. Acta Psychiatrica et Neurologica Scandinavica Supplementum 106:1–160, 1956

Evans DL, Funkenstein H, Albert MS, et al: Prevalence of Alzheimer's disease in a community population of older persons. JAMA 262:2551–2556, 1989

Farris RE, Dunham HW: Mental Disorders in Urban Areas. Chicago, IL, University of Chicago Press, 1939

Folstein MF, Breitner JCS: Language disorder predicts familial Alzheimer's disease. Johns Hopkins Medical Journal 149:145–147, 1981

Folstein MF, Folstein SE, McHugh PR: Mini-Mental State: a practical method for grading the cognitive state of patients for the clinician. J Psychiatr Res 12:189–198, 1975

Folstein MF, Anthony JC, Parhad I, et al: The meaning of cognitive impairment in the elderly. J Am Geriatr Soc 33:228–235, 1985

Fowles DG: A Profile of Older Americans: 1990 (DHHS Publ No. PF3029[1290] D996). Washington, DC, American Association of Retired Persons, Administration on Aging, 1990, pp 1–2

German PS, Shapiro S, Skinner EA: Mental health of the elderly: use of health and mental health services. J Am Geriatr Soc 33:246–252, 1985

Goodwin DW, Guze SB: Psychiatric Diagnosis, 2nd Edition. New York, Oxford University Press, 1979

Goodwin JS, Goodwin JM, Garry PJ: Association between nutritional status and cognitive functioning in a healthy elderly population. JAMA 249:2917–2921, 1983

Gruenberg EM: Epidemiology of senile dementia, in Neurological Epidemiology. Edited by Schoenberg BS. New York, Raven, 1978, pp 437–457

Haas AP, Hendin H: Suicide among older people: projections for the future. Suicide Life Threat Behav 13:147–154, 1983

Hanlon JT, Fillenbaum GG, Burchett B, et al: Drug-use patterns among black and nonblack community-dwelling elderly. Annals of Pharmacology 26:679–685, 1992

Hathaway SR, McKinley JC: Minnesota Multiphasic Personality Inventory, Revised. Minneapolis, University of Minnesota, 1970

Henderson AS, Jorm AF, Konten AE, et al: Environmental risk factors for Alzheimer's disease: the relationship to age of onset and to familial or sporadic types. Psychol Med 22:429–436, 1992

Heren TJ, Lagaay AM, Hijmans W, et al: Prevalence of dementia in the "oldest old" of a Dutch community. J Am Geriatr Soc 39:755–759, 1991

Heston LL, Mastri AR, Anderson E, et al: Dementia of the Alzheimer's type: clinical genetics, natural history, and associated conditions. Arch Gen Psychiatry 38:1085–1090, 1981

Heyman A, Wilkinson WE, Hurwitz BJ, et al: Alzheimer's disease: genetic aspects and associated clinical disorders. Ann Neurol 14:507–515, 1983

Hilliard JR, Holland JM, Ramm D: Christmas and psychopathology: data from a psychiatric emergency room population. Arch Gen Psychiatry 38:377–381, 1981

Holmes TH, Rahe RH: The social readjustment rating scale. Journal of Psychosometric Research 11:213–218, 1967

Huntley J, Brock DB, Ostfeld AM, et al: Established Populations for Epidemiologic Studies of the Elderly: Resource Data Book (NIH Publ No 86-2443). Washington, DC, National Institute on Aging, 1986

Kahn RL, Goldfarb AI, Pollack M, et al: Brief objective measures for the determination of mental status in the aged. Am J Psychiatry 117:326–328, 1960

Kay DWK, Beamish P, Roth M: Old age mental disorders in Newcastle-Upon-Tyne, I: a study of prevalence. Br J Psychiatry 110:146–158, 1964

Kay DWK, Bergmann K, Foster EM, et al: Mental illness and hospital usage in the elderly: a random sample followed up. Compr Psychiatry 11:26–35, 1970

Kleinbaum DL, Fupper LL, Morgenstern H: Epidemiologic Research. Belmont, CA, Lifetime Learning Publications, 1982

Klerman GL, Lavori PW, Rice J, et al: Birth-cohort trends in rates of major depression among relatives of patients with affective disorder. Arch Gen Psychiatry 42:689–694, 1985

Koenig HG, Meador KG, Cohen HJ, et al: Depression in elderly hospitalized patients with medical illness. Arch Intern Med 148:1929–1936, 1988

Lester D: Temporal variation in suicide and homicide. Am J Epidemiol 109:517–520, 1979

Lowenthal MF, Berkman PL: Aging and Mental Disorders in San Francisco: A Social Psychiatric Study. San Francisco, CA, Jossey-Bass, 1967

MacMahon B, Pugh TF: Epidemiology: Principles and Methods. Boston, Little, Brown, 1970

Meehan PJ, Saltzman LE, Sattin RW: Suicides among older United States Residents: epidemiologic characteristics and trends. Am J Public Health 81:1198–1200, 1991

Mellinger GD, Balter MB, Manheimer DI, et al: Psychic distress, life crisis, and use of psychotherapeutic medications: national household survey data. Arch Gen Psychiatry 35:1045–1052, 1978

Morris JN: Uses of Epidemiology, 3rd Edition. Edinburgh, Churchill Livingstone, 1975

Murphy E, Lindesay J, Grundy E: Sixty years of suicide in England and Wales. Arch Gen Psychiatry 43:969–977, 1986

Murphy GE, Wetzel RD: Suicide risk by birth cohort in the United States, 1949–1974. Arch Gen Psychiatry 37:519–523, 1980

Murrell SA, Himmelfarb S, Wright K: Prevalence of depression and its correlates in older adults. Am J Epidemiol 117:173–185, 1983

New York State Department of Mental Hygiene, Mental Health Research Unit: Mental Health Survey of Older People. Utica, NY, State Hospital Press, 1960

Parker DA, Parker ES, Brody JA, et al: Alcohol use and cognitive loss among employed men and women. Am J Public Health 73:521–526, 1983

Parmelee PA, Katz IR, Lawton MP: Depression among institutionalized aged: assessment and prevalence estimation. J Gerontol 44:M22–M29, 1989

Pasamanick B, Roberts DW, Lemkau PW, et al: A survey of mental disease in an urban population: prevalence by race and income, in Epidemiology of Mental Disorder. Edited by Pasamanick B. Washington, DC, American Association for the Advancement of Science, 1959, pp 183–202

Pfeiffer E: A Short Portable Mental Status Questionnaire for the assessment of organic brain deficit in elderly patients. J Am Geriatr Soc 23:433–441, 1975

Pifer A, Bronte DL: Introduction: squaring the pyramid. Daedalus 115:1–12, 1986

Platt R: Wisdom is not enough: reflections on the art and science of medicine. Lancet 2:977–980, 1952

Radloff LS: The CES-D scale: a self-report depression scale for research in the general population. Applied Psychological Measurement 1:385–401, 1977

Ray WA, Federspiel CF, Schaffner W: A study of antipsychotic drug use in nursing homes: epidemiologic evidence suggesting misuse. Am J Public Health 70:485–491, 1980

Regier DA, Boyd JH, Burke JD, et al: One-month prevalence of mental disorders in the United States. Arch Gen Psychiatry 45:977–986, 1988

Roberts CJ: Epidemiology for Clinicians. London, Pitman Medical, 1977

Robins LN, Helzer JE, Croughan J, et al: National Institute of Mental Health Diagnostic Interview Schedule: its history, characteristics, and validity. Arch Gen Psychiatry 38:381–389, 1981

Rosch E: Principles of categorization, in Cognition and Categorization. Edited by Rosch E, Lloyd BB. Hillsdale, NJ, Lawrence Erlbaum, 1978, pp 3–27

Rosenwaike I: A demographic portrait of the oldest old. Milbank Memorial Fund Quarterly 63:187–205, 1985

Rossiter LF: Prescribed medicines: findings from the National Medical Care Expenditure Survey. Am J Public Health 73:1312–1315, 1983

Rovner BW, Kafonek S, Fillipp L, et al: Prevalence of mental illness in a community nursing home. Am J Psychiatry 143:1446–1449, 1986

Schoenberg DS, Kokmen E, Okozaki HS: Alzheimer's disease and other dementing illnesses in a defined United States population: incidence rates and clinical features. Ann Neurol 22:724–729, 1987

Shapiro S, Skinner EA, Kessler LG, et al: Utilization of health and mental health services. Arch Gen Psychiatry 41:971–982, 1984

Spitzer RL, Endicott J: Schedule for Affective Disorders and Schizophrenia (Lifetime Version), 3rd Edition. New York, New York State Psychiatric Institute, 1978

Spitzer RL, Endicott J, Robins E: Research Diagnostic Criteria: rationale and reliability. Arch Gen Psychiatry 35:773–782, 1978

Srole L, Fischer AK: The Midtown Manhattan Longitudinal Study vs. "The Mental Paradise Lost" doctrine. Arch Gen Psychiatry 37:209–221, 1981

Strauss JS, Gabriel KR, Kokes R, et al: Do psychiatric patients fit their diagnoses? patterns of symptomatology as described with a biplot. J Nerv Ment Dis 167:105–113, 1979

Swartz M, Blazer D, Woodbury M, et al: Somatization disorder in a US southern community: use of a new procedure for analysis of medical classification. Psychol Med 16:595–609, 1986

Teeter RB, Garetz FK, Miller WR, et al: Psychiatric disturbances of aged patients in skilled nursing homes. Am J Psychiatry 133:1430–1434, 1976

Warheit GJ, Hodzer CE, Schwart JJ: An analysis of social class and racial differences in depressive symptomatology: a community study. J Health Soc Behav 14:291–299, 1973

Weinstein MC, Feinberg HV: Clinical Decision Analysis. Philadelphia, PA, WB Saunders, 1980

Weissman MM, Klerman GL: Epidemiology of mental disorders. Arch Gen Psychiatry 25:705–715, 1978

Wing JK: Patients with psychiatric disorders, in Community Mental Health: An International Perspective. Edited by Williams RN, Ozarin LD. San Francisco, Jossey-Bass, 1968

Wing JK, Cooper JE, Sartorius N: The Description and Classification of Psychiatric Symptoms: An Instruction Manual for the PSE and CATEGO System. London, Cambridge University Press, 1974

The Diagnostic Interview
in Late Life

The Psychiatric Interview
of the Geriatric Patient

Dan G. Blazer, M.D., Ph.D.

The foundation of the diagnostic workup of the older adult suffering from a psychiatric disorder is the diagnostic interview. Unfortunately, in this age of increasing technology in the laboratory and of standardization of interview techniques, the art of the clinical interview has suffered. In this chapter the core of the psychiatric interview, including history taking, assessment of the family, and the mental status examination, is reviewed. To supplement the clinical interview, structured interview schedules and rating scales of value in the assessment of older adults are described as well. Finally, techniques for communicating effectively with older adults are outlined.

History

The elements of a diagnostic workup of the elderly patient are presented in Table 10–1. To obtain historical information, the clinician should first interview the older adult, if this is feasible. Then permission can be asked of the patient to interview family members. If available, family members from at least two generations can expand the perspective of the older adult's impairment. If the patient has difficulty providing an accurate or understandable history, the clinician should concentrate especially on eliciting those symptoms or problems perceived as being most disabling by the older adult and fill the historical gap with data from the family.

DSM-IV (American Psychiatric Association 1994) provides the clinician with a useful catalogue of symptoms and behaviors of psychiatric interest. Symptoms are bits of data, the most visible part of the clinical picture and generally the part that is most easily agreed on among clinicians. Given that clinicians obtain equivalent information, symptoms should be defined in such a way that minimal disagreement arises as to the presence or absence of a symptom. The decision as to whether those symptoms form a syndrome or derive from a particular etiology must be determined independently of the data collection on symptoms.

Even so, the clinical interaction may be confounded by bias when a clinician communicates with an older adult regarding psychiatric symptoms. As many insightful clinicians, such as Eisen-

Table 10–1.   Psychiatric interview of the geriatric patient

History
Symptoms
Present episode, including onset, duration, and
    change in symptoms over time
Past history of medical and psychiatric disorders
Family history of depression, alcohol abuse/
    dependence, psychoses, and suicide

Physical examination
Evaluation of neurologic deficits, possible endocrine
    disorders, occult malignancy, cardiac dysfunction,
    and occult infections

Mental status examination
Disturbance of consciousness
Disturbance of mood and affect
Disturbance of motor behavior
Disturbance of perception (hallucinations, illusions)
Disturbance of cognition (delusions)
Disturbance of self-esteem and guilt
Suicidal ideation
Disturbance of memory and intelligence (memory,
    abstraction, calculation, aphasia, and knowledge)

berg (1977), have recognized, physicians diagnose and treat diseases—that is, abnormalities in the structure and function of body organs and systems. Patients suffer illnesses—experiences of disvalued changes in states of being and in social function. Disease and illness do not maintain a one-to-one relationship. Factors that determine who becomes a patient and who does not can only be understood by expanding horizons beyond symptoms. In other words, *patienthood* is a social state (Eisenberg and Kleinman 1981). During the process of becoming a patient, the older adult, usually with the advice of others, forms a self-diagnosis of his or her problem and makes a judgment regarding the degree of ill-being. For some, illness is perceived when a specific discomfort is experienced. For others, illness reflects a general perception of physical or social alienation and despair. Given that few uniform, satisfactory definitions of illness (or ill-being) exist, it is not surprising that terms for wellness (or well-being) also mean different things to different people. The historical background and the values of the older adult within a social class and culture contribute to the formation of constructs regarding the nature of the problem, the cause, and the possibility for recovery.

For this reason, the clinician must take care to avoid accepting the patient's explanation for a given problem or set of problems. Statements such as "I guess I'm just getting old and there's nothing really to worry about" or "Most people slow down when they get to be my age" can lull the clinician into complacency in the face of a treatable psychiatric disorder. On the other hand, the advent of new and disturbing symptoms in an older adult between each office visit can exhaust the clinician's patience to the point at which adequate pursuit of the problem is derailed. For example, the hypochondriacal older adult who suffers from increased difficulty with awakenings during the night may insist that this symptom be treated with a sedative and plead with the clinician not to allow continual suffering. In the clinician's view, however, the symptom is a normal accompaniment of old age and therefore should be accepted. Distress over a change in functioning, such as changes in sexual functioning, may overwhelm the elder and, especially if the clinician is perceived as unconcerned, precipitate self-medication or even a suicide attempt.

To prevent attitudinal biases when eliciting reports by the older adult (and therefore missing the symptoms and signs of a treatable psychiatric disorder), the clinician must include in the initial interview with the older adult a review of the more important psychiatric symptoms in a relatively structured format. Common symptoms that should be reviewed include excessive weakness or lethargy, depressed mood or the blues, memory problems, difficulty concentrating, helplessness, hopelessness, uselessness, isolation, suspicion of others, anxiety and agitation, sleep problems, and appetite problems. Critical symptoms that should be reviewed include the presence or absence of suicidal thoughts, profound anhedonia, impulsive behavior, delusions and hallucinations, and confusion.

The review of symptoms is most valuable when it is considered within the context of symptom presentation. When did the symptoms begin? How long have they lasted? Has their severity changed over time? Are there physical or environmental events that precipitate the symptoms? What means, if any, have been taken to try to correct the symptoms? Have any of these interventions proved successful? Do the symptoms vary during the day (diurnal variation)? Do they vary during the week or with seasons of the year? Do the symptoms form clusters—that is, are they associated with one another? Which symptoms appear ego-syntonic and which symptoms appear ego-dystonic? As symptoms are reviewed, a specific time frame facilitates focus on the present illness. Having a 1-month or 6-month window enables the patient to review symptoms and events temporally, an approach not usually taken by distressed elders, who tend to concentrate on immediate sufferings.

Next, the clinician must review the past history of symptoms and episodes. The patient should be asked if he or she has suffered from similar episode(s) in the past. How long did the episode(s) last? When did it (they) occur? How many times in the patient's lifetime has such an episode occurred? Unfortunately, the older adult may not equate present distress with past episodes that are symptomatically similar, and so the perspective of the family is especially valuable in the attempt to link current and past episodes. Other psychiatric and medical problems should be reviewed as well, especially medical illnesses that have led to hospitalization and the use of medication. Not infrequently, the older adult has experienced a major illness or trauma in childhood or as a younger adult, but he or she views this information as being of no relevance to the present episode and therefore dismisses it. Probes to elicit these data are essential. Older adults do not spontaneously connect their present distress with past problems. They may ignore or even forget past psychiatric difficulties, especially if these difficulties were disguised. For example, mood swings in early or middle life may have been covered by periods of excessive and productive activity, by episodes of excessive alcohol intake, or by vague, undiagnosed physical problems. Periods of overt disability in usual activities may flag those previous episodes. Elders sometimes become angry or irritated when the clinician continues to probe. Reassurance regarding the importance of obtaining this information will generally suffice, except when dealing with a patient who cannot tolerate the discomfort and distress, even for brief periods. Elders with chronic and moderately severe anxiety who have a hysterical personality style, as well as distressed Alzheimer's patients, tolerate their symptoms poorly.

The distribution of psychiatric symptoms and illnesses within the family should be determined next. The older person with symptoms consistent with senile dementia or primary degenerative dementia is highly likely to have a family history of dementia. The genogram remains one of the best means for evaluating the distribution of mental illness and other relevant behaviors through the family tree. This genogram should include both parents, blood-related aunts and uncles, brothers and sisters, spouse(s), children, grandchildren, and great-grandchildren. A history should be obtained of institutionalization, significant memory problems in family members, hospitalization for a nervous breakdown or depressive disorder, suicide, alcohol abuse and dependence, electroconvulsive therapy, long-term residence in a mental health facility (and possibly a diagnosis of schizophrenia), and mental health services use by family members (Blazer 1984). Of relevance to the pharmacological treatment of certain disorders in older adults (especially depression) is the tendency of individuals within a family to respond therapeutically to the same pharmacological agent. If the older adult suffers from a depressive disorder and biological relatives have been treated effectively for depression, the clinician should determine what pharmacological agent was used to treat the depression. For example, a positive response to nortriptyline in a family member of the depressed elder could make nortriptyline the drug of choice in treating that depressed elder, assuming side effects to this particular drug are not at issue (Ayd 1975).

Mendlewicz and colleagues (1975) remind us that accurate genetic information can be better obtained when family members from more than one generation are interviewed. Many psychiatric disorders are characterized by a variety of symptoms, and so asking the patient or one family member for a history of depression would be insufficient. Research of the genetic expression of psychiatric disorders in families requires the investigator to interview directly as many family members as possible to obtain a true determination of case distribution through the family. Such detailed family assessment is not feasible for clinicians, yet a telephone call to more than one affected relative may become a standard of clinical assessment as the genetics of psychiatric disorders are clarified.

Psychiatric disorders occur within a biomedical and psychosocial context. The clinician naturally will determine what medical problems the patient has experienced, but could overlook a variation in the relative contribution of these medical disorders to psychopathology. The psychosocial contribution to the onset and continuance of the problem is just as likely to be overlooked. Has the spouse of the older adult undergone a change? Are the middle-aged children managing stress, such as the stress of caring for a disabled parent and financing their children through college simultaneously? Are the grandchildren placing emotional stress on the elderly patient and family because of adjustment problems in adolescence and young adulthood? Has the economic status of the older adult deteriorated? Has the availability of medical care changed? Though many psychiatric disorders are biologically driven, they do not occur in a psychosocial vacuum. Environmental precipitants remain important in the web of causation leading to the onset of an episode of emotional distress.

Next, it is essential to evaluate the medication history of the older adult. Most elderly persons take a variety of medicines simultaneously, and the potential for drug–drug interaction is high. For example, concomitant use of fluoxetine and warfarin has been associated with increased half-life of warfarin, which could lead to severe bruising (although this finding is not well documented). Some medications prescribed for older persons—such as the beta-blocker propranolol and the antihypertensive drug alpha-methyldopa—can exacerbate or produce depressive symptoms. Antianxiety agents and sedative-hypnotics can precipitate episodes of confusion and depression. Antidepressants, such as the tricyclics, may adversely interact with other drugs, including the antihypertensive agent clonidine. Simultaneous administration of clonidine and a tricyclic may lead to poorly controlled episodes of hypertension with confusional episodes, and possibly an exacerbation of a multi-infarct dementia. The physician, a nurse, a social worker, or a paraprofessional should carefully determine present and past medication use through an historical inventory and a review of the patient's medicine containers brought to the office.

Family Assessment

Clinicians working with older adults must be equipped to evaluate the dysfunctional family. Just as an elevated white blood cell count is not pathognomonic for a particular infectious agent yet is critical to the diagnosis, the complaint that "my family no longer loves me" does not reveal the specific problems within the family but does highlight the need to assess the potential of that family to provide care and support for the older adult (Blazer 1984). Determination of the nature of the family structure in interaction, the presence or absence of a crisis within the family, and the type and amount of support available to the older adult are the basic goals of a comprehensive diagnostic family workup.

The genogram detailing the distribution of illnesses across a family has already been described. A family-tree review for roles of individuals in the family, and the availability of members to provide care to the older adult, is equally important. For clinical purposes, the family consists of not only individuals genetically related but also those who have developed relationships and are living together as if they were related (Miller and Miller 1979). Many older adults, especially those who have been widowed, have close relationships with friends that are virtually familial. Garetz (1979) has described certain roles filled by family members when the older adult suffers from a mental or physical illness. These roles are helpful in evaluating and planning individual and family intervention. Modified somewhat (Blazer and Kaplan 1983), they include the following:

1. **Facilitator**—that individual in the family who resists medical or psychiatric treatment in order to maintain the stability achieved within a family secondary to the older adult's dysfunction. Facilitators can present obstacles to therapeutic intervention even though they may believe that they are being helpful. For example, children wishing to obtain financial control of a family business for a parent may facilitate organic brain dysfunction.
2. **Victim**—the individual in a family who perceive the disorder of the older adult as a threat to self. The victim is usually in frequent contact with the disabled elder and therefore is in frequent contact with the clinician. The clinician may be criticized by the victim because of the burden of the illness. A sibling, forced for economic reasons to care for a disabled and demanding elder, may assume the victim role and, in turn, will often place demands on the clinician.
3. **Manager**—that family member who takes charge of a family during a crisis. He or she is usually calm, may be overly intellectual, and tends to organize and orchestrate family activi-

ties, often from a distance. The manager can be most helpful to the clinician in arranging tangible supports, but is less able to provide the emotional support to the older adult or family members suffering as a result of a psychiatric disorder.

4. **Caregiver**—the family member who nurture the disabled older adult. Such a person may provide inexhaustible help to a severely disturbed elder, sometimes maintaining an older adult in the home far beyond the point at which institutionalization is indicated—such as in cases of advanced primary degenerative dementia. Often avoiding opportunities for respite, caregivers may wear themselves to exhaustion and have few meaningful activities beyond caregiving. If the older adult dies, these individuals often suffer a tremendous void that may manifest itself in a severe and prolonged grief reaction.

5. **Escapee**—a family member who may withdraw from usual interactions within the family and who is, therefore, blamed for not demonstrating care and concern for the older person. A child frequently fills the role of escapee, especially if he or she has moved a good distance from the family. The escapee may become involved in altruistic endeavors, such as religious or civic activities locally, or may become devoted to his or her own nuclear family, and may, therefore, have little or no time and energy for the impaired elder. Families faced with the prospect of caring for a previously independent parent are often seized with conflict and use the escapee to diffuse tensions within. In turn, the escapee may function well outside the family and as a result may resist being drawn back into that stressed and conflicted network, despite a desire to be of help to the older adult.

6. **Identified patient**—the older person with the problem, who is perceived to be the cause of a family crisis. The identified patient may suffer only minimal problems and may be content with his or her current state, and yet the older adult may provide an admission pass for the entire family to seek help from the clinician. The needs and problems of the older adult may quickly be set aside as family conflicts emerge during the diagnostic interview.

A primary goal of the clinician, as advocate for the psychiatrically disturbed older adult, is to facili-

tate family support for the elder during a time of disability. At least four parameters of support are important for the clinician to evaluate as the treatment plan evolves. These include 1) availability of family members to the older person over time, 2) the tangible services provided by the family to the disturbed elder, 3) the perception of family support by the older adult (and subsequently the willingness of the elder to cooperate and accept support), and 4) tolerance by the family for specific behaviors that derive from the psychiatric disorder.

The clinician should ask the older person, "If you become ill, is there a family member who will take care of you for a short period of time?" Next, the availability of family members who can care for the older adult over an extended period of time can be determined. If a particular member is designated as the primary caregiver, plans for respite should be discussed. Given the increased focus on short hospital stays and documented levels of greater impairment on discharge, the availability of family members becomes essential to the effective care of the older adult after hospitalization for a psychiatric, or combined medical and psychiatric, disorder.

What specific, tangible services can be provided to the older adult by family members? Even the most devoted spouse is limited in the delivery of certain services because he or she may not drive a car (and therefore cannot provide transportation) or is not physically strong enough to provide certain types of nursing care. Generic services of special importance in the support of the psychiatrically impaired older adult at home include transportation; nursing services (such as administering medications at home); physical therapy; checking services or continual supervision; homemaker and household services; meal preparation; administrative, legal, and protective services; financial assistance; living quarters; and coordination of the delivery of services. These services have been termed *generic* because they can be defined in terms of their activities, regardless of who provides the service. Assessing the range and extent of service delivery by the family to the functionally impaired elder provides a convenient barometer of the economic, social, and emotional burdens of the geropsychiatric patient on the family.

Regardless of the level of service provided by the family to the older person, for these services to be effective it is beneficial for the older person to perceive that he or she lives in a supportive environment. These intangible supports include the perception of a dependable network, participation or interaction in the network, a sense of belonging to the network, intimacy with network members, and a sense of usefulness to the family (Blazer and Kaplan 1983). Usefulness may be of less importance to some older adults in that they believe they have contributed to the family for many years and, therefore, deserve reciprocal service delivery in their waning years. Unfortunately, family members, frequently stressed across generations, may not recognize this reciprocal responsibility.

Family tolerance of specific behaviors may not correlate with overall support. Every person has a level of tolerance for specific behaviors that are especially difficult. Sanford (1975) found that the following behaviors were tolerated in decreasing frequency by families of impaired elders: incontinence of urine (81%), personality conflicts (54%), falls (52%), physically aggressive behavior (44%), inability to walk unaided (33%), daytime wandering (33%), and sleep disturbance (16%). This frequency may appear counterintuitive, for incontinence is generally considered particularly aversive to family members. Yet the outcome of incontinence can be corrected easily enough. A few nights of no sleep, however, can easily extend family members beyond their capabilities of serving a parent, sibling, or spouse.

The Mental Status Examination

Physicians and other clinicians are at times hesitant to perform a structured mental status examination, fearing the effort will insult or irritate the patient. Perhaps the exam is also viewed as an unnecessary waste of time. Nevertheless, the mental status examination of the psychiatric patient in later life is central to the diagnostic workup (Blazer 1982). Affect and mood can usually be assessed by observing the patient during the interview. Affect is the feeling tone, pleasurable or unpleasurable, that accompanies the patient's cognitive output (Linn 1980). Affect may fluctuate during the interview; however, the older person is more likely to demonstrate a constriction of affect. Mood, the state that underlies overt affect and is sustained over time, is usually apparent by the completion of the interview. For ex-

ample, the affect of a depressed older adult may not reach the degree of dysphoria seen in younger persons (as evidenced by crying spells or protestations of uncontrollable despair), yet the depressed mood is usually sustained and discernible from beginning to end.

Psychomotor retardation or underactivity is characteristic of major depression and severe schizophreniform symptomatology, as well as some variants of primary degenerative dementia. Psychiatrically impaired elders (except some who have more advanced dementia) are more likely to exhibit hyperactivity or agitation. Those who are depressed will appear uneasy, move their hands frequently, and have difficulty remaining seated through the interview. Mild to moderately demented patients, especially those suffering from multi-infarct dementia, are easily distracted, arise from a seated position, and walk around the room or even out of the room. Pacing is often observed when the older adult is admitted to a hospital ward. Agitation can usually be distinguished from anxiety, for the agitated individual does not complain of a sense of impending doom or dread. Movement generally relieves the immediate discomfort—yet does not correct the underlying disturbance—in patients with psychomotor dysfunction. Occasionally, the older adult with motor retardation may, in fact, be suffering from a disturbance in consciousness, having reached an almost stuporous state. He or she may not be easily aroused, but when aroused, will respond by grimacing or withdrawal.

Perception is the awareness of objects in relations that follows stimulation of peripheral sense organs (Linn 1980). Disturbances of perception include hallucinations—that is, false sensory perceptions not associated with real or external stimuli. For example, the paranoid older adult may perceive invasion of her house at night by individuals who disarrange her belongings and abuse her sexually. Hallucinations often take the form of false auditory perceptions, false perceptions of movement or body sensation (such as palpitations), and false perceptions of smell, taste, and touch. The severely depressed elder may suffer from frank auditory hallucinations that condemn or encourage self-destructive behavior.

Disturbances in thought content are the most common disturbances of cognition noted in the psychiatrically impaired elder. The depressed patient often develops beliefs that are inconsistent with the objective information obtained from family members about the patient's abilities and social resources. In a series of studies, Meyers and co-workers (Meyers and Greenberg 1986; Meyers et al. 1985) found delusional depression to be more prevalent among older depressed patients. Forty-five percent of 161 patients with endogenous depression as determined by Research Diagnostic Criteria (RDC; Spitzer et al. 1978a) were found to be delusional. These delusions included beliefs such as "I've lost my mind," "My body is deteriorating," "I have an incurable illness," and "I have caused some great harm." Even after elderly persons recover from the depression, they may still experience periodic recurrences of delusional thoughts, which can be most disturbing to an otherwise rational older adult. Elders appear less likely to suffer from delusions of self-remorse, guilt, or persecution.

Even if delusions are not obvious, preoccupation with a particular thought or idea is common among depressed elderly persons. Such preoccupation is closely associated with obsessional thinking or irresistible intrusion of thoughts into the conscious mind. Although the older adult rarely acts on these thoughts compulsively, the guilt-provoking or self-accusing thoughts may occasionally become so difficult to bear that the person considers, attempts, or succeeds in committing suicide.

Evaluation of the content and process of cognition may uncover disturbances such as problems with structure of associations, the speed of associations, and the content of thought. Thinking is a goal-directed flow of ideas, symbols, and associations initiated in response to environmental stimuli, a perceived problem, or a task that requires progression to a logical or reality-based conclusion (Linn 1980). The compulsive or schizophrenic older adult may pathologically repeat the same word or idea in response to a variety of probes, as may the patient who has primary degenerative dementia. Some demented older adults exhibit circumstantiality—that is, the introduction of many apparently irrelevant details to cover a lack of clarity and memory problems. Such interviews can be most frustrating because they proceed at such a slow pace. On other occasions, elders appear incoherent, with no logical connection to their thought, or they may produce irrelevant answers. The intrusion of thoughts from previous conversations into current conversation is

a prime example of the disturbance in association found in patients with primary degenerative dementia (for example, Alzheimer's disease). This symptom is not typical of other dementias, such as the dementia of Huntington's disease. However, in the absence of dementia, even paranoid older adults generally do not demonstrate a significant disturbance in the structure of associations.

Although thoughts of death are common in late life, spontaneous revelations of suicidal thoughts are rare. A stepwise probe is the best means of assessing the presence of suicidal ideation (Blazer 1982). First, the clinician should ask the patient if he or she has ever thought that life was not worth living. If so, has the patient considered acting on that thought? If so, how would the patient attempt to inflict such harm? When definite plans are revealed, the clinician should probe to determine if the implements for a suicide attempt are available. For example, if the patient has considered shooting himself, the clinician should ask, "Do you have a gun available and loaded at home?" Suicidal ideation in an older adult is always of concern, but intervention is necessary when suicide has been considered seriously and the implements are available.

Although older adults may not complain of memory dysfunction, they are more likely to suffer problems with memory, concentration, and intellect. Formal testing of cognitive status, as described below, is usually indicated. Yet there are brief, informal means of testing cognitive functioning that should be included in the diagnostic workup. As the clinician proceeds through an evaluation of memory and intellect, it must be remembered that poor performance may reflect psychic distress or a lack of education as opposed to mental retardation or dementia. To rule out the potential confounding of agitation and anxiety, testing can be performed on more than one occasion.

Testing of memory is based on three essential processes: 1) registration (the ability to record an experience in the central nervous system), 2) retention (the persistence and permanence of a registered experience), and 3) recall (the ability to summon consciously the registered experience and report it) (Linn 1980). Registration, apart from recall, is difficult to evaluate directly. Occasionally, events or information that the older adult denies remembering will appear spontaneously during other parts of the interview. Otherwise, techniques such as hypnosis, narcoanalysis, and psychoanalysis are the usual means of determining if registration has occurred. Registration usually is not impaired, except in patients with one of the more severely dementing illnesses.

Retention, on the other hand, can be blocked by both psychic distress and brain dysfunction. Lack of retention is especially relevant to the unimportant data often asked for on a mental status examination. For example, requesting the older adult to remember three objects for 5 minutes will frequently reveal a deficit if the older adult has little motivation to attempt the task. Disturbances of recall can be tested directly in a number of ways. The most common are tests of orientation to time, place, person, and situation. Most persons continually orient themselves via radio, television, and reading material, as well as through conversations with others. Some elders may be isolated through sensory impairment or social isolation, and so poor orientation in these patients may represent deficits in the physical and social environment rather than brain dysfunction. Immediate recall can be tested by asking the older person to repeat a word, phrase, or series of numbers, but may also be tested in conjunction with cognitive skills by requesting that a word be spelled backward or that elements of a story be recalled.

During the mental status examination, intelligence can be assessed only superficially. Tests of simple arithmetic calculation and fund of knowledge, supplemented by portions of well-known psychiatric tests, are helpful. A capacity for abstract thinking is often tested by asking the patient to interpret a well-known proverb, such as "A rolling stone gathers no moss." A more accurate test of abstraction, however, is the request to classify objects into a common category. For example, the elder is asked to state the similarity between an apple and a pear. Whereas naming objects from a category (such as fruits) is retained despite moderate and sometimes marked declines in cognition, the opposite process of classifying two different objects into a common category is not retained as well. The classic test for calculation is to ask a patient to subtract 7 from 100, and to repeat this operation on the succession of remainders. Usually five calculations are sufficient to determine the ability of the older adult to complete this task. If the older adult fails this task, a less exacting test is to request the patient to subtract 3 from 20, and to repeat this operation on the succession of remainders

until 0 is reached. These examinations must not be rushed, for elders may not perform as well when they perceive a pressure in time.

Rating Scales and Standardized Interviews

Rating scales and standardized or structured interviews have progressively been incorporated into the diagnostic assessment of the psychiatric patient. Such rating procedures have increased in popularity as the need has increased for systematic, reproducible diagnoses for third-party carriers (part of the impetus for the dramatic change in nomenclature evidenced in DSM-IV), and for a standard means of assessing change in clinical status. A thorough review of all instruments that are used is not possible. Therefore, selected instruments are presented and evaluated in this section, chosen either because they have special relevance to the geriatric patient or because they are widely used.

Cognitive Dysfunction and Dementia Schedules

Two interviewer-administered cognitive screens have been popular in both clinical and community studies. The first is the Short Portable Mental Status Questionnaire (SPMSQ; Pfeiffer 1975), a derivative of the Mental Status Questionnaire developed by Kahn et al. in 1960. The SPMSQ consists of 10 questions designed to assess orientation, memory, fund of knowledge, and calculation. For most community-dwelling older adults, two or fewer errors indicate intact functioning; three or four errors, mild impairment; five to seven errors, moderate impairment; and eight or more errors, severe impairment. The ease of administration and the reliability of this instrument, as supported by accumulated epidemiological data, make it useful for both clinical and community screens. The Mini-Mental State Examination (Folstein et al. 1975) is a 30-item instrument that is used to assess orientation, registration, attention and calculation, recall, and language. It requires 5–10 minutes to administer and includes more items of clinical significance than does the SPMSQ. Seven to 12 errors suggest mild to moderate cognitive impairment; 13 or more errors, severe impairment.

A number of clinical assessment procedures for dementia have emerged in recent years. The most widely used, and one of the first to appear, is the scale suggested by Blessed et al. (1968), usually referred to as the Blessed Dementia Index. In contrast to what can be gleaned by use of the screening scales, clinical judgment is required in using the Blessed Dementia Index to assess changes in performance of everyday activities (such as handling money, household tasks, and shopping); changes in eating and dressing habits; changes in personality, interests, and drive; tests of information (orientation and recognition of persons); memory (of past information, such as occupation, place of birth, and town where the individual worked); and concentration (calculation task). A score is assigned to each of these tasks, and a summary score is tabulated. The score has been shown to correlate well with the cerebral changes of primary degenerative dementia.

A dementia scale for assessing the probability that the dementia is secondary to multiple infarcts is that suggested by Hachinski et al. (1975). In a study of cerebral blood flow in patients with primary degenerative dementia compared with those who had multi-infarct dementia, certain clinical features were determined to be more associated with multi-infarct dementia, and each of these was assigned a score. These items, along with their scores, are as follows: abrupt onset = 2, stepwise deterioration = 1, fluctuating course = 2, nocturnal confusion = 1, relative preservation of personality = 1, depression = 1, somatic complaints = 1, emotional incontinence = 1, history of hypertension = 1, history of strokes = 2, evidence of associated atherosclerosis = 1, focal neurological symptoms = 2, and focal neurological signs = 2. A score of 7 or greater was highly suggestive of multi-infarct dementia. Given the frequent overlap of multiple small infarcts and primary degenerative dementia, as well as the difficulty of assessing these items effectively, most investigators have ceased to rely on the Hachinski scale for clinical use.

Depression Schedules

A number of self-rating depression scales have been used to screen for depression in patients at all stages of the life cycle; most of these scales have been studied in older populations. The Zung Self-Rating Depression Scale (Zung 1965) was the most widely used until recent years. The initial popularity of the Zung scale was probably due to the availability of data for persons throughout the life cycle, especially the elderly (Zung 1967). Few randomly sampled community populations have been surveyed with the Zung Self-Rating Depression Scale, and so a deficit exists in normative community standards. With this 20-item scale, each of the 20 symptoms is ranked from 0 ("none") to 3 ("all or about all the time"), according to severity. Most older adults can use the Zung scale, although the four choices may create problems for some elders with mild cognitive impairment. Using the Zung scale, Freedman and colleagues (1982) found peak symptom levels in 65- to 69-year-old females and 70- to 74-year-old males.

The most widely used of the current instruments in community studies is the Center for Epidemiologic Studies Depression Scale (CES-D; Radloff 1977). This instrument, because of the normative population data available on it, has replaced the Zung scale in recent years as a common instrument for screening for depression. The CES-D scale is similar in format to the Zung scale. In a factor-analytic study of the CES-D in a community population, three factors were identified: an enervation factor, a positive affect factor, and an interpersonal relationship factor (Ross and Mirowsky 1984). The disaggregation of these factors and the exploration of their interaction is a significant step forward in understanding the results derived from symptom scales like the CES-D in older populations. For example, are the enervation items (e.g., loss of interest, poor appetite) truly associated with a course of depressive episodes similar to that described for major depression with melancholia, and the positive affect items more associated with life satisfaction scores?

A scale that has been widely used in clinical studies, but which has been less studied in community populations, is the Beck Depression Inventory (BDI; Beck et al. 1961). The reliability of the BDI has been demonstrated to be good in both depressed and nondepressed older samples (Gallagher et al. 1982). The instrument consists of 21 symptoms and attitudes that are rated on a scale of 0 to 3 in terms of intensity. In another study by Gallagher et al. (1983), the BDI misclassified only 16.7% of subjects diagnosed based on RDC as suffering from a major depression.

The Geriatric Depression Scale (GDS) was developed because of problems the above scales present to older persons who have difficulty selecting one of four forced-response items (Yesavage et al. 1983). The GDS is a 30-item scale that permits patients to rate items as either present or absent, and includes questions about symptoms such as cognitive complaints, self-image, and losses. Items selected were thought to have relevance to late-life depression. The GDS has not been used in community populations and is not yet well standardized.

Another instrument, similar to the GDS, is the Carroll Rating Scale for Depression (Carroll et al. 1981). This instrument consists of 52 items, scored either as "Yes" or "No," which follow those areas assessed for the Hamilton Rating Scale for Depression (see below). Although it has not been used extensively in older populations, the Carroll scale has the same advantage as the GDS in being the forced-response type with yes/no answers.

Of the interviewer-rated scales, the Hamilton Rating Scale for Depression (Hamilton 1960) is by far the most commonly used. Although no formal normative data exist, the advantage of having ratings based on clinical judgment has made this scale a popular instrument for rating outcome in clinical trials. For example, a reduction in the Hamilton score to one-half the initial score or to below a certain value would indicate partial or complete recovery from an episode of depression. In one study of this scale in older adults, Hodern et al. (1963) found that among depressed women, agitation, delayed insomnia, loss of weight, and depressed mood were more severe in the elderly compared with younger age groups.

A newer scale that is receiving considerable attention clinically, but which remains to be standardized in both clinical and community populations, is the Montgomery-Åsberg Rating Scale for Depression (Montgomery and Åsberg 1979). This scale follows the pattern of the Hamilton scale and concentrates on 10 symptoms of depression; it calls for the clinician to rate each of these symptoms on a scale of 0 to 6 (for a range of scores between 0 and 60). The symptoms that are rated include apparent sadness, reported sadness, inattention, reduced sleep, reduced appetite, concentration difficulties, lassitude, inability to feel, pessimistic thoughts, and suicidal thoughts. This scale, theoretically, is an improvement over the Hamilton scale in that it appears to better differentiate between responders and nonresponders to intervention for depression. The in-

strument does not include many somatic symptoms that tend to be more common in older adults, and therefore it may be of greater value in tracking the symptoms of depressive illness that would be expected to change with therapy.

General Assessment Scales

A number of general assessment scales of psychiatric status (occasionally combined with functioning in other areas) have been found to be useful in both community and clinical populations.

One of the more frequently used scales is the Global Assessment Scale (GAS; Spitzer et al. 1978b). Using this scale, the rater makes a single rating, ranging from 0 to 100, that best describes—on the basis of his or her clinical judgment—the lowest level of the subject's functioning in the week before the rating. The scale has not been standardized for older adults, but its common use in psychiatric studies suggests the need for standardization. The scale has been incorporated as Axis V in DSM-IV to measure overall functioning.

A similar scale is the Brief Psychiatric Rating Scale (BPRS; Overall and Gorham 1962). With this scale, 16 relatively independent symptom areas—including somatic concern, anxiety, depressive mood, unusual thought content, and suspiciousness—are rated from "not present" to "extremely severe." A summary score is obtained. Symptom profiles on the BPRS have been shown to be different in older populations. Among older adults, depressive mood more often occurs in association with motor retardation, emotional withdrawal, and blunted affect, whereas depressive mood is usually accompanied by anxiety in younger patients (Beller and Overall 1984). In another study, Overall and Beller (1984) found five distinct phenomenological types in a geriatric population: agitated dementia, retarded dementia, anxious depression, withdrawn depression, and paranoid psychosis.

Shader et al. (1974) developed the Sandoz Clinical Assessment—Geriatric (SCAG) scale, an 18-symptom scale with each symptom rated along a 7-point scale. The SCAG has been shown to identify the existence of psychopathology in older persons, but the discrimination between subgroups of psychiatrically disturbed older adults remains to be tested. This scale has not been used as frequently as other scales in recent years. The Geriatric Mental

State Schedule (Copeland et al. 1976) is an adaptation of the Present State Examination (PSE; Wing et al. 1974) and the Psychiatric Status Schedule (Spitzer et al. 1968); the Geriatric Mental State Schedule is a semistructured interviewing guide that allows the rater to inventory symptoms associated with psychiatric disorders. More than 500 ratings are made on the basis of information obtained by a highly trained interviewer, who elicits symptoms from the month preceding the evaluation. Data are computerized in order to derive psychiatric diagnoses (Copeland et al. 1986). The instrument measures depression, impaired memory, selected neurological symptoms (such as aphasia), and disorientation.

The Comprehensive Assessment and Referral Evaluation (CARE; Gurland et al. 1977) is a hybridized assessment procedure developed for older adults. Dimensional scores are obtained in memory–disorientation, depression–anxiety, immobility–incapacity, isolation, physical–perceptual difficulty, and poor housing–income. The goal of CARE is to provide a comprehensive assessment of the older adult that bridges the professional disciplines. The instrument has not been used extensively, though it has been used in cross-national studies. For example, Herbst and Humphrey (1980) used CARE in a study examining how hearing impairment relates to mental status. The investigators found a relationship between deafness and depression that was independent of age and socioeconomic status.

The Older Americans Resources and Services (OARS) Multidimensional Functional Assessment Questionnaire (Duke University Center for the Study of Aging and Human Development 1978) is administered by a lay interviewer, and is used to gather data in order to produce functional impairment ratings in five dimensions: mental health, physical health, social functioning, economic functioning, and activities of daily living. In one community survey (Blazer 1978a), 13% of persons in the community suffered from mental health impairment. The OARS instrument was developed in order to integrate functional measures across a series of parameters relevant to older adults; it has been used widely in both community and clinical surveys. With the recent emphasis that has been placed on discrete psychiatric disorders, however, the instrument has not been as widely used by mental health workers as it might otherwise have been.

Any discussion of clinical rating scales is not complete without the Abnormal Involuntary Movements Scale (AIMS; National Institute of Mental Health 1975). Given the increased incidence of tardive dyskinesia among older adults, coupled with the need for better documentation for this dreaded outcome of prolonged use of antipsychotic agents, regular ratings on the AIMS by clinicians are becoming essential for the practice of inpatient and outpatient geriatric psychiatry. The scale consists of a list of seven movement disorders, the presence and severity of each of which is rated from "none" to "severe." Three items are devoted to a global judgment: severity of abnormal movements, incapacitation due to abnormal movements, and the patient's awareness of abnormal movements. Current problems with teeth or dentures are also assessed. Procedures are described to increase the reliability of this rating scale.

Structured Interviews

A number of structured interview schedules are now available for both clinical and community diagnosis. These interview schedules have allowed increased reliability of the identification of particular symptoms and psychiatric diagnoses. Unfortunately, the richness inherent in the unstructured interview tends to be lost if one adheres closely to the structured interview. Comments made by the patient during the evaluation that could be used to trace relevant associations must be ignored in order to push through the interview schedule. Most of these interviews require more time than the traditional, unstructured first session with the patient.

The oldest of the currently used interview schedules is the PSE (Wing et al. 1974). As noted above, the Geriatric Mental State Schedule is a variant of the PSE. The PSE is actually not an interview at all, but a list of definitions of behaviors or symptoms of psychiatric interest, ranging from specific delusions to general changes in affect. The clinician scores whether or not the symptom is present, and a computer algorithm provides a diagnosis. Suggested questions for eliciting the symptoms are available, but not obligatory. Only 54 questions are required during the interview, though many additional probes are provided to track positive responses. The interview schedule provides an excellent education for many psychiatrists in the meaning of various symptoms of relevance to working with older adults. Nevertheless, the focus on 1 month before the evaluation date and the association of the symptoms with the World Health Organization's International Classification of Diseases (ICD)—instead of the American Psychiatric Association's DSM—make the PSE less popular with American investigators.

The most frequently used instrument in the United States is the Structured Clinical Interview for DSM-III-R (SCID; Spitzer et al. 1992). This instrument is easily adaptable to the RDC and DSM-IV. Although specific questions are suggested for probing most areas of interest, the interviewer using the SCID has the flexibility to ask additional questions and can use whatever data are available in order to assign a diagnosis. The interviewer must have clinical training but does not have to be a psychiatrist. Many of the symptoms may not be relevant to older adults (especially the extensive probes for psychotic symptoms), and the interview frequently takes 2½–3 hours to administer. Nevertheless, the experience gained by the clinician in using this instrument can be translated into a more effective clinical practice.

A relatively recent addition to the schedules available is the Diagnostic Interview Schedule (DIS; Robins et al. 1981). This highly structured, computer-scored interview, which can be administered by a lay interviewer, allows psychiatric diagnoses to be made according to DSM-IV criteria, Feighner criteria (Feighner et al. 1972), and RDC. The DIS questions probe for the presence or absence of symptoms or behaviors relevant to a series of psychiatric disorders, the severity of these symptoms, and the putative cause of the symptoms. Diagnoses of cognitive impairment, schizophrenia or schizophreniform disorder, major depression, generalized anxiety, panic disorder, agoraphobia, obsessive-compulsive disorder, dysthymic disorder, somatization disorder, alcohol abuse and/or dependence, and other substance abuse and/or dependence can be made from Axis I of DSM-IV. A diagnosis of antisocial personality disorder, from Axis II, can also be made. The instrument has proved reasonably reliable in clinic populations for both current and lifetime diagnoses.

The range of disorders probed by the DIS questions, coupled with this instrument's relative ease of administration (it generally takes 45–90 minutes to administer to an older adult), has made it popular for use in clinical studies. In addition, community-based comparative data are available on a large sample from the Epidemiologic Catchment Area study (Regier et al. 1984; Myers et al. 1984). The DIS can be supplemented with additional questions to probe for specific symptoms (such as probing for melancholic symptoms and additional data regarding sleep disorders for depressed older adults). No problems have arisen when the instrument is used among older adults in the community. The memory decay that occurs in the elderly in general is no more of a problem with this instrument than with other instruments. Nevertheless, the DIS is of less value in the study of institutional populations and reconstruction of lifetime history regardless of setting, because memory problems cannot be circumvented by clinical judgment. Supplementary data can be added to the instrument for developing a standardized diagnosis. A shortened versions of the DIS, which has been used in recent epidemiological surveys, is the Composite International Diagnostic Interview (CIDI; World Health Organization 1989).

Communicating with the Older Patient

The clinician who works with the older adult should be cognizant of those factors relating to both the patient and the clinician that may produce barriers to effective communication (Blazer 1978b). Many older persons experience a relatively high level of anxiety, yet do not complain of this symptom. Stress deriving from a new situation, such as visiting a clinician's office or being interviewed in a hospital, may intensify the anxiety and subsequently impair effective communication. Perceptual problems, such as hearing and visual impairment, may exacerbate disorientation and complicate the communication of problems to the clinician. Elderly persons are more likely to withhold information than to hazard answers that may be incorrect. In other words, older persons tend to be more cautious. They frequently take longer to respond to inquiries and resist the clinician who attempts to rush through the history-taking interview.

The elderly patient may perceive the physician unrealistically, on the basis of previous life experiences (that is, transference may occur). Although the older patient will sometimes accept the role of a child, viewing the physician as parent, he or she is initially more likely to view the clinician as the idealized child who can provide reciprocal care to the previously capable but now impaired parent. Splitting between the physician and children of the patient may subsequently occur. The clinician can perceive the older adult patient incorrectly because of preconceived fears of aging and death, or because of previous negative experiences with his or her own parents. For a clinician to work effectively with older adults, these personal feelings should be discussed during training (and afterward).

Once physician and patient attitudes have been recognized and acknowledged, certain techniques have proved to be valuable, in general, in communicating with the elderly patient. These techniques should not be implemented indiscriminately, however, for the variation among the population of older adults is significant. First, the older person should be approached with respect. The clinician should knock before entering a patient's room, and should greet the patient by surname (Mr. Jones, Mrs. Smith) rather than by given names, unless the clinician also wishes to be addressed by a given name.

After taking a position near the older person—near enough to reach out and touch the patient—the clinician should speak clearly and slowly and use simple sentences in case the person's hearing is impaired. Because of hearing problems, older patients may understand conversation better over the telephone than in person. By placing the receiver against the mastoid bone, the patient with otosclerosis can take advantage of preserved bone conduction.

The interview should be paced so that the older person has time enough to respond to questions. Most elders are not uncomfortable with silence, because it gives them an opportunity to formulate their answers to questions and elaborate certain points they wish to emphasize. Nonverbal communication is frequently a key to effective communication with elders, because the older person may be reticent to reveal affect verbally. Changes in facial expression, gestures, postures, and long silences may provide clues to the clinician concerning issues that are unspoken.

One key to successful communication with an older adult is a willingness to continue working as a professional with that person. Older adults in the 1990s—possibly unlike some of their children and grandchildren—place a great deal of stress on loyalty and continuity. Most elders do not require large amounts of time from clinicians. Those who are more demanding can usually be controlled through structure in the interview.

References

American Psychiatric Association: Diagnostic and Statistical Manual of Mental Disorders, 4th Edition. Washington, DC, American Psychiatric Association, 1994

Ayd FJ: Treatment-resistant patients: a moral, legal and therapeutic challenge, in Rational Psychopharmacotherapy and the Right to Treatment. Edited by Ayd FJ. Baltimore, MD, Ayd Medical Communications, 1975

Beck AT, Ward CH, Mendelson M, et al: An inventory for measuring depression. Arch Gen Psychiatry 4:561–571, 1961

Beller SA, Overall JE: The Brief Psychiatric Rating Scale in geropsychiatric research, II: representative profile patterns. J Gerontol 39:194–200, 1984

Blazer DG: The OARS Durham surveys: description and application, in Multidimensional Functional Assessment: The OARS Methodology—A Manual, 2nd Edition. Durham, NC, Duke University Center for the Study of Aging and Human Development, 1978a, pp 75–88

Blazer DG: Techniques for communicating with your elderly patient. Geriatrics 33:79–80, 83–84, 1978b

Blazer DG: Depression in Late Life. St Louis, MO, CV Mosby, 1982

Blazer DG: Evaluating the family of the elderly patient, in A Family Approach to Health Care in the Elderly. Edited by Blazer D, Siegler IC. Menlo Park, CA, Addison-Wesley, 1984, pp 13–32

Blazer DG, Kaplan BH: The assessment of social support in an elderly community population. American Journal of Social Psychiatry 3:29–36, 1983

Blessed G, Tomlinson BE, Roth M: The association between quantitative measures of dementia and of senile change in the cerebral gray matter of elderly subjects. Br J Psychiatry 114:797–811, 1968

Carroll BJ, Feinberg M, Smouse PE, et al: The Carroll Rating Scale for Depression, I: development, reliability and validation. Br J Psychiatry 138:194–200, 1981

Copeland JRM, Kelleher MJ, Kellet JM, et al: A semistructured clinical interview for the assessment and diagnosis of mental state in the elderly: the Geriatric Mental State Schedule. Psychol Med 6:439–449, 1976

Copeland JRM, Dewey ME, Griffiths-Jones HM, et al: A computerized psychiatric diagnostic system and case nomenclature for elderly subjects: GMS and AGECAT. Psychol Med 16:89–99, 1986

Eisenberg L: Disease and illness: distinctions between professional and popular ideas of sickness. Cult Med Psychiatry 1:9–23, 1977

Eisenberg L, Kleinman A: Clinical social science, in The Relevance of Social Science for Medicine. Edited by Eisenberg L, Kleinman A. Boston, MA, D Reidel, 1981, pp 1–26

Feighner JP, Robins E, Guze SB, et al: Diagnostic criteria for use in psychiatric research. Arch Gen Psychiatry 26:57–63, 1972

Folstein MF, Folstein SE, McHugh PR: Mini-Mental State: a practical method for grading the cognitive state of patients for the clinician. J Psychiatr Res 12:189–198, 1975

Freedman N, Bucci W, Elkowitz E: Depression in a family practice elderly population. J Am Geriatr Soc 30:372–377, 1982

Gallagher D, Nies G, Thompson LW: Reliability of the Beck Depression Inventory with older adults. J Consult Clin Psychol 50:152–153, 1982

Gallagher D, Breckenridge J, Steinmetz J, et al: The Beck Depression Inventory and Research Diagnostic Criteria: congruence in an older population. J Consult Clin Psychol 51:945–946, 1983

Garetz FR: Responses of families to health problems in the elderly. Paper presented at the annual meeting of the American Geriatrics Society, New York, May 1979

Gurland B, Kuriansky J, Sharpe L, et al: The Comprehensive Assessment and Referral Evaluation (CARE)—rationale, development and reliability. Int J Aging Hum Dev 8:9–42, 1977

Hachinski VC, Iliff LD, Zilhka E, et al: Cerebral blood flow in dementia. Arch Neurol 32:632–637, 1975

Hamilton M: A rating scale for depression. J Neurol Neurosurg Psychiatry 23:56–62, 1960

Herbst KG, Humphrey C: Hearing impairment and mental state in the elderly living at home. BMJ 281:903–905, 1980

Hodern A, Holt NF, Burt CE, et al: Amitriptyline in depressive states: phenomenology and prognostic considerations. Br J Psychiatry 109:815–825, 1963

Kahn RL, Goldfarb AI, Pollack M, et al: Brief objective measures for the determination of mental status in the aged. Am J Psychiatry 117:326–328, 1960

Linn L: Clinical manifestations of psychiatric disorders, in Comprehensive Textbook of Psychiatry, 3rd Edition, Vol 1. Edited by Kaplan HI, Freedman AM, Sadock BJ. Baltimore, MD, Williams & Wilkins, 1980, pp 990–1034

Mendlewicz J, Fleiss JL, Cataldo M, et al: Accuracy of the family history method in affective illness: comparison with direct interviews in family studies. Arch Gen Psychiatry 32:309–314, 1975

Meyers BS, Greenberg R: Late-life delusional depression. J Affect Disord 11:133–137, 1986

Meyers BS, Greenberg R, Varda M: Delusional depression in the elderly, in Treatment of Affective Disorders in the Elderly. Edited by Shamoian CA. Washington, DC, American Psychiatric Press, 1985, pp 37–63

Miller KT, Miller JL: The family as a system. Paper presented at the annual meeting of the American College of Psychiatrists, New York, February 1979

Montgomery SA, Åsberg M: A new depression scale designed to be sensitive to change. Br J Psychiatry 134:382–389, 1979

Myers JK, Weissman MM, Tischler GL, et al: Six-month prevalence of psychiatric disorders in three communities: 1980 to 1982. Arch Gen Psychiatry 41:959–967, 1984

National Institute of Mental Health: Development of a Dyskinetic Movement Scale (Publ No 4). Rockville, MD, National Institute of Mental Health, Psychopharmacology Research Branch, 1975

Older Americans Resources and Services: Multidimensional Functional Assessment: The OARS Methodology—A Manual, 2nd Edition. Durham, NC, Duke University Center for the Study of Aging and Human Development, 1978

Overall JE, Beller SA: The Brief Psychiatric Rating Scale (BPRS) in geropsychiatric research, I: factor structure on an inpatient unit. J Gerontol 39:187–193, 1984

Overall JE, Gorham DR: The Brief Psychiatric Rating Scale. Psychol Rep 10:799–812, 1962

Pfeiffer E: A Short Portable Mental Status Questionnaire for the assessment of organic brain deficit in elderly patients. J Am Geriatr Soc 23:433–441, 1975

Radloff LS: The CES-D Scale: a self-report depression scale for research in the general population. Applied Psychological Measurement 1:385–401, 1977

Regier DA, Myers JK, Kramer M, et al: The NIMH Epidemiologic Catchment Area program: historical context, major objectives, and study population characteristics. Arch Gen Psychiatry 41:934–941, 1984

Robins LN, Helzer JE, Croughan J, et al: National Institute of Mental Health Diagnostic Interview Schedule: its history, characteristics, and validity. Arch Gen Psychiatry 38:381–389, 1981

Ross CE, Mirowsky J: Components of depressed mood in married men and women: the CES-D. Am J Epidemiol 119:997–1004, 1984

Sanford JRA: Tolerance of debility in elderly dependents by supporters at home: its significance for hospital practice. BMJ 3:471–473, 1975

Shader RI, Harmatz JS, Salzman C: A new scale for clinical assessment in geriatric populations: Sandoz Clinical Assessment—Geriatric (SCAG). J Am Geriatr Soc 22:107–113, 1974

Spitzer RL, Endicott J, Cohen GM: Psychiatric Status Schedule, 2nd Edition. New York, New York State Department of Mental Hygiene, Evaluation Unit, Biometrics Research, 1968

Spitzer RL, Endicott J, Robins E: Research Diagnostic Criteria: rationale and reliability. Arch Gen Psychiatry 35:773–782, 1978a

Spitzer RL, Gibbon M, Endicott J: The Global Assessment Scale (GAS). New York, New York State Department of Mental Hygiene, Evaluation Unit, Biometrics Research, 1978b

Spitzer RL, Williams JB, Gibbon M, et al: The structured clinical interview for DSM-III-R (SCID): history, rationale and description. Arch Gen Psychiatry 49:624-629, 1992

Wing JK, Cooper JE, Sartorius N: The Measurement and Classification of Psychiatric Symptoms. London, Cambridge University Press, 1974

World Health Organization: Composite International Diagnostic Interview. Geneva, Switzerland, World Health Organization, 1989

Yesavage JA, Brink TL, Rose TL, et al: Development and validation of a geriatric depression screening scale: a preliminary report. J Psychiatr Res 17:37–49, 1983

Zung WWK: A self-rating depression scale. Arch Gen Psychiatry 12:63–70, 1965

Zung WWK: Depression in the normal aged. Psychosomatics 8:287–292, 1967

CHAPTER 11

Use of the Laboratory in the Diagnostic Workup of Older Adults

Dan G. Blazer, M.D., Ph.D.
Ewald W. Busse, M.D.
W. Edward Craighead, Ph.D.
Don Evans, Ph.D.

In this chapter, we consider the usefulness of a series of biomedical and psychological laboratory tests for diagnosis and evaluation of the treatment of psychiatric disorders in late life. (Other evaluation procedures, especially diagnostic interviews and self-rated and clinician-rated symptom screens, are discussed in Chapter 10 of this text.) Technological advances have led to, and will continue to result in, rapid changes in virtually all of these laboratory diagnostic procedures. Consequently, the reader must be alert to the relative value of these tests within the clinical setting, as well as to their limitations.

Some tests that were once used mainly in research settings now have an almost uniformly accepted role in general clinical practice. For example, the therapeutic monitoring of tricyclic antidepressant (TCA) plasma levels is now a standard diagnostic test available to virtually all clinicians practicing in developed and some developing countries. Other tests, such as magnetic resonance imaging (MRI), are in transition from research use to clinical use. Limitations in widespread use of these tests include cost and lack of objective data regarding their utility. All of these tests will come under closer scrutiny with emerging health care reform. In all cases, the "yield" in terms of data that shape therapy will be balanced against the cost.

As yet there is no test that is pathognomonic for a primary psychiatric illness, although many laboratory tests provide the information needed to diagnose a physical illness that presents primarily with psychiatric symptoms. For example, an abnormal thyroid panel and elevated thyroid-stimulating hormone document hypothyroidism as a cause of lethargy and depression. For this reason, a routine medical laboratory screen is indicated for all seriously ill elderly psychiatric patients. Most test results are indirect "markers" of pathophysiology, including an abnormal dexamethasone suppression test (DST), an abnormal electroencephalogram (EEG), a shortened rapid eye movement (REM) latency shown on a polysomnogram, decreased cerebral blood flow, and a high score on the Minnesota Multiphasic Personality Inventory (MMPI). These markers can be of value in the clinical setting by providing data complementary to the history and physical examination.

Psychiatrists and other mental health care providers must become informed users of the laboratory in the future if they are to perform effectively as diagnosticians. Laboratory test results are subject to the same bias as clinical diagnostic procedures—a lack of reliability and validity. Therefore, for most diagnostic tests, such as the DST, certain methodological criteria must be met if the test is to prove useful as a marker of an illness. Shelps and Schechter (1984) suggest a series of methodological criteria, which are listed below in slightly modified form.

1. Is there a well-defined gold standard?
2. Are "positive" and "negative" results clearly defined for the diagnostic tests?
3. Is the test an "independent test"? For example, is the interpretation of performance of the diagnostic test blind to other clinical information?
4. In presentation of the usefulness of the test, are the data clearly displayed in tabular form?
5. Are sensitivity and specificity defined and used correctly in the presentation?
6. Are limitations for use of the test clearly stated?
7. Are guidelines provided for appropriate use?
8. Has the cost/benefit ratio or cost-effectiveness of the test been discussed?
9. Have the procedures for performing the test been described in sufficient detail to permit replication?

The above questions relate primarily to the usefulness of a test in establishing a diagnosis of a psychiatric disorder in a setting where the clinical decision is to determine the appropriate clinical management of an individual patient. With the advent of DSM-III and DSM-III-R (American Psychiatric Association 1980, 1987)—and, subsequently, of DSM-IV (American Psychiatric Association 1994)—establishing the "presence or absence" of a specific psychiatric disorder determines the course of therapy. With the advent of clinical practice guidelines, therapies will more uniformly derive from objective

clinical data contributing to diagnosis (Agency for Health Care Policy and Research [AHCPR] 1993). The value of a test will ultimately depend upon what the results contribute to clinical decisions regarding therapy through the intermediary of diagnosis.

To assess validity, a test is compared to a gold standard (such as a clinical diagnosis) that highlights four characteristics of the test. These characteristics are outlined in Figure 11–1.

Sensitivity is defined as the number of persons who have a disorder and who exhibit a positive test result, divided by the total number of individuals who have the disorder: $a \div (a + c)$. *Specificity* is defined as the number of individuals who do not have a disorder and who exhibit a negative test result, divided by the total number of individuals who do not have the disorder: $d \div (b + d)$. The *positive predictive value* is the proportion of patients with positive test results who have the disorder: $a \div (a + b)$. The *negative predictive value* is the proportion of individuals who exhibit a negative test result and who do not have the disorder: $d \div (c + d)$. Obviously, the percentage of individuals in the study population who actually have the disorder will affect these values. For example, as prevalence falls in the study population, the positive predictive value must fall along with it, and the negative predictive value must rise.

When diagnostic tests are sensitive, relatively easy to administer, and not costly, they can be used as screening procedures. To date, there are no useful

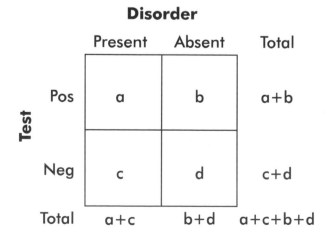

Figure 11–1.   Data required to evaluate the usefulness of a diagnostic test.

biomedical screens for primary psychiatric disorders. Nevertheless, screening scales—such as the Center for Epidemiology Studies Depression Scale (CES-D), discussed in detail later in this text (see Chapter 13, "Mood Disorders")—may be implemented with such populations as patients in a geriatric evaluation and treatment clinic. If the test results raise the suspicion that a disorder is present but further information is required to justify a course of therapy, a laboratory test may be indicated. Such tests may be expensive, and so abnormal results on laboratory tests should confirm the presence of the disease (for example, confirmation of the presence of multi-infarct dementia on MRI scanning). In the future, however, mere confirmation of the presence of a suspected disease may not be enough to justify routine use of expensive tests; it will be necessary to prove that the test is of value in shaping clinical management.

The evaluation of the usefulness of a test is a complex process. One factor to consider is that diagnostic tests are usually not performed in isolation. When multiple tests are used, the accumulation of abnormal results may confirm the presence of a disorder or may provide data relevant to comorbid medical conditions that may alter therapy. (For example, rapid-cycling depression in the presence of hypothyroidism may render thyroid replacement therapy the first choice of therapies.) These tests are least helpful when the result of one test is positive and the results of the others are normal. Laboratory tests are more likely to be appropriate if 1) unusual symptoms and signs emerge during the examination, 2) the patient is older, 3) the disorder first occurs after age 40–45, and 4) the disorder does not fully respond to routine treatment (AHCPR 1993).

Biomedical tests are subject to another bias: a lack of reliability that directly affects validity. The modern geriatric psychiatrist has become familiar with the laboratory procedures for performing assays of hormones, metabolites of neurotransmitters, and concentrations of pharmacological agents. Adequate laboratory assays that are reliable must be available to the clinician if these tests are to be useful. In addition, the range of normality and abnormality may vary from one laboratory to another. Therefore, it is essential that test results be interpreted within the framework of the laboratory in which they are performed. Additional sources of variability must be explored in the future, because many of these tests

for pathophysiology are complex. For example, the variation in metabolism of dexamethasone across subjects may significantly alter the results of the DST.

The use of laboratory tests is not limited to screening and confirming diagnoses. Other uses include prediction of a patient's response to therapy. For example, abnormalities in a thyroid function test—even in the absence of overt hyperthyroidism or hypothyroidism—may indicate an increased potential benefit of using a supplemental thyroid preparation like liothyronine sodium as an adjunct to TCA therapy in the treatment-resistant depressed older adult. Tests may also predict clinical course. For example, there is an increased likelihood of rapid relapse (Schweitzer et al. 1987) if a DST abnormal during the initial phases of an episode fails to normalize in the presence of improved clinical function.

Given the variety of laboratory tests available and the increasing restrictions on the overall cost of a diagnostic workup, geriatric psychiatrists and other clinicians working with psychiatrically impaired older adults must select appropriate batteries of tests that can provide optimal complementary information at a reasonable cost. Which tests are justified in the routine workup of a depressed or demented older adult? What are the relative costs of tests, both in terms of money and in terms of burden upon patients who have already been subjected to multiple diagnostic procedures? To what extent do diagnostic tests contribute to clinical decision making?

The following discussion of specific diagnostic tests is cursory, because an exhaustive review is beyond the scope of this text. Nevertheless, we hope that these discussions will be of value in helping clinicians to select an appropriate array of tests in the diagnostic workup of the psychiatrically impaired older adult.

Polysomnography

The development of multiple monitoring of sleep and somatic function, coupled with the increased flexibility that is now possible in the use of these methods, has ushered in a new era in the diagnosis of sleep disorders. Diagnostic units for the investigation of sleep complaints are now available in almost every major metropolitan area. The core diagnostic procedure used in sleep disorders units is the polysomnogram. This all-night, multiple monitoring of cerebral and somatic function during sleep has proved both reliable and sensitive for recording the stages of sleep and concomitant physiological functioning. Three basic recording variables are included in the polysomnogram: the sleep EEG, the electrooculogram (to measure eye movements during sleep), and the submental electromyogram (to measure ventilatory air exchange and respiratory effort). Additional monitors can be used for more specialized investigation, such as the electrocardiogram (ECG), electrodes placed over the anterior tibialis muscles (to measure leg movements), and venous catheterization to measure blood oxygen saturation. In specialized laboratories, video recording of sleep behaviors and postures and measurement of penile tumescence are also included.

For years, the availability of the sleep laboratory to the clinician was limited because of logistic difficulties. In the past, it was necessary for a patient to sleep in the laboratory for 2–3 nights (with constant monitoring by a laboratory technician) so that adequate data could be collected. The relatively recent development of portable units has permitted data collection in the patient's home or hospital room. These new units are no larger than a portable tape recorder, and collect data by means of electrodes attached to the scalp. The resulting sleep tracings are later evaluated by computer-assisted monitoring.

Despite the recent technological advances, the polysomnogram remains of limited use in the general diagnostic workup of the depressed and/or demented older adult. An adequate polysomnogram requires that the patient be drug-free for at least 7 days, and preferably for 10–14 days, before the study begins. The more severely depressed and demented older adult, especially one who is difficult to control behaviorally, requires ongoing medication. Although medication in such a case could be withheld within a hospital setting, the advent of capitation to hospital care reimbursement has limited the time available for hospitalization of older adults. Nevertheless, the polysomnogram is and will continue to be a valuable diagnostic procedure for the study of the psychiatrically impaired older adult with persistent and unexplained sleep problems. The use of polysomnography in the diagnosis of affective disorders and sleep disorders is discussed in Chapters 13 and 18.

Electrocardiogram

The ECG in combination with a recording of blood pressure is the most frequently used screen of cardiovascular disease. The ECG provides a graphic description of the electrical activity of the heart, which is recorded from the body surface by electrodes positioned to reflect activity from a variety of spatial perspectives. Cardiovascular disease can have psychiatric manifestations in the older adult. For example, confusion and agitation may be present in patients with congestive heart failure or pulmonary edema. Acute confusion may be a sign of transient ischemic attacks or cardiac arrhythmias. However, the most valuable use of electrocardiography in the diagnostic workup of the older adult is as a screening method for identifying cardiovascular disease that would preclude the use of certain biological therapies such as antidepressant medications or electroconvulsive therapy, and, in those persons for whom use of such therapies is not precluded, for monitoring the effect of these therapies on cardiovascular function.

The TCAs are known to be cardiotoxic in overdose, and their use has been considered unsafe—even at therapeutic doses—in patients with cardiovascular disease. Glassman and Bigger (1981), however, documented that the most common cardiovascular complication associated with the tricyclics is orthostatic hypotension, and that patients with ventricular arrhythmias are likely to experience improvement in their symptoms with TCA therapy. Veith and colleagues (1982) found that tricyclic drugs had no effect on left-ventricular ejection fractions at rest or during maximal exercise and that premature ventricular contractions were reduced by imipramine.

It is a common observation that near- or above-therapeutic plasma levels of tricyclics are frequently associated with a prolonged PR interval and QRS complex. Although these ECG findings do not represent a cardiac hazard, tricyclic levels should be monitored by an ECG both before drug therapy is instituted and periodically during therapy. Individuals with preexisting bundle branch block are at some danger for increased AV or HV block. Therefore, these elderly adults should be monitored frequently, probably in the hospital, when initially prescribed TCAs.

Cardiovascular toxicity is occasionally a problem with antipsychotic agents as well. Orthostatic hypertension is the most common difficulty and can be induced by the less potent phenothiazines, such as thioridazine. Neuroleptic drugs also produce nonspecific T wave changes on ECG, but, once again, these changes are not known to be of clinical significance. Nevertheless, it is generally recommended that low-potency neuroleptics not be used with individuals in whom conduction defects are identified initially on the ECG. When a patient who is taking TCAs or a neuroleptic agent is referred for a routine ECG, the medication history should be communicated so that the ECG can be interpreted correctly.

Clinical Chemistry Screen

A clinical chemistry screen is routine for virtually all hospital admissions and for many outpatient visits. The yield from these screens is usually low for identifying the cause of psychiatric disorder, but the low cost and potential for correcting a previously undetected medical illness may make routine laboratory screenings valuable to the psychiatrist. However, with capitation, such screenings will probably no longer be routine, and psychiatrists will, therefore, be forced to choose tests with the highest yield.

Clinical chemistry screening may be of most value in the diagnostic workup of the patient with cognitive impairment. The clinician must search for potentially reversible dementias—that is, dementias secondary to thyroid dysfunction, vitamin B_{12} deficiency, substance abuse, and infection. The American Medical Association's Council on Scientific Affairs (1986) published a consensus report on those laboratory tests that should be included in the diagnostic workup of the dementia patient, and recommended a blood count, electrolytes, blood sugar, blood urea nitrogen, creatinine, liver function tests, thyroid function tests, serologic tests for syphilis, toxicology screen, B_{12} and folate concentrations, sedimentation rate, and urinalysis. When a toxicology screen is not available, it is often helpful to obtain blood concentrations of all the medicines the patient is taking.

Abnormal sodium and chloride levels can lead to dehydration that can progress to delirium, lethargy, and convulsions. Overhydration may also evoke delirium and lethargy, as well as weakness and muscular twitching. Respiratory or metabolic acidosis (an increased CO_2 level) may lead to drowsiness and weakness, which may be mistaken for a chronic depression or dementia. Respiratory alkalosis secondary to hyperventilation may lead to symptoms of light-headedness, feelings of unreality, and paresthesias.

Among the electrolyte abnormalities, potassium disorders are the most critical to identify. Though they rarely manifest psychiatric symptoms, the presence of a flaccid paralysis and paresthesias or muscular twitching may signify the onset of a severe cardiac arrhythmia and cardiac failure. Increased calcium resulting from hyperparathyroidism can lead to paranoid ideation and a variety of mental changes, as can hypocalcemia secondary to hypoparathyroidism. The mental changes associated with hypoparathyroidism may range from agitation to frank psychosis. Hyperinsulinism, causing hypoglycemia, may initially be manifested by anxiety, perspiration, weakness, and shortness of breath. The symptoms of hyperglycemia (usually adult-onset diabetes) include lethargy, which may lead to diabetic coma and ketoacidosis.

The monitoring of thyroid function is especially important. Three tests are available in most laboratories, and, for the psychiatric patient, a fourth test is generally suggested. The three traditional components of the thyroid panel are a direct assay of thyroxine (T_4) by radioimmunoassay, triiodothyronine (T_3) uptake, and the calculation of a free thyroxin index. The fourth test that may be helpful in assessing the psychiatric patient is an assay of thyroid-stimulating hormone (TSH). A combination of results of the thyroid panel and TSH assists in the diagnosis of both clinical and subclinical hypothyroidism. Subclinical hypothyroidism is not an uncommon cause of depressive symptoms in older adults, and it is a condition that may respond to supplemental thyroid replacement.

Thyrotropin-Releasing/ Thyroid-Stimulating Hormone Test

The thyrotropin-releasing hormone (TRH) stimulation test is the most sensitive of the clinical tests for thyroid disorder. The test assesses the functional state of the TSH-secretory mechanism. The interpretation of this test as it relates to the diagnosis of depression is described in Chapter 13. Patients who undergo this test must be drug-free for the previous 7 days and must fast from the night before. The test begins at 9:00 A.M.; with the patient in the recumbent position, the clinician performing the test administers 0.5 mg of TRH, and TSH is recorded at 30-minute intervals for 3 hours. In addition to its value in identifying depression, a blunted TSH response to TRH is seen in functionally euthyroid patients with toxic goiters, and is also observed occasionally in patients with pituitary hypothyroidism. Davies and co-workers (1985) found a blunted TSH response to TRH common in sick elderly patients but, contrary to the group's initial hypothesis, did not find that patients with cardiac arrhythmias were more likely to exhibit a blunted response. Factors that may influence TSH response in normal subjects are thought to be relatively uncommon (Loosen and Prange 1982), but poor nutrition clearly contributes to an abnormal response. Elevated serum cortisol also appears to reduce TSH response, both in patients with endocrine disorders and in normal subjects, although there is no evidence that serum cortisol elevation accounts for the TSH blunting seen in depressed patients. The test, however, is of little use for the routine clinical workup of the depressed or demented older adult.

Dexamethasone Suppression Test

Because it is valuable in the diagnoses of dementia and depression, the DST is discussed in detail in Chapters 12 and 13, respectively. This test, which has been used for the diagnosis of Cushing's syndrome for years, has only recently been applied to the diagnosis of psychiatric disorders, specifically depression. The DST became more valuable in psychiatry when the dose of dexamethasone was decreased from that usually recommended for the Cushing's syndrome test to detect more subtle changes in the hypothalamic-pituitary-adrenal axis. The test procedure is to administer 1 mg of dexamethasone orally at 11:00 P.M. Venous blood samples are drawn for cortisol at 3:00 P.M. and 10:00 P.M. the next day, although 8:00 A.M. or 3:00 P.M. single cortisol levels have also been used. An abnormal

DST result is defined as a plasma cortisol level greater than 5 µg/dL after dexamethasone administration.

The laboratory assay is critical to the reliability of the test results. Good precision and accuracy, particularly at the low end of plasma cortisol levels, are essential, in that the differences between normal and abnormal are found at the lower end of the possible values of cortisol. A number of exogenous factors may lead to a false-positive result. These include the use of certain medications such as phenytoin, barbiturates, and carbamazepine; endocrine factors such as Cushing's disease or pregnancy; major medical problems such as serious infections or cancer; metabolic problems (e.g., recent withdrawal from alcohol, rapid weight loss, malnutrition, or nausea and vomiting); neurological problems such as multi-infarct dementia; increased intracranial pressure; and other factors, including the questionable effect of an unstable circadian rhythm. False-negative results may occur in patients taking synthetic corticosteriods and, possibly, in those taking certain benzodiazepines. Of all laboratory tests, the DST has been the one most carefully scrutinized for its sensitivity and specificity, as well as for its clinical usefulness in psychiatry. There is little evidence that the test adds significantly to the diagnostic process and initial therapeutic decisions. Nevertheless, the DST is useful in predicting outcome.

Cerebrospinal Fluid

Cerebrospinal fluid (CSF) investigations associated with geriatric mental disorders have focused on biochemical components in the CSF, including neurotransmitters and neuropeptides, that may correlate with alterations within the brain. These investigations have been enhanced by modern biochemical methods that can measure constituents using small amounts of CSF. Such studies are complicated by the fact that the content of lumbar spinal fluid may be quite different from that of intracranial CSF; furthermore, changes in CSF obtained at the lumbar level may not reflect what is transpiring within the brain (Gottfries 1983). The central nervous system (CNS) proteins of the CSF are of particular interest in the study of degenerative diseases (Harrington et al. 1986). Again, the variation in the site of origin that is within the blood or brain complicates the interpretation of these findings. For example, aluminum is believed to accumulate in the brains of persons with Alzheimer's disease, but increased aluminum is not consistently found in the CSF of Alzheimer's patients.

The American Medical Association's Council on Scientific Affairs (1986) reports that in the workup of patients with dementia, some clinicians do a lumbar puncture routinely, whereas others do it selectively. We recommend that lumbar puncture should be done if the geriatric psychiatrist suspects a brain infection, trauma, or bleeding from an intracranial blood vessel.

Imaging

Plain radiographs continue to constitute a significant portion of diagnostic imaging performed today in the practice of psychiatry. Clinicians often request plain skull films because they are useful in revealing the presence of intracranial masses, skull fractures, and bone changes.

During the last decade, a number of new imaging techniques have enhanced the research and diagnostic capabilities of the geriatric psychiatrist. These procedures provide "windows into the brain." The following discussion will be limited to four diagnostic procedures: computed tomography (CT), MRI, positron-emission tomography (PET), and single-photon emission computed tomography (SPECT). Because discussions of specific clinical applications of these procedures appear throughout this book, we limit the discussion in this chapter to the historical backgrounds and scientific bases of these procedures. We hope this presentation provides clinicians with an appreciation for and understanding of procedures that are not only helpful in diagnosis and treatment decisions but also useful in providing the patient with sufficient information to ensure informed consent.

The architecture of the brain plays an important role in this organ's functional imaging. The cerebral cortex has approximately four times the blood flow and the glucose metabolism of the white matter. Consequently, tracers that measure blood flow or glucose metabolism are all taken up predominantly by the cerebral cortex. Because the cortex is so thin (4–8 mm) and because of the deep invaginations that carry two layers of cortex deep into the cerebrum, images obtained with these tracers reflect both the cerebral architecture and the limitations of the spatial resolution of the instrumentation (Holman 1985). As a result, the cerebral cortex appears much thicker on the images than it really is. The deep invaginations of gray matter create large "islands" of image that must be taken into consideration when interpreting pictures.

Computed Tomography

CT, originally called computerized axial tomography (CAT), was developed in England in 1972 by Hounsfield (1973) and was introduced into clinical use by Ambrose (1973). This radiological scanning procedure has proved to be of considerable value for viewing the body, including the skull and its contents. CT is often said to be the "ultimate X ray." Actually, CT is a general term for several X-ray techniques that result in pictures of designated layers or slices of an organ such as the brain. The CT scanner uses a small X ray that rotates around the patient's skull (or other part of the body) in a fixed plane. A computer converts the information generated by the beam into a cross-sectional X-ray picture. The resulting picture, which looks like a slice through the brain, permits many parts of the brain to be easily identified.

CT imaging is essentially structural, whereas other types of imaging that will be discussed add a functional dimension. Pictures obtained on CT permit evaluation of cerebral atrophy, ventricular size, and an estimation of the amount of CSF, and distinguish between gray and white matter. Measures based on CT images have been used to determine the effect of normal aging and to contrast these effects with those found in patients who have diseases of the brain. The CT scans of so-called normal elderly subjects often indicate cortical cerebral atrophy. It appears that this loss of gray matter is an integral aspect of normal aging and is especially evident in the very old (Goldstein et al. 1985). Such atrophy is not consistently related to intellectual decline; consequently, its significance is unclear. Similarly, mild to moderate ventricular dilatation is common in the elderly. Only when these two findings exceed mild to moderate levels can they be related to dementia.

Ventricular dilatation, increase in CSF, and reduced brain tissue volume in the elderly are well documented by CT scan. Such gross anatomical changes would logically be reflected in a reduction of cerebral metabolic rates of glucose and oxygen; however, when these measures are carried out by PET, no reduction is reported. One explanation for this lack of observed effect has been offered: that some brain tissue is actually redundant and is essentially nonfunctioning. Such an explanation may also be relevant to the poor correlation of PET results with intellectual changes.

Magnetic Resonance Imaging

MRI was originally called nuclear magnetic resonance (NMR) imaging. The name was changed because the term "nuclear" produced some apprehension in patients who falsely expected that the procedure would expose them to harmful radiation. Actually, the principle underlying MRI has been used by chemists for three decades. The nuclei of certain identifiable atoms (isotopes) behave like tiny spinning magnets. This permits identification of these atoms by MRI scanning. The scanner designed for clinical use is a large, doughnut-shaped magnet with a magnetic field that is 3,000–25,000 times the strength of the earth's natural magnetic field.

The stable isotopes of hydrogen and phosphorus are commonly used in MRI. Isotopes are forms of a single element that differ only in weight, owing to a different number of neutrons in the nuclei. Such isotopes have identical chemical properties of the common atom. For example, the hydrogen isotope reacts with oxygen to form water, and the phosphorus isotope is incorporated into the metabolic processes that transpire in various tissues. When these isotopes, acting as tiny spinning magnets, are placed in a static magnetic field generated by the MRI apparatus, the nuclei will line up in the direction of that field. However, the nuclei are spinning, and therefore they also wobble. Different molecules can be identified because their nuclei wobble at different frequencies.

The second step in magnetic resonance imaging is the use of an alternating field applied at right angles to the first field. This moves some nuclei into a new alignment. Only the nuclei in resonance with this oscillating field—that is, only the nuclei wobbling at the same frequency as the field—will be realigned. When the second field is turned off, the realigned nuclei return to their original positions, releasing detectable signals that a computer can pro-

cess and display either as numerical data or as an image. This tells how much of a certain substance is present, and also what kind of chemical and physical environment surrounds it.

To further clarify, during the first exposure to a strong magnetic field the nuclei align themselves parallel to the field and their axes wobble randomly around it. When the second right angle magnetic field is applied, it is an oscillating one that makes the nuclei in the continuous field wobble or move in unison. When the second oscillating field is turned off, the synchronized movement introduces a voltage that can be picked up and recorded. Gradually, on the order of milliseconds, the synchrony of the nuclei spin diminishes and the nuclei once again resume their random wobble, but they continue to be aligned with the first continuous magnetic field.

Measurements may be taken at various intervals during the MRI procedure (Bensen et al. 1985). For example, a measure can be taken at t_1, the spin-lattice relaxation time (i.e., the time needed for protons to resume their previous positions). t_1 is the time constant for the longitudinal component of magnetization to reach its equilibrium; it measures the difference between gray and white matter. This is possible because the two tissue types have different fat-to-water ratios. It has been observed that there is a significant difference between the t_1 of patients with Alzheimer's disease and that of normal control subjects. Furthermore, t_1 is altered by both multi-infarct dementia and Alzheimer's disease. It permits recognition of pathology in both white and gray matter. t_2 represents spin-spin relaxation time; it is the time constant for the transverse component of magnetization to reach its equilibrium.

MRI has several advantages. No radiation is involved and no contrast dye is needed. MRI produces high-resolution images and distinguishes normal from abnormal tissues. It can be used to obtain pictures from parts of the body that are usually not accessible by the CT scan. The disadvantages include the fact that the MRI procedure is limited by the patient's condition, because the patient must remain perfectly motionless for extended periods of time and is surrounded by the previously described large, doughnut-like structure (which produces claustrophobic responses in some patients). In addition, this massive magnetic device must be housed in a large area devoid of iron and lined with copper. The copper shield is necessary to block any external interference. The intense large magnetic field used in the procedure requires that personnel, as well as patients, do not carry, wear, or have embedded within their bodies certain metals.

Positron–Emission Tomography

PET is an exciting research technique and clinical evaluation procedure. In vivo studies of cerebral perfusion and metabolism and identification of their anatomical distribution are possible with PET. The quantitative PET technique requires the integration of three components:

1. **Compounds labeled with positron-emitting radioisotopes (unstable isotopes).** The isotopes, which are either injected or inhaled by the patient, serve as tracers for physiological processes.
2. **A position tomograph.** This is a scanner for detecting tissue distribution of the tracer; emissions produced by the positrons are measured by a circular array of radiation detectors and are recorded by a computer.
3. **A tracer kinetic model.** This is a mathematical model that follows the labeled compounds through various so-called compartments, noting when the tracer is in a certain compartment of a metabolic sequence. It is a way to quantify a physiological process. An example of a compartment model is that of oxygen metabolism. The first compartment is oxygen in the plasma; the second is the oxygen metabolic processes that take place within the tissue.

Positrons are relatively short lived (unstable isotopes). Frequently used are the radioisotopes of carbon (^{11}C, which has a high half-life of 20 minutes), nitrogen (^{13}N, with a half-life of 10 minutes), oxygen (^{15}O, with a half-life of 2 minutes), and fluoride (^{18}F).

Fluoride (^{18}F), a positron-emitter tracer that does not naturally occur in the body, is often preferred over other isotopes because of its long half-life—110 minutes. The ^{18}F tracer is first produced by a cyclotron and is then incorporated into a molecule. The tracer compound that is often used to study the rate of glucose utilization is ^{18}F-labeled 2-deoxy-2-fluoro-D-glucose. Other labeled compounds are used for measuring specific processes (Ferris et al. 1981).

To understand how PET works, one must first understand what a positron is. It is often held to be one of the fundamental fragments that compose anatomic nuclei. An emitted positron is an antielectron and antimatter. When it strikes an electron, annihilation takes place and two photons are formed. The photons (gamma rays) strike the detectors and the event is recorded (Phelps 1983). The data collected in this manner are used to form a tomographic image. These images are cross-sectional and form a picture of the distribution of tissue concentrations. The pictures are developed in accordance with the principles of CT (Phelps and Mazziotta 1985). PET has been used to observe the physiological processes associated with perception, learning, recall, and so forth. The technique has been used to study patients with epilepsy, Parkinson's disease, senile dementia, schizophrenia, affective disorders, and Down's syndrome, among others.

It is generally agreed that patients with Alzheimer's disease have a decrease in metabolic activity in the temporal and parietal regions (D. Sullivan, personal communication, June 1987). In some cases, hypometabolism is widespread. Some decrease is seen in the thalamus and in the striatum, but the decrease is less than what occurs in the cortex.

Phelps (1983) has reported a number of other observations concerning PET. One is that in 70% of patients with partial seizure disorders, the epileptogenic focus shows a decrease in glucose utilization while dormant, but very high glucose utilization during seizure switches. Another observation, from studies involving patients with depression, is that during a depressive phase the entire brain shows a reduction in glucose metabolism. Studies of patients during manic episodes could not be satisfactorily completed because the patients could not be sufficiently controlled (Phelps and Mazziotta 1985). This same group has reported that symptomatic patients with Huntington's disease have reduced glucose metabolism in the caudate nuclei. It is possible that this reduction can be detected before the onset of symptoms (Mazziotta et al. 1987). This study needs further attention.

Rapaport (1986) reported that age differences are not found for the regional cerebral metabolic rates for glucose metabolism measured by PET. Right and left asymmetries appear early in Alzheimer's disease and are likely to be consistent with changes in specific brain function.

Single Photon Emission Computed Tomography

SPECT is similar to PET in that it provides information concerning the function of the brain and other organs of the body. The usual procedure is to inject into a vein a small amount of a radioactive compound (such as ^{123}I or ^{133}Xe), which is used to label a number of compounds. The patient lies on a table between two SPECT cameras, which are similar to Geiger counters. The cameras encircle the target site for 10–20 minutes and record the amount of radioactivity given off. A computer converts this information into color or black-and-white cross-sectional images (Drayer 1986).

Although it is claimed that the information produced by SPECT is less detailed than that produced by PET or CT, the procedure is considerably less costly. Further, if its clinical value can be clearly demonstrated, its use can be extended to such sites as community hospitals and not confined to major medical centers (Drayer and Friedman 1983).

In the SPECT procedure, the emitting substance is a photon. A photon is a mass of energy, not a particle such as a neutron, proton, or electron. When a photon decays, it creates a positron and an electron as well as other fragments. The notion of the existence of a photon that is not a particle was originated by Max Planck (1858–1947), who first discovered that heat radiation is absorbed or given out in the form of tiny packets of energy called quanta. This is known as Planck's quantum theory. In 1905, Albert Einstein (1879–1955) expressed the conviction that light must behave in the same way, since each color of light is made of up packets containing different amounts of energy. Later, after further study, these light quanta were named photons.

Radioisotopes that are commercially available often emit only one photon per disintegration. Dual-photon–emitting isotopes are also available. Dual-photon isotopes are positron emitters. They are short lived, technologically complex, and costly (Lassen 1985).

Electroencephalography

Brain wave changes are associated with alteration of brain function. Abnormalities occur on EEG that have diagnostic implications; some of these are described below.

Electroencephalographic Sleep in Psychotic Depression

Psychotic depression is considered a distinct subtype of major affective disorder, according to both the Research Diagnostic Criteria (RDC; Spitzer et al. 1978) and DSM-III-R. Persons with psychotic depression tend to be middle aged or older, and their severe depression is accompanied by evidence of psychomotor disturbances as well as many other signs of depression. They often show a poorer clinical response to treatment with TCAs. A familial factor is not uncommon. Thase et al. (1986) compared 27 patients with psychotic depression with 79 nonpsychotic subjects. Sleep in those with psychotic depression was characterized by increased wakefulness, decreased REM sleep percentage, and decreased REM activity. Patients with psychosis were more likely to have extremely short sleep-onset REM latency. These EEG abnormalities tended to increase with the duration of the illness. The test results from patients with recent-onset depressions were characterized by marked initial insomnia, increased stage 1 sleep percentage, and long REM latencies. This is in contrast to patients with illnesses of longer duration, who had extremely short REM latencies.

To summarize, patients with psychotic depression were found to have a significantly decreased generation of REM sleep. It is generally accepted that endogenous depressions are accompanied by characteristic EEG sleep abnormalities, including sleep continuity disturbances, diminished slow-wave sleep, shortened REM latency, and altered distribution of REM density and time. On the basis of these studies, we believe that there is a difference between psychotic depression and nonpsychotic depressive reactions.

Electroencephalogram Findings in Mixed Depression and Dementia

A frequent diagnostic and therapeutic problem involves the elderly person who manifests mixed symptoms of depression and dementia. It is estimated that 20% of elderly persons with depression also have deficits suggesting the presence of organic dementia. Depressive symptoms are not uncommon in patients with Alzheimer's disease. Routine EEG findings do not appear to differentiate between those who will show clinical improvement and those who will deteriorate. In seven of eight patients who showed clinical improvement in one study (Reynolds et al. 1986), EEGs were found to be normal or only mildly abnormal. Of the eight patients who deteriorated, five were found to have normal or mildly abnormal EEGs. One depressed patient with a markedly abnormal EEG showed an infarct on CT scan. Sleep EEGs were not studied.

Rae-Grant and colleagues (1987) pointed out that many studies have been done in which investigators examined EEG changes in patients with dementing disorders. However, these studies have been marked by serious methodological problems, such as the lack of a well-defined diagnostic classification and the presence of pathological variation at autopsy. Aside from the resolution of these problems, it is important to study such patients and subjects over a period of years, and to correlate the EEG studies with clinical, psychological, and laboratory observations. Correlations must be done at regular intervals throughout the study.

Although one would expect a progressive change in the EEG paralleling the progression of the dementia, this does not always happen. Furthermore, there are some patients who remain at a plateau for long periods of time (Gordon 1968). Rae-Grant et al. (1987) studied 318 patients with dementia and 159 control subjects. The subjects were matched for gender and age. The sample of those with dementia was reduced to 139 patients with disease of the Alzheimer's type. Under this broad classification the researchers included patients with dementia of the Alzheimer's type, those with senile dementia of the Alzheimer's type, and those with a mixed type of dementia (the latter being identified by an ischemic score of 4–7). On a qualitative basis, the EEG findings in this study were not unlike those from previous reports—that is, there was a general slowing of the alpha rhythm, with the appearance of slow waves and the presence of focal abnormalities. The EEG results among the patients were significantly more abnormal than those obtained for the control subjects. Temporal lobe focal abnormalities of the type often associated with aging were not significantly different between patients and control subjects. Focal abnormalities characteristic of the subjects' ages appeared in the first EEGs of 13% of patients and 14% of control subjects. Over a span of 4 years, it appears that the survivors of the dementia group had an increasing tendency to have EEGs that remained relatively unchanged. In fact, a small per-

centage of EEGs from patients with dementia showed improvement. It was concluded that EEGs do not show a consistent progression to slower and more malignant rhythms, but do vary in progression and pattern. There was a parallel between the worsening of the EEG and mental deterioration as measured by psychological testing. The EEGs did not discriminate between those with early-onset dementia (that is, dementia of the Alzheimer's type) and those with senile dementia of the Alzheimer's type. At autopsy, severe EEG alterations correlated well with the presence of more severe neuronal loss in the hippocampi and with an increase in granulovacuolar ratio.

The Psychodiagnostics Laboratory

The psychodiagnostics laboratory may be used for a number of valuable clinical activities. The primary services provided by a psychodiagnostics laboratory include neuropsychological testing, intelligence testing, personality testing, and testing for presence and level of severity of specific disorders. These services provide information pertinent to both Axis I and Axis II diagnoses, as well as to the patient's status on various personality constructs.

The most effective use of the psychodiagnostics laboratory is achieved when the question to be answered from the assessment is formulated properly and clearly. The referring clinician needs to know what he or she wants from the clinical assessment and the report of that assessment. The diagnostician must receive the proper question regarding the patient in order to know what assessment instrument to use and how best to report back the obtained information to the referring clinician. The proper formulation of the question also assists the diagnostician in determining the testability of the patient. A clear statement of the purpose of the diagnostic evaluation allows the evaluator to determine if the patient is capable of completing the psychodiagnostic process necessary to obtain the requested assessment information. For example, the clinician requesting an evaluation for a hearing- or sight-impaired or extremely confused person should note those limitations.

The effective use of the psychodiagnostics laboratory can also be facilitated by developing an ongoing working relationship with a specific laboratory and/or the specific person doing the assessments and reports. This relationship will provide for efficient and effective communication. It will allow for clear communication of the question being asked of the assessment and will, over time, provide for the expedient transfer of information, formatting of reports, and scheduling of patients.

The following material provides a sampling and brief overview of some of the instruments that are generally available in a psychodiagnostics laboratory. The listing is in no way exhaustive, and it is beyond the scope of this chapter to provide a detailed description of the assessment instruments or a thorough evaluation of their usefulness and psychometric properties.

Neuropsychological and Intelligence Testing

The major contributions of a neuropsychological evaluation fall into three broad categories (Golden 1983, 1992). The first of these is diagnosis. Included in this category are 1) identification of the presence of brain injury or related disorder, including differentiation between emotional problems and brain dysfunction; 2) specification of the nature of the deficits caused by brain damage, including localization of the injury to specific areas of the brain; and 3) assistance in determining the cause of the brain dysfunction.

The second important contribution is the tracking of changes in functioning over time. Through the establishment of a baseline level of functioning and periodic reevaluations, clinicians can accurately determine the efficacy of a particular course of treatment or monitor the course of a progressive illness.

The third area is assistance in the planning and evaluation of a rehabilitation program. This relatively new area holds considerable promise. Both the knowledge of brain function and the ability to assess it are rapidly increasing. As the understanding of brain-behavior relationships improves, so will efforts to provide specific rehabilitative procedures that maximally benefit the individual.

As outlined previously, neuropsychological assessment may address a variety of questions. A selected sample of common types of evaluation and typical instruments used are described below. In ad-

dition, two of the most widely used comprehensive neuropsychological batteries are briefly reviewed.

Screening.   The Mini-Mental State Examination (MMSE; Folstein et al. 1975) is an abbreviated mental status examination in which each area to be evaluated is represented by only a few questions (Lezak 1995). Areas evaluated include orientation, verbal reception, attention and calculation, language, and figure construction. It is quite brief and can be administered in 5–10 minutes. Because of its brevity, the MMSE can be especially useful in initial diagnostic screening or in following the course of a condition. Both administration and scoring are standardized, and its use is easily learned. More comprehensive mental status examination information—assessing attention, memory, language, visual-spatial skills, calculation skills, apraxia, agnosia, and so forth—can be obtained through the use of instruments such as the Mattis Dementia Rating Scale (Mattis 1976), the Neurobehavioral Cognitive Status Examination (Kiernan et al. 1987), the Neurobehavioral Rating Scale (Levin et al. 1987), the Global Deterioration Scale (Reisberg et al. 1988), and the Alzheimer's Disease Assessment Scale (Rosen et al. 1984). For brief reviews of these instruments, see Schmitt and Ranseen (1989).

Intellectual assessment.   One of the most widely used intelligence tests is the Wechsler Adult Intelligence Scale—Revised (WAIS-R; Wechsler 1981), an updated version of the original published in 1955 (Lezak 1995). Another frequently used test is the Stanford-Binet Intelligence Scale (Thorndike et al. 1986). Although both tests have proven to be of value for intellectual assessment, the WAIS-R is described here because of its inclusion in the Halstead-Reitan Neuropsychological Test Battery (Reitan 1979).

The WAIS was initially designed as a measure of "general" intelligence; it is actually a composite test consisting of a number of subtasks. A review of intellectual functioning in which the WAIS or WAIS-R serves as the major instrument is often sufficient to demonstrate adequate intellectual functioning or to provide an indication of the nature of altered function. For all but the most severely impaired adults, the WAIS-R can constitute a substantial portion of the neuropsychological examination.

The WAIS-R is composed of 11 different subtests divided into two categories, verbal and performance. The six verbal tests are Information, Comprehension, Arithmetic, Similarities, Digit Span, and Vocabulary. The five performance tests include Digit Symbol, Picture Completion, Block Design, Picture Arrangement, and Object Assembly. After each subtest is administered and scored, it is adjusted for age effects on the basis of established norms. Although the usual norms extend to age 75, Ivnik and colleagues (1992) published norms up to age 90. The results of the test consist of 11 age-corrected subscale scores and age-corrected composite scores for Verbal IQ, Performance IQ, and Overall IQ. Additionally, the results can be used to provide both an estimate of premorbid functioning and useful information regarding the possible nature and location of observed deficits.

Proper use of the WAIS-R as a neuropsychological assessment tool requires a combination of skills. In addition to knowing how specific aspects of brain functioning affect test performance, the clinician must take other potential influences into account by using available behavioral, historical, and psychological information.

Memory assessment. Memory is essential for an individual's adequate functioning. One test that evaluates several important aspects of memory is the Wechsler Memory Scale—Revised (WMS-R; Russell 1975; Wechsler 1987). It consists of the Logical Memory and Visual Reproduction subtests of the original instrument, and an additional recall trial after a half-hour delay. Together, the tests provide indices of both immediate and delayed recall for verbal and figural material. Severity-of-impairment scores are easily derived from available norms, and these scores have been found to be useful in discriminating between normal control subjects and patients with organic cognitive impairment (Lezak 1995).

Neuropsychological batteries. A vast number of tests are available to evaluate specific cognitive functions. In many instances, the selective use of a small number of these tests is adequate to answer a given referral question. However, another approach is the use of general neuropsychological test batteries, which provide a comprehensive evaluation of cognitive functioning. The Halstead-Reitan Neuropsychological Test Battery (Reitan 1979), which consists of a number of independent tests, continues to be the most widely used and most extensively validated battery (Meier 1985). Several versions exist

(Golden and Maruish 1986); however, most consist of the following:

1. WAIS-R
2. WMS-R
3. Halstead Category Test
4. Speech Sounds Perception Test
5. Seashore Rhythm Test
6. Tactual Performance Test
7. Trail Making Test
8. Reitan–Klove Sensory–Perceptual Examination
9. Reitan–Indiana Aphasia Examination
10. Lateral Dominance Examination
11. Halstead Finger Tapping Test
12. Strength of Grip Test
13. Tactile Form Recognition Test
14. MMPI

The MMPI (discussed below in more detail) is included to evaluate emotional factors that could contribute to deficits in test performance.

The Luria–Nebraska Neuropsychological Battery differs from the Halstead-Reitan in several ways (Anastasi 1988). The Luria–Nebraska battery generally requires less time to administer—2 hours, as opposed to 6 or more hours for the Halstead-Reitan battery. However, in elderly patients, the administration time for the Luria–Nebraska battery can extend to as much as 4 hours or longer (Schmitt and Ranseen 1989). Its content, materials, administration, and scoring are more highly standardized. Although the Luria–Nebraska is less established and not as thoroughly researched, thus far its clinical utility compares favorably with that of the Halstead-Reitan (Lezak 1995). Further modifications will undoubtedly be forthcoming to address problems such as a weakness in the memory function evaluation. Primary summary scores are provided in the following areas: motor functions, rhythm, tactile functions, visual function, receptive speech, expressive speech, writing, reading, arithmetic, memory, and intellectual processes. It is also possible to use a short form (about 1 hour) of the Luria–Nebraska, which may be more practically useful with the elderly (McCue et al. 1989).

Personality Assessment

Information for personality assessments is usually obtained from the patient via one or more of the following three formats: paper-and-pencil instruments, interviews, and projective procedures. In the sections below, we discuss the most widely used personality assessment instruments in each of these formats, and then note assessment procedures that have become available for evaluating a patient's status on a specific personality trait or disorder.

Paper-and-pencil instruments. The most widely used personality assessment instrument is the MMPI, developed by Hathaway and McKinley of the University of Minnesota in the 1940s (Hathaway and McKinley 1943). It is composed of 566 items, to which the patient responds in a true-false format. If a statement does not apply, the patient simply makes no answer.

The MMPI is a criterion-keyed, empirically developed instrument originally designed to allow discrimination among various clinical groups (Axis I diagnoses) and a control group of about 700 "normals." It provides scores on a number of clinical scales that correspond to the equivalent of the Axis I diagnoses current at the time the instrument was developed. It also includes various correction scales for lying, faking, and similar deceptive or misleading responses. Over the many years of its use in the clinical setting, The MMPI has gradually come to be seen as being of less value for aiding in specific clinical judgment and of more value in providing information regarding a patient's status on scales or patterns of scales of personality traits. It is probably most valuable to the clinician when the diagnostician reports on the various patterns of personality scales or traits for which the individual achieves a deviant score or set of scores. Major modifications of the MMPI have been completed, and the most recent revision is available as the MMPI-2 (Hathaway and McKinley 1989). An extensive manual is also available (Butcher et al. 1989), and descriptions and suggestions regarding its clinical usefulness are already available (Butcher 1990; Graham 1990; Greene 1991).

The MMPI may serve several useful functions for the clinician. It is most helpful as a diagnostic aid for the trained clinician. The pattern of abnormal clinical scales may suggest both the general form and the level of severity of pathology, which can be evaluated further in clinical work. In some cases, the MMPI report may call attention to pathology that the clinician otherwise might not note, or at least

might not note early on in the work with a specific patient. Thus, so long as the clinician does not take either a clinical report or a computerized report of clinical diagnostic scales as representing valid clinical classification data, the MMPI may continue to be of clinical usefulness.

The other paper-and-pencil personality inventory that may be useful in clinical practice is the Millon Clinical Multiaxial Inventory–II (MCMI-II; National Computer Systems 1987). This is a 1987 revision of the personality assessment scale that was developed by Theodore Millon in the mid-1970s (Millon 1982). The MCMI-II is designed to be used with individuals age 17 and older, is written at an eighth-grade reading level, and takes about 30 minutes to complete. The MCMI-II is composed of 175 items requiring responses in a true-false format. The instrument provides scores for 9 clinical syndromes (Axis I diagnoses) and 13 personality disorders (Axis II diagnoses). The reliabilities of the individual scales are generally adequate, although in some cases reliability is marginal (National Computer Systems 1987). In addition to the 22 clinical and personality scales, the MCMI-II also has corrective scales for deceptive-type responses and a validity index that is designed to detect random or confused response patterns. The instrument's distributor, National Computer Systems, also makes available computerized reports that either simply summarize the individual scale scores or provide a more exhaustive clinical interpretive report.

The MCMI-II is not as exhaustive as the MMPI with regard to Axis I diagnoses. It probably does not go far beyond the information gathered in standard clinical interviews and intervention sessions. The MCMI-I was of questionable validity in regard to Axis I diagnoses because of an overlap of items, intercorrelations, and the multidimensional nature of the clinical syndrome scales (Choca et al. 1986); because it is quite similar to MCMI-I, the MCMI-II is likely to suffer the same problems with validity. On the other hand, it may be considerably useful for Axis II diagnosis. The MCMI-II probably can best be used as an efficient "first pass" at personality psychopathological diagnoses. Its ultimate validity relative to clinical diagnosis of Axis II disorders remains to be adequately demonstrated. Furthermore, clinical outcome studies have not yet been published demonstrating the prognostic capabilities of either the MCMI-I or the MCMI-II.

Interviews. Several structured interviews have been developed to assess personality disorders. An excellent example of this type of instrument is the Structured Interview for DSM-III Personality Disorders (SIDP; Pfohl et al. 1982) and its 1989 revision to reflect DSM-III-R criteria (Pfohl et al. 1989).

The SIDP-R consists of 159 questions grouped around 17 themes (such as self-esteem and social interaction skills), as opposed to being grouped around the DSM-III-R personality disorders themselves. The interviewer asks each question on the structured interview and records the response. When the interview is completed, the interviewer rates the presence or absence of each of the DSM-III-R personality disorder criteria and uses these ratings to determine whether the patient meets the necessary criteria for any of the personality disorders.

The interview takes between 60 and 90 minutes to complete. Zimmerman et al. (1986) have demonstrated that the reliability and validity of the SIDP can be enhanced by briefly interviewing an informant regarding the patient and his or her behavior. Stangl et al. (1985) report kappas (i.e., results of tests of validity; κ) for many of the personality disorders included in the SIDP. Most of the kappas were indicative of adequate reliabilities for the scales. However, a few of them were below .70, indicating that they were barely acceptable or even unacceptable— for example, .45 for avoidant personality disorder. Thus, many of the specific Axis II categories are of questionable validity, even with younger patients, and virtually nothing is known about the psychometric properties of the instruments used for their diagnosis among the elderly. Other structured interviews that take a similar approach include the Structured Clinical Interview for DSM-III (SCID; Spitzer et al. 1992) and the Personality Disorders Examination (Loranger et al. 1987).

There are a number of other interviews available to assess personality disorders. Perhaps the most promising of these (but less developed than the SIDP) is the Tridimensional Interview of Personality Style (TIPS) developed by Cloninger (1987). This interview is built around his recent model of personality and personality disorders, and it very likely will prove to be of clinical and theoretical significance. Cloninger (1987) also has developed the Tridimensional Personality Questionnaire, which is a self-report instrument developed from the TIPS and designed to assess personality disorders via the pa-

per-and-pencil format. Cloninger's instruments need further psychometric refinement before they will be of general clinical and research usefulness.

Projectives. Projective assessment techniques can be distinguished from other forms of psychodiagnostic testing by the use of a relatively unstructured task. Test stimuli are usually vague, and only general instructions are given. Projective tests are based on the fact that the lack of structure present in the task requires the individual to provide the structure. The projections from the person are observed by the examiner and assumed to reflect the characteristic thought processes and other aspects of personality organization. Although the person being tested is aware of being evaluated, the projective tests are generally less transparent than other forms of inquiry (Anastasi 1988).

Projective techniques for assessing individuals are available in a wide variety of forms. Only two of the major instruments will be described here. In general, when the psychometric properties of this class of instruments are evaluated, they are quite weak (Cronbach 1984). However, they may be clinically useful when administered and interpreted by an experienced and skilled examiner. They continue to enjoy popular and widespread use, even though they possess poor psychometric properties.

Hermann Rorschach (1884–1922), a Swiss psychiatrist, was the first to demonstrate that patients of differing types respond to inkblots differently (Cronbach 1984). The task of the respondent is to describe what he or she sees in the inkblot. The materials consist of a set of 10 cards, each with a symmetric blot so irregular as to allow a wide range of interpretations. Some of the cards are black-and-white and others include colors.

Several scoring systems have been developed in an attempt to address the criticisms regarding the poor psychometric properties of projectives. Most share counting the number of responses, location, determinants, and content. Beyond these there is considerable variability in the scoring procedures.

The Thematic Apperception Test (TAT) elicits open or disguised statements about beliefs, attitudes, and motives (Anastasi 1988). This task requires the subject to tell a story based on a picture presented by the examiner. The person is instructed to describe what is happening, what led up to the scene, and the outcome. It is presumed that persons taking the test project themselves into the scene, identifying with a character. The TAT consists of 19 pictures in black-and-white and one blank, white card. Some of the cards are suggested for one gender or the other. Usually a subset (approximately 10) of the cards is administered. Although formal scoring systems are available, the most common method of interpretation is the impressionistic approach (Cronbach 1984). The interpreter considers recurrent themes, reflected attitudes, stylistic issues, and concern for detail and accuracy. This information is used to form hypotheses to describe the person's personality, motives, drives, defenses, and emotional conflicts.

Assessment of specific disorders. During recent years there has been an increasing emphasis in psychological assessment on the evaluation of specific disorders. Thus, a number of assessment batteries have been developed that focus on the clinical evaluation of disorders such as major depression, anxiety, and antisocial behavior. Although it is beyond the scope of this chapter to review the various assessment instruments available, a quick overview of a possible depression assessment battery will illustrate the potential utility of the psychodiagnostics laboratory as a resource for obtaining pertinent clinical information for specific disorders.

The major interview available to evaluate the presence of a major depressive disorder is the Schedule of Affective Disorders and Schizophrenia, Lifetime Version (SADS-L; Endicott and Spitzer 1978). Clinical rating scales that can be based on this interview include the Hamilton Rating Scale for Depression (Hamilton 1960) and the Montgomery-Åsberg Rating Scale for Depression (Montgomery and Åsberg 1979). Both of these scales have demonstrated adequate reliability and therefore are good indicators of the clinician's judgment of the level of the severity of the depression.

In addition to these instruments, there are several self-report instruments that give a good measure of the patient's experienced level of depression. Perhaps the two most useful scales in this regard are the Beck Depression Inventory (Beck et al. 1961) and the Carroll Rating Scale for Depression (Carroll et al. 1981).

Information from these three types of personality assessments provides the clinician with a very thorough indication of the presence or absence of a major depressive episode and the level of severity of that disorder. Similar instruments are also available for the specific assessment of most other types of psychiatric disorders.

References

Agency for Health Care Policy and Research: Depression in Primary Care (AHCPR Publ No. 93-0550). Washington, DC, AHCPR, 1993

Ambrose J: Computerized transverse axial scanning—clinical application. Br J Radiol 46:1023–1047, 1973

American Medical Association, Council on Scientific Affairs: Dementia. JAMA 256:2234–2238, 1986

American Psychiatric Association: Diagnostic and Statistical Manual of Mental Disorders, 3rd Edition. Washington, DC, American Psychiatric Association, 1980

American Psychiatric Association: Diagnostic and Statistical Manual of Mental Disorders, 4th Edition. Washington, DC, American Psychiatric Association, 1994

Anastasi A: Psychological Testing. New York, Collier Macmillan, 1988

Beck AT, Ward CH, Mendelson M, et al: An inventory for measuring depression. Arch Gen Psychiatry 4:561–571, 1961

Bensen J, Mutch W, Smith F, et al: The relationship between Parkinson's disease and dementia: a study using proton NMR imaging parameters. Br J Psychiatry 147:380–382, 1985

Butcher J: The MMPI-2 in Psychological Treatments. New York, Oxford University Press, 1990

Butcher J, Dahlstrom WG, Graham J, et al: Minnesota Multiphasic Personality Inventory—2 (MMPI-2): Manual for Administration and Scoring. Minneapolis, University of Minnesota Press, 1989

Carroll BJ, Feinberg M, Smouse PE, et al: The Carroll Rating Scale for Depression, I: development, reliability and validation. Br J Psychiatry 138:194–200, 1981

Choca JP, Peterson CA, Shanley LA: Factor analysis of the Millon Clinical Multiaxial Inventory. J Consult Clin Psychol 54:253–255, 1986

Cloninger CR: A systematic method for clinical description and classification of personality variants: a proposal. Arch Gen Psychiatry 44:573–588, 1987

Cronbach LJ: Essentials of Psychological Testing. New York, Harper & Row, 1984

Davies AB, Williams J, John R, et al: Diagnostic value of thyrotropin-releasing hormone test in elderly patients with atrial fibrillation. BMJ 291: 773–777, 1985

Drayer B: Radiology—"windows" into the living body. Duke Health Line, Spring 1986, pp 4–6

Drayer B, Friedman JR: In vivo quantification of regional cerebral blood flow: validation of the HIPDm SPECT. American Journal of Neural Radiology 4:572–576, 1983

Endicott J, Spitzer R: Schedule for Affective Disorders and Schizophrenia (Lifetime Version), 3rd Edition. New York, New York State Psychiatric Institute, 1978

Ferris S, Mony J, Wolf A, et al: Positron emission tomography in the study of aging and senile dementia. Neurobiol Aging 1:127–131, 1981

Folstein MF, Folstein SE, McHugh PR: Mini-Mental State: a practical method for grading the cognitive state of patients for the clinician. J Psychiatr Res 12:189–198, 1975

Glassman AH, Bigger JT: Cardiovascular effects of therapeutic doses of tricyclic antidepressants: a review. Arch Gen Psychiatry 38:815–820, 1981

Golden CJ: The neuropsychologist in neurological and psychological populations, in Foundations of Clinical Neuropsychology. Edited by Golden CJ, Vincente PJ. New York, Plenum, 1983, pp 1–38

Golden CJ: Neuropsychological Assessment and Intervention. Springfield, IL, Charles C Thomas, 1992

Golden CJ, Maruish M: The Luria–Nebraska Neuropsychological Battery, in Neuropsychological Test Batteries. Edited by Incagnoli T, Goldstein G, Golden CJ. New York, Plenum, 1986, pp 193–227

Goldstein SJ, Wekstein D, Kirkpatrick C, et al: Imaging the centenarian brain: a computed tomographic study. J Am Geriatr Soc 33:579–584, 1985

Gordon EB: Serial EEG studies in presenile dementia. Br J Psychiatry 114:779–780, 1968

Gottfries C-G: Biochemical changes in blood and cerebrospinal fluid, in Alzheimer's Disease. Edited by Reisberg B. New York, Free Press, 1983

Graham J: MMPI-2: Assessing Personality and Psychopathology. New York, Oxford University Press, 1990

Greene R: The MMPI-2/MMPI: An Interpretive Manual. Boston, MA, Allyn & Bacon, 1991

Hamilton M: A rating scale for depression. J Neurol Neurosurg Psychiatry 23:56–62, 1960

Harrington MG, Merril CR, Asher DM, et al: Abnormal proteins in the cerebrospinal fluid of patients with Creutzfeldt-Jakob disease. N Engl J Med 315:279–283, 1986

Hathaway SR, McKinley JC: Minnesota Multiphasic Personality Inventory. Minneapolis, University of Minnesota, 1943

Hathaway SR, McKinley JC: Minnesota Multiphasic Personality Inventory—2. Minneapolis, University of Minnesota, 1989

Holman BL: Anatomy and function of the brain, in Radionuclide Imaging of the Brain: Contemporary Issues in Nuclear Imaging, Vol 1. Edited by Holman BL. New York, Churchill Livingstone, 1985

Hounsfield CN: Computerized transverse axial scanning (tomography): description of a system. Br J Radiol 46:1016–1022, 1973

Ivnik RV, Malex JF, Smith GE, et al: Mayo's older-American study. Clinical Neuropsychologist 6:1–30, 1992

Kiernan RJ, Mueller J, Langston JW, et al: The Neurobehavioral Cognitive Status Examination: a brief but differentiated approach to cognitive assessment. Ann Intern Med 107:481–485, 1987

Lassen NA: Measurement of regional cerebral blood flow in humans with single–photon emitting radioisotope, in Brain Imaging and Brain Function. Edited by Sokoloff L. New York, Raven, 1985, pp 94–98

Levin HS, High WM, Goethe KE, et al: The Neurobehavioral Rating Scale: assessment of the behavioral sequelae of head injury by the clinician. J Neurol Neurosurg Psychiatry 50:183–193, 1987

Lezak MD: Neuropsychological Assessment, 3rd Edition. New York, Oxford University Press, 1995

Loosen PT, Prange AJ: Serum thyrotropin response to thyrotropin-releasing hormone in psychiatric patients: a review. Am J Psychiatry 139:405–416, 1982

Loranger AW, Susman VL, Oldham JM, et al: The Personality Disorder Examination: a preliminary report. Journal of Personality Disorders 1:1–13, 1987

Mattis S: Mental status examination for organic mental syndrome in the elderly patient, in Geriatric Psychiatry: A Handbook for Psychiatrists and Primary Care Physicians. Edited by Bellak L, Karasu TB. New York, Grune & Stratton, 1976, pp 77–121

Mazziotta JC, Phelps ME, Pahl JJ, et al: Glucose metabolism and Huntington's disease. N Engl J Med 316:357–362, 1987

McCue M, Goldstein G, Shelly C: The application of a short form of the Luria–Nebraska Neuropsychological Battery to discrimination between dementia and depression in the elderly. International Journal of Clinical Neuropsychology 2:21–29, 1989

Meier MJ: Review of the Halstead-Reitan neuropsychological test battery, in The Ninth Mental Measurements Yearbook, Vol 1. Edited by Mitchel JV Jr. Lincoln, NE, University of Nebraska Press, 1985

Millon T: Millon Clinical Multiaxial Inventory Manual. Minneapolis, MN, National Computer Systems, 1982

Montgomery SA, Åsberg M: A new depression scale designed to be sensitive to change. Br J Psychiatry 134:382–389, 1979

National Computer Systems: Millon Clinical Multiaxial Inventory–II. Minneapolis, MN, National Computer Systems, 1987

Pfohl B, Stangl D, Zimmerman M: The Structured Interview for DSM-III Personality Disorders (SIDP), Iowa City, University of Iowa Department of Psychiatry, 1982[1]

Pfohl B, Blum N, Zimmerman M: Structured Interview for DSM-III-R Personality Disorders—Revised (SIDP-R), Iowa City, University of Iowa Department of Psychiatry, 1989

Phelps ME: Positron computed tomography for studies of myocardial and cerebral function. Ann Intern Med 98:339–359, 1983

Phelps ME, Mazziotta JC: Positron emission tomography: human brain function and biochemistry. Science 228:799–809, 1985

Rae-Grant A, Blume W, Lau C, et al: The electroencephalogram in Alzheimer-type dementia. Arch Neurol 50–54, 1987

Rapaport SI: Positron emission tomography in normal aging and Alzheimer's disease. Gerontology 32 (suppl 1):6–13, 1986

Reisberg B, Ferris SH, deLeon MJ, et al: Global deterioration scale. Psychopharmacol Bull 24:661–663, 1988

Reitan RM: Halstead-Reitan Neuropsychological Test Battery. Tucson, AZ, Neuropsychology Laboratory, University of Arizona, 1979

Reynolds CF III, Kupfer DJ, Hoch CC, et al: Two-year follow-up of elderly patients with mixed depression and dementia. J Am Geriatr Soc 34:793–799, 1986

Rosen WG, Mohs RC, Davis KL: A new rating scale for Alzheimer's disease. Am J Psychiatry 141:1356–1364, 1984

Russell EW: A multiple scoring method for the assessment of complex memory functions. J Consult Clin Psychol 43:800–809, 1975

Schweitzer I, McGuire KP, Gee AH, et al: Prediction of outcome in depressed patients by weekly monitoring with the dexamethasone suppression test. Br J Psychiatry 151:780–784, 1987

Schmitt FA, Ranseen JD: Neuropsychological assessment of older adults, in Testing Older Adults: A Reference Guide for Geropsychological Assessments. Edited by Hunt T, Lindley CJ. Austin, TX, Pro-Ed, 1989, pp 51–69

Shelps SB, Schecter MT: The assessment of diagnostic tests: a survey of current medical research. JAMA 252:2418–2422, 1984

Spitzer RL, Endicott J, Robins E: Research Diagnostic Criteria: rationale and reliability. Arch Gen Psychiatry 35:773–782, 1978

Spitzer RL, Williams JB, Gibbon M, et al: The structured clinical interview for DSM-III-R (SCID): history, rationale and description. Arch Gen Psychiatry 49:624–629, 1992[2]

Stangl D, Pfohl B, Zimmerman M, et al: A structured interview for DSM-III personality disorders: a preliminary report. Arch Gen Psychiatry 42:591–596, 1985

Thase ME, Kupfer DJ, Ulrich RF: Electroencephalographic sleep in psychotic depression. Arch Gen Psychiatry 43:886–893, 1986

Thorndike R, Kagen E, Sattler J: Stanford-Binet Intelligence Scale, 4th Edition. Chicago, IL, Riverside, 1986

Veith RC, Raskind MA, Caldwell JH, et al: Cardiovascular effects of tricyclic antidepressants in depressed patients with chronic heart disease. N Engl J Med 306:954–959, 1982

Wechsler D: Wechsler Adult Intelligence Scale—Re-

---

[1] Available from B. Pfohl, M.D., Department of Psychiatry, University of Iowa, 500 Newton Road, Iowa City, IA 52242.

[2] Available from Biometrics Research Department, New York Psychiatric Institute, 722 West 168th Street, New York, NY 10032.

vised Manual. New York, Psychological Corporation, 1981

Wechsler D: Wechsler Memory Scale—Revised Manual. New York, Psychological Corporation, 1987

Zimmerman M, Pfohl B, Stangl D, et al: Assessment of DSM-III personality disorders: the importance of interviewing an informant. J Clin Psychiatry 47:261–263, 1986

Psychiatric Disorders
in Late Life

CHAPTER 12

Cognitive Disorders

Elaine R. Peskind, M.D.
Murray A. Raskind, M.D.

The cognitive disorders are the most prevalent psychiatric disorders of later life. The predominant problem in these disorders is a clinically meaningful deficit in memory and/or other cognitive functions that represents a significant change from a previous level of functioning. The cognitive disorders to be discussed in this chapter are dementia, delirium, and amnestic disorders. We attempt to use nomenclature in this chapter that is consistent with DSM-IV (American Psychiatric Association 1994). DSM-IV contains substantial changes in nomenclature relevant to these disorders. Perhaps foremost among these changes is the use of the broad term *cognitive disorder* as opposed to the term *organic mental disorder* used in DSM-III-R (American Psychiatric Association 1987). Although use of the term organic mental disorder has a long historic tradition, the authors of DSM-IV recognized that this term implied that "nonorganic" mental disorders do not have a biological basis. It is becoming increasingly clear that all behavioral disorders have some biological components, be it a genetic diathesis or a physiological change in brain function. Therefore, such terms as *functional* and *organic* are confusing and have become obsolete. Other terms that are now obsolete include *organic brain syndrome* and *senility*, the latter of which has been used both by laypersons and some health care professionals as a synonym for dementia.

Dementia and the other cognitive disorders of later life are extremely costly to society, both in terms of financial resources dedicated to patient care and in terms of morbidity, mortality, and the stress that patients place on caregivers and the broader community. One-half of the beds in community long-term care facilities are devoted to patients with dementia, predominantly dementia of the Alzheimer's type (DAT); the other cognitive disorders also consume large amounts of public health resources. The prevalence and burden of the cognitive disorders of later life will further increase as the proportion of elderly persons in the United States population increases over the next 50 years.

Dr. Peskind's research was supported in part by the Department of Veterans Affairs and by National Institute on Aging Alzheimer's Disease Research Center (ADRC) Grant AG05316.

Dementia

Dementia is a syndrome—that is, a group of signs and symptoms that cluster together but can be caused by a number of underlying diseases. Most, if not all, of these diseases produce neuronal loss or other structural brain damage. The central feature of dementia is acquired impairment of memory. In addition, the dementia syndrome includes at least one other of the following cognitive deficits: aphasia (language impairment secondary to disruption of brain function), apraxia (inability to perform complex motor activities despite intact motor abilities), agnosia (failure to recognize or identify objects despite intact sensory function), and disturbance in executive functions such as planning, organizing, sequencing, and abstracting. All specific dementia disorders have the above features in common. In addition, DSM-IV assigns distinguishing criteria to each of the specific dementia disorders.

Clinical Features of Dementia

Although all disorders causing dementia must produce acquired impairment of memory and impairment of other cognitive function sufficient to interfere substantially with occupational functioning, and must represent a substantial decline from a previous level of functioning, the features of the specific dementia disorders are quite variable, reflecting the nature of the underlying disease that causes such disruption in brain function. An example of this variability is the course of the syndrome among specific dementia disorders. Because DAT is the most common dementia disorder of later life, the course of DAT is often assumed to be the course of dementia in general. In fact, the course of DAT is a relatively specific diagnostic feature of that disorder. The typical course of DAT is one of insidious onset, with gradual but inexorable progression of cognitive deficits over a period ranging from 5 to 15 years. Other dementia disorders may have quite different clinical courses. For example, dementia due to head trauma has a sudden onset, and the course is either stable or can improve over time. Dementia due to anoxia (such as in older persons resuscitated from cardiac arrest but not soon enough to prevent hypoxic brain damage) may have a similar course. Vascular dementia can manifest a stepwise progression,

reflecting new episodes of ischemic stroke. If persons with dementia due to alcohol can be kept free of alcohol, a substantial number will show meaningful improvements in cognitive function (Victor and Adams 1971).

Differential Diagnosis of Dementia

Dementia and delirium.   A common problem in the differential diagnosis of the dementia syndrome is mistaking a delirium for dementia. An even more common problem is missing a delirium superimposed on an underlying dementia disorder. Both delirium and dementia manifest as impairment in cognitive functions, but the two conditions differ in the pattern of deficits and the cognitive domains primarily involved. In at least the early and middle stages of dementia, the patient is alert and attentive, whereas in delirium the patient shows decreased attention to the environment and altered level of arousal. The delirious patient's cognitive deficits fluctuate broadly, whereas those of the dementia patient are usually stable. Unfortunately, in the more advanced stages of progressive dementing disorders of late life such as DAT, attention is impaired. However, even in the late stages of DAT, a fluctuating level of consciousness is cause for concern that a superimposed delirium may exist.

Dementia and depression.   A differential diagnostic problem that has received much attention is the differentiation of a major depressive episode from dementia in the cognitively impaired older person. Although the term *depressive pseudodementia* (Kiloh 1961) has been justly criticized by Reifler (1982), it remains a concept that continues to have some heuristic value. It is unusual for a major depressive episode to produce such severe cognitive impairment that its distinction from a specific dementia disorder such as DAT is persistently difficult. Depressive pseudodementia secondary to a primary major depressive episode usually begins with dysphoric mood, loss of interest and pleasure, and other typical signs and symptoms of primary depression. Depressive signs and symptoms precede cognitive impairment in this syndrome. Furthermore, patients with depressive pseudodementia often have a history of primary affective disorder in earlier life. The clinical examination is helpful in this differential diagnostic problem. The patient with a primary depression is much more likely to exhibit poor motivation during mental status examination, and frequently gives "don't know" answers to questions probing memory function. Aphasia, apraxia, and anomia are not present in the patient with cognitive symptoms secondary to a primary depression.

More common than depressive pseudodementia are depressive signs and symptoms complicating a preexisting dementia disorder. Such depressive signs and symptoms, as well as a diagnosable major depressive episode, complicate the clinical picture of vascular dementia, dementia secondary to Parkinson's disease, and DAT. Vigorous treatment of a major depressive episode with standard antidepressant therapeutic modalities is clearly appropriate for patients with depressive pseudodementia. The management of patients with depressive signs and symptoms or with a diagnosable major depressive episode complicating specific dementia disorders is more controversial and is discussed later in this chapter (see "Serotonergic Abnormalities in DAT: Implications for Antidepressant Therapy").

More than a decade ago it appeared that identification of neuroendocrine changes that occur in patients with a major depressive episode would be helpful in the differential diagnosis of dementia disorders and depression. Specifically, it was hypothesized that the dexamethasone suppression test (DST) would be useful in this regard (McAllister et al. 1982; Rudorfer and Clayton 1981). Because resistance to suppression of the hypothalamic-pituitary-adrenal (HPA) axis by the potent synthetic glucocorticoid dexamethasone was demonstrated in patients with a major depressive episode (Carroll et al. 1981), it was suggested that a "positive DST"—failure of a late-evening dose of dexamethasone to suppress plasma cortisol below a predetermined level the following day—in a patient with acquired cognitive impairment and depressive signs and symptoms would favor the diagnosis of either primary major depressive episode or secondary major depressive episode complicating a primary dementia disorder. Unfortunately, it soon became apparent that a positive DST occurred as frequently in patients with DAT uncomplicated by depression as in those with a primary major depressive episode (Raskind et al. 1982; Spar and Gerner 1982). Although the demonstrations of increased HPA axis activity in DAT per se negated the diagnostic utility of the DST in differentiating DAT and depression, it remains possible that this neuroendocrine abnormality might play a role in the pathophysiology of DAT. A growing body of evidence suggests that increased HPA-axis activity in normal aging (Raskind et al. 1994)—a phenomenon that is exaggerated in patients with DAT (Davis et al. 1986)—may lower the threshold for neuronal loss in later life (reviewed in Sapolsky 1987).

The differential diagnosis of dementia does not end with the exclusion of delirium and depression. It is also important to make the diagnosis of a specific dementia disorder with as great a degree of certainty as possible, given that prognosis varies among dementia disorders and that specific treatments for dementia disorders are now available. The essential elements of the clinical evaluation of the older patient with acquired cognitive impairment are listed in Table 12–1. By far the most important part of the evaluation is a careful history, obtained not only from the patient but also from friends, relatives, or other persons familiar with the patient's premorbid status. Without corroborative history, an accurate description of the onset, progression, and nature of changes in cognitive and other domains cannot be obtained. A careful mental status exam focusing on the patient's level of awareness and attention, memory, calculation, language, praxis, and visual-spatial skills should be included. Observation of the pa-

Table 12–1. Evaluation of cognitive impairment in later life

History from patient and relative or friend

Mental status exam

Physical and neurologic exam

Medication inventory/urine toxicology

Head CT or MRI scan

Complete blood count

Serum VDRL

Serum sodium, potassium, chloride, bicarbonate, calcium

Serum blood urea nitrogen, creatinine, bilirubin, albumin/globulin

Serum B_{12}

Serum triiodothyronine/thyroxine, thyroid-stimulating hormone

Brief cognitive test (e.g., Mini-Mental State Examination)

Note. CT = computed tomography; MRI = magnetic resonance imaging; VDRL = venereal disease research laboratory (test).

tient's affect during the examination is more helpful in evaluating the presence of depression than is the patient's subjective response to questions about his or her mood status in the recent past. A physical examination, including a screening neurological evaluation with special attention to localizing neurological signs, is also essential. An inventory of current medications, either prescribed or obtained without a prescription, should be routinely included in the evaluation, and a urine specimen should be obtained and analyzed for the presence of drugs if there is a question about the reliability of the drug history. This part of the evaluation is particularly important if the clinical picture suggests delirium. Behavioral toxicity from a variety of medications is probably the most common etiology of reversible cognitive and behavioral impairments in the elderly patient (Larson et al. 1984). Serum electrolytes and blood urea nitrogen (BUN) levels should be measured to rule out correctable causes of delirium either as the primary problem or as a complicating factor in a dementia disorder. Thyroid function tests, including a thyroid-stimulating hormone (TSH) test and a serum B_{12} level also should be obtained. Early in their course, both thyroid deficiency and B_{12} deficiency can manifest as a reversible delirium. However, if thyroid deficiency or B_{12} deficiency persists chronically, neuronal loss ensues and full recovery of cognitive function is unusual despite aggressive replacement therapy.

Although the routine inclusion of either a computed tomography (CT) or a magnetic resonance imaging (MRI) scan of the brain in the evaluation of late-life cognitive impairment has been debated since Larson and colleagues' (1986) evaluation of the cost effectiveness of these neuroimaging diagnostic procedures, they continue to be part of the standard diagnostic evaluation in most centers, particularly in the evaluation of patients with an early onset of cognitive impairment or with an atypical presentation. These brain neuroimaging examinations can detect potentially treatable intracranial mass lesions such as tumors or subdural hematomas, and also can suggest the presence of normal-pressure hydrocephalus. Although the presence of clearly defined infarcts revealed by CT or MRI supports the diagnosis of vascular dementia or combined vascular dementia and DAT, the frequently observed periventricular hyperintensities on t_2-weighted images obtained with high-resolution MRI scanners con-

tinue to be of unknown significance. These periventricular changes have not been clearly demonstrated to be attributable to "microvascular disease," and their usefulness in differential diagnosis is unclear (Chui et al. 1992).

A formal cognitive rating scale should be part of the standard evaluation of the older patient with acquired cognitive impairment. The Mini-Mental State Exam (MMSE; Folstein et al. 1975) is a brief and easily performed tool that has proved to be widely useful. The MMSE assesses orientation, registration and recall of information, attention, calculation, language, praxis, and visual-spatial skills. Although it is not designed for the differential diagnosis of the various specific dementia disorders, it provides an excellent "snapshot" of overall cognitive function and has gained extremely wide acceptance as a means both of estimating cognitive function and of following changes in cognitive function over time. Longer cognitive evaluation instruments such as the Mattis Dementia Rating Scale (Mattis 1976) provide a more comprehensive evaluation of cognitive function and are useful if neuropsychological testing resources are available. The Mattis Dementia Rating Scale is a reliable instrument that correlates well with the functional capacity of patients with DAT (Vitaliano et al. 1984).

The search for correctable causes of cognitive impairment in the older patient must be pursued vigorously, but a completely reversible cognitive disorder is, unfortunately, the exception rather than the rule. Although early reports suggested that potentially correctable disorders causing cognitive impairment would be detected by a careful evaluation in up to 30% of patients with acquired cognitive loss (Fox et al. 1975; Freeman 1976; Victoratos et al. 1977), Larson and co-workers (1984) have reported a more realistic yield of truly correctable disorders impairing cognitive function after comprehensive diagnostic evaluation in patients with late-onset cognitive disorders in the outpatient setting. In this study, among 107 unselected elderly outpatients referred for evaluation of global cognitive impairment of at least 3 months' duration, only 15 had potentially reversible disorders possibly related to their cognitive loss. Six patients with apparent cognitive loss secondary to adverse behavioral effects of medications formed the largest single group. Other potentially reversible causes of cognitive loss that were identified included hypothyroidism, subdural hematoma, and rheumatoid cerebrovasculitis. Only 3 of the 107 patients evaluated actually proved to have a reversible cause of cognitive loss, as demonstrated by return to normal cognitive function after treatment. One of these patients had a subdural hematoma, another had mixed-drug toxicity, and the third had rheumatoid cerebrovasculitis. Two of these 3 patients presented with only subtle and mild cognitive deficits. Of the 13 patients who were judged to have potentially reversible cognitive deficits at intake evaluation and who were available for follow-up over a 2-year period, 3 of the 4 with hypothyroidism, 1 with subdural hematoma, and 4 of 6 with behavioral toxicity from medications subsequently developed progressive cognitive deterioration consistent with DAT. The results of this study suggest that the most important part of the diagnostic evaluation of the cognitively impaired older person is the attempt to delineate the specific type of dementia disorder and to uncover treatable or general medical and psychiatric disorders that may be exacerbating the cognitive deficits caused by a primary dementia disorder.

Specific Dementia Disorders

Dementia of the Alzheimer's Type

The majority of patients with late-life dementia of insidious onset and a progressive deteriorating course have DAT (Katzman 1976). The term *primary degenerative dementia of the Alzheimer's type* used in DSM-III-R has been changed in DSM-IV to *dementia of the Alzheimer's type*. The new criteria for DAT are presented in Table 12–2. DAT is a combined clinical and neuropathological diagnosis that can be made definitively only when a patient meeting antemortem clinical criteria for DAT is found on brain biopsy or at postmortem examination to have the histopathological changes of DAT: numerous neuritic plaques and neurofibrillary tangles in the hippocampus and neocortex. If a clinician practicing in the 1950s were to examine the current DAT literature, he or she would be mystified at the emphasis placed on what was considered 30 years ago to be a relatively uncommon "presenile" dementia disorder. That DAT would be considered the most important neuropsychiatric disorder of later life would be difficult to comprehend. This "epidemic" of DAT

can be attributed largely to increased knowledge of the correct etiology of dementia in later life. Before the landmark studies of Blessed et al. (1968), the large number of persons who developed the dementia syndrome after age 65—so called "senile dementia"—were believed to be suffering from some form of cerebrovascular insufficiency. Blessed et al. (1968) performed a careful neuropathological and neurohistological study of elderly patients with "senile dementia." In 70% of these patients, the only neuropathological lesions found were the neuritic plaques and neurofibrillary tangles described by Dr. Alzhei-

---

Table 12–2. DSM-IV diagnostic criteria for dementia of the Alzheimer's type

A. The development of multiple cognitive deficits manifested by both:
  1. memory impairment (impaired ability to learn new information or to recall previously learned information)
  2. one (or more) of the following cognitive disturbances:
    a. aphasia (language disturbance)
    b. apraxia (impaired ability to carry out motor activities despite intact motor function)
    c. agnosia (failure to recognize or identify objects despite intact sensory function)
    d. disturbance in executive functioning (i.e., planning, organizing, sequencing, abstracting)

B. The cognitive deficits in criteria A1 and A2 each cause significant impairment in social or occupational functioning and represent a significant decline from a previous level of functioning.

C. The course is characterized by gradual onset and continuing cognitive decline.

D. The cognitive deficits in criteria A1 and A2 are not due to any of the following:
  1. other central nervous system conditions that cause progressive deficits in memory and cognition (e.g., cerebrovascular disease, Parkinson's disease, Huntington's disease, subdural hematoma, normal-pressure hydrocephalus, brain tumor)
  2. systemic conditions that are known to cause dementia (e.g., hypothyroidism, vitamin B_{12} or folic acid deficiency, niacin deficiency, hypercalcemia, neurosyphilis, human immunodeficiency virus [HIV] infection)
  3. substance-induced conditions

E. The deficits do not occur exclusively during the course of a delirium.

F. The disturbance is not better accounted for by another Axis I disorder (e.g., major depressive disorder, schizophrenia)

Source. American Psychiatric Association 1994, pp. 142–143.

mer in 1907 in his patient with early-onset dementia (Alzheimer 1907/1987). Furthermore, there was no difference in the degree of cerebrovascular atherosclerosis between patients with late-onset dementia and cognitively intact elderly persons. Only in approximately 15% of patients with late-onset dementia could cognitive impairment be attributed to sequelae of cerebrovascular disease—specifically, infarcted brain tissue. Multiple studies have confirmed that a dementia of insidious onset and with a gradually progressive course—whether beginning before or after the age of 65—is usually DAT (Katzman 1986).

Course of DAT. DAT begins insidiously. Subtle difficulties in recent memory are almost always the first sign. Personality changes also occur early and most often are manifested by apathy and loss of interest in persons and activities. Memory impairment gradually becomes more severe and deficits in other cognitive domains, such as executive function and visual-spatial skills, appear. Usually after several years of cognitive impairment, a fluent type of aphasia begins, characterized by difficulty naming objects or choosing the right word to express an idea. Apraxia often occurs concurrently, and the loss of ability to perform often routine motor activities, such as eating with utensils or dressing, can pose tremendous care burdens on the patient's family and other care providers. In the later stages of DAT, patients develop disrupted sleep/wake cycles, begin to wander, have episodes of irritability and motor hyperactivity, and lose their ability to attend to personal care needs such as dressing, feeding, and personal hygiene. Motor signs, such as rigidity and myoclonic jerks and seizures, occur in subgroups of patients (Risse et al. 1990a). The course of the illness is rarely less than 5 years and may extend to more than 15 years. Prevalence studies suggest that approximately 5% of persons over age 65 and 20% of persons over age 80 suffer from dementia severe enough to impair their ability to live independently (Mortimer 1983). It can be assumed that most of these persons suffer from DAT. The results of a study performed in East Boston, Massachusetts, suggest that the prevalence of Alzheimer's disease in later life may be even higher (Evans et al. 1989). Evaluation of all noninstitutionalized persons 65 or older in this geographically defined community of 32,000 persons revealed an estimated prevalence rate for DAT of 10% among those older than 65 and of 47% for those over age 85. Even when persons with mild cognitive impairment were excluded from the data, fully 8% of the persons over age 65 and 36% of those over age 85 had moderate to severe cognitive impairment sufficient to limit their ability to live independently.

Accuracy of antemortem diagnosis of DAT. The likelihood that an antemortem diagnosis of DAT by currently proposed DSM-IV criteria or by similar criteria proposed earlier (McKhann et al. 1984) will be confirmed at postmortem examination is at least 85% (Morris et al. 1988; Joachim et al. 1988; Tierney 1988). This is an excellent rate of antemortem diagnostic accuracy, and it compares favorably with that of many common general medical disorders in which the high probability of an accurate antemortem clinical diagnosis is widely accepted. The clinician should not feel that DAT is a difficult diagnosis that can be made only after exclusion of a long list of both common and uncommon disorders that have the potential to produce the dementia syndrome. In an older person in whom dementia begins insidiously and progresses gradually but inexorably, the diagnosis of DAT is highly likely to be confirmed neuropathologically. Diagnostic certainty is further enhanced if the patient did not suffer from alcoholism, preexistent Parkinson's disease, or multiple cerebrovascular accidents and poorly controlled hypertension.

A specific chemical antemortem diagnostic marker for DAT that would be measurable in blood or cerebrospinal fluid (CSF) would be useful in both clinical care and research. Such an in vivo test might prove extremely valuable in the management of patients in the early stages of DAT, in patients with atypical presentations of DAT, and in monitoring the effectiveness of future therapeutic interventions in DAT. Unfortunately, studies in which an attempt has been made to identify a protein or neurotransmitter with high sensitivity and specificity in the diagnosis of DAT have yielded disappointing results to date. Results of a recent study (Wagner et al. 1994) suggest that the measurement in CSF of soluble beta-amyloid precursor protein (sβPP) may have some diagnostic utility in DAT. This protein is a cleavage product of the same amyloid precursor protein (APP) that contains the beta-amyloid peptide, the major constituent of the senile plaques in DAT

(Rosenberg 1993). Low concentrations of sβPP in CSF are highly specific for DAT in its later stages but lack sufficient sensitivity to be more than supplementary to the standard clinical examination. The diagnostic usefulness of peripheral changes purported to occur in DAT, such as abnormal platelet membrane fluidity (Zubenko 1992), are currently under investigation.

Pathophysiology of DAT. Attempts to understand basic neurobiological mechanisms underlying the clinical deficits in DAT have focused on several areas. These include attempts to understand the biochemical nature and potential neurotoxic effects of neuritic plaques and neurofibrillary tangles—the histopathological hallmarks of DAT—and to understand changes in brain neurotransmitter systems that may underlie cognitive and noncognitive behavioral deficits in patients with DAT. Obviously these areas interrelate and are not mutually exclusive. An extensive discussion of these areas is beyond the scope of this chapter, but we review some aspects of this research that are pertinent to a general understanding of DAT.

Abnormalities of Brain Proteins in DAT

Efforts in multiple laboratories have been directed toward understanding the possible role of the beta-amyloid protein (the major protein constituent of neuritic plaques) in the pathophysiology of DAT. The beta-amyloid protein was first sequenced by Glenner and Wong (1984) from congophilic angiopathic deposits in postmortem brain tissue from patients with DAT. It has become clear that beta-amyloid protein is a normal product of APP (Rosenberg 1993). Unfortunately, the role of APP and its cleavage products remains mysterious. Furthermore, it is unclear whether the beta-amyloid protein is neurotoxic. Demonstrations of neurotoxic properties of beta-amyloid protein in vitro or in vivo in some laboratories (Kowall et al. 1991) have been very difficult to replicate in other laboratories (Busciglio et al. 1992; Podlisny et al. 1992). That beta-amyloid protein or another product of APP is involved in the pathogenesis of some familial forms of DAT has received the most convincing support from the rare families in whom point mutations in the APP gene on chromosome 21 segregate with DAT in these families (for further explanation, see "Molecular Genetics of DAT," below). Studies undertaken to examine the nature of neurofibrillary tangles in the DAT disease process also have been frustrating. The major constituent of neurofibrillary tangles is a hyperphosphorylated form of the microtubule-associated phosphoprotein tau (Selkoe 1986). The protein chemistry of tau and its role in neuronal degeneration in DAT remain poorly understood.

Abnormalities of Brain Neurotransmitters in DAT

Attempts to discover abnormalities in brain neurotransmitter systems in DAT that might be correctable by pharmacological treatments (that would result in subsequent symptomatic improvement) received impetus from the successful application of such a strategy to Parkinson's disease. In this degenerative neurological disorder, which affects motor function predominantly, the discovery of a deficit in brain dopamine systems has led to effective symptomatic treatment with dopaminergic-enhancing drugs. That such a strategy might succeed in DAT became a plausible hypothesis in the late 1970s with the discovery of a deficit in the brain cholinergic system in postmortem tissue of patients with DAT (Davies and Maloney 1976; E. K. Perry et al. 1978). This cholinergic-deficiency hypothesis received further support when Whitehouse and colleagues (1982) demonstrated extensive neuronal loss in the cholinergic nucleus basalis of Meynert in patients with DAT. The basal forebrain magnocellular nucleus is the primary source of cholinergic projections to the neocortex and hippocampus. A brain presynaptic cholinergic deficit in patients with DAT has been confirmed by many other investigators. Unfortunately, therapeutic attempts to compensate for the cholinergic deficit in patients with DAT have been less successful than analogous attempts to compensate for the central nervous system (CNS) dopaminergic deficit in Parkinson's disease. However, the recent approval by the U.S. Food and Drug Administration of the drug tacrine hydrochloride for the symptomatic treatment of cognitive deficits in DAT is an encouraging result of extensive work in this area (Farlow et al. 1992; Knapp et al. 1994). It has been demonstrated that tacrine produces modest but clinically meaningful cognitive improvement in a subgroup of patients with DAT. One possible reason for the difficulty in demonstrating marked efficacy of cholinergic replacement or enhancement in the majority of patients with DAT is the possibility that the cholinergic lesion may not be restricted to presynaptic cholinergic neurons. Flynn and co-workers (1991) demonstrated that postsynaptic muscarinic receptors, previously believed to be reasonably intact in patients with DAT, may in fact be severely impaired. These investigators demonstrated that there was reduced ability of the M_1 muscarinic receptor subtype to form a high-affinity agonist state in patients with DAT, and speculated that the failure of many cholinergic replacement strategies to improve specific features of memory and other cognitive functions in patients with DAT might be a function of postsynaptic cholinergic receptor abnormalities.

Abnormalities in noncholinergic neurotransmitter systems also may contribute to the difficulty in finding a markedly effective neurotransmitter enhancement therapeutic strategy that is applicable to the majority of patients with DAT. For example, in patients with DAT there is a clear deficiency in brain serotonin systems, manifested by loss of serotonergic neurons in the brain stem raphe nuclei (Mann and Yates 1983; Yamamoto and Hirano 1985), decreased concentrations of serotonin and its metabolite in brain tissue (Arai et al. 1984; D'Amato et al. 1987) and CSF (Volicer et al. 1985; Blenow et al. 1991), and decreased—probably postsynaptic—serotonin receptor concentrations (Cross et al. 1984). This serotonin deficiency may be relevant to both the cognitive and the depressive signs and symptoms seen in patients with DAT (see "Serotonergic Abnormalities in DAT: Implications for Antidepressant Therapy," below).

The other major neurotransmitter system affected in DAT is the brain noradrenergic system. Studies in postmortem brain tissue have consistently demonstrated neuronal loss in the locus coeruleus (the major source of noradrenergic neurons innervating the CNS) in patients with DAT (Bondareff et al. 1982; Mann et al. 1980; Tomlinson et al. 1981). Such locus coeruleus atrophy suggests a brain noradrenergic deficiency in DAT. On the other hand, studies involving brain noradrenergic systems in which measures have been made of norepinephrine (NE)—or of its metabolite, 3-methoxy-4-hydroxyphenylglycol (MHPG)—either in brain tissue obtained postmortem or in the CSF of living patients with Alzheimer's disease have suggested that the nature of the noradrenergic abnormalities associated with DAT may be more complex than is sug-

gested by studies of locus coeruleus neuron counts alone. Specifically, several studies have shown an increased ratio of MHPG to NE in brain tissue, suggesting increased NE turnover in locus coeruleus projection areas (Francis et al. 1985; Palmer 1987; Winblad et al. 1982). Furthermore, measurements of NE or MHPG in CSF demonstrate normal or even increased concentrations in patients with DAT, particularly in those who are in the later stages of the disease (Gibson et al. 1985; Raskind et al. 1984). The implications of these seemingly paradoxical findings of decreased locus coeruleus neuronal counts but normal or even enhanced brain noradrenergic functional activity in the living patient with DAT must remain speculative. It is possible that both reduced and increased CNS noradrenergic activity occur at different times and in different parts of CNS noradrenergic systems in patients with DAT.

Pharmacological Treatment Implications of Neurotransmitter Abnormalities in DAT

The cholinergic deficit observed in DAT has been the focus of numerous studies in which investigators have attempted to improve cognitive function by enhancing brain cholinergic activity. These efforts have yielded disappointing results in the past, but some benefit now appears achievable with oral cholinesterase therapy. The strategy of administering acetylcholine precursors such as choline or lecithin has proved ineffective (Brinkman et al. 1982; Thal et al. 1981). The administration of muscarinic cholinergic agonists also has been ineffective (Christie et al. 1981; Harbaugh 1984). The only strategy that has shown some success has been the administration of centrally active cholinesterase-inhibiting drugs, which prolong the intrasynaptic presence of acetylcholine released from presynaptic cholinergic neurons. Intravenous physostigmine produced modest, albeit short-lasting, gains in cognitive function in mildly demented patients with DAT (Davis et al. 1979). Orally administered physostigmine also has been reported to be modestly helpful in several studies (Harrell et al. 1990; Mohs et al. 1985; Stern et al. 1988; Thal et al. 1983), although not all reports have been positive (Jenike et al. 1990; Schmechel et al. 1984).

The only approach that has led to a clinically available treatment for cognitive deficits in DAT has resulted from studies of the orally administered cholinesterase inhibitor tetrahydroaminoacridine

(THA), also called tacrine. In an open study, Summers et al. (1986) reported a substantial positive effect on cognitive function in patients with DAT who were treated chronically with tacrine. Although most of these initially reported cognitive improvements with tacrine therapy have not been replicated in subsequent large-scale, parallel-group, placebo-controlled trials, the efficacy of tacrine in at least a subgroup of patients with DAT has been clearly established. Farlow et al. (1992) compared the efficacy and safety of tacrine with placebo in a 12-week, double-blind, parallel-group study of 468 patients with DAT who had mild to moderate cognitive impairments. After 12 weeks, a dose-related significant improvement was demonstrated on the Alzheimer's Disease Assessment Scale (ADAS; Rosen et al. 1984) and on both clinician-rated and caregiver-rated global improvement measures. Reversible transaminase elevations greater than three times normal occurred in 25% of patients. Knapp et al. (1994) evaluated the efficacy and safety of higher-dose tacrine administered over 30 weeks to 653 patients with DAT at 33 sites in the United States. Subjects were randomized to groups receiving placebo, 80 mg/day of tacrine, 120 mg/day of tacrine, or 160 mg/day of tacrine. These final doses were achieved after gradual titration protocols. Again, cognitive function was rated using the ADAS, and overall function was rated by both clinicians and caregivers using global rating instruments. In the evaluable patient population, 42% of patients in the tacrine group, compared with 18% of patients in the placebo group, demonstrated improvement on the clinician's global impression. There were significant dose-response trends and between-group comparisons on both the ADAS and the global ratings. Primary reasons for withdrawal of tacrine-treated patients from the study were asymptomatic liver transaminase elevations (28%) and gastrointestinal complaints (16%). Although it has become clear that tacrine produces modest but clinically meaningful improvement and cognitive function in a minority of patients with DAT, the clinical parameters identifying this subgroup remain unclear.

Serotonergic Abnormalities in DAT: Implications for Antidepressant Therapy

The identification of abnormalities in CNS noradrenergic and serotonergic systems in patients with DAT carries implications for the treatment of major depressive episodes or depressive signs and symptoms complicating DAT. That the noradrenergic abnormalities in DAT may play a role in the pathophysiology of depression complicating Alzheimer's disease is a hypothesis supported by a number of studies in which investigators have demonstrated greater locus coeruleus neuronal loss or damage in patients with DAT who have a history of depression than in patients with DAT who are free of substantial depressive signs and symptoms (Chan-Palay and Asan 1989; Zubenko and Moossy 1988; Zweig et al. 1988). Zweig and colleagues (1988) also found a trend toward increased evidence of serotonergic damage in patients with DAT who had a past history of depression. Taken together, these combined noradrenergic and serotonergic abnormalities in patients with Alzheimer's disease suggest that a drug active on both of these systems would be a rational choice for the treatment of depression complicating Alzheimer's disease. In fact, the only placebo-controlled treatment trial of depression complicating DAT involved use of such an agent, albeit not specifically with that original intent. Reifler and co-workers (1989) compared the tricyclic antidepressant imipramine, which blocks the neuronal reuptake of both norepinephrine and serotonin, with placebo in patients with DAT complicated by major depressive episode. Patients in the treatment group received a mean dose of 83 mg/day of imipramine. Depressive signs and symptoms improved significantly in both the treated and the placebo groups, but response to drug therapy was not different between the two active treatment groups. However, imipramine doses could be titrated only to 100 mg/day before patients developed clinically meaningful adverse effects such as orthostatic hypotension and peripheral, anticholinergically mediated constipation and urinary retention. It is possible that achieving optimal therapeutic plasma concentrations of imipramine and its active metabolite desipramine can rarely be accomplished in the DAT patient without incurring unacceptable adverse effects.

The antiadrenergic and anticholinergic effects of the tricyclic antidepressants often make their use problematic in patients with DAT. A potentially attractive drug for the treatment of depression complicating DAT is venlafaxine. This drug blocks the reuptake of both norepinephrine and serotonin without affecting cholinergic or noradrenergic receptors, and therefore is not associated with anticholinergic adverse effects or orthostatic hypotension. A study in nondemented depressed older patients showed that venlafaxine appears to be effective and well tolerated in this population (Khan et al. 1994). A placebo-controlled outcome trial of this compound in depressed patients with DAT would be of interest.

Pharmacological management of disruptive agitated behaviors in DAT. Agitated disruptive behaviors frequently complicate the course of DAT (Reisberg et al. 1987), and their occurrence is often the precipitating event for institutionalization. With some license, the term "agitated behaviors" will be used to describe diverse but often coexistent problems, such as hyperactive pacing, violent outbursts, disturbing delusions and hallucinations, and irritability. Although antipsychotic drugs are widely prescribed for elderly patients with DAT who manifest these problems (Prien and Caffe 1977), the efficacy of the antipsychotics for disruptive agitation in such patients appears to be substantially lower than their efficacy in younger patients with acute schizophrenia and other psychotic illnesses.

The results of open, uncontrolled studies often have been reported as positive (reviewed in Raskind et al. 1987; Salzman 1987), but the small number of interpretable, placebo-controlled trials of antipsychotic drugs in patients with DAT suggests that efficacy is modest, and adverse effects often are problematic. Only three placebo-controlled trials of antipsychotic drugs in patients with DAT (with DAT defined according to reasonable criteria) have been reported. Petrie and colleagues (1982) compared haloperidol, loxapine, and placebo in 64 chronically hospitalized patients with dementia, many of whom probably would meet current criteria for DAT. Although the antipsychotic drugs were significantly more effective than placebo for controlling suspiciousness, hallucinatory behavior, excitement, hostility, and uncooperativeness, only one-third of the patients treated with an antipsychotic drug were globally rated as moderately or markedly improved. Similar results were reported by Barnes and coworkers (1982) in a group of patients, most of whom had DAT, who were studied in a community nursing home. The investigators compared thioridazine, loxapine, and placebo in 53 patients whose mean age was 83 years. Again, antipsychotic medication

was superior to placebo for controlling anxiety, excitement, and uncooperativeness. However, suspiciousness and hostility improved as much with placebo as with active medication. As in the study by Petrie's group (1982), only one-third of patients treated with antipsychotic medication were rated as either markedly or moderately improved upon rating with a global measurement instrument. The study by Barnes and colleagues also suggests that the components of what can be called "placebo effect" in this population need closer examination to provide clues to nonpharmacological factors that may ameliorate suspiciousness and hostility in elderly patients with DAT who reside in nursing homes. Finally, in a placebo-controlled crossover trial, Devanand (1989) prescribed haloperidol to eight patients with DAT who clearly had delusions and hallucinations. Although haloperidol proved superior to placebo in reducing these symptoms, the investigators found that it was difficult to increase haloperidol beyond a dosage of 3 mg/day without producing unacceptable extrapyramidal adverse effects. Patients' cognitive function also was impaired modestly by haloperidol therapy.

The use of psychoactive drugs other than antipsychotics to treat patients with DAT for disruptive agitated behaviors has been reviewed (Raskind 1993). Anecdotal reports suggest possible efficacy for a broad range of compounds, including trazodone, valproate, carbamazepine, benzodiazepines, and buspirone. The role of these compounds in the management of patients with disruptive agitated behaviors complicating DAT cannot be defined without well-designed, placebo-controlled outcome trials.

Molecular genetics of DAT. The clinical genetics of DAT, suggesting the existence of autosomal-dominant transmission in at least subgroups of patients, has been discussed elsewhere in this volume (see Chapter 6). Attempts to map and eventually clone a gene or genes for DAT focused first on chromosome 21. This focus resulted from the discovery that persons with Down's syndrome (trisomy 21) express the neurohistological lesions of Alzheimer's disease in middle life (Lai and Williams 1989). Further enhancing interest in chromosome 21 was the mapping of the gene for APP to chromosome 21 (Goldgarber et al. 1987). In 1987, St. George-Hyslop and co-workers reported positive linkage results in four familial

DAT kindreds with two anonymous markers close to the centromere on the long arm of chromosome 21. Unfortunately, several attempts to replicate this chromosome 21 linkage in familial DAT were unsuccessful (Pericak-Vance 1988; Schellenberg et al. 1988). Very rare point mutations in the APP gene on chromosome 21 do occur in some families with autosomal-dominant early-onset DAT (Goate et al. 1989). Furthermore, it has been demonstrated that these point mutations can affect APP metabolism (Hardy 1992; Mullan et al. 1992). Thus, these unusual mutations provide the strongest evidence that the association of beta-amyloid with Alzheimer's disease is not an epiphenomenon, but rather that beta-amyloid is involved in the pathogenesis of this disease.

A gene for early-onset familial DAT has been mapped to chromosome 14 (Schellenberg et al. 1992). This finding was rapidly confirmed by several groups and appears to account for up to 80% of cases of familial early-onset DAT. This gene has recently been identified (Sherrington et al. 1995). Another major advance in the molecular genetics of DAT was the discovery that apolipoprotein E genotype is a genetic risk factor for DAT (Corder et al. 1993). It has been repeatedly confirmed that the apolipoprotein E-4 allele increases the likelihood of both late-onset familial and sporadic DAT. These studies have recently been reviewed by Strittmatter et al. (1994).

Vascular Dementia ("Multi-Infarct Dementia")

The authors of DSM-IV have changed the terminology for dementia attributable to cerebrovascular disease from *multi-infarct dementia* to *vascular dementia*. This change is consistent with the uncertainty about the role that vascular deficiency plays in the etiology of dementia in late life. Blessed et al. (1968) definitively demonstrated that DAT was the principal cause of late-onset dementia. However, when Tomlinson et al. (1970) examined the same neuropathological material, they demonstrated that cerebrovascular dementia—defined as dementia resulting from enough loss of brain tissue, secondary to repeated episodes of cerebral infarction, to impair cognitive function globally—was still an important cause of late-onset dementia.

The DSM-IV diagnostic criteria for vascular dementia are presented in Table 12–3. The important differential diagnostic features separating vascular dementia from other dementia disorders are the presence of focal neurological signs and symptoms and laboratory evidence indicative of cerebrovascular disease. It should be noted that the stepwise deteriorating course included in the criteria for multi-infarct dementia in DSM-III-R is not included in DSM-IV. This change appears to be reasonable in light of Zubenko's (1990) demonstration that the existence of such a stepwise deteriorating course may not be extremely useful as an indicator in differentiating vascular dementia from DAT.

The DSM-IV criterion that evidence indicative of cerebrovascular disease should include multiple infarctions involving both cortex and underlying white matter also is prudent, given the controversy concerning the pathophysiological significance of periventricular white-matter hyperintensities that are often seen on t_2-weighted MRI images both in healthy older persons and in those with dementia.

Table 12–3. DSM-IV diagnostic criteria for vascular dementia

A. The development of multiple cognitive deficits manifested by both:

   1. memory impairment (impaired ability to learn new information or to recall previously learned information).

   2. one (or more) of the following cognitive disturbances:

      a. aphasia (language disturbance)

      b. apraxia (impaired ability to carry out motor activities despite intact motor function)

      c. agnosia (failure to recognize or identify objects despite intact sensory function)

      d. disturbance in executive functioning (i.e., planning, organizing, sequencing, abstracting)

B. The cognitive deficits in criteria A1 and A2 each cause significant impairment in social or occupational functioning and represent a significant decline from a previous level of functioning.

C. Focal neurological signs and symptoms (e.g., exaggeration of deep tendon reflexes, extensor plantar response, pseudobulbar palsy, gait abnormalities, weakness of an extremity) or laboratory evidence indicative of cerebrovascular disease (e.g., multiple infarctions involving cortex and underlying white matter) that are judged to be etiologically related to the disturbance.

D. The deficits do not occur exclusively during the course of a delirium.

Source. American Psychiatric Association 1994, p. 146.

Although the radiologic appearance of these periventricular white-matter changes is interpreted by some neurologists as being compatible with ischemia or microvascular disease, neuropathological documentation of actual ischemic lesions correlating with these antemortem neuroimaging findings has been scanty. George et al. (1986a) reviewed the CT scans of 275 normal and demented subjects. The incidence and severity of white-matter changes increased significantly with age but did not differ significantly between patients and healthy elderly persons. Furthermore, within the group of subjects with dementia, the severity of white-matter changes did not correlate with severity of cognitive impairment. In a similar study using MRI scans (George et al. 1986b), this group of investigators demonstrated that the MRI was more sensitive than the CT scan for demonstrating periventricular white-matter changes, but that such changes were equally common in patients with Alzheimer's disease and age-matched control subjects. Although the extent of white-matter involvement was greater in the DAT group, the configuration of the patches of increased signal intensity were similar for both healthy elderly subjects and those with Alzheimer's disease.

It is still possible that periventricular white-matter changes are involved in the pathophysiology of late-life dementia in both DAT and vascular dementia. However, investigators who have noted correlations between periventricular white-matter changes and severity of dementia differ as to whether these changes indicate increased water content in the brain (Bondareff et al. 1988) or reflect ischemic lesions (Braffman et al. 1988; Brun and Englund 1986). Erkinjuntti et al. (1987) reported that white-matter changes on MRI and CT scans actually were more common in patients with DAT than in patients with vascular dementia, thereby further calling into question the relevance of vascular disease to these neuroradiologic findings. It also is possible that the white-matter lesions detected by MRI scans may be benign. Fein and colleagues (1990) reported the case of an elderly patient with extensive and progressive deep white-matter brain lesions demonstrated on MRI over a 7-year period; they found no association between either the extent or the progression of these lesions and the patient's cognitive, behavioral, and neurological functioning. These investigators concluded that periventricular white-matter lesions do not necessarily indicate a clinically significant disease process. The question of the significance of these lesions will only be resolved by careful clinicopathological correlation studies.

Despite the uncertainties described above, clearly there are patients in whom the course of dementia is related to the occurrence of cerebrovascular accidents. Usually these patients have a history of poorly controlled hypertension and demonstrate "patchy" cognitive deficits in the early stages of their illness. In addition to displaying focal neurological signs, these patients often manifest rigidity, pseudobulbar palsy, emotional incontinence, and paucity of speech and motor activity. Retention of insight is more common in patients with vascular dementia than in those with DAT, and patients with vascular dementia may be more prone to episodes of secondary major depression than are persons with DAT.

To resolve the very difficult issue of the accurate diagnosis of vascular dementia and the delineation of the boundaries of the disorder, the State of California Alzheimer's Disease Diagnostic and Treatment Centers have proposed criteria for the diagnosis of ischemic vascular dementia (Chui et al. 1992). These criteria broaden the conceptualization of vascular dementia—that is, they extend the concept beyond multiple infarctions as the only etiology for vascular dementia; in addition, the criteria refine nosology and identify areas that require further research.

Identification of vascular dementia is important, given that prevention of further infarctions or other ischemic damage (by blood pressure control, institution of aspirin therapy, cessation of smoking, or other means) offers at least the potential for slowing or arresting the progression of the disorder.

Dementia Due to Other Disorders

DSM-IV codes dementia due to other disorders by using the same A and B criteria as in DAT and vascular dementia and adding a criterion C: "there is evidence from the history, physical examination, or laboratory findings that the disturbance is the direct physiological consequence of one of the general medical conditions listed below." This list includes human immunodeficiency virus (HIV) disease, head trauma, Parkinson's disease, Huntington's disease, Pick's disease, Creutzfeldt-Jakob disease, normal-pressure hydrocephalus, hypothyroidism, vitamin B_{12} deficiency, brain tumor, and intracranial radiation. The most common of these dementia disorders are discussed below.

Dementia due to Parkinson's disease and the spectrum of Lewy body diseases. The dementia that occurs in the later stages of illness of a subgroup of patients with Parkinson's disease is associated with impaired memory and slowness of thinking. In general, language function and praxis are preserved, although aphasia and apraxia also may occur (E. K. Perry et al. 1985). In an extensive review of the prevalence of dementia among patients with Parkinson's disease, Brown and Marsden (1984) conservatively estimated that some degree of dementia occurs in 20% of such patients. Mayeux and colleagues (1988), using standardized criteria for dementia and idiopathic Parkinson's disease, found a dementia prevalence of 11% in 339 patients with idiopathic Parkinson's disease. In this study, dementia was associated with older age, later onset of motor manifestations, more rapid progression of physical disability, and relatively poor response to L-dopa therapy. Regardless of the estimate of the prevalence of dementia in Parkinson's disease, dementia is clearly more common among such patients than among neurologically intact adults of the same age (Rajput 1987).

Although the plaques and tangles of DAT have been reported in some patients with Parkinson's disease dementia (Boller et al. 1980; Hakim and Mathieson 1979), it is also clear that the dementia of Parkinson's disease can occur in patients who show only the classic neurohistological lesions of Parkinson's disease but no neuritic plaques and neurofibrillary tangles (Chui et al. 1984). E. K. Perry and co-workers (1985) and Ball (1984) have demonstrated that the dementia associated with Parkinson's disease usually occurs in the absence of substantial neurohistological evidence of DAT in the neocortex and hippocampus.

Just as most investigators were reaching consensus that the dementia associated with Parkinson's disease is not usually the result of the coincident presence of the neurohistological stigmata of DAT, a number of investigators reported the unexpected finding of the classic neurohistological change of Parkinson's disease—that is, Lewy bodies—in patients meeting criteria for DAT. Leverenz and Sumi (1986) noted pathology—either neuronal loss or Lewy bodies—suggestive of Parkinson's disease in the substantia nigra of 18 of 40 patients meeting antemortem as well as postmortem criteria for DAT. Ditter and Mirra (1987) found Lewy bodies in the substantia nigra in 11 of 20 consecutive cases of pathologically confirmed DAT. Three of these 11 subjects also had Lewy bodies in the neocortex. Although 80% of their 11 subjects with Parkinson's disease pathology had rigidity in later stages of their dementing illness, tremor had not been observed in any patient at any time before death.

In addition to these findings of classic Parkinson's disease pathology in patients meeting both antemortem and postmortem criteria for DAT, another syndrome involving Lewy bodies and dementia has been described (Kosaka et al. 1988). In this disorder, Lewy bodies are present in the brain stem and also are widespread throughout the cerebral cortex (Okazaki et al. 1961). This syndrome, *diffuse Lewy body disease*, may be a relatively common cause of dementia in later life. The diffuse Lewy bodies can occur with or without the neuritic plaques of Alzheimer's disease. The clinical neurological presentation of diffuse Lewy body disease differs markedly from that of Parkinson's disease in that dementia in the former is prominent, and motor signs are usually limited to rigidity. Bradykinesia and tremor are uncommon in diffuse Lewy body disease, and when tremor occurs it often is described as transient or mild. Patients with this disorder may be more likely to demonstrate delirium and psychotic symptoms such as visual hallucinations (R. H. Perry et al. 1990). (For a recent review and further discussion of the Lewy body spectrum of diseases, see Raskind and Peskind 1992.)

Dementia due to Pick's disease. Pick's disease is a progressive disorder of middle and late life that is often difficult to distinguish from DAT. Although rare in most neuropathological series, it may account for up to 5% of the cases of late-life progressive dementia that occurred in series from Scandinavia (Sjogren et al. 1952) and Minnesota (Heston et al. 1987). Both clinical and neuropathological dissimilarities seem to exist between DAT and Pick's disease. The marked cholinergic deficit in DAT does not appear to occur in Pick's disease (Wood et al. 1983). Frontotemporal atrophy and microscopic changes are present in Pick's disease; the latter include neuronal cell loss, gliosis, and the presence of massed cytoskeletal elements called "Pick's bodies." Although affective lability and excessive eating and other oral behaviors have been described in Pick's disease (Cummings and Duchen 1981), Heston et al. (1987) could not easily clinically distinguish patients with Pick's from those with DAT.

Dementia due to normal-pressure hydrocephalus. Normal-pressure hydrocephalus (NPH) was described by Adams et al. (1965) as an acquired disorder characterized by a triad of signs—dementia, gait disturbance, and urinary incontinence associated with dilatation of the cerebral ventricles—but no evidence of persistently elevated intracranial pressure. Although NPH is an unusual disorder, it is an important one to identify because of the potential for neurosurgical treatment and reversibility of the dementia. In most cases, the etiology of NPH is unclear, but previous subarachnoid hemorrhage or meningitis probably account for a sizable proportion of cases. A cerebroventricular shunting procedure can markedly improve cognitive function in some cases (Friedland 1989).

Factors associated with a good postoperative outcome are a brief history of dementia and other signs and symptoms, absence of gyral atrophy, and a known etiology (Thomasen et al. 1986). Despite these prognostic factors, it is difficult to predict which patients with NPH will respond well to a neurosurgical approach and which will not. Wikkelso et al. (1982) have suggested that drainage of 20–40 mL of CSF by lumbar puncture followed by transient clinical improvement may be an indication that the patient is likely to respond to neurosurgical intervention. Of course, this suggestion requires evaluation by controlled clinical trials, as does the cerebroventricular shunting procedure itself. The fact that such trials have not been done is understandable, given the invasive nature of this surgical procedure, but lack of such interpretable studies limits the ability to accurately evaluate the actual therapeutic benefits of neurosurgical shunting (Clarfield 1989).

Disorders secondary to metabolic disease (hypothyroidism and vitamin B$_{12}$ deficiency). Although early in their course, hypothyroidism and vitamin B$_{12}$ deficiency produce a syndrome more appropriately described as a delirium, persistent deficiencies result in neuronal loss and can produce a

dementia that is then irreversible. Hypothyroidism classically produces a cognitive syndrome of dementia accompanied by irritability, paranoid ideation, and depression. Unfortunately, it appears that once dementia is established, even aggressive thyroid replacement does not result in the return of the patient to his or her previous level of function (Larson et al. 1984). Vitamin B$_{12}$ deficiency can produce dementia even in the absence of anemia or megaloblastic bone marrow changes (Strachan and Henderson 1965). Anecdotal reports suggest that B$_{12}$ replacement in dementia that is apparently secondary to B$_{12}$ deficiency can produce some cognitive improvement (Gross et al. 1986; Wieland 1986) but that dementia persists. It also has been suggested that B$_{12}$ deficiency complicated by cognitive and other neuropsychiatric problems may be responsive to treatment with exogenous vitamin B$_{12}$. The retrospective study (Lindenbaum et al. 1988) from which this suggestion was drawn was performed in a predominantly African-American population, and these results may not be completely generalizable to other ethnic groups.

Dementia due to HIV infection. HIV, the virus that has been identified as the cause of acquired immunodeficiency syndrome (AIDS), attacks brain neurons as well as the immune system. AIDS occurs in the geriatric population, but not nearly as frequently as in younger persons (Kendig and Adler 1990). The cognitive disorders caused by HIV infection have recently been reviewed (S. W. Perry 1990). HIV appears to enter the brain shortly after initial infection (Price et al. 1988), causing an acute clinical or subclinical meningoencephalitis. Patients usually recover from the cognitive and other behavioral manifestations of this initial infection. As immunosuppression progresses, virus replication within the CNS occurs, and a progressive multifocal leukoencephalopathy can result. Approximately two-thirds of all patients who develop AIDS will have clinical evidence of a neurodegenerative disorder termed the *AIDS dementia complex* (Price et al. 1988). However, expression of an overt dementia as the primary clinical presentation of HIV infection is unusual (Jansen et al. 1989). Early signs and symptoms of the AIDS dementia complex include impaired attention and concentration, as well as a slowing of information processing—symptoms compatible with a delirium. The patient often appears apathetic and withdrawn, and may meet criteria for depression. Later cognitive deficits include severe dementia and mutism; these are often accompanied by motor signs such as weakness, bradykinesia, ataxia, incontinence, and paraplegia (Navia et al. 1987). Increased age appears to be associated with more rapid disease progression and shorter survival time (Bacchetti et al. 1988; Rothenberg et al. 1987).

Dementia due to Creutzfeldt-Jakob disease. Creutzfeldt-Jakob disease is caused by a nonnucleic acid protein called a *prion body*. The disease, which affects multiple neurological systems, is characterized by a prolonged latency from exposure to expression of the disease (Prusiner et al. 1990). It is rapidly fatal—death usually occurs within 2 years of the time symptoms first appear. It is rare in the elderly population, mainly occurring among persons in middle to late middle life. Dementia—an almost universal feature of this infection—is rapidly progressive and is accompanied by myoclonus, seizures, ataxia, rigidity, and other signs of widespread CNS involvement. Because patients with DAT may also demonstrate myoclonic jerks and seizures in the late stages of their disease, the rapid clinical course and multiple motor system involvement that is characteristic of Creutzfeldt-Jakob disease helps to differentiate between this infection and DAT (Mayeux et al. 1985; Risse et al. 1990b). Neurohistological changes include spongiform encephalopathy, neuronal loss, and gliosis.

Dementia secondary to neurosyphilis. Although neurosyphilis was once a common cause of dementia in later life, it has become almost unknown since the advent of widespread use of antibiotics. Given the recent increase in sexually transmitted diseases, however, neurosyphilis should be considered in the differential diagnosis of dementia. The latency from infection to development of paralytic dementia can be as much as 20 years. Because venereal disease research laboratory (VDRL) test results are negative in nearly one-third of patients with late syphilitic infection, the more sensitive fluorescent treponemal antibody absorption test is more likely to be diagnostic. Unfortunately, neurosyphilis may progress despite what appears to be adequate antibiotic therapy with ultra-high-dose penicillin (Wilner and Brody 1968).

Delirium

The criteria for delirium in DSM-IV (see Table 12–4) emphasize disturbance of consciousness, impairment of attention, and fluctuation during the course of the day. Delirium usually is due to disturbance of brain physiology by a medical disorder or an ingested substance. In contrast, diseases that produce dementia usually cause neuronal loss. One aspect of the new DSM-IV criteria should be applied cautiously: the requirement that the disturbance must have developed over a short period of time—usually hours to days. In the elderly patient, a delirium secondary to drugs such as long-acting benzodiazepines or illnesses such as renal failure may have a longer prodromal period.

It is commendable that DSM-IV does not specify brief duration as a criterion for delirium. In a careful study at the Beth-Israel Hospital in Boston, Levkoff et al. (1992) demonstrated that incident delirium in elderly persons hospitalized for medical or surgical reasons usually persists for months. Full resolution of symptoms of delirium in a short period of time was the exception rather than the rule in this study.

It is important to keep in mind that the disturbance in level of consciousness can range from reduced wakefulness or even stupor to severe insomnia and hyperarousal. Etiological factors for delirium are numerous and include systemic medical illnesses, toxic effects of both prescribed and nonprescribed medications, metabolic disorders, and a

---

Table 12–4. DSM-IV diagnostic criteria for delirium due to a general medical condition

A. Disturbance of consciousness (i.e., reduced clarity of awareness of the environment) with reduced ability to focus, sustain, or shift attention.

B. A change in cognition (such as memory deficit, disorientation, language disturbance) or the development of a perceptual disturbance that is not better accounted for by a preexisting, established, or evolving dementia.

C. The disturbance develops over a short period of time (usually hours to days) and tends to fluctuate during the course of the day.

D. There is evidence from the history, physical examination, or laboratory findings that the disturbance is caused by the direct physiological consequences of a general medical condition.

Source. American Psychiatric Association 1994, p. 129.

host of other illnesses and environmental stressors (e.g., intensive care unit syndrome) (see Table 12–5). It must not be forgotten that withdrawal from addiction to alcohol and/or sedative-hypnotic drugs can occur in older persons, and denial of drug abuse is not restricted to the young.

Treatment of delirium should be directed toward correcting the underlying disorder when that disorder can be detected. Frequently, however, symptomatic treatment becomes necessary if disruptive behaviors such as agitation, delusions, hallucinations, or angry outbursts interfere with patient management or threaten the safety of the patient or others in the environment. Reassurance from a family member or a health care professional can sometimes be helpful in managing the manifestations of delirium; however, pharmacological intervention to resolve an acute crisis may be necessary. Low doses of neuroleptic medication can be helpful. Delirium secondary to withdrawal from a CNS-depressive drug such as ethanol or a benzodiazepine should be treated with a cross-tolerant sedative-hypnotic drug.

Table 12–5.   Etiologies of delirium

Systemic illness
  Congestive heart failure
  Pulmonary insufficiency
  Renal insufficiency
  Hepatic insufficiency
  Lupus erythematosus
  Infection
  Burns and multiple trauma
  Acquired immunodeficiency syndrome

Metabolic disorders
  Hypothyroidism
  Hyperadrenocorticism
  Hypoadrenocorticism
  Hypercalcemia
  Hypoglycemia

Miscellaneous
  Withdrawal from addiction to alcohol, sedatives, hypnotics
  Postoperative state (particularly cardiac surgery and cataract surgery)
  Intensive care unit syndrome

Neurological disorders
  Cerebrovascular accident
  Head trauma
  Subarachnoid hemorrhage
  Meningitis (acute and chronic)
  Intracranial mass lesion
  Neurosyphilis
  Seizure

Pharmacological adverse effects
  Bromide
  Digitalis
  Anticholinergic drugs
  Antipsychotics (e.g., phenothiazines)
  Tricyclic antidepressants
  Antispasmodics (e.g., belladonna)
  Antiparkinsonian agents
  Corticosteroids
  Cimetidine
  Sedatives, hypnotics

Amnestic Disorder

The primary deficit in amnestic disorder is the development of memory impairment as manifested by the inability to learn new information or to recall previously learned information. Although acquired impairment of memory is a central feature of dementia, the diagnosis of amnestic disorder implies a much more discrete deficit that is limited—at least in terms of substantial impairment—to memory function. Of course, careful neuropsychological evaluation often reveals deficits in other cognitive domains in persons who meet criteria for amnestic disorder.

The etiology of an amnestic disorder is usually damage to diencephalic and medial temporal lobe structures, which are important in memory function. Such damage can occur from head trauma, hypoxia, posterior cerebral artery distribution infarction, and herpes simplex encephalitis. However, the most common cause of amnestic disorder is alcoholism. The amnestic disorder caused by alcohol would be diagnosed, according to the DSM-IV criteria, as *alcohol-induced persisting amnestic disorder.* Synonymous terms are *Korsakoff's psychosis* and *Wernicke-Korsakoff syndrome.* The etiology of this disorder is generally considered to be multiple episodes of encephalopathy caused by thiamine deficiency in the context of severe binge alcoholism. However, it is highly probable that alcohol is directly toxic to brain neurons in susceptible individuals (Riley and Walker 1978), and the clear distinction between alcohol-induced persisting amnestic disorder and alcohol-induced persisting dementia is problematic.

The acute thiamine deficiency encephalopathy described by Wernicke is manifested by confusion, lateral gaze palsy, nystagmus, and ataxia. These clinical signs and symptoms reflect damage to brain areas adjacent to the third and fourth ventricles and in the medial temporal lobes. Thiamine is specifically therapeutic if instituted promptly, but this treatable cause of eventual amnestic disorder may be underdiagnosed. Of 51 patients showing the neuropathological stigmata of Wernicke's encephalopathy at postmortem examination, only 7 had been diagnosed as such antemortem (Harper 1979). Although it is widely believed that alcohol-induced amnestic disorder produces permanent cognitive deficits, the actual prognosis for improvement may not be so poor. Victor and colleagues (1971) reported complete recovery in 21% of 104 patients, and some degree of recovery of cognitive function occurred in an additional 53% of patients who were kept free of alcohol use. This classic study suggests that alcohol-induced amnestic disorder is one of the most treatable of the cognitive disorders.

References

Adams RD, Fisher CM, Hakim S: Symptomatic occult hydrocephalus with normal cerebrospinal fluid pressure: a treatable syndrome. N Engl J Med 273:117–126, 1965

Alzheimer A: About a peculiar disease of the cerebral cortex (1907). Translated by Jarvik L, Greenson H. Alzheimer Dis Assoc Disord 1:7–8, 1987

American Psychiatric Association: Diagnostic and Statistical Manual of Mental Disorders, 3rd Edition, Revised. Washington, DC, American Psychiatric Association, 1987

American Psychiatric Association: Diagnostic and Statistical Manual of Mental Disorders, 4th Edition. Washington, DC, American Psychiatric Association, 1994

Arai H, Kosaka K, Iizuka R: Changes in biogenic amines and their metabolites in postmortem brains from patients with Alzheimer-type dementia. J Neurochem 43:388–393, 1984

Bacchetti P, Osmond I, Chaisson RE, et al: Survival patterns of the first 500 patients with AIDS in San Francisco. J Infect Dis 157:1044–1047, 1988

Ball MJ: The morphological basis of dementia in Parkinson's disease. Can J Neurol Sci 11:180–184, 1984

Barnes R, Veith R, Okimoto J, et al: Efficacy of antipsychotic medications in behaviorally disturbed dementia patients. Am J Psychiatry 139:1170–1174, 1982

Blenow KAH, Wallin A, Gottfries CG, et al: Significance of decreased lumbar CSF levels of HVA and 5-HIAA in Alzheimer's disease. Neurobiol Aging 13:107–113, 1991

Blessed G, Tomlinson BE, Roth M: The association between quantitative measures of dementia and of senile change in the cerebral gray matter of elderly subjects. Br J Psychiatry 114:797–811, 1968

Boller F, Mizutani T, Roessman U, et al: Parkinson's disease, dementia, and Alzheimer's disease: clinicopathological correlations. Ann Neurol 7:329–335, 1980

Bondareff W, Mountjoy CQ, Roth M: Loss of neurons of origin of the adrenergic projection to cerebral cortex (nucleus locus coeruleus) in senile dementia. Neurology 32:164–168, 1982

Bondareff W, Raval J, Colletti PM, et al: Quantitative magnetic resonance imaging and the severity of dementia in Alzheimer's disease. Am J Psychiatry 145:853–856, 1988

Braffman BH, Zimmerman RA, Trojanowski JQ, et al: Brain MR: pathologic correlation with gross and histopathology, II: hyperintense white-matter foci in the elderly. American Journal of Radiology 151:559–566, 1988

Brinkman SD, Smith RC, Meyer JS, et al: Lecithin and memory training in suspected Alzheimer's disease. J Gerontol 37:4–9, 1982

Brown RG, Marsden CD: How common is dementia in Parkinson's disease? Lancet 2:1262–1265, 1984

Brun A, Englund E: A white matter disorder in dementia of the Alzheimer type: a pathoanatomic study. Ann Neurol 19:253–262, 1986

Busciglio J, Lorenzo A, Yankner B: Methodological variables in the assessment of beta-amyloid neurotoxicity. Neurobiol Aging 13:609–612, 1992

Carroll BJ, Feinberg M, Greden JF, et al: A specific laboratory test for the diagnosis of melancholia: standardization, validity, and clinical utility. Arch Gen Psychiatry 38:15–22, 1981

Chan-Palay V, Asan E: Alterations in catecholamine neurons of the locus coeruleus in senile dementia of the Alzheimer type and Parkinson's disease with and without dementia and depression. J Comp Neurol 287:373–392, 1989

Christie JE, Shering A, Ferguson J, et al: Physostig-mine and arecoline: effects of intravenous infu-sions in Alzheimer's presenile dementia. Br J Psychiatry 138:46–50, 1981

Chui HC, Mortimer JA, Slager U, et al: Pathological correlates of dementia in Parkinson's disease. Pa-per presented at the annual scientific meeting of the Gerontological Society, San Francisco, CA, November 1984

Chui HC, Victoroff MD, Margolin DJ, et al: Criteria for the diagnosis of ischemic vascular dementia pro-posed by the State of California Alzheimer's Dis-ease Diagnostic and Treatment Centers. Neurology 42:473–480, 1992

Clarfield AM: Normal-pressure hydrocephalus: saga or swamp? JAMA 262:2592–2593, 1989

Corder EH, Saunders AM, Strittmatter WJ, et al: Gene dose of apolipoprotein E type 4 allele and the risk of Alzheimer's disease in late onset fami-lies. Science 261:921–923, 1993

Cross AJ, Crow TJ, Ferrier IN, et al: Serotonin recep-tor changes in dementia of the Alzheimer type. J Neurochem 43:1574–1581, 1984

Cummings JL, Duchen LW: Klüver-Bucy syndrome in Pick's disease: clinical and pathologic correla-tions. Neurology 31:1415–1422, 1981

D'Amato RJ, Zweig RM, Whitehouse PJ, et al: Aminergic systems in Alzheimer's disease and Parkinson's disease. Ann Neurol 22:229–236, 1987

Davies P, Maloney AJ: Selective loss of central cholinergic neurons in Alzheimer's disease (let-ter). Lancet 2:1403, 1976

Davis KL, Mohs RC, Tinklenberg JR: Enhancement of memory by physostigmine (letter). N Engl J Med 301:946, 1979

Davis KL, Davis BM, Greenwald BS, et al: Cortisol and Alzheimer's disease, I: basal studies. Am J Psychiatry 143:300–305, 1986

Devanand DP, Sackheim HA, Brown RP, et al: A pilot study of haloperidol treatment of psychosis and behavioral disturbance in Alzheimer's disease. Arch Neurol 46:854–857, 1989

Ditter SM, Mirra SS: Neuropathologic and clinical features of Parkinson's disease in Alzheimer's disease patients. Neurology 37:754–760, 1987

Erkinjuntti T, Ketonen L, Sulkava R, et al: Do white matter changes on MRI and CT differentiate vascular dementia from Alzheimer's disease? J Neurol Neurosurg Psychiatry 50:37–42, 1987

Evans IA, Funkenstein H, Albert MS, et al: Preva-lence of Alzheimer's disease in a community population of older persons: higher than pre-viously reported. JAMA 262:2551–2556, 1989

Farlow M, Gracon SI, Hershey LA, et al., for the Tac-rine Study Group: a controlled trial of tacrine in Alzheimer's disease. JAMA 268:2523–2529, 1992

Fein G, Van Dyke C, Davenport L, et al: Preservation of normal cognitive functioning in elderly sub-jects with extensive white-matter lesions of long duration. Arch Gen Psychiatry 47:220–223, 1990

Flynn DD, Weinstein DA, Mash DC: Loss of high-af-finity agonist binding to M1 muscarinic recep-tors in Alzheimer's disease: implications for the failure of cholinergic replacement therapies. Ann Neurol 29:256–262, 1991

Folstein MF, Folstein SE, McHugh PR: Mini-Mental State: a practical method for grading the cogni-tive state of patients for the clinician. J Psychiatr Res 12:189–198, 1975

Fox JH, Topel JL, Huckman MS: Dementia in the el-derly: a search for treatable illnesses. J Gerontol 30:557–564, 1975

Francis PT, Palmer AM, Sims NR, et al: Neurochemi-cal studies of early onset Alzheimer's disease. N Engl J Med 313:7–11, 1985

Freeman FR: Evaluation of patients with progres-sive intellectual deterioration. Arch Neurol 33:658–659, 1976

Friedland RP: "Normal"-pressure hydrocephalus and the saga of the treatable dementias. JAMA 262:2577–2581, 1989

George AE, De Leon MJ, Gentes CI, et al: Leukoen-cephalopathy in normal and pathologic aging, I: CT of brain lucencies. AJNR Am J Neuroradiol 7:561–566, 1986a

George AE, De Leon MJ, Kalnin A, et al: Leukoen-cephalopathy in normal and pathologic aging, II: MRI of brain lucencies. AJNR Am J Neuroradiol 7:567–570, 1986b

Gibson CJ, Logue M, Growdon JH: CSF monoamine metabolite levels in Alzheimer's and Parkinson's disease. Arch Neurol 42:489–492, 1985

Glenner GG, Wong CW: Alzheimer's disease: initial report of the purification and characterization of a novel cerebrovascular amyloid protein. Bio-chem Biophys Res Commun 120:885–890, 1984

Goate AM, Haynes AR, Owen MJ, et al: Predispos-ing locus for Alzheimer's disease on chromo-some 21. Lancet 1:352–355, 1989

Goldgarber D, Lerman MI, McBride OW, et al: Characterization and chromosomal localization of a cDNA encoding brain amyloid of Alzheimer's disease. Science 235:877–879, 1987

Gross JS, Weintraub NT, Neufeld RR, et al: Pernicious anemia in the demented patient without anemia or macrocytosis: a case for early recognition. J Am Geriatr Soc 34:612–614, 1986

Hakim AM, Mathieson I: Dementia in Parkinson's disease: a neuropathologic study. Neurology 29:1209–1214, 1979

Harbaugh RE, Roberts DW, Coombs DW, et al: Preliminary report: intracranial cholinergic drug infusion in patients with Alzheimer's disease. Neurosurgery 15:514–518, 1984

Hardy J: Framing beta-amyloid. Nature Genetics 1:233–234, 1992

Harper C: Wernicke's encephalopathy: a more common disease than realized. J Neurol Neurosurg Psychiatry 42:226–231, 1979

Harrell LE, Jope RS, Falgout J, et al: Biological and neuropsychological characterization of physostigmine responders and non-responders in Alzheimer's disease. J Am Geriatr Soc 38:112–113, 1990

Heston LL, White JA, Mastri AR: Pick's disease: clinical genetics and natural history. Arch Gen Psychiatry 44:409–411, 1987

Jansen R, Stehr-Green J, Starcher T: Epidemiology of HIV encephalopathy in the United States, in Abstracts of the Fifth International Conference on AIDS. Montreal, Canada, International Development Research Centre, 1989

Jenike MA, Albert MS, Heller H, et al: Oral physostigmine treatment for patients with presenile and senile dementia of the Alzheimer's type: a double-blind placebo-controlled trial. J Clin Psychiatry 51:3–7, 1990

Joachim CL, Morris JH, Selkoe DJ: Clinically diagnosed Alzheimer's disease: autopsy results in 150 cases. Ann Neurol 24:50–56, 1988

Katzman R: The prevalence and malignancy of Alzheimer disease: a major killer. Arch Neurol 33:217–218, 1976

Katzman R: Alzheimer's disease. N Engl J Med 314:964–973, 1986

Kendig NE, Adler WH: The implications of the acquired immunodeficiency syndrome for gerontology research and geriatric medicine. J Gerontol [Med Sci] 45:M77–M81, 1990

Khan A, Rudolph R, Baumel B, et al: Venlafaxine in depressed geriatric outpatients: an open-label clinical study. Paper presented at Collegium Internationale Neuro-Psychopharmacologium, Washington, DC, June 1994

Kiloh LG: Pseudo-dementia. Acta Psychiatr Scand 37:336–351, 1961

Knapp MJ, Knopman DS, Solomon PR, et al., for the Tacrine Study Group: A 30-week randomized controlled trial of high-dose tacrine in patients with Alzheimer's disease. JAMA 271:985 991, 1994

Kosaka K, Tsuchiya K, Yoshimura M: Lewy body disease with and without dementia: a clinico-pathological study of 35 cases. Clin Neuropathol 7:299–305, 1988

Kowall N, Beal M, Busciglio J, et al: An in vivo model for the neurodegenerative effects of beta-amyloid and protection by substance P. Proc Natl Acad Sci USA 88:7247–7251, 1991

Lai F, Williams RS: A prospective study of Alzheimer's disease in Down's syndrome. Arch Neurol 46:849–853, 1989

Larson EB, Reifler BV, Featherstone HJ, et al: Dementia in elderly outpatients: a prospective study. Ann Intern Med 100:417–423, 1984

Larson EB, Reifler BV, Sumi SM, et al: Diagnostic tests in the evaluation of dementia: a prospective study of 200 elderly outpatients. Arch Intern Med 146:1917–1922, 1986

Leverenz J, Sumi SM: Parkinson's disease in patients with Alzheimer's disease. Arch Neurol 43:662–664, 1986

Levkoff SE, Evans DA, Liptzin B, et al: Delirium: the occurrence and persistence of symptoms among elderly hospitalized patients. Arch Intern Med 152:334–340, 1992

Lindenbaum J, Healton EB, Savage DG, et al: Neuropsychiatric disorders caused by cobalamin deficiency in the absence of anemia or macrocytosis. N Engl J Med 318:1720–1728, 1988

Mann DMA, Yates PO: Serotonin nerve cells in Alzheimer's disease. J Neurol Neurosurg Psychiatry 46:96–98, 1983

Mann DMA, Lincoln J, Yates PO, et al: Changes in the monoamine-containing neurons of the human CNS in senile dementia. Br J Psychiatry 136:533–541, 1980

Mattis S: Mental status examination for organic mental syndrome in the elderly patient, in Geriatric Psychiatry: A Handbook for Psychiatrists and Primary Care Physicians. Edited by Bellack L, Karasu TB. New York, Grune & Stratton, 1976, pp 77–121

Mayeux R, Stern Y, Spanton S: Heterogeneity in dementia of the Alzheimer type: evidence of subgroups. Neurology 35:453–461, 1985

Mayeux R, Stern Y, Rosenstein R, et al: An estimate of the prevalence of dementia in idiopathic Parkinson disease. Arch Neurol 45:260–262, 1988

McAllister TW, Ferrell RB, Price TRP, et al: The dexamethasone suppression test in two patients with severe depressive pseudodementia. Am J Psychiatry 139:479–481, 1982

McKhann G, Drachman D, Folstein M, et al: Clinical diagnosis of Alzheimer's disease: report of the NINCDS–ADRDA work group under the auspices of Department of Health and Human Services Task Force on Alzheimer's disease. Neurology 34:939–944, 1984

Mohs RC, Davis BM, Johns CA, et al: Oral physostigmine treatment of patients with Alzheimer's disease. Am J Psychiatry 142:28–33, 1985

Morris JC, McKeel DW, Fulling K, et al: Validation of clinical diagnostic criteria for Alzheimer's disease. Ann Neurol 24:17–22, 1988

Mortimer JA: Alzheimer's disease and senile dementia: prevalence and incidence, in Alzheimer's Disease: The Standard Reference. Edited by Reisberg B. New York, Free Press, 1983, pp 141–148

Mullan M, Crawford F, Axelman K, et al: A pathogenic mutation for probable Alzheimer's disease in the APP gene at the *N*-terminus of beta-amyloid. Nature Genetics 1:345–347, 1992

Navia BA, Price RW: The acquired immunodeficiency syndrome dementia complex as the presenting or sole manifestation of human immunodeficiency virus infection. Arch Neurol 44:65–69, 1987

Okazaki H, Lipin LE, Aronson SM: Diffuse intracytoplasmic ganglionic inclusions (Lewy type) associated with progressive dementia and quadriparesis in flexion. J Neuropathol Exp Neurol 20:237–244, 1961

Palmer AM, Francis PT, Bowen DE, et al: Catecholaminergic neurons assessed ante-mortem in Alzheimer's disease. Brain Res 414:365–375, 1987

Pericak-Vance MA, Yamoaka LH, Haynes CS, et al: Genetic linkage studies in Alzheimer's disease families. Exp Neurol 102:271–279, 1988

Perry EK, Tomlinson BE, Blessed G, et al: Correlation of cholinergic abnormalities with senile plaques and mental test scores in senile dementia. BMJ 2:1457–1459, 1978

Perry EK, Curtis M, Dick DJ, et al: Cholinergic correlates of cognitive impairment in Parkinson's disease: comparisons with Alzheimer's disease. J Neurol Neurosurg Psychiatry 48:413–421, 1985

Perry RH, Irving D, Blessed G, et al: Senile dementia of Lewy body type: a clinically and neuropathologically distinct form of Lewy body dementia in the elderly. J Neurol Sci 95:119–139, 1990

Perry SW: Organic mental disorders caused by HIV: update on early diagnosis and treatment. Am J Psychiatry 147:696–710, 1990

Petrie WM, Ban TA, Berry S, et al: Loxapine in psychogeriatrics: a placebo- and standard-controlled clinical-investigation. J Clin Psychopharmacol 2:122–126, 1982

Podlisny M, Stephenson D, Frosch M, et al: Synthetic amyloid beta-protein fails to produce specific neurotoxicity in monkey cerebral cortex. Neurobiol Aging 13:561–567, 1992

Price RW, Brew B, Sidtis J, et al: The brain in AIDS: central nervous system HIV-1 infection and AIDS dementia complex. Science 239:586–592, 1988

Prien F, Caffe EM: Pharmacologic treatment of elderly patients with organic brain syndrome: a survey of twelve Veterans Administration hospitals. Compr Psychiatry 18:551–560, 1977

Prusiner SB, DeArmond SJ: Prion disease of the central nervous system. Monogr Pathol 32:86–122, 1990

Rajput AH, Offord K, Beard CM, et al: A case-control study of smoking habits, dementia, and other illnesses in idiopathic Parkinson's disease. Neurology 37:266–232, 1987

Raskind MA: Geriatric psychopharmacology: management of late life depression and the noncognitive behavioral disturbance of Alzheimer's disease. Psychiatr Clin North Am 16:815–827, 1993

Raskind MA, Peskind ER: Alzheimer's disease and other dementing disorders, in Handbook of Mental Health and Aging, 2nd Edition. Edited by Birren JE, Sloane RB, Cohen GD. San Diego, CA, Academic Press, 1992, pp 487–490

Raskind MA, Peskind E, Rivard MR, et al: Dexamethasone suppression test and cortical circadian rhythm in primary degenerative dementia. Am J Psychiatry 139:1468–1471, 1982

Raskind MA, Peskind ER, Halter JB, et al: Norepinephrine and MHPG levels in CSF and plasma in Alzheimer's disease. Arch Gen Psychiatry 4:343–346, 1984

Raskind MA, Risse SC, Lampe TH: Dementia and antipsychotic drugs. J Clin Psychiatry 48:16–18, 1987

Raskind MA, Peskind ER, Wilkinson CW: Hypothalamic-pituitary-adrenal axis regulation and human aging. Ann N Y Acad Sci 746:327–335, 1994

Reifler BV: Arguments for abandoning the term pseudodementia. J Am Geriatr Soc 30:665–668, 1982

Reifler BV, Teri L, Raskind M, et al: Double-blind trial of imipramine in Alzheimer's disease patients with and without depression. Am J Psychiatry 146:45–49, 1989

Reisberg B, Borenstein J, Salob SP, et al: Behavioral symptoms in Alzheimer's disease: phenomenology and treatment. J Clin Psychiatry 48:9–15, 1987

Riley JN, Walker DW: Morphological alterations in hippocampus after long-term alcohol consumption in mice. Science 201:646–648, 1978

Risse SC, Lampe TH, Bird TD, et al: Myoclonus, seizures and rigidity in Alzheimer's disease. Alzheimer Dis Assoc Disord 4:217–225, 1990a

Risse SC, Raskind MA, Nochlin D, et al: Neuropathological findings in patients with clinical diagnosis of probable Alzheimer's disease. Am J Psychiatry 147:168–172, 1990b

Rosen WG, Mohs RC, Davis KL: A new rating scale for Alzheimer's disease. Am J Psychiatry 141:1356–1364, 1984

Rosenberg RN: A causal role for amyloid in Alzheimer's disease: the end of the beginning. Neurology 43:851–856, 1993

Rothenberg R, Woelfel M, Stoneburner R, et al: Survival with the acquired immunodeficiency syndrome: experience with 5,833 cases in New York City. N Engl J Med 317:1297–1302, 1987

Rudorfer MV, Clayton PV: Depression, dementia and dexamethasone suppression (letter to editor). Am J Psychiatry 138:701, 1981

Salzman C: Treatment of the elderly agitated patient. J Clin Psychiatry 48 (suppl):19–22, 1987

Sapolsky R, Armanini M, Packan D, et al: Stress and glucocorticoids in aging. Endocrinol Metab Clin North Am 16:965–980, 1987

Schellenberg GD, Bird TD, Wijsman EM, et al: Absence of linkage of chromosome 21q21 markers to familial Alzheimer's disease. Science 241:1507–1510, 1988

Schellenberg GD, Bird T, Wijsman E, et al: Genetic linkage evidence for a familial Alzheimer's disease locus on chromosome 14. Science 258:668–671, 1992

Schmechel DR, Schmitt I, Horner J, et al: Lack of effect of oral physostigmine and lecithin in patients with Alzheimer's disease. Neurology 34:280, 1984

Selkoe DJ: Altered structural proteins in plaques and tangles: what do they tell us about Alzheimer's disease? Neurobiology Aging 7:425–432, 1986

Sherrington R, Rogaev EI, Llang Y, et al: Cloning of a gene bearing mis-sense mutations in early-onset familial Alzheimer's disease. Nature 375:754–760, 1995

Sjogren T, Sjogren H, Lindgren AGH: Morbus Alzheimer and morbus Pick. Acta Psychiatr Scand Suppl 82:1–66, 1952

Spar JE, Gerner R: Does the dexamethasone suppression test distinguish dementia from depression? Am J Psychiatry 139:238–240, 1982

St. George-Hyslop G, Tanzi R, Polinsky R, et al: The genetic defect causing familial Alzheimer disease maps on chromosome 21. Science 235:885–889, 1987

Stern Y, Sano M, Mayeux R: Long-term administration of oral physostigmine in Alzheimer's disease. Neurology 38:1837–1841, 1988

Strachan RW, Henderson JG: Psychiatric syndromes due to avitaminosis B_{12} with normal blood and bone arrow. Q J Med 34:303–309, 1965

Strittmatter WJ, Weisgraber KH, Goedert M, et al: Hypothesis: microtubule instability and paired helical filament formation in the Alzheimer disease brain are related to apolipoprotein E genotype. Exp Neurol 125:163–171, 1994

Summers WK, Machovski LV, Marsh GM, et al: Oral tetrahydroaminoacridine in long-term treatment of senile dementia, Alzheimer type. N Engl J Med 315:1241–1245, 1986

Thal IJ, Rosen W, Sharpless NS: Choline chloride fails to improve cognition in Alzheimer's disease. Neurobiol Aging 2:205–208, 1981

Thal IJ, Fuld PA, Masur DM, et al: Oral physostigmine and lecithin improve memory in Alzheimer's disease. Ann Neurol 13:491–496, 1983

Thomasen AM, Borgesen SE, Bruhn P, et al: Prognosis of dementia in normal-pressure hydrocephalus after a shunt operation. Ann Neurol 20:304–310, 1986

Tierney MC, Fisher RH, Lewis AJ, et al: The NINCDS-ADRDA Work Group criteria for the clinical diagnosis of probable Alzheimer's disease: a clinicopathologic study of 57 cases. Neurology 38:359–364, 1988

Tomlinson BE, Blessed G, Roth M: Observations on the brains of demented old people. J Neurol Sci 11:205–242, 1970

Tomlinson BE, Irving D, Blessed G: Cell loss in the locus coeruleus in senile dementia of Alzheimer type. J Neurol Sci 49:419–428, 1981

Victor M, Adams RD: The Wernicke-Korsakoff Syndrome. Philadelphia, PA, FA Davis, 1971

Victoratos GC, Lonman JAR, Herzberg L: Neurological investigation of dementia. Br J Psychiatry 130:131–133, 1977

Vitaliano PP, Breen AR, Russo J, et al: The clinical utility of the dementia rating scale for assessing Alzheimer patients. Journal of Chronic Diseases 37:743–753, 1984

Volicer L, Direnfeld LK, Freedman M, et al: Serotonin and 5-hydroxyindoleacetic acid in CSF: differences in Parkinson's disease and dementia of the Alzheimer's type. Arch Neurol 42:127–129, 1985

Wagner SL, Leverenz J, Ito RK, et al: Clinicopathologic correlations of soluble amyloid beta-protein in cerebrospinal fluid in Alzheimer's disease patients and controls (abstract), in Proceedings of the 25th annual meeting of the International Society of Psychoneuroendocrinology, Seattle, WA, 1994, p 24

Whitehouse PJ, Price DL, Struble RG, et al: Alzheimer's disease and senile dementia: loss of neurons in the basal forebrain. Science 215:1237–1239, 1982

Wieland RG: Vitamin B_{12} deficiency in the nonanemic elderly. J Am Geriatr Soc 34:618–619, 1986

Wikkelso C, Anderson H, Blomstrand C, et al: The clinical effect of lumbar puncture in normal-pressure hydrocephalus. J Neurol Neurosurg Psychiatry 45:64–69, 1982

Wilner E, Brody JA: Prognosis of general paresis after treatment. Lancet 2:1370–1371, 1968

Winblad B, Adolfsson R, Carlsson A, et al: Biogenic amines in brains of patients with Alzheimer's disease, in Alzheimer's Disease: A Report of Progress. Edited by Corkin S. New York, Raven, 1982, pp 25–33

Wood PL, Nair NP, Etienne P, et al: Lack of cholinergic deficit in the neocortex in Pick's disease. Prog Neuropsychopharmacol Biol Psychiatry 7:725–727, 1983

Yamamoto T, Hirano A: Nucleus raphe dorsalis in Alzheimer's disease: neurofibrillary tangles and loss of large neurons. Ann Neurol 17:573–577, 1985

Zubenko GS: Progression of illness in the differential diagnosis of primary depression. Am J Psychiatry 147:435–438, 1990

Zubenko GS: Biological correlates of clinical heterogeneity in primary dementia. Neuropsychopharmacology 6:77–93, 1992

Zubenko GS, Moossy J: Major depression in primary dementia. Arch Neurol 45:1182–1186, 1988

Zweig RM, Ross CA, Hedreen JC, et al: The neuropathology of aminergic nuclei in Alzheimer's disease. Ann Neurol 24:233–242, 1988

CHAPTER 13

Mood Disorders

Dan G. Blazer, M.D., Ph.D.
Harold G. Koenig, M.D., M.H.Sc.

The themes of aging and depression often coalesce. Frequent questions surrounding these themes include the following: Do persons become more depressed as they grow older? Does depression become more difficult to treat with increased age? Is depression more difficult to identify in the older adult? The answers to these questions rest in part with the definition of late-life depression. Depression in late life is not a unitary construct. Depending on how depression is defined, the answers to questions regarding late-life depression will change.

Depression can be construed in at least three ways, each of which has clinical relevance for older adults. First, depression can be viewed as a unitary phenomenon, with the various manifestations of depression forming a continuum. Sir Aubrey Lewis (1934) noted that the various classifications of depression are "nothing more than attempts to distinguish between acute and chronic, mild and severe" (p. 1). In more recent years, Kendell (1976) has argued for the unitary view. Although the extremes of the continuum are different, precise boundaries can be found between these extremes. Depression symptom checklists, such as the Zung Self-Rating Depression Scale (Zung 1965), the Center for Epidemiologic Studies Depression Scale (CES-D; Radloff 1977), and the Geriatric Depression Scale (Yesavage et al. 1983), would therefore be useful in distinguishing the degree to which an individual suffers from depression in late life.

Most modern investigators, however, find it difficult to conceive of depression as phenomenologically homogeneous. Rather, a categorical approach, as exemplified in DSM-III-R and DSM-IV (American Psychiatric Association 1987, 1994), has been of more interest to modern clinicians. If one views the affective disorders as a group of distinct entities or independent syndromes, with each of the categories mutually exclusive, the diagnosis and management of depression are allied with the traditional medical model. Given the availability of excellent, but potentially dangerous, biological therapies, the use of the categorical approach has been adopted by most geriatric psychiatrists. Specific therapies can be prescribed for distinct diagnostic entities.

The third approach to the conceptualization of the depressed elder is a functional approach, by which depressive symptoms become severe enough to be identified as a case worth clinical attention when function is impaired. Social function, especially the performance of role responsibilities, has been targeted as a critical variable in monitoring treatment. An example of the functional approach can be found in many surveys of community subjects (Langner and Michael 1963; Multidimensional Functional Assessment 1978). For the family, function is a critical element because they do not view symptom remission alone as an essential marker of improvement, but they also consider a return to social involvement and improved life satisfaction as critical signs. An older adult who sleeps better, has a better appetite, and ceases to be suicidal may be determined improved by the clinician but little improved by the family if social isolation and disinterest in the social environment persist after appropriate therapy. Axis V of DSM-III-R partially assesses the impact of a disorder on social functioning.

The categorical approach to diagnosis—that is, a focus on Axis I of DSM-III-R—is adopted, for the most part, through the remainder of this chapter. Nevertheless, the reader must recognize that other constructs of depression must complement the categorical approach if it is to be effective in the diagnosis and treatment of older adults. Depressive symptoms that do not cluster in such a way as to fit the procrustean bed of a given diagnostic system may nevertheless be of clinical significance. Social and physical functioning, both during and after therapy, are at least as important in assessing the success of therapeutic intervention as is the remission of a series of symptoms.

There have been few changes in the categorization of major depression and other affective disorders in the transition from DSM-III-R to DSM-IV; where changes are relevant, we will point them out.

Epidemiology of Late-Life Depression

Prevalence

General comments on the epidemiology of psychiatric disorders in late life have been reported in Chapter 9. Investigators at Duke University Medical Center attempted to untangle the different subtypes of depression in late life in a community survey (Blazer et al. 1987a). More than 1,300 older adults living in both urban and rural communities who were 60 years of age or older were screened for depressive symptomatology. Of the 27% reporting depressive symptoms, 19% had mild dysphoria only. Persons with symptomatic depression—that is, subjects with more severe depressive symptoms—made up 4% of the population. These individuals were primarily experiencing stressors, such as physical illness and stressful life events. Only 2% had a dysthymic disorder, and 0.8% were experiencing a current major depressive episode. No cases of current manic episodes were identified. Finally, 1.2% had a mixed depression and anxiety syndrome. These data suggest that the traditional DSM-III-R depressive categories do not capture most depressed older adults in the community population.

In a study of psychiatric inpatients (Blazer et al. 1987b), subjects in both middle life and late life were identified as experiencing a major depressive episode with melancholia. Criteria symptoms for depression and symptoms specifically associated with melancholic or endogenous depression did not differ across age groups. The syndrome of major depression with melancholia is relatively common in inpatient service among older adults and is easily enough recognized.

How does one reconcile these seemingly disparate results? *Depression in late life* remains a generic term that captures many constructs, some of which are well defined and others of which are ill defined. The burden of depression in the elderly, as noted above in the frequency of significant depressive symptoms in community populations, is unquestioned. Many older persons with atypical presentations of depression do not meet criteria for major depression. Nevertheless, the usual reasons given for not identifying a severely depressed older adult in the clinical setting—pseudodementia, somatization, denial of depressive symptomatology, poor response to antidepressant medication, or masked depression—do not apply to most severely depressed elders, such as the melancholic older adult. DSM-III-R and similar nomenclatures may therefore apply to some, but not all, depressive syndromes in late life.

Because of the association between medical illness and depression, many depressed elders may be either in acute-care settings or in nursing homes and thus be unavailable for (or be unable to participate in) community surveys. In contrast to low rates of major depression found among older adults in the community (>1%), it has been estimated that 12% of hospitalized elders fulfill criteria for a major depressive episode, and an additional 20%–25% have a minor depression (Koenig et al. 1988a). Likewise, rates of major depression in elderly nursing home patients are even higher, in the range of 12%–16% (Parmelee et al. 1989; Rovner et al. 1991; Weissman et al. 1991).

Manic episodes in late life are uncommon but not unseen. In a study of 6-month prevalence of psychiatric disorders in three communities (Myers et al. 1984), out of more than 3,000 elders interviewed, no person over the age of 65 was found to suffer from a current manic episode. One reason for the very low prevalence in community populations may be the inability of structured instruments to identify the atypical presentation of manic episodes among the elderly. When mania does occur, the syndrome may be so severe that the elder is hospitalized and therefore would not be located during a community inquiry. Alternatively, manic episodes in later life may present with a mixture of manic, dysphoric, and cognitive symptoms, with euphoria less common (Post 1978). When mania is associated with significant changes in cognitive function—so-called manic delirium—it may be difficult to distinguish from organic conditions or schizophrenia (Shulman 1986). Thus, manic episodes may present in an atypical manner that does not allow easy categorization, especially when they have been diagnosed using structured psychiatric interviews administered by lay interviewers as in the Epidemiologic Catchment Area (ECA) surveys. Despite such considerations, however, the ECA surveys did diagnose bipolar disorder in 9.7% of nursing home patients, suggesting that this setting may have become a dumping ground for such patients (Weissman et al. 1991).

Snapshot prevalence studies do not adequately represent late-life depression within the context of historical trends. The 20-year follow-up of the Midtown Manhattan study in New York illustrates the importance of cohort analysis (Srole and Fischer 1980). Nearly 700 of the original 1,660 adults between the ages of 20 and 59 who were initially interviewed were reinterviewed 20 years later using an identical instrument. This mental health impairment scale actually assessed primarily depressive symptomatology. Although in the assessments in both 1954 and 1974 the highest rates of mental health impairment were found among the elderly (22% for the 50- to 59-year-olds, compared with 7% for the 20- to 29-year-olds in 1954), the prevalence of mental health impairment did not increase longitudinally with age. For example, from age 50–59 to age 70–79, depression remained almost constant (22% in 1954 vs. 18% in 1974). How can these findings be explained? Cohort effects may influence the distribution of depressive symptoms across the life cycle more than do the effects of aging. The burden of depressive symptoms within a birth cohort may remain relatively constant through the life cycle.

Mortality

An additional parameter of late-life affective disorders is the outcome from these disorders. The epidemiology of suicide has already been discussed in Chapter 9. The association between depressive symptoms and all-cause mortality among older participants in the ECA study in North Carolina did not reveal a relationship between depressive symptoms and mortality when other known causes of mortality were included in a logistic analysis (Fredman et al. 1989). When age, activities of daily living, gender, and cognitive impairment were controlled, neither the diagnosis of major depression nor the accumulation of significant depressive symptoms at baseline predicted mortality 2 years after the initial interview of more than 1,600 community respondents 60+ years of age. Long-term follow-up of this elderly cohort, however, will produce interesting and important findings in the future.

The association between late-life depression and mortality is intuitively attractive, for older persons are thought to experience loss of meaningful roles and emotional support through retirement, widowhood, death of friends, low economic and material well-being, and increased isolation and loneliness (Atchley 1972; Fassler and Gavira 1978). In other community-based prospective longitudinal studies, depressed persons did have a significantly higher mortality rate than the nondepressed, but in most of these studies only age was controlled as a potential confounder (Enzell 1984; Kay and Bergmann 1966; Markush et al. 1977; Persson 1981).

More recently, Murphy and colleagues (1988) examined all-cause mortality in a 4-year follow-up study of 120 depressed elderly psychiatric inpatients, comparing them with 197 age- and gender-matched control subjects. Among the depressed women, mortality was twice the expected rate; among the men, it was three times the expected rate. After stratification by health status, older men with physical health problems and depression were significantly more likely to die compared with similarly aged, physically ill nondepressed men. Likewise, a study of elderly veterans hospitalized with medical illness found a significantly higher mortality during hospitalization for 41 patients who were depressed, compared with 41 nondepressed patients matched for age, sex, and severity and type of medical illness (Koenig et al. 1989). Rovner and colleagues (1991) also found greater death rates among elderly nursing home patients with depression. These studies indicate higher rates of mortality for depressed elderly patients—men in particular—with concurrent physical health problems; this relationship in clinical samples has persisted after important covariates have been controlled.

Prognosis

Until recently, long-term psychiatric follow-up investigations of survivors of severe episodes of late-life depression have been relatively scarce, given the frequency and clinical importance of the disorder. The typical course of major depression throughout the life cycle is remission and relapse. In patients who have a history of recurrent episodes, new episodes tend to be associated with similar symptoms and last for about as long as prior episodes. Classic studies of depression suggest the duration of major depression throughout the life cycle to be approximately 9 months, if untreated (Dunner 1985). As individuals age, however, they may experience episodes more frequently, and these episodes can merge into a chronic condition.

Post (1972) argued that the episodes of depression in late life may last longer than at earlier stages of the life cycle. After following 92 depressed elders for 3 years, he found that only 26% had completely recovered from their index episode, whereas 37% had further attacks with good recoveries and 37% experienced recurrent attacks on a baseline of chronic depression or remained continuously ill. Murphy (1983) and co-workers, following 124 depressed elders for 1 year, found that 35% experienced a complete recovery, 19% recovered but later relapsed, 29% were continuously ill, and 17% were

either demented or dead. Patients with delusional depression had particularly poor outcomes, with only 1 in 10 recovering.

In contrast, Cole (1983) found that older adults with primary depression with onset after the age of 60 were more likely to remain well if they recovered. Baldwin and Jolley (1986) followed 100 elderly psychiatric inpatients with severe unipolar depression for 3–8 years; 60% remained well throughout or had relapses with complete recovery and only 7% had continuous depression. Likewise, in a direct comparison of middle-aged and elderly patients hospitalized for major depression, little difference was found between middle-aged and older adults in recovery (Blazer et al. 1992). Of the 44 older adults (60+ years of age), 48% had not recovered from the depressive episode leading to hospitalization, 27% had recovered completely from the index episode but experienced a recurrence of another episode of major depression, and 25% had recovered completely without a recurrence. Of the 35 middle-aged patients, 46% had not recovered from the index episode, 45% had recovered completely but experienced a recurrence of another episode, and 9% had recovered completely and remained recovered. Significant depressive symptoms at the time of follow-up (a score of 16 or higher on the CES-D) were reported by 59% of the elderly but only 43% of the middle-aged subjects. This 1- to 2-year follow-up suggests that, in terms of recovery and remission, older adults do not differ from their middle-aged counterparts. If they do recover, however, elders appear to experience residual depressive symptoms. Whether these symptoms result from the major depressive episode or whether they were present before the onset of the depressive episode is unknown.

Most clinicians and clinical investigators report that more than 70% of elderly patients with major depression who are treated with antidepressant medications (at an adequate dose for a sufficient time period) will recover from the index episode of depression. Reynolds and colleagues (1992) reported that treatment of healthy depressed elders with combined interpersonal psychotherapy and nortriptyline achieved response rates nearing 80%. Even long-term outcome studies of treatment-resistant depression in older adults have reported that 15 months after treatment with an antidepressant or electroconvulsive therapy (ECT), 47% were clinically improved; at 4 years of follow-up, that percentage had increased to 71% (Stoudemire et al. 1993). These optimistic results must be tempered by the fact that physical illness and impaired cognition may complicate both the course of depression and its response to treatment (Baldwin and Jolley 1986; Cole 1983; Koenig et al. 1992a; Murphy et al. 1988). Once an older patient has experienced one or more moderate to severe episodes of major depression, he or she may need to continue on antidepressant therapy permanently to minimize the risk of relapse (Greden 1993; Old Age Depression Interest Group 1993).

Prediction of recovery from a depressive episode may also be enhanced through use of the dexamethasone suppression test (DST; Carroll et al. 1981; Greden et al. 1983). Return to normal suppression of cortisol from a nonsuppression state often precedes clinical improvement and therefore bodes a good prognosis. In contrast, if nonsuppression persists, even if patients improve clinically, they are more likely to experience an early relapse (Greden et al. 1980). For predicting long-term follow-up, however, the DST has proved to be of less value (Zimmerman et al. 1987). Authors of a recent meta-analysis on pooled data from 144 studies concluded that 1) baseline DST status does not predict response to antidepressant treatment or outcome after hospital discharge; 2) nonsuppression of cortisol on baseline DST does predict a poorer response to placebo; and 3) persistent nonsuppression on DST after treatment is associated with a high risk of early relapse and poor outcome after discharge (Ribeiro et al. 1993).

Persons with a dysthymic disorder (depressive neurosis) experience a more chronic course than do persons with major depression. By DSM-III-R definition, an individual's depressive symptoms must last for at least 2 years to receive a dysthymic disorder diagnosis. An undetermined percentage of community-dwelling (and possibly institutionalized) elders—as high as 4%–8%—experience moderately severe depressive symptoms for longer than 2 years, although they report intermittent periods lasting longer than a few days when they are relatively free of depressive symptoms. The severity of their symptoms is not so great as to meet the criteria for a diagnosis of major depression, and the intermittent symptom-free periods disqualify them from the diagnosis of dysthymic disorder. Nevertheless, these individuals experience a chronic depression. Other older adults experience chronic depressions secon-

dary to medical or even psychiatric disease—for example, alcoholism and anxiety disorders such as obsessive-compulsive disorder. Each of these disorders contributes to residual depression in the ambulatory elderly.

Factors associated with an improved outcome in late-life depression include a history of recovery from previous episodes, family history of depression, female sex, extroverted personality, current or recent employment, absence of substance abuse, no history of major psychiatric disorder, less severe depressive symptomatology, and absence of major life events (Baldwin and Jolley 1986; Post 1972). The results of a number of studies have suggested a relationship between social support during an index episode and outcome from psychological distress and depression. Intuition suggests that the availability of adequate support should enhance the recovery from a severe or moderately severe psychiatric disorder such as major depression. In a study of 493 community respondents, Holahan and Moos (1981) found that decreases in social support from family and work environments were related to increases in psychological maladjustment over a 1-year follow-up period. In a longitudinal study, however, Henderson and Moran (1983) found no relationship between objective measures of support and the onset or the remission of substantial neurotic symptoms in community-dwelling elders.

In a similar study (George et al. 1989), 104 inpatients diagnosed as having major depression were followed for 1–2 years after their hospitalization. Fifty-three of these patients were age 60 or older. Thirty-three reported that they had recovered from the index episode and scored lower than 10 on the CES-D at follow-up. Subjects who reported an adequate social support network at the time of the index depressive episode were 2.3 times more likely to have recovered than those who reported an impaired social network (44% vs. 19%). In a multiple regression analysis, social support remained a predictor of recovery from major depression when age, gender, and the initial CES-D score were controlled.

Coping behavior may also affect the prognosis of late-life depression. One of the most common coping behaviors used by this generation of older adults is religion. In a study of 100 middle-aged or elderly adults, one-third of men and nearly two-thirds of women used religious cognitions or behaviors to help them cope with a stressful period in life

(Koenig et al. 1988b). A number of investigators have reported inverse associations between religious coping and depressive symptoms in older adults with acute and chronic medical illness (Idler 1987; Idler and Kasl 1992; Koenig et al. 1992b; Pressman et al. 1990). A study of 850 medically ill hospitalized elders found that those using religion as a coping behavior were less likely to be depressed and more likely to experience improvement in depressive symptoms over time (Koenig et al. 1992b).

Personality pathology is another measurable phenomenon that is known to affect the outcome of major depression (Weissman et al. 1978). Unfortunately, there are no published reports of personality as a predictor of major depression outcome in the elderly. In addition, studies done so far in mixed-aged samples have generally been confounded by the interaction of depressive symptomatology and personality variables at baseline assessment—that is, a depressed affect may influence the underlying personality. Given the stability of personality in late life, longitudinal studies of personality relationships to both the onset and outcome of major depression would be most helpful.

The outcome of bipolar disorder in the elderly remains virtually unknown. Winokur (1975), in a long-term follow-up study of 500 patients in Iowa, found a tendency for bipolar disorder to occur in clusters over time and speculated that early-onset bipolar illness may "burn itself out" with time. Shulman and Post (1980), in a study of elderly patients with bipolar disorder, found that only 8% had their first episode of mania before age 40. In a review of a small number of untreated patients with severe and prolonged bipolar disorder, Cutler and Post (1982) found a tendency for more rapid recurrences late in the history of the illness, with decreasing periods of normality. In other words, if bipolar disorder reemerges in the later years, then the episodes of mania—or mania mixed with depression—may once again tend to cluster, as the disorder typically clusters at earlier periods of life. Most clinicians who have worked with patients with bipolar disorder in late life recognize the tendency for these disorders to recur frequently for periods of time, only to remit for an extended period.

Ameblas (1987) emphasized a relationship between life events and onset of mania, noting that stressful events were more likely to precede early- rather than late-onset mania. Likewise, Shulman

(1989) stressed that increased cerebral vulnerability due to organic insults (stroke, head trauma, other brain insults) played a stronger role than life events in precipitating late-onset mania (a factor that may also play a role in treatment resistance).

Controversy exists over whether age at onset of first manic episode affects response to treatment. Whereas Glasser and Rabins (1984) described no significant age-related differences in presentation or treatment response, Young and Falk (1989) reported that late-onset mania was associated with less intense activity level, lower sexual drive, and less disturbed thought processes; despite this, however, they found that older age was also associated with longer hospitalization, greater residual psychopathology, and poorer response to pharmacotherapy.

Risk Factors

The etiology of late-life affective disorders is undoubtedly multifactorial. Twin and family studies, along with studies of molecular genetics, provide strong evidence for a heritable contribution to the etiology of major depression and bipolar disorder (Egeland et al. 1987; Slater and Cowie 1971). Evidence that these genetic factors weigh heavily in the etiology of bipolar disorders in late life is virtually nonexistent, although the biological nature of this disorder would suggest some genetic contribution. Evidence from studies of unipolar depression in late life suggests that the genetic contribution is weaker in late-life depression than it is at earlier stages of the life cycle (Hopkinson 1964; Mendlewicz 1976; Schulz 1951). For example, Hopkinson (1964) found the risk for immediate relatives of patients with onset of depression after age 50 to be 8.3%, compared with 20.1% for relatives of patients with onset before age 50. Stenstedt (1959) found the risk for affective disorder among relatives of probands falling ill for the first time at the age of 60 or over to be 4%–5%, higher than expected but lower than the risk among relatives of manic-depressive probands earlier in life.

Associated with the genetic predisposition for depression is the observation that major depression is more common in women (Myers et al. 1984). Most studies that consider the distribution of major depression across the life span confirm the persistence of the 2:1 ratio of women to men into late life. However, there is no evidence for a genetic predisposition—that is, a sex-linked mode of inheritance—that would favor women in the onset of major depression. Nevertheless, even in the best-controlled studies, the gender difference in the prevalence of the more severe depressions persists. The operable factor or factors persist into the later years. It is possible, however, that women are more likely to admit and complain about their dysphoric feelings than are men, who are more likely to deny feelings and instead act them out (such as through alcoholism or suicide).

Another contributing factor to late-life depression may be selective changes that occur in the activity and metabolism of neurotransmitters with aging. For example, Robinson et al. (1971) analyzed the concentrations of norepinephrine and serotonin in the hindbrains of 55 psychiatrically normal subjects who died at various ages. The concentrations of both neurotransmitters decreased with age, but the metabolite 5-hydroxyindoleacetic acid and the enzyme monoamine oxidase were found to increase with age.

Dysregulation of the hypothalamic-pituitary-adrenal (HPA) axis is also thought to contribute to a predisposition for depression. An association between increased cortisol concentrations and depression has been recognized for many years: there is an increase throughout the 24-hour circadian excretion of cortisol in depressed patients (Sachar 1975). This led Carroll et al. (1981) to propose the DST as a laboratory test for melancholic depression. In a large study of men and women between the ages of 20 and 78, Rosenbaum et al. (1984) found that 18% of persons over the age of 65 were nonsuppressors of cortisol after administration of DST, compared with 9.1% of younger subjects. Whether this higher prevalence of nonsuppression reflects an increased propensity of older persons to suffer dysregulation of the HPA axis, or whether it may result from difficulty in absorbing or metabolizing dexamethasone, remains to be discovered.

Dysregulation of the thyroid axis as well as in growth hormone release has also been implicated in the etiology of depression in later life. Blunted responses of thyroid-stimulating hormone (TSH) to the administration of thyrotropin-releasing hormone (TRH) are found in many normal elderly subjects (Snyder and Utiger 1972) and in depressed patients (Targum et al. 1982). Secretion of growth hormone in the elderly occurs only during sleep, and may cease altogether (Finkelstein et al. 1972).

Drugs known to stimulate alpha-adrenergic receptors, such as clonidine, also affect the release of growth hormone, a response that has been shown to be blunted in patients with endogenous depression (Checkley et al. 1981).

Despite these numerous neurotransmitter and neuroendocrine changes that are common to old age and depressive illness, the relatively low prevalence of major depression and bipolar disorder in late life militates against the assumption that older persons are uniquely predisposed to the onset of melancholic or endogenous depressions. Thus, protective factors that are yet to be discovered may also be operative in late life.

A relatively new putative contributor to the etiology of depressive disorders is desynchronization of circadian rhythms. The cyclicity of depressive disorders suggests an underlying disruption of the normal biochemical and physiological circadian rhythms. Vogel et al. (1980) noted that the clinical features of depression, especially insomnia and diurnal variation of mood, suggest abnormalities in biological rhythms. The disruption of the sleep cycle with age (though this is the only circadian rhythm known to be dramatically affected by age) suggests the possibility that circadian problems contribute to the etiology of depression in late life. As age increases, there is a gradual diminution in total sleep time and a decrease in sleep continuity (Kupfer 1984; Ulrich et al. 1980). Endocrine secretion patterns, also associated with depression, are known to be less affected by the aging process (Lakatua et al. 1984).

Finally, social factors must be considered in the development of a risk model for depression in late life. Pfifer and Murrell (1986) examined the additive and interactive roles of six sociodemographic factors—three being from the domain of social resources and three being categories of life events—in the development of depressive symptoms. In a probability sample of more than 1,200 persons age 55 and older, 66 developed significant depressive symptoms (as measured by the CES-D scale) 6 months after an initial evaluation. Health and social support played both an additive and an interactive role in the onset of depressive symptoms, life events had weak effects, and sociodemographic factors did not contribute to depression onset. A weak support network in the presence of poor physical health placed older persons at an especially high risk for the onset of depressive symptoms. It must be recognized, however, that the occurrence of depressive symptoms is not analogous to the onset of a major depressive episode. Although the relationship between stressful life events and the onset of major depression across the life cycle has been established in a number of cross-sectional studies (Lloyd 1980), the relationship weakens when persons are studied longitudinally, as was observed in the Pfifer and Murrell study.

The interaction of social support and depression is more complex. Social support may contribute to the onset of major depression, it may contribute to the outcome of major depression, or it may in turn be affected by the depressive symptoms. Blazer (1983) tested the hypothesis that a major depressive disorder contributes to a decline in social support by studying 331 community subjects selected at random. Impaired support was associated with the presence of major depressive disorder at baseline. Thirty months later, however, the surviving subjects whose social supports had improved were nearly three times more likely to have been depressed earlier than were those whose social supports did not improve. In other words, major depressive disorder was a significant predictor of improvement in supports at follow-up.

Diagnosis and Differential Diagnosis of Late-Life Affective Disorders

Four clinical entities listed under the mood disorders in DSM-III-R are relevant to depression in the elderly: 1) bipolar disorder (manic, depressed, and mixed), 2) major depression (single episode, recurrent, with or without melancholia, with or without psychotic features), 3) dysthymic disorder (depressive neurosis), and 4) depression not otherwise specified (NOS), previously called "atypical depression"). Other DSM-III-R disorders, such as bereavement, adjustment disorder with depressed mood, and the organic mood syndrome, are likewise manifested by a depressive symptom picture. Still other psychiatric disorders are associated with depressive symptomatology as a central component of the clinical picture on occasions, such as organic mental disorders, paranoid disorders, sleep disorders, and hypochondriasis.

Bipolar Disorder

For a patient to qualify for a diagnosis of manic episode, DSM-III-R requires the inclusion of at least three classic manic symptoms, such as overactivity, pressure of speech, distractibility, decreased sleep (without feeling a need for sleep), overspending, and grandiosity. Mood, however, can be either elevated or irritable and may be labile or mixed in the affective presentation. Post (1978) found that most elderly patients with a bipolar disorder exhibited a depressive admixture with manic symptomatology. Spar et al. (1979) reported that manic elders are atypical in presentation, with dysphoric mood and denial of classic manic symptoms. As noted earlier, Shulman (1986) described the special problem of manic delirium. When an individual is experiencing a full-blown manic episode, cognitive functioning is difficult to test, yet perseverative behavior, catatonia-like symptoms, and even negativistic symptoms may emerge. The patient in manic delirium can demonstrate the delirium-like symptom of picking at imaginary objects. The differential diagnosis between a manic episode and an agitated depressive episode often cannot be disentangled except by virtue of a thorough examination of the longitudinal course and therapeutic response to medications.

Major Depressive Disorder

First-onset episodes of major depression in late life are common and often go untreated for months or even years. For this reason, many investigators have suggested that late-life depression is "masked" (Davies 1965; Lesse 1974; Salzman and Shader 1972). Some studies, however, suggest that older persons admit many feelings of sadness on self-rating scales for depression (Epstein 1976; Zung and Green 1972). In a more recent study (Blazer et al. 1987b) of hospitalized patients diagnosed as having major depressive episodes with melancholia, the criteria symptoms for depression and symptoms specifically associated with melancholia (or endogenous depression) did not differ between individuals in middle life and late life. Melancholic depression was a relatively frequent syndrome identified in the elderly and was symptomatically similar to that found among persons in middle age. Community surveys confirm that major depressive disorder is identified among the elderly when usual case-finding methods are applied across the life cycle (Meyers et al. 1984). Nevertheless, there is still some concern, based on poor correlations between observer- and self-rated symptom scores, that the elderly (African-American men, in particular) may conceal or deny symptoms on self-report (Koenig et al. 1992c; J. Lyness, personal communication, October 1993). Thus, considerable effort at symptom elicitation may be required to obtain an accurate assessment.

Seasonal Affective Disorder

Variants of classic major depression also occur among the elderly. One is seasonal affective disorder (Jacobsen et al. 1987). Diagnostic criteria for seasonal affective disorder include 1) a history of depression fulfilling Research Diagnostic Criteria (RDC; Spitzer et al. 1978) or DSM-III-R criteria for major depression, 2) a history of at least 2 consecutive years of fall/winter depressive episodes remitting in the spring or summer, and 3) the absence of other major psychiatric disorder or psychosocial explanations for the seasonal mood changes. These disorders are most difficult to treat with usual therapies and may be perpetuated by the use of tricyclic antidepressants. Specifically, tricyclic antidepressants are thought to increase the likelihood of rapid cycling. In contrast, lithium carbonate or carbamazepine may be of some benefit in preventing the cyclic episodes. Light therapy, using high-intensity light to approximate the visual experience of a sunny day (usually in the morning), has been proved to be of some value in the treatment of patients with these disorders.

Psychotic Depression

Late-onset psychotic depression deserves special attention. Meyers et al. (1984) compared the prevalence of delusions between individuals who suffered the onset of depression before and after the age of 60 in 50 patients hospitalized for endogenous major depression. Depressive patients with onset after age 60 had delusions more frequently than did those with earlier onset. Individuals with delusional depression tended to be older and to respond to ECT as opposed to tricyclic antidepressants. Delusions of persecution or of having an incurable illness are more common than delusions associated with guilt. If guilt predominates the delusional picture, it usually involves some relatively trivial episode that oc-

curred many years before the onset of the depressive episode, forgotten over time, but presently viewed as a major problem (Bridges 1986). For example, a one-time sexual liaison, forgotten or forgiven by the spouse, is resurrected by the patient with a fear of an ongoing venereal disease or cancer, or is associated with chronic and severe pain. Nihilistic delusions (delusions of nothingness) may occur more commonly in late life. Focus on the abdomen is common in the elderly patient with a delusional or psychotic depression. Hallucinations are uncommon, however.

Dysthymic Disorder

Every clinician who has worked with elderly patients has observed significant and unremitting depressive symptoms associated with apparently psychosocial causes. Verwoerdt (1976) suggested that "reactive depressions" become more frequent with aging (such as the depression associated with bereavement), whereas dysthymic disorder (depressive neurosis) seems to be less frequent in the later part of the life cycle. More recent community data, however, suggest that the prevalence of dysthymic disorder in the elderly is lower, but not dramatically lower, in contrast to what is seen with major depression (Myers et al. 1984).

The psychological mechanisms of late-life dysthymic disorder usually do not include the classic mechanism of dysthymia—that is, self-reproach, guilt, and the turning inward of hostile feelings toward loss. Cath (1965) noted that manifest guilt in older persons is less prevalent, although reaction to loss is a common factor. Busse et al. (1954) suggested that among the elderly, introjection is seldom a mechanism for developing depression. Instead, late-life depression is associated with a loss of self-esteem that results from the older adult's inability to supply needs and drives or to defend himself or herself against threats to security. Levin (1965) noted the role of restraint as a mechanism in the neurotic depressions of later life. Although sexual satisfaction and interest in sexuality continue to be important for the older adult, sexual drive, though persistent, may not at times be as easily mobilized into behavior. Restraint may derive from either physical problems or lack of an available partner.

Other investigators have emphasized the cultural factors that may contribute to a dysthymic disorder in late life. Wigdor (1980) noted that the major resources in our culture lead to the development of habit patterns that emphasize activity and productivity—that is, ours is an achievement-oriented society. With retirement from the work force and cessation of parenting responsibilities, recognition, self-esteem, and confidence for many are withdrawn. These needs are not easily substituted. Erikson (1950) suggested that the primary developmental task for late life is the acquisition of integrity, and that the means for achieving integrity is to resolve previous developmental crises that have persisted through the life cycle. In other words, striving for industry and generativity may continue to be important for the older adult. If the opportunities for realizing these productive urges are unavailable or the elder cannot reconcile previous generative disappointments, then despair will ensue.

Lazarus and Weinberg (1980), emphasizing the role of narcissistic pathology in the etiology of late-life depression, note that narcissism may manifest itself in

> recurring depressions or defensive grandiosity in response to minor slights or disappointments, self-consciousness, overdependence on approval from others for maintenance of self-esteem, and the transitory periods of fragmentation and discohesiveness of the self. (p. 435)

Associated with the depressive symptoms are an overconcern with physical appearance, possessions, and past accomplishments, and the seeking of approval and reassurance from others.

In summary, dysthymic disorders in the elderly, although no more common than at other stages of the life cycle, are to be expected, given the psychological tasks that older adults face, along with a social environment that may restrain and devalue elders. That the elder maintains a sense of satisfaction and fulfillment given these inevitable losses and responses from others is a testimony to the resilience of older adults and a psychological integration that permits a mature completion of life's developmental tasks.

Depression NOS

Another subtype of depression in the elderly is codified under DSM-III-R nomenclature as "depression not otherwise specified" (depression NOS). This subtype of depression (in DSM-III called "atypical depression") is more often intermittent and unexplained by psychosocial or clear biological factors. Two subcategories for depression NOS empirically capture the symptom pattern frequently seen by clinicians who work with depressed elders. First, the syndrome may fulfill the criteria for dysthymic disorder; however, there are intermittent periods of normal mood lasting more than a few months. The dysphoric older adult reports prolonged periods of depression, usually lasting a period of months but not extending for the entire 2 years required for DSM-III-R dysthymic disorder. Other elders fill the second criterion for depression NOS: a brief episode of depression that does not meet the criteria for major depression and is apparently not reactive to psychosocial stress (so that it cannot be classified as an adjustment disorder). These episodes do not meet criteria, for they do not last the full 2 weeks required for DSM-III-R diagnosis of major depression. Nevertheless, the symptoms can be moderately severe and most troubling to the older adult. The possibility that pharmacological intervention will be effective in treating elders with depression NOS cannot be eliminated. Nevertheless, the difficulty in describing the heterogeneous phenomenology of the depressive syndromes subsumed under this category must be overcome if effective drug trials can be implemented.

Bereavement

Bereavement is a universal human experience and therefore cannot be properly classified as a psychiatric disorder. Primary care physicians are likely to encounter the normal symptoms of grief, but these may be poorly recognized as such by the bereaved elder. Lindemann (1944), for example, suggested that the normal symptoms of bereavement include sensations of somatic distress such as tightness in the throat, shortness of breath, sighing respirations, lassitude, and loss of appetite. The bereaved are preoccupied with the image of the deceased and frequently can identify events from which they report guilt (often guilt at not having met the needs of the deceased). The grieving are often irritable and hostile, and change their usual patterns of conduct. These behavior changes are disturbing to the family and include a pressure of speech, restlessness, an inability to sit still, and a lack of capacity to initiate and maintain usual activities. Pathological grief, in contrast, is delayed (an apparent denial of the loss) and/or distorted. Overactivity without a sense of loss, acquisition of symptoms belonging to the last illness of the deceased, frank psychosomatic illness, an alteration of relationships with family and friends, hostility toward specific persons (not uncommonly, family members), and persistent loss of patterns of social interaction can be seen.

The DSM-III-R description of uncomplicated bereavement has not improved on Lindemann's classic description. Uncomplicated bereavement is usually characterized by a symptom picture of major depression, yet the syndrome is recognized by the older adult as normal to the occasion and does not seriously interfere with necessary function. DSM-IV designates the category of uncomplicated bereavement to virtually all symptoms of depression experienced during the first 2 months after the loss, with the possible exception of extreme feelings of worthlessness or active suicidal ideation; any person fulfilling the full symptom picture of major depression at or beyond 2 months from the death is recognized as having a major depressive disorder warranting treatment (American Psychiatric Association 1994). For additional discussion of bereavement, see Chapter 17, "Bereavement and Adjustment Disorders."

Adjustment Disorder With Depressed Mood

Among the common presentations of depression in late life is the onset of a depressed mood and expressions of hopelessness as a reaction to an identifiable stressor. The DSM-III-R category of adjustment disorder with depressed mood is reserved for those individuals who exhibit a maladaptive reaction to an identifiable stressor, yet the relationship of the syndrome to the stressful event is clear. Stressors for older adults include life events such as marital problems, difficulty with children, loss of a social role, and an ill-advised change of residence. Retirement is usually not a source of excessive stress for the older adult. Therefore, the onset of significant depressive symptomatology and withdrawal from activities after retirement may indicate a true adjustment disorder. Of much greater frequency, however, is the development of depressive symptomatology secondary to a physical illness. When an episode of de-

pression accompanies a physical illness and exceeds dramatically the level of symptoms expected, then the diagnosis of adjustment disorder is indicated.

Organic Mood Syndrome

The final depressive category of relevance is the organic mood syndrome (in DSM-IV called "mood disorder due to a general medical condition" or "substance-induced mood disorder"). The essential feature of this syndrome is a disturbance in mood resembling a major depressive episode due to a specific organic factor. The most common toxic factors that cause depressive symptoms in older adults are medications. Agents frequently prescribed to older adults that can precipitate depressive symptoms include beta-blockers, benzodiazepines, clonidine, reserpine, methyldopa, and even tricyclic antidepressants. Withdrawal of these agents produces a dramatic improvement in symptoms, although both patient and clinician may not associate these medications with the onset of the symptoms. Mild cognitive impairment is often observed in conjunction with the change in mood. Fearfulness, anxiety, irritability, and excessive somatic concerns may accompany the depressive symptoms as well. Metabolic disorders induce appreciable depressive symptoms, and these are properly classified in DSM-III-R under the category of the organic mood syndrome. For example, hyperthyroidism and hypothyroidism are known to be associated with depressive features. These disorders are included below in the discussion of physical illnesses that may contribute to a depressive episode.

Depression and Medical Illness

Depressive disorders have been documented to be associated with a variety of physical illnesses, including cardiovascular disease (Dovenmuehle and Verwoerdt 1962), endocrine disturbances (Relkin 1969), Parkinson's disease (Mayeux et al. 1986), stroke (Robinson et al. 1990), diabetes (Lustman et al. 1988), cancer (Massie and Holland 1990), chronic pain (Krishnan et al. 1985), chronic fatigue syndrome (Kruesi et al. 1989), and fibromyalgia (Hudson et al. 1985). As noted previously, depressive symptoms and disorders are common findings in surveys of general medical inpatients (Koenig et al. 1988a, 1991; Schwab et al. 1965). Controversy continues over the degree to which acute or chronic medical illnesses cause depression because of direct physiological effects on the brain or because of a psychological reaction to the disability and other life changes evoked by these illnesses (Koenig 1991).

The association between depression and *hypothyroidism* has been well established. Although the profoundly life-threatening symptoms of myxedema—stupor or coma—are rarely missed in diagnosis, less severe symptoms and signs are common with normal aging and major depression. These include constipation, cold intolerance, psychomotor retardation, decreased exercise tolerance, and cognitive changes, as well as a depressed affect. Laboratory evaluation will generally reveal a depressed thyroxine and elevated serum TSH concentration. When this laboratory finding is identified, intervention for the thyroid difficulty must precede intervention for the depressive affect.

Depressive symptoms have also been associated with both the development and outcome of *cancer*. Early in modern medicine, Guy (1759) published his opinion that women with melancholia were more prone to develop breast cancer. Whitlock and Siskind (1979) studied 39 men and 90 women age 40 and older who had a primary diagnosis of depression. The subjects were followed from 28 months to 4 years. During the follow-up period, 9 men and 9 women died, 6 from cancer—a significantly higher number than would have been expected. Depression may also result from a direct effect on the brain of neurohumoral substances released from the tumor (pancreatic cancer), or as a reaction to the diagnosis of cancer and the morbidity that ensues.

Massie and Holland (1990) note that at least 25% of hospitalized patients with cancer meet the criteria for major depression disorder or adjustment disorder with depressed mood. Physical function is highly correlated with depression in such patients. In one study (Bukberg et al. 1984), among patients with a Karnofsky score of 40 or less (most disabled), almost 80% had major depression, whereas among those who scored 60 or better (moderate to good function), only 23% had major depression. Lower rates of depression are found in ambulatory outpatients with cancer (5%–13%) (Koenig and Blazer 1992). Many studies documenting high rates of depression in patients with cancer are controversial because they often involve patients referred for treatment of cancer, who may have more advanced

or complicated cases. Massie and Holland (1990) admit, however, that depression is no more common in patients with cancer than in patients with other severe medical illnesses. Thus, certain myths about depression and cancer must be dispelled: first, that "all cancer patients are depressed" and second, that "physicians should not bother to treat depression, because such patients *should* be depressed." Among hospitalized elders with cancer, at least one study has shown substantially higher mortality in cancer patients with major depression compared with nondepressed cancer patients (Koenig et al. 1989).

Dovenmuehle and Verwoerdt (1962) found that 64% of 62 patients with *cardiac disease,* 41 of whom were more than 60 years of age, developed moderate to severe depressive symptoms. More recently, Schleifer and colleagues (1989) conducted structured psychiatric interviews (Schedule for Affective Disorders and Schizophrenia [SADS; Endicott and Spitzer 1978]) in 283 patients (mean age 64 years) admitted to the coronary care unit for myocardial infarction 8–10 days after infarction and then again 3–4 months later. Initially, 45% met the diagnostic criteria for minor or major depression, including 18% with major depression. By 3–4 months later, 33% of patients continued to meet the criteria for depression, including 77% of those who had initially met the criteria for major depression. In another study, Frasure-Smith et al. (1993) followed 222 patients for 6 months after myocardial infarction; depression was a significant predictor of mortality (hazard ratio 5.7; $P < .001$), even after other relevant risk factors were controlled.

The impact of physical illness on emotion can be more direct. Evidence is emerging that a neurology of depression exists (Coffey 1987). The right hemisphere may be uniquely specialized for the perception, experience, and expression of emotion. Consistent differences have been observed in the emotional behavior of individuals who have suffered either left- or right-hemispheric *stroke.* A left-sided stroke may be associated with depressive and even catastrophic responses manifested by combinations of dysphoria, episodes of crying, feelings of despair, hopelessness, anger, and self-depreciation (Gainotti 1972; Robinson et al. 1990; Sackheim et al. 1982). A lesion of the right cerebral hemisphere is more often followed by a neutral or indifferent—or even euphoric—response, with denial of deficits and social disinhibition. Although exceptions exist to the findings from these studies, the recognition that selective lesions of the brain may contribute to specific syndromes that are closely associated with the depressive disorders implies, in some cases, an anatomy of depression rather than generalized neurochemical abnormalities.

Depression is a frequent accompaniment of *Parkinson's disease,* with prevalence rates ranging from 20%–90%; Mayeux (1990) determined a rate of 50% after reviewing the medical records of 339 patients with the disease. Most older persons differ little in the physical symptoms and signs of paralysis agitans from persons observed at earlier ages. The major problems encountered in treating the older adult with Parkinson's disease are secondary to either undue sensitivity to medications or the emotional state of the patient. The older adult with parkinsonism may become disoriented and aggressive and experience ideas of persecution. More commonly, the elder withdraws socially and expresses helplessness and hopelessness regarding the future and considerable anger regarding the difficulties in adjusting doses of medication (Carter 1986). Slow movement, weakness, rigidity, and masked and unexpressive facial expressions suggest to the clinician a depressed affect associated with the progression of Parkinson's disease. However, the appearance of depression may be more severe than the actual affect indicates. Clinicians must be judicious in determining the necessity of pharmacological intervention in the patient with Parkinson's disease.

Nevertheless, depression in patients with Parkinson's disease seldom disappears spontaneously, and many patients improve with treatment. Recent studies indicate that serotonin metabolism may be affected in such patients (Mayeux 1990). Not only is there profound loss of dopamine-containing neurons in the substantia nigra, there is also cell loss in the serotonin pathway into the limbic and diencephalon areas in the nucleus of the dorsal raphe. Other work has shown a decreased level of serotonin metabolites (5-hydroxyindoleacetic acid [5-HIAA]) in the cerebrospinal fluid of some depressed patients with Parkinson's disease, although this finding is controversial (Mayeux et al. 1984). Also, ECT has been shown to produce a transient relief of both depression and motor symptoms in patients with Parkinson's disease. It is likely that the etiology of depression in these patients is multifactorial, depending on the patient's premorbid personality

characteristics, on the history of depression, on the degree of functional disability induced by the disease, and on biological changes in the brain that are induced by Parkinson's disease.

Vitamin B_{12} (cobalamin) deficiency has long been associated with depressive symptoms. In a study (Lindenbaum et al. 1988) of 141 patients with neuropsychiatric abnormalities due to cobalamin deficiency, 28% had no anemia or microcytosis on the initial evaluation. Characteristic features of cobalamin deficiency in these patients included a variety of neurological symptoms (neurosensory loss, ataxia, and memory loss) as well as weakness, fatigue, and depressive symptoms. Most of these patients were over the age of 65, and the distribution between men and women was equal. All but one of the patients in this study responded to cobalamin therapy with improvement in their neuropsychiatric symptoms, including depressed mood. Bell and colleagues (1991) compared B-complex vitamin status at time of admission in 20 geriatric and 16 young adult nonalcoholic inpatients with major depression. Twenty-eight percent of all of these subjects were deficient in B_2 (riboflavin), B_6 (pyridoxine), and/or B_{12}. None were deficient in B_1 (thiamine) or folate. Patients with psychotic depression had lower B_{12} levels than did patients with nonpsychotic depression.

The association between *chronic pain* and depression has been established for many years (Blumer and Heilbronn 1982; Kraemlinger et al. 1983). The evidence for this association is based on the increased frequency of depression among patients with chronic pain and the frequent reports of pain by depressed patients, coupled with the high concurrence of biological markers of depression and markers for chronic pain. Krishnan et al. (1985) found that most items on a typical depression rating scale, such as the Hamilton Rating Scale for Depression (Hamilton 1960), did not discriminate patients with major depression from those with chronic low back pain. Nevertheless, the items discriminated well between patients with and without depression. France et al. (1984) studied a group of 42 patients with chronic pain in an attempt to unravel the relationship between chronic pain and depression. These investigators found that 41% of those with major depression were nonsuppressors of cortisol in response to a challenge with dexamethasone, yet all patients without major depression had normal

DST. In general, chronic pain does not become more prevalent with aging, but many older persons do suffer from specific and rather severe chronic pain syndromes, such as pain from cancer or severe osteoarthritis. The clinician must distinguish the patient with chronic pain from the individual with hypochondriasis (in which the interrelationship with depressive symptoms may be different).

Normal Aging

The differential diagnosis of late-life depression must include not only other psychiatric and physical disorders but also the changes of normal aging. Some investigators associate a depressed mood with aging. However, most longitudinal studies of depression and life satisfaction do not validate this assumption. Although Busse et al. (1954) found that elderly subjects were aware of more frequent and more annoying depressive periods than they had experienced earlier in life, only a small number admitted to severe and protracted periods of depression. Approximately 85% of the subjects in this study were able to trace the onset of these depressive episodes to specific stimuli. Epidemiological data (see Chapter 9) confirm that the frequency of severe late-life depression (major depression) is lower than at earlier stages of the life cycle.

Life satisfaction, morale, and adjustment were not found to decline in a 4-year longitudinal study of an elderly cohort (Palmore and Kivett 1977). Rather, life satisfaction is associated with health status, socioeconomic status, social participation, income, and living arrangements (Thomae 1980). Poor life satisfaction may be correlated with depressive symptoms, yet these two constructs must be considered independently. Severe clinical depression can occur within the context of satisfaction with one's life and adjustment to one's situation. On the other hand, dissatisfaction with life and demoralization may be manifested as poor self-esteem, helplessness and hopelessness, sadness, confused thinking, and so forth, yet never progress to the point at which the syndrome could adequately be described as meeting criteria for a psychiatric disorder. Rather, discouragement and dissatisfaction are typical of the elder who, as described by Frank (1973), "finds that he cannot meet the demands placed on him by the environment, and cannot extricate himself from his predicament" (p. 312).

The normal biological changes of aging may interact with depressive symptomatology as well. Older persons, for example, spend more time lying in bed at night either without attempting to sleep or unsuccessfully trying to sleep, and therefore complain of decreased sleep efficiency. Rapid eye movement (REM) sleep latency, a marker that has been associated with depression (see "Primary Sleep Disorder," below), is also known to decrease slightly throughout life in both sexes (Dement et al. 1982). Elderly persons are notorious for complaining of poor appetite and reduced food intake. Munro (1981) found that caloric intake falls with aging. Poor dentition may contribute to decreased food intake as well. Taste acuity also decreases with increasing years (Schiffman 1979). Lethargy is another common complaint of older adults.

Organic Mental Disorders

Among the psychiatric disorders, the most common problem in the differential diagnosis of depression is presented by the organic mental disorders. Pseudodementia is a syndrome in which dementia is mimicked or caricatured by a functional psychiatric illness, most commonly depression (Wells 1979). Patients with pseudodementia respond on the mental status examination similarly to those who suffer from true degenerative brain disease. Although the condition is not rare among elderly persons, Kiloh (1961) reminded clinicians that the term pseudodementia is "purely descriptive and carries no diagnostic weight," and yet patients with pseudodementia are in danger of inaccurate diagnosis and therapeutic neglect. Wells (1979) distinguished depression presenting as pseudodementia from true dementia by the rapid onset of the cognitive problems in depression, the relatively short duration of symptoms, the consistent depressed mood associated with cognitive difficulties, and a tendency among depressed patients to highlight disabilities as opposed to concealing (or attempting to conceal) them. The depressed older adult is more likely to respond with "I don't know" on the mental status exam, whereas the demented elder is more likely to attempt answers or to attempt to deflect the questions. Cognitive impairment in depression fluctuates from one exam to another, whereas cognitive impairment in dementia is relatively stable.

Of greater clinical importance, however, is the

frequent overlap of depressive symptoms and symptoms of the organic mental disorders. Grinker et al. (1961) noted impaired recent memory in 21% and poor remote memory in 14% of persons of all ages with depressive disorders who were studied. Reifler et al. (1982) studied 88 cognitively impaired elderly outpatients and found that depression was superimposed on dementia in 17 (19%). Patients with greater cognitive impairment exhibited fewer symptoms of depression. When treated with an antidepressant, patients responded with a remission of the depressive symptoms, yet the cognitive dysfunction persisted. Likewise, Alexopoulos and colleagues (1993) followed 23 elderly depressed patients with "reversible dementia" and 34 depressed elders without dementia for an average of 34 months after treatment; irreversible dementia developed significantly more often in the depressed group with reversible dementia (43%) than in the group with depression alone (12%). These researchers concluded that depression and a reversible dementia in elderly patients often indicates the presence of an early dementing illness.

Work done specifically with Alzheimer's patients has shown a concurrent diagnosis of major depression in 20%–30% (Reifler et al. 1986). Both depressed and nondepressed Alzheimer's patients were treated with the relatively potent anticholinergic antidepressant imipramine; patients improved whether or not they were in the treatment group, and cognitive function did not decline (Reifler et al. 1989). Greenwald and colleagues (1989) reported that the treatment of both nondemented and demented depressed elderly individuals resulted in an improvement of both depression and cognitive impairment.

The diagnostic problems may be more complex, however. Specifically, there may be actual cerebral changes in depression that contribute to the dementia-like syndromes that are seen in some depressed older adults (Thielman and Blazer 1986). Although, in the presence of significant depressive symptoms, older adults may not spontaneously complain of difficulty with memory and concentration more frequently than do persons at earlier stages of the life cycle, they do have more difficulty performing on mental status examinations (Blazer et al. 1986).

Schizophrenia

Given the propensity of older adults to exhibit more psychotic features during an episode of major depression, the appearance of an overt psychosis with delusional thinking suggests for many clinicians the onset of a major depressive episode. The discovery of paranoid ideation and delusions, however, may be evidence of a late-life schizophrenic disorder. Older adults with late-life schizophrenia-like symptoms generally do not become profoundly depressed. Rather, they are distressed and focus all of their difficulties on a perceived hostile environment. Although family members or physicians are often surprised to discover these symptoms, paranoid ideation and delusional thinking in a schizophrenia-like illness rarely begin suddenly but instead evolve gradually. An inquiry into the history of the disorder uncovers gradual withdrawal, bizarre comments, and often elaborate preparations to ensure safety (such as multiple locks on the door, bars on the windows, or stockpiling of food). The source of threat gradually moves from outside to within, such as a perception of being sexually molested, yet the paranoid elder rarely has a sense of poor self-worth.

Primary Sleep Disorder

Idiopathic sleep problems are often accompanied by depressive symptoms. The normal changes in sleep that mimic depressive sleep problems were reviewed previously. A number of sleep disorders also contribute to symptoms that mimic major depression. Delayed or advanced sleep phase syndrome—that is, the shift of the normal sleep cycle to later or earlier in the evening—is most disturbing to older persons who have previously viewed their sleep as a habitual given. The elder who, because of boredom or other conditions, begins a night's sleep at 8:00 or 9:00 P.M. will awaken at 2:00 or 3:00 in the morning and thus complain of "early-morning awakening." In addition, the anxiety inherent in awakening to a darkened home with no activity exacerbates the discomfort associated with a sleep phase syndrome.

Sleep apnea syndrome, which is more common with aging, may not be recognized by the older adult (especially if he or she lives alone; a spouse or sleeping partner cannot spend many nights with an apneic elder without recognizing that something is abnormal about the sleep pattern). However, the elder who suffers from sleep apnea typically will only complain of lethargy and vague concerns regarding sleep, including excessive sleep.

Hypochondriasis

Hypochondriasis is a frequent confounder of the differential diagnosis of the depressed older adult. Although the hypochondriacal elder may experience a depressed mood, the essential feature of hypochondriasis is an unrealistic interpretation of physical signs or sensations as abnormal, which in turn leads to a preoccupation with the fear or belief that one is suffering from a serious illness (American Psychiatric Association 1980). A number of investigators have reported the prevalence of "hypochondriacal symptoms" to be elevated among depressed elderly patients. De Alarcon (1964) found that, of 152 patients with depression, 65% of the men and 62% of the women reported concomitant hypochondriacal symptoms, the most common being constipation. Nevertheless, caution should be used when attributing presumed hypochondriacal complaints to depression in older adults with medical illness. Recent work suggests that among medically ill hospitalized patients, hypochondriacal and somatic complaints are equally common among depressed younger and depressed elderly patients when severity of medical illness is controlled (Koenig et al. 1993).

The concurrence of depressive and hypochondriacal symptoms may increase the risk of suicide. In de Alarcon's study (1964), 24.8% of individuals with hypochondriacal symptoms attempted suicide, whereas only 7.3% of those without such symptoms did so. Hypochondriasis as a disorder differs from hypochondriacal symptoms. True hypochondriasis usually can be distinguished from depression by the duration of the episode (hypochondriasis usually persists from middle life); the degree to which the patient appears to suffer from symptoms (the depressed appear to suffer more); and the cyclicity of symptoms (atypical of hypochondriasis but typical of depression). The endogenously depressed older adult with many somatic complaints will generally tolerate antidepressant medications as well as do other elders, whereas the hypochondriacal patient generally does not tolerate an antidepressant medication because of the anticholinergic side effects (Blazer 1984).

Anxiety

The differentiation of depression from primary anxiety syndromes such as generalized anxiety disorder and adjustment disorder with anxious mood is difficult because of the frequent coexistence of anxiety in late-life depression. Blazer and colleagues (1989) determined that early-morning anxiety was a symptom in nearly one-third of the elderly and middle-aged patients surveyed between 12 and 24 months after psychiatric admission for depression. Anxiety is a common symptom in persons with medical illness, especially cancer (Derogatis et al. 1983). Anxiety as a primary disorder can usually be distinguished from primary depression by the time course of symptom onset—anxiety precedes depressive symptoms. In addition, the patient with anxiety usually has a less depressed mood and more motor tension, autonomic hyperactivity, feelings of apprehension or worry, and hypervigilance.

Alcoholism

Alcoholism peaks in middle age and becomes less frequent in late life; nevertheless, between 3% and 10% of older persons fulfill criteria for a diagnosis of alcohol abuse or dependence. Symptoms of alcoholism that may mimic depression include cognitive changes, disturbed sleep, chronic fatigue, weight loss, and suicidal thoughts. Alcohol abuse or dependence may also coexist with depression, and many elders with late-onset alcoholism may actually use alcohol as a form of self-medication for their depressive symptoms. However, a diagnosis of depression in an alcoholic patient should not be made until the patient has been sober for at least 2 weeks, because alcohol withdrawal may include dysphoria and other depressive symptoms.

Diagnostic Workup of the Depressed Older Adult

Of special importance in evaluating the depressed elder is the assessment of the duration of the current depressive episode; the history of previous episodes; the history of drug and alcohol abuse; response to previous therapeutic interventions for the depressive illness; a family history of depression, suicide, and/or alcohol abuse; and the degree to which the older adult appears to be suffering from the depressive symptoms. Establishing some indication of the risk for suicide is essential, for suicidal risk may determine the location of treatment. The physical examination must include a thorough neurological examination to detect the presence of soft neurological signs (e.g., frontal release signs) or laterality. Weight loss and psychomotor retardation in the depressed older adult may lead, in some individuals, to a peroneal palsy, documented by electromyography and nerve conduction abnormalities (Massey and Bullock 1978). Because the older adult is less occupied with physical activities and therefore tends to be sedentary, the peroneal nerve is subject to chronic trauma.

The laboratory workup of the depressed older adult should include a thyroid panel (triiodothyronine, thyroxine, and radioactive iodine uptake) and TSH. If a supersensitive test is used, TSH levels can be relied on to detect both hypothyroidism and hyperthyroidism. TSH values between 5 and 10 μU/mL are suggestive of—and those above 10 μU/mL near-diagnostic for—hypothyroidism. TSH values below 1.0 μU/mL, and especially below 0.5 μU/mL, are suggestive of hyperthyroidism.

A blood screen enables the clinician to detect the presence of an anemia. Usually the evaluation of red cell size and abnormalities on the smear enables recognition of a potential deficit in vitamin B_{12} or folate. Although dementing illness is the most prominent outcome of a B_{12} deficiency, depressive symptoms may also result.

The use of psychological testing can assist the clinician in distinguishing permanent from temporary cognitive deficits, as well as in identifying potential laterality of cognitive abnormalities. Nevertheless, in the midst of severe depressive illness, psychological testing may be of less value. Therefore, timing the use of psychological testing is essential to maximize the value of test results in clinical decision making.

The laboratory evaluation of depression has entered a new era in the 1980s and 1990s. Depressive disorders that were once identified exclusively by clinical signs and symptoms can now be delineated by a combination of these signs and symptoms and so-called biological markers. Although no true laboratory test is available for the diagnosis of major depression (or even the subtypes of major depression), the use of the laboratory by clinicians as well as clinical investigators has increased dramatically.

The most-used—and the topic of most debate—of these laboratory tests is the DST. Based on the recognition of hyperactivity of the HPA axis in patients with depressive disorders, Carroll et al. (1981) sug-

gested a modified DST as a diagnostic aid for endogenous depression or melancholia. One milligram of dexamethasone is administered at 11:00 P.M. The next day, blood samples for the determination of plasma cortisol are drawn at 4:00 P.M. and 11:00 P.M. For outpatients, only the 4:00 sample would be drawn. An increased plasma concentration of cortisol in either of the blood samples signifies an abnormal, or positive, result. The cutoff in most laboratories for normal plasma cortisol concentration after dexamethasone administration is 5 g/dL with competitive protein-binding assays. In the original study by Carroll and colleagues, the test was nearly 50% sensitive and more than 90% specific for endogenous depression. Since the initial introduction of the DST, many investigators have replicated these results. Two factors have emerged from these investigations, however, that bear attention. First, the DST may not be as specific as originally believed, since persons with other psychiatric disorders also exhibited a positive DST. In addition, a number of conditions may contribute to false-positive results, such as physical illness (Cushing's disease, pregnancy, diabetes mellitus), medications (barbiturates, meprobamate, phenytoin), low body weight, ongoing weight loss (which frequently accompanies depressive illness), and acute infectious illnesses with fever and dehydration.

The DST has been studied extensively in elderly populations. Magni et al. (1986) found a sensitivity of 73% for major depressive disorder among hospitalized depressed elders, with only 11% of the control subjects and 11% of the persons with dysthymic disorder having an abnormal DST. Jenike and Albert (1984) found that among persons with mild cognitive impairment secondary to Alzheimer's disease, the DST was useful in distinguishing the depressed from the nondepressed patients. When they included the more severely demented subjects, however, the DST was less specific. Tourigny-Rivard et al. (1981) did not find that advanced age affected the overnight DST in healthy normal adults, and they therefore suggested that the test would be equally useful for the young and the elderly. In general, however, investigators believe that nonsuppression after dexamethasone increases gradually with age, and so the usefulness of the DST probably diminishes with increasing age, especially in persons over age 75.

A second biological marker that has received

increased attention is the use of sleep electro-encephalogram (EEG) results to identify depression. Generally, 2 nights of sleep recording are obtained after patients have been drug free for 14 days, and mean data from the 2 nights are used for the study. REM density and REM latency have both been proposed as potential markers for depression (Kupfer et al. 1978). Compared with control subjects, endogenously depressed patients appear to show increased sleep discontinuity (that is, a disruption of the sleep architecture); reduced slow-wave sleep (stages 3 and 4); shortened REM latency (the time between the onset of sleep and the first REM period); and increased REM density (the ratio of the sum of eye movements to the length of time of REM sleep). Those trends in the sleep EEG that appear to mark endogenous depression are, as described above, trends that often accompany the normal aging process. However, the combined use of sleep EEG tracings and other markers may help to increase the probability of identifying the more biologically derived depressive disorders.

Attention has been directed in recent years to platelet-binding density of tritiated imipramine as a marker of depressive illness. A number of reports have suggested that the maximal density (B_{max}) of platelet imipramine-binding sites is lowered in unmedicated subjects who have a unipolar affective disorder (Asarch et al. 1981; Briley et al. 1980). In contrast to the DST, which is associated with decreased specificity with aging, tritiated imipramine binding may actually be a more specific test for endogenous depression in the elderly than in younger control subjects (Knight et al. 1986; Schneider et al. 1985). In the study by Knight and colleagues, in which subjects between the ages of 35 and 50 were compared with subjects 60+ years of age, the number of tritiated imipramine platelet binding sites was reduced in patients with major depression. Imipramine binding was particularly well correlated with depression in elderly patients, and it remained normal in subjects with other neuropsychiatric disorders such as Alzheimer's disease and schizophrenia.

Another marker that has been associated with depression throughout the life cycle is platelet mono-amine oxidase activity. In a study by Schneider et al. (1986), platelet monoamine oxidase activity was found to be significantly higher in elderly depressed women than in gender- and age-comparable control subjects. There were no significant relationships between monoamine oxidase activity and duration of the current depressive episode, lifetime duration of the illness, or family history.

Another potential marker for biological depression is platelet alpha$_2$-adrenoceptors. This marker may also be of value in studying depression in late life, as neither binding capacity nor affinity of alpha$_2$-adrenoceptors on platelets is known to be correlated specifically with age (Buckley et al. 1986).

A more thoroughly studied marker that may have both diagnostic and therapeutic implications is the blunted TSH response to TRH. TRH stimulates the release of TSH from the anterior pituitary gland. The TRH test—the measurement of serum TSH concentration after administration of TRH—has become a standard test in endocrinology. Administration of synthetic TRH challenges the anterior pituitary to respond. Differential response in the serum TSH may characterize disorders of the HPA axis. Although TSH blunting is not specific to depression, a number of studies have shown that TSH is blunted in patients with depression (Gregoire et al. 1977; Loosen and Prange 1982). However, increasing age is also known to be associated with a blunted TSH response to TRH (Snyder and Utiger 1972). Because of this abnormality, supplemental thyroid has been prescribed to depressed persons, with occasional beneficial response. For example, liothyronine sodium, 25 g/day, could augment the therapeutic effects of the traditional tricyclic antidepressants. This augmentation may be valuable in the treatment of some elders, since subclinical hypothyroidism occasionally contributes to depression in older adults. The first step, however, is a more thorough workup and the use of thyroid agents alone to determine if the depressive symptoms are solely determined by hypothyroidism.

Given the emergence of an ever-increasing list of potential markers—some to be investigated further, some yet to be discovered, and some that will be dropped from the list because they are not useful for clinical purposes—what is the best way for the clinician to integrate these markers into clinical practice? First, clinicians should recognize that the primary utility of such markers is in probing the biological contribution to the depressive disorders of late life. None of these biochemical, neuroendocrinological, or circadian abnormalities qualifies as a biological test for a psychiatric disorder at present. They may never reach this status, because the etiology of late-life depression is multidetermined, with no clear evidence that one factor is necessary for symptoms to emerge. Nevertheless, these markers may be considered analogous to symptoms, in that they can be included in the data collected to increase the probability of delineating a real psychopathological entity that can be effectively diagnosed and treated, and the outcome of which can be predicted.

Treatment

The treatment of depression in late life is four-pronged, and includes psychotherapy, pharmacotherapy, ECT, and family therapy. Because pharmacotherapy is covered in some detail in Chapter 20 ("Pharmacological Treatment in the Elderly"), we emphasize the remaining three therapeutic approaches here.

Psychotherapy

Cognitive-behavior therapy is the only psychotherapy that has been designed specifically to treat depression (Beck et al. 1979). Even the more recent technique of interpersonal therapy (Klerman et al. 1984) is primarily a cognitive-behavioral orientation to improving interpersonal relationships. The advantage of cognitive-behavior therapy in treating the older adult is that it is directive and time limited, usually requiring between 10 and 25 sessions for completion. Cognitive-behavior therapy has been studied specifically in the elderly (Gallagher and Thompson 1982; Steuer et al. 1984).

The goal of the behavioral and cognitive therapies is to change behavior and modes of thinking. This change is accomplished through behavioral interventions such as weekly activity schedules, mastery and pleasure logs, and graded task assignments. Cognitive approaches to restructuring negative cognitions or automatic thoughts include subjecting these cognitions to empirical reality testing, examining distortions (such as overgeneralizations, catastrophizing, and dichotomous thinking), and generating new ways of viewing one's life (Steuer et al. 1984). Depressed patients typically regard themselves and their present and future in somewhat idiosyncratic or negative ways. Such patients believe themselves to be inadequate or defec-

tive and believe that unpleasant experiences are caused by a problem with themselves, and that they are, therefore, worthless, helpless, and hopeless. This cognitive triad leads the older adult to believe that he or she has a never-ending depression and that nothing pleasant will ever happen again. The cognitive model presupposes that these symptoms of depression are consequences of negative thinking patterns.

Thompson and colleagues (1987) randomly assigned 91 elders with major depression to either cognitive therapy, behavioral therapy, or brief dynamic therapy (a treatment that stresses the importance of the patient-therapist relationship and that emphasizes realistic collaborative aspects of the therapeutic alliance). Patients in each group received 16–20 sessions of therapy by expert clinicians; 20 additional patients were assigned to a waiting-list control group. By the end of 6 weeks, 52% of the patients in therapy were in complete remission, and 18% showed significant improvement. All therapies were equally efficacious and superior to no treatment.

Results from empirical studies (including the work of Gallagher and Thompson 1982; Thompson et al. 1987; Steuer et al. 1984) suggest that, compared with control subjects, those engaging in psychotherapy exhibit incremental improvement. Not only does the percentage of elders who respond to these treatments compare favorably with that of younger samples, the degree of improvement appears equal to that obtained with medications, especially with milder forms of depression. Because drug therapy is not appropriate for some elders, cognitive, behavioral, or brief dynamic psychotherapy provide viable alternatives. In addition, evidence has emerged that suggests that the long-term benefit of cognitive-behavior therapy may be greater than that of medications, especially if the medications are discontinued during the first year of treatment.

Older adults with minor depression or adjustment disorders, or those experiencing dysphoria because of losses of various types, often require less intensive forms of psychotherapy. Active listening and simple support may be sufficient to help distressed elders to better cope with their situation. Because religion is an important factor in the lives of many older adults, referral to a pastoral counselor may be particularly helpful and acceptable (Koenig 1993).

Pharmacotherapy

The tricyclic antidepressants remain the agents of choice for patients with the more severe forms of major depression. Medications that are effective yet relatively free of side effects (especially cardiovascular effects) are preferred. Nortriptyline and desipramine have become the more popular medications in recent years for treating older adults with endogenous or melancholic major depression, yet doxepin remains a favorite among many practitioners. It is recommended that all elderly patients have an electrocardiogram (ECG) before initiation of treatment and again after therapeutic blood levels have been achieved. Treatment with tricyclic antidepressants should not be initiated—or should be withdrawn in patients who are taking these medications—if the ECG shows a second-degree block or higher, a bifascicular bundle-branch block, a left bundle-branch block, or a QTc interval of greater than 480 milliseconds.

Although experience with newer antidepressants, such as the selective serotonin reuptake inhibitors (SSRIs) and bupropion, is relatively limited in elderly patients (especially in those with concurrent medical illness), these agents are quickly becoming the drugs of first choice for mild to moderate forms of depression. Their lack of anticholinergic, orthostatic, and cardiac side effects; lack of sedation; and safety in overdose are important advantages for use in the elderly. Nevertheless, for a significant number of older adults, the newer antidepressants cause other unacceptable effects, including excessive activation and disturbance of sleep, tremor, headache, significant gastrointestinal side effects, and weight loss.

The dosage of antidepressant medication for persons in late life should be case specific, but generally is less than for persons in middle life. For example, 25–50 mg of nortriptyline orally at bedtime or 25 mg of desipramine orally twice a day are frequently adequate in relieving depressive symptoms. Plasma levels of the medications can be helpful in determining dosing: nortriptyline levels between 50 and 150 ng/mL and desipramine levels greater than 125 ng/mL have been found to be therapeutic. Also found to be therapeutic in some patients—with the benefit of avoiding many side effects that might be experienced at higher doses—are fluoxetine doses as low as 5 mg every other day; sertraline, 25–

50 mg/day; paroxetine, 10 mg/day; or bupropion, 75 mg twice a day.

Trazodone is an alternative in patients who cannot tolerate tricyclics or one of the newer antidepressants. Trazodone has advantages over the tricyclic antidepressants in that it is virtually free of anticholinergic effects, and it has advantages over the newer antidepressants because of its strong sedative effects. Nevertheless, the drug is not without side effects, including excessive daytime sedation, priapism (occasionally), and significant orthostatic hypotension. Monoamine oxidase inhibitors (MAOIs) provide another alternative to tricyclics and the newer antidepressants. If MAOIs are considered when intolerance to side effects of other antidepressants ensues, it should be noted that older adults usually do not tolerate the MAOIs any better. If therapy with an MAOI is to follow therapy with an SSRI, a minimum of 1 or 2 weeks (for fluoxetine, 2–4 weeks) must elapse after discontinuing the SSRI before starting the MAOI to avoid a serotonergic syndrome. If a patient's depression is severe and ECT is contemplated, the use of an MAOI also precludes initiation of ECT until 10 days to 2 weeks after the drug is discontinued. Such a delay may seriously impede effective clinical management of the suicidal elder.

Some clinicians prescribe low morning doses of stimulant medications, such as 5 mg of methylphenidate, to improve the mood of the apathetic older adult. The effectiveness of stimulants has not been conclusively demonstrated. Nevertheless, these agents are generally safe at low doses, and rarely does the clinician encounter an elder with a propensity to abuse stimulants or to become addicted when these drugs are given on a once-a-day basis.

For further details regarding the treatment of the older adult with psychopharmacological agents, see Chapter 20.

Electroconvulsive Therapy

ECT continues as the most effective form of treatment available for patients with more severe major depressive episodes (Scovern and Kilmann 1980). The induction of a seizure appears to be the factor that is effective in reversing a major depression. ECT was first established as a treatment in 1938, but it is no longer used as much as it was immediately after its development (Weiner 1982). Despite its effectiveness, ECT is not the first-line treatment of choice for a patient with major depression and should be prescribed only because other therapeutic modalities have been ineffective. ECT has been shown to be effective in selected individuals, primarily those having major depression with melancholia, and especially those having major depression with psychotic symptoms associated with agitation or withdrawal. Many older adults with such syndromes either do not respond to antidepressant medications or experience toxicity (usually postural hypotension) when taking antidepressants. The presence of self-destructive behavior, such as a suicide attempt or refusal to eat, increases the necessity for intervening effectively; in such situations, ECT may be the treatment of choice.

If ECT is selected as an intervention, the clinician must first discuss in detail with the patient and the family the nature of the treatment and the reasons for this recommendation. Why is ECT necessary? What are the procedures that the patient will undergo during a course of ECT? How many treatments can be expected, and how long will the hospitalization continue? Can ECT be performed on an outpatient basis? What are the risks and side effects of ECT? What results, both immediate and long term, can be expected from the treatment? Even when the elderly patient is severely depressed, careful and thoughtful discussion with the patient and family will usually result in a willingness by the patient (often with encouragement from the family) to undergo the course of treatments. Once treatment is begun, the fears of ECT usually remit.

The medical workup before ECT includes a complete medical history, physical examination, and consultation with a cardiologist if any cardiac abnormalities are recognized. A family history of a psychiatric disorder, suicide, or treatment of a family member with ECT is helpful in predicting a successful response to treatment. Laboratory examination includes a complete blood count, a urinalysis, routine chemistries, chest and spinal X rays (the latter to document previous compression fractures), an electrocardiogram, and a computed tomography (CT) scan or magnetic resonance imaging (MRI). With CT or MRI available, an EEG and skull X ray are not routinely required. The presence of some abnormalities on MRI does not militate against the use of ECT, however. For example, a series of older adults with major depression were found to have subcor-

tical arteriosclerotic encephalopathy on MRI but promptly improved after undergoing ECT (Coffey et al. 1987).

To prepare the older adult for ECT, all medications should be withdrawn, if possible. As noted above, any MAOI must be withdrawn 10 days to 2 weeks before the procedure to prevent any toxic interactions or effects of this drug with the anesthetic used during ECT. Reserpine and anticholinesterase drugs should also be withdrawn for at least 1 week. Lithium carbonate, tricyclic antidepressants, antipsychotics, or antianxiety agents (including the sedative-hypnotics) are not absolutely contraindicated in patients who are to have ECT. Benzodiazepines, however, increase the seizure threshold and should be avoided. Generally, a short-acting barbiturate, such as 500 mg of chloral hydrate orally at bedtime, is the most appropriate sedative-hypnotic, although this drug should not be given on the night preceding ECT, if possible. The use of low-dose haloperidol or thiothixene is probably the most appropriate means of controlling severe agitation or psychotic symptoms.

The basic techniques for ECT are well described. Thirty minutes before treatment, an anticholinergic agent is administered intramuscularly to prevent complications of cardiac arrhythmias and aspiration. Directly before treatment, a short-acting anesthetic, such as thiopental or methohexital, is administered until an eyelash response is no longer present. Then a muscle relaxant, such as succinylcholine, is administered to prevent severe muscle contractions. Investigators now are increasingly using a unilateral electrode placement to the non-dominant cerebral hemisphere, since evidence has accumulated that there is less confusion after treatment with unilateral versus bilateral treatment. Nevertheless, unilateral electrode placement does not preclude the development of memory difficulties. (Some question the efficacy of unilateral versus bilateral electrode placement, but no evidence has accumulated that clearly establishes bilateral electrode placement as therapeutically superior to unilateral placement.) The electrical stimulus is applied, and the seizure is monitored either by applying a tourniquet to one arm and observing the tonic and clonic movements in the extremity peripheral to the tourniquet or by direct EEG monitoring. Direct EEG monitoring is preferred, and a seizure lasting 25 seconds or more is required for optimal results.

Seizure duration varies with age. In a study of 228 patients treated with ECT, Hinkle et al. (1986) found that of patients over the age of 60, a greater percentage were likely to have a seizure of 30 seconds or less. The use of caffeine may increase the likelihood of inducing a seizure without the necessity of restimulation with higher electrical parameters (which could lead to increased central nervous system toxicity).

ECT treatments are generally administered three times per week, and usually 6–12 treatments are necessary for an adequate therapeutic response. A clear improvement is often noted after one of the treatments, with the patient reporting a remarkable improvement in mood and functioning after that treatment. Two or three treatments are generally given after the ECT administration leading to improvement.

The risks and side effects of ECT in the elderly are similar to those in the general population. Cardiovascular effects are of most concern and include premature ventricular contractions, ventricular arrhythmias, and transient systolic hypertension. Multiple monitoring during treatment decreases the risk of one of these side effects leading (albeit infrequently) to permanent problems. Confusion and amnesia often result after a treatment, but the length of this confusional episode is brief. Even with the use of unilateral nondominant treatment, however, some patients suffer from prolonged memory difficulties. Headaches are a common symptom with ECT, but usually respond to nonnarcotic analgesics. Status epilepticus and vertebral compression fractures are some of the rare but more serious adverse effects. Compression fractures are a particular risk in older women because of the high incidence of osteoporosis in the postmenopausal population.

What can the clinician expect in terms of outcome from the use of ECT in older adults? The overall success rate of ECT in drug nonresponders is usually 80% or greater, and there is no evidence that effectiveness is lower for older adults (Avery and Lubrano 1979). Wesner and Winokur (1989) examined the influence of age on the natural history of major depressive disorder and found that ECT reduced the rate of chronicity when it was used in patients age 40 or over, but, surprisingly, not in those under age 40.

Unfortunately, the relapse rate with no prophylactic intervention after treatment may exceed 50%

in the year after a course of ECT. This relapse rate can be lowered if antidepressants or lithium carbonate is prescribed after the treatment. In some patients who exhibit a high likelihood of recurrence despite the use of prophylactic medication and/or who experience high toxicity and therefore cannot tolerate prophylactic medications, the use of maintenance ECT may be necessary. For such patients, weekly or monthly treatments (usually on an outpatient basis) are prescribed, with careful monitoring of response and side effects.

Despite the effectiveness of ECT, few deny that treatment may lead to memory difficulties. In a study by Frith et al. (1983), 70 severely depressed patients were randomly assigned to receive eight real or sham ECT treatments, and were divided on the basis of the degree of recovery from depression afterward. Compared with nondepressed control subjects, the depressed patients were impaired on a wide range of tests of memory and concentration before treatment, but afterward performance on most tests had improved. Real ECT induced impairments of concentration, short-term memory, and learning, but significantly facilitated access to remote memories. At 6-month follow-up, all differences between real and sham ECT groups had disappeared.

Price and McAllister (1989) have examined the efficacy of ECT in elderly depressed patients with dementia. Overall, their patients achieved an 86% response rate, with only 21% experiencing a significant worsening of cognition; the cognition problems were transient in most cases. Of particular importance is that 49% of the patients treated with ECT showed improvement in memory function after treatment. Although data on the safety and efficacy of ECT in patients with concurrent medical illness come primarily from retrospective studies of psychiatric patients with stable disease, these data do support the use of ECT in patients with cardiovascular, neurological, endocrine, metabolic, and a variety of other conditions (Weiner and Coffey 1987). For more information on the efficacy and safety of ECT in patients with late-life depressions, see Benlow's (1989) comprehensive review.

Family Therapy

The final component of therapy for the elderly depressed patient is work with the family. Not only may family dysfunction contribute to the depressive symptoms experienced by the older adult, but family support is critical to a successful outcome in the treatment of the depressed elder. A clinician must attend to 1) those members of the family who will be available to the elder, 2) the interaction of the older adult with family members and the interactions among other family members (both frequency and quality of interaction), 3) the overall family atmosphere, 4) family values regarding psychiatric disorders, 5) family support and tolerance of symptoms (such as expressions of wishing not to live), and 6) stressors encountered by the family other than the depression experienced by the elder (Blazer 1993).

Most depressed elders do not resist interaction between the clinician and family members. With the permission of the patient, the family should be instructed as to the nature of the depressive disorder and the potential risks resulting from depression in late life, especially suicide. Family members can assist the clinician in observing changes in behavior, such as an increase in discomfort (either physical or emotional), increased withdrawal and decreased verbalization, preoccupation with medications or weapons, and so forth. The family can assist by removing possible implements of suicide from easy access. The family can also take responsibility for administering medications to an older adult who is unreliable or whose potential for suicide is high.

Family members can also benefit from simple instructions regarding means by which they may communicate with the elderly depressed patient. Methods of responding to expressions of low self-esteem and pessimism, such as paraphrase and expression of understanding without a sense of responsibility to intervene, can be especially effective. Families can be taught, for example, to acknowledge to the patient that "I hear what you are saying, and I understand." Behavioral techniques for dealing with demanding or overly dependent elders can be taught to families as well. A demand for constant attention by a family member from a depressed elder may require "weaning" the patient from continued contact.

When the symptoms of depression become so severe that hospitalization is required, family members are valuable in facilitating hospitalization. Without a proper alliance between the clinician and family, families may be resistant to hospitalization and undermine the attempts of the clinician to treat the older adult appropriately. It is usually necessary for the clinician to take responsibility for saying that hospitalization is essential, that the situation has reached the point at which the family has no choice. In such a situation, the clinician informs the patient of the necessity of hospitalization in the presence of the family, and the family in turn can support the clinician's position. In such a situation, the patient rarely resists hospitalization for long.

References

Alexopoulos GS, Meyers BS, Young RC, et al: The course of geriatric depression with "reversible dementia": a controlled study. Am J Psychiatry 150:1693–1699, 1993

Ameblas A: Life events and mania. Br J Psychiatry 150:235–240, 1987

American Psychiatric Association: Diagnostic and Statistical Manual of Mental Disorders, 3rd Edition. Washington, DC, American Psychiatric Association, 1980

American Psychiatric Association: Diagnostic and Statistical Manual of Mental Disorders, 3rd Edition, Revised. Washington, DC, American Psychiatric Association, 1987

American Psychiatric Association: Diagnostic and Statistical Manual of Mental Disorders, 4th Edition. Washington, DC, American Psychiatric Association, 1994

Asarch KB, Shih JC, Kulscar A: Decreased 3H-imipramine binding in depressed males and females. Communications in Psychopharmacology 4:425–432, 1981

Atchley RC: Social Forces in Later Life. Belmont, CA, Wadsworth, 1972

Avery D, Lubrano A: Depression treated with imipramine and ECT: the DeCarolis study reconsidered. Am J Psychiatry 136:559–562, 1979

Baldwin JC, Jolley DJ: The prognosis of depression in old age. Br J Psychiatry 149:574–583, 1986

Beck AT, Rush AJ, Shaw BF, et al: Cognitive Therapy of Depression. New York, Guilford, 1979

Bell IR, Edman JS, Maroow FD, et al: B complex vitamin patterns in geriatric and young adult inpatients with major depression. J Am Geriatr Soc 39:252–257, 1991

Benlow SM: The role of ECT in the treatment of depressive illness in old age. Br J Psychiatry 155:147–152, 1989

Blazer DG: Impact of late-life depression on the social network. Am J Psychiatry 140:162–166, 1983

Blazer DG: Hypochondriasis, in A Family Approach to Health Care in the Elderly. Edited by Blazer D, Siegler IC. Menlo Park, CA, Addison-Wesley, 1984, pp 140–156

Blazer DG: Depression in Late Life, 2nd Edition. St. Louis, MO, CV Mosby, 1993

Blazer DG, George LK, Landerman R: The phenomenology of late life depression, in Psychiatric Disorders in the Elderly. Edited by Bebbington PE, Jacoby R. London, Mental Health Foundation, 1986, pp 143–152

Blazer DG, Hughes DC, George LK: The epidemiology of depression in an elderly community population. Gerontologist 27:281–287, 1987a

Blazer DG, Bachar JR, Hughes DC: Major depression with melancholia: a comparison of middle-aged and elderly adults. J Am Geriatr Soc 35:927–932, 1987b

Blazer DG, Hughes DC, Fowler N: Anxiety as an outcome symptom of depression in elderly and middle-aged adults. International Journal of Geriatric Psychiatry 27:281–287, 1989

Blazer DG, Hughes DC, George LK: Age and impaired subjective support: predictors of symptoms at one-year follow-up. J Nerv Ment Dis 180:172–178, 1992

Blumer D, Heilbronn M: Chronic pain as a variant of depressive disease: the pain-prone disorder. J Nerv Ment Dis 170:381–394, 1982

Bridges P: The drug treatment of depression in old age, in Affective Disorders in the Elderly. Edited by Murphy E. Edinburgh, Churchill Livingstone, 1986, pp 97–149

Briley MS, Raisman R, Sechter D, et al: [^{H}]Imipramine binding in human platelets: a new biochemical parameter in depression. Neuropharmacology 19:1209–1210, 1980

Buckley C, Curtin D, Walsh T, et al: Aging and platelet alpha$_2$-adrenoceptors (letter). Br J Clin Pharmacol 21:721–722, 1986

Bukberg J, Penman D, Holland JC: Depression in hospitalized cancer patients. Psychosom Med 46:199–210, 1984

Busse EW, Barnes RH, Silverman AJ, et al: Studies of the processes of aging, VI: factors that influence the psyche of elderly persons. Am J Psychiatry 110:897–903, 1954

Carroll BJ, Feinberg M, Greden JF, et al: A specific laboratory test for the diagnosis of melancholia: standardization, validity, and clinical utility. Arch Gen Psychiatry 38:15–22, 1981

Carter AB: The neurologic aspects of aging, in Clinical Geriatrics, 3rd Edition. Edited by Rossman I. Philadelphia, PA, JB Lippincott, 1986, pp 326–351

Cath SH: Some dynamics of middle and later years: a study in depletion and restitution, in Geriatric Psychiatry: Grief, Loss, and Emotional Disorders in the Aging Process. Edited by Berezin MA, Cath SH. New York, International Universities Press, 1965, pp 21–72

Checkley SA, Slade AP, Schur E: Growth hormone and other responses to clonidine in patients with endogenous depression. Br J Psychiatry 138:51–55, 1981

Coffey CE: Cerebral laterality and emotion: the neurology of depression. Compr Psychiatry 28:197–219, 1987

Coffey CE, Hinkle PE, Weiner RD, et al: Electroconvulsive therapy of depression in patients with white matter hyperintensity. Biol Psychiatry 22:626–629, 1987

Cole MG: Age, age of onset and course of primary depressive illness in the elderly. Can J Psychiatry 28:102–104, 1983

Cutler NR, Post RM: Life course of illness in untreated manic-depressive patients. Compr Psychiatry 23:101–115, 1982

Davies BM: Depressive illness in the elderly patient. Postgrad Med 38:314–320, 1965

de Alarcon R: Hypochondriasis and depression in the aged. Gerontologia Clinica 6:266–277, 1964

Dement WC, Miles LE, Carskadon MA: "White paper" on sleep and aging. J Am Geriatr Soc 30:25–50, 1982

Derogatis LR, Morrow GR, Fetting J, et al: The prevalence of psychiatric disorders among cancer patients. JAMA 249:751–757, 1983

Dovenmuehle RH, Verwoerdt A: Physical illness and depressive symptomatology, I: incidence of depressive symptoms in hospitalized cardiac patients. J Am Geriatr Soc 10:932–947, 1962

Dunner DL: Affective disorder: clinical features, in Psychiatry, Vol 1. Edited by Michels R, Cavenar JO. Philadelphia, PA, JB Lippincott, 1985, pp 59–60

Egeland JA, Gerhard DS, Pauls DL, et al: Bipolar affective disorders linked to DNA markers on chromosome 11. Nature 325:783–787, 1987

Endicott J, Spitzer RL: A diagnostic interview: the Schedule for Affective Disorders and Schizophrenia. Arch Gen Psychiatry 35:837–844, 1978

Enzell K: Mortality among persons with depressive symptoms and among responders in a health checkup. Acta Psychiatr Scand 69:89–102, 1984

Epstein LJ: Depression in the elderly. J Gerontol 3:278–282, 1976

Erikson EH: Childhood and Society. New York, WW Norton, 1950

Fassler LB, Gavira M: Depression in old age. J Am Geriatr Soc 26:471–475, 1978

Finkelstein JW, Roffwarg HP, Boyar RM, et al: Age-related change in the twenty-four-hour spontaneous secretion of growth hormone. J Clin Endocrinol Metab 35:665–670, 1972

France RD, Krishnan KRR, Houpt JL, et al: Differentiation of depression from chronic pain with the dexamethasone suppression test and DSM-III. Am J Psychiatry 141:1577–1578, 1984

Frank JD: Persuasion and Healing. Baltimore, MD, Johns Hopkins University Press, 1973

Frasure-Smith N, Lesperance F, Talajic M: Depression following myocardial infarction: impact on 6-month survival. JAMA 270:1819–1825, 1993

Fredman L, Schoenbach VJ, Kaplan BH, et al: The association between depressive symptoms and mortality among older participants in the Epidemiologic Catchment Area–Piedmont Health Survey. J Gerontol 44:S149–S156, 1989

Frith CD, Stevens M, Johnstone EC, et al: Effects of ECT and depression on various aspects of memory. Br J Psychiatry 142:610–617, 1983

Gainotti G: Emotional behavior and hemispheric side of lesion. Cortex 8:41–55, 1972

Gallagher D, Thompson LW: Differential effectiveness of psychotherapies for the treatment of major depressive disorder in older adult patients. Psychotherapy: Theory, Research and Practice 19:42–49, 1982

George LK, Blazer DG, Hughes DC, et al: Social support and the outcome of major depression. Br J Psychiatry 154:478–485, 1989

Glasser M, Rabins P: Mania in the elderly. Age Ageing 13:210–213, 1984

Greden JF: Antidepressant maintenance medications: when to discontinue and how to stop. J Clin Psychiatry 54 (suppl 8):39–45, 1993

Greden JF, Albala AA, Haskett RF, et al: Normalization of dexamethasone suppression test: a laboratory index of recovery from endogenous depression. Biol Psychiatry 15:449–458, 1980

Greden JF, Gardner R, King D, et al: dexamethasone suppression test and antidepressant treatment of melancholia. Arch Gen Psychiatry 40:493–500, 1983

Greenwald BS, Kramer-Binsberg E, Marin DB, et al: Dementia with coexistent major depression. Am J Psychiatry 146:1472–1477, 1989

Gregoire F, Brauman H, de Buck R, et al: Hormone release in depressed patients before and after recovery. Psychoneuroendocrinology 2:303–312, 1977

Grinker RR, Miller J, Sabshin M, et al: The Phenomena of Depressions. New York, Harper & Row, 1961

Guy R: An Essay on Scirrhous Tumors and Cancer. London, J & A Churchill, 1759

Hamilton M: A rating scale for depression. J Neurol Neurosurg Psychiatry 23:56-62, 1960

Henderson AS, Moran PAP: Social relationships during the onset and remission of neurotic symptoms: a prospective community study. Br J Psychiatry 143:467–472, 1983

Hinkle P, Coffey CE, Weiner R, et al: ECT seizure duration varies with age. Paper presented at the annual meeting of the American Geriatrics Society, Chicago, IL, 1986

Holahan CJ, Moos RH: Social support and psychological distress: a longitudinal analysis. J Abnorm Psychol 90:365–370, 1981

Hopkinson G: A genetic study of affective illness in patients over 50. Br J Psychiatry 110:244–254, 1964

Hudson JI, Hudson MS, Pliner LF, et al: Fibromyalgia and major affective disorder. Am J Psychiatry 142:441–446, 1985

Idler EL: Religious involvement and the health of the elderly: some hypotheses and an initial test. Social Forces 66:226–238, 1987

Idler EL, Kasl S: Religion, disability, depression, and the timing of death. American Journal of Sociology 97:1052–1079, 1992

Jacobsen FM, Wehr TA, Sack DA, et al: Seasonal affective disorder: a review of the syndrome and its public health implications. Am J Public Health 77:57–60, 1987

Jenike MA, Albert MS: The dexamethasone suppression test in patients with presenile and senile dementia of the Alzheimer's type. J Am Geriatr Soc 32:441–444, 1984

Kay DWK, Bergmann K: Physical disability and mental health in old age: a follow-up of a random sample of elderly people seen at home. J Psychosom Res 10:3–12, 1966

Kendell RE: The classification of depressions: a review of contemporary confusion. Br J Psychiatry 129:15–28, 1976

Kiloh LG: Pseudo-dementia. Acta Psychiatr Scand 37:336–351, 1961

Klerman GL, Weissman MM, Rounsaville BJ, et al: Interpersonal Psychotherapy of Depression. New York, Basic Books, 1984

Knight DL, Krishnan KRR, Blazer DG, et al: Tritiated imipramine binding to platelets is markedly reduced in elderly depressed patients. Society for Neuroscience Abstracts 12:1251, 1986

Koenig HG: Treatment considerations for the depressed geriatric medical patient. Drugs and Aging 1:266–278, 1991

Koenig HG: Aging and God: Spiritual Pathways to Mental Health in Mid-Life and the Later Years. Binghamton, NY, Haworth Press, 1993

Koenig HG, Blazer DG: Epidemiology of geriatric affective disorders. Clin Geriatr Med 8:235–251, 1992

Koenig HG, Meador KG, Cohen HJ, et al: Depression in elderly hospitalized patients with medical illness. Arch Intern Med 148:1929–1936, 1988a

Koenig HG, George LK, Siegler IC: The use of religion and other emotion-regulating coping strategies among older adults. Gerontologist 28:303–310, 1988b

Koenig HG, Shelp F, Goli V, et al: Survival and healthcare utilization in elderly medical inpatients with major depression. J Am Geriatr Soc 37:599-607, 1989

Koenig HG, Meador KG, Shelp F, et al: Depressive disorders in hospitalized medically ill patients: a comparison of young and elderly men. J Am Geriatr Soc 39:881–890, 1991

Koenig HG, Goli V, Shelp F, et al: Major depression in hospitalized medically ill older patients: documentation, management, and prognosis. International Journal of Geriatric Psychiatry 7:25–34, 1992a

Koenig HG, Cohen HJ, Blazer DG, et al: Religious coping and depression in hospitalized medically ill older men. Am J Psychiatry 149:1693–1700, 1992b

Koenig HG, Meador KG, Goli V, et al: Self-rated depressive symptoms in medical inpatients: age and racial differences. Int J Psychiatry Med 22:11–31, 1992c

Koenig HG, Cohen HJ, Blazer DG, et al: Profile of depressive symptoms in younger and older medical inpatients with major depression. J Am Geriatr Soc 41:1169–1176, 1993

Kraemlinger KG, Swanson DW, Maruta T: Are patients with chronic pain depressed? Am J Psychiatry 140:747–749, 1983

Krishnan KRR, France RD, Pelton S, et al: Chronic pain and depression, I: classification of depression in chronic low back pain patients. Pain 22:279–287, 1985

Kruesi MJ, Dale J, Straus SE: Psychiatric diagnoses in patients who have chronic fatigue syndrome. J Clin Psychiatry 40:53–56, 1989

Kupfer DJ: Neurophysiological markers: EEG sleep measures. J Psychiatr Res 18:467–495, 1984

Kupfer DJ, Foster FG, Coble P, et al: The application of EEG sleep for the differential diagnosis of affective disorders. Am J Psychiatry 135:69–74, 1978

Lakatua DJ, Nicolau GY, Bogdan C, et al: Circadian endocrine time structure in humans above 80 years of age. J Gerontol 39:648–654, 1984

Langner TS, Michael ST: Life Stress and Mental Health. Toronto, Canada, Free Press of Glencoe, 1963

Lazarus LW, Weinberg J: Treatment in the ambulatory care setting, in Handbook of Geriatric Psychiatry. Edited by Busse EW, Blazer DG. New York, Van Nostrand Reinhold, 1980, pp 427–452

Lesse S: Masked Depression. New York, Jason Aronson, 1974

Levin S: Depression in the aged, in Geriatric Psychiatry: Grief, Loss, and Emotional Disorders in the Aging Process. Edited by Berezin MA, Cath SH. New York, International Universities Press, 1965, pp 203–225

Lewis AJ: Melancholia: a historical review. Journal of Mental Science 80:1–42, 1934

Lindemann E: Symptomatology and management of acute grief. Am J Psychiatry 101:141–148, 1944

Lindenbaum J, Healton EB, Savage DG, et al: Neuropsychiatric disorders caused by cobalamin deficiency in the absence of anemia or macrocytosis. N Engl J Med 318:1720–1728, 1988

Lloyd C: Life events and depressive disorder reviewed, I: events as predisposing factors. Arch Gen Psychiatry 37:529–535, 1980

Loosen PT, Prange AJ: Serum thyrotropin response to thyrotropin-releasing hormone in psychiatric patients: a review. Am J Psychiatry 139:405–416, 1982

Lustman PJ, Griffith LS, Clouse RE: Depression in adults with diabetes. Diabetes Care 11:605–612, 1988

Magni G, Schifano F, De Leo D, et al: The dexamethasone suppression test in depressed and nondepressed geriatric medical inpatients. Acta Psychiatr Scand 73:511–514, 1986

Markush RE, Schwab JJ, Farris P, et al: Mortality and community mental health: the Alachua County, Florida, mortality study. Arch Gen Psychiatry 34:1393–1401, 1977

Massey EW, Bullock R: Peroneal palsy in depression. J Clin Psychiatry 28:291–292, 1978

Massie J, Holland J: Depression and the cancer patient. J Clin Psychiatry 51 (suppl 7):12–17, 1990

Mayeux R: Depression in the patient with Parkinson's disease. J Clin Psychiatry 51 (suppl 7):20–23, 1990

Mayeux R, Stern Y, Cote L, et al: Altered serotonin metabolism in depressed patients with Parkinson's disease. Neurology 34:642–646, 1984

Mayeux R, Stern Y, Williams JBW, et al: Clinical and biochemical features of depression in Parkinson's disease. Am J Psychiatry 143:756–759, 1986

Mendlewicz J: The age factor in depressive illness: some genetic considerations. J Gerontol 31:300–303, 1976

Meyers BS, Kalayam B, Mei-Tal V: Late-onset delusional depression: a distinct clinical entity? J Clin Psychiatry 45:347–349, 1984

Multidimensional Functional Assessment: The OARS Methodology—A Manual, 2nd Edition. Durham, NC, Duke University Center for the Study of Aging and Human Development, 1978

Munro HN: Nutrition and aging. Br Med Bull 37:83–88, 1981

Murphy E: The prognosis of depression in old age. Br J Psychiatry 142:111–119, 1983

Murphy E, Smith R, Lindsay J, et al: Increased mortality rates in late-life depression. Br J Psychiatry 152:347–353, 1988

Myers JK, Weissman MM, Tischler GL, et al: Six-month prevalence of psychiatric disorders in three communities, 1980–1982. Arch Gen Psychiatry 41:959–967, 1984

Old Age Depression Interest Group: How long should the elderly take antidepressants? a double-blind placebo-controlled study of continuation/prophylaxis therapy. Br J Psychiatry 162:175–182, 1993

Palmore E, Kivett V: Change in life satisfaction: a longitudinal study of persons aged 46–70. J Gerontol 32:311–316, 1977

Parmelee PA, Katz IR, Lawton MP: Depression among institutionalized aged: assessment and prevalence estimation. J Gerontol 44:M22–M29, 1989

Persson G: Five-year mortality in a 70-year-old urban population in relation to psychiatric diagnosis, personality, sexuality, and early parental death. Acta Psychiatr Scand 64:244–253, 1981

Pfifer JF, Murrell SA: Etiologic factors in the onset of depressive symptoms in older adults. J Abnorm Psychol 95:282–291, 1986

Post F: The management and nature of depressive illnesses in late life: a follow-through study. Br J Psychiatry 121:393–404, 1972

Post F: The functional psychoses, in Studies in Geriatric Psychiatry. Edited by Isaacs AD, Post F. New York, Wiley, 1978, pp 77–98

Pressman P, Lyons JS, Larson DB, et al: Religious belief, depression, and ambulation status in elderly women with broken hips. Am J Psychiatry 147:758–760, 1990

Price TRP, McAllister TW: Safety and efficacy of ECT in depressed patients with dementia: a review of clinical experience. Convulsive Therapy 5:61–74, 1989

Radloff LS: The CES-D scale: a self-report depression scale for research in the general population. Applied Psychological Measurement 1:385–401, 1977

Reifler BV, Larson E, Henley R: Coexistence of cognitive impairment and depression in geriatric outpatients. Am J Psychiatry 39:623–626, 1982

Reifler BV, Larson E, Teri L, et al: Dementia of the Alzheimer's type and depression. J Am Geriatr Soc 34:855–859, 1986

Reifler BV, Teri L, Raskind M, et al: Double-blind trial of imipramine in Alzheimer's disease patients with and without depression. Am J Psychiatry 146:45–49, 1989

Relkin R: Effect of endocrines on central nervous system, I. N Y State J Med 69:2133–2145, 1969

Reynolds CF III, Frank E, Perel JM, et al: Combined pharmacotherapy and psychotherapy in the acute and continuation treatment of elderly patients with recurrent major depression: a preliminary report. Am J Psychiatry 149:1687–1692, 1992

Ribeiro SCM, Tandon R, Grunhaus L, et al: The DST as a predictor of outcome in depression: a meta-analysis. Am J Psychiatry 150:1618–1629, 1993

Robinson DS, Davies JM, Nies A, et al: Relation of sex and aging to monoamine oxidase activity of human plasma and platelets. Arch Gen Psychiatry 24:536–541, 1971

Robinson RG, Morris PLP, Fedoroff P: Depression and cerebrovascular disease. J Clin Psychiatry 51 (suppl 7):26–31, 1990

Rosenbaum AH, Schatzberg AF, MacLaughlin MS, et al: The DST in normal control subjects: a comparison of two assays and the effects of age. Am J Psychiatry 141:1550–1555, 1984

Rovner BW, Perman PS, Brant LJ, et al: Depression and mortality in nursing homes. JAMA 265:993–996, 1991

Sachar EJ: Neuroendocrine abnormalities in depressive illness, in Topics in Psychoendocrinology. Edited by Sachar EJ. New York, Grune & Stratton, 1975, pp 135–156

Sackheim HA, Greenberg MS, Wiman AL, et al: Hemispheric asymmetry in the expression of positive and negative emotions. Arch Neurol 39:210–218, 1982

Salzman C, Shader RI: Responses to psychotropic drugs in the normal elderly, in Psychopharmacology in Aging. Edited by Eisdorfer C, Fann WE. New York, Plenum, 1972, pp 159–168

Schiffman S: Changes in taste and smell with age: psychophysiological aspects, in Aging: Sensory Systems and Communication in the Elderly, Vol 10. Edited by Ordy JM, Brizzee K. New York, Raven, 1979

Schleifer SJ, Macari-Hinson MM, Coyle DA, et al: The nature and course of depression following myocardial infarction. Arch Intern Med 149:1785–1789, 1989

Schneider LS, Severson JA, Sloane RB: Platelet H-imipramine binding in depressed elderly patients. Biol Psychiatry 20:1234–1237, 1985

Schneider LS, Severson JA, Pollock V, et al: Platelet monoamine oxidase activity in elderly depressed outpatients. Biol Psychiatry 21:1360–1364, 1986

Schulz B: Auszahlungen in der Verwandtschaft von nach Erkrankungsalter und Geschlecht gruppierten Manisch-Depressiven. Archiv fur Psychiatrie und Nervenkrankheiten 186:560–576, 1951

Schwab JJ, Clemmons RS, Bialow M, et al: A study of the somatic symptomatology of depression in medical inpatients. Psychosomatics 6:273–276, 1965

Scovern AW, Kilmann PR: Status of electroconvulsive therapy: review of the outcome literature. Psychol Bull 87:260–303, 1980

Shulman KI: Mania in old age, in Affective Disorders in the Elderly. Edited by Murphy E. Edinburgh, Churchill Livingstone, 1986, pp 203–216

Shulman KI: The influence of age and aging on manic disorder. International Journal of Geriatric Psychiatry 4:63–65, 1989

Shulman KI, Post F: Bipolar affective disorder in old age. Br J Psychiatry 136:26–32, 1980

Slater E, Cowie V: The Genetics of Mental Disorder. London, Oxford University Press, 1971

Snyder PJ, Utiger RD: Response to thyrotropin releasing hormone (TRH) in normal man. J Clin Endocrinol Metab 34:380–385, 1972

Spar JE, Ford CV, Liston EH: Bipolar affective disorder in aged patients. J Clin Psychiatry 40:504–507, 1979

Spitzer RL, Endicott J, Robins E: Research Diagnostic Criteria: rationale and reliability. Arch Gen Psychiatry 35:773–782, 1978

Srole L, Fischer AK: The Midtown Manhattan Longitudinal Study vs "The Mental Paradise Lost" doctrine: a controversy joined. Arch Gen Psychiatry 37:209–221, 1980

Stenstedt A: Involutional melancholia: an etiologic, clinical and social study of endogenous depression in later life, with special reference to genetic factors. Acta Psychiatrica et Neurologica Scandinavica Supplementum 127:5–71, 1959

Steuer JL, Mintz J, Hammen CL, et al: Cognitive-behavioral and psychodynamic group psychotherapy in treatment of geriatric depression. J Consult Clin Psychol 52:180–189, 1984

Stoudemire A, Hill CD, Morris R, et al: Long-term outcome of treatment-resistant depression in older adults. Am J Psychiatry 150:1539–1540, 1993

Targum SD, Sullivan AC, Byrnes SM: Neuroendocrine relationships in major depressive disorder. Am J Psychiatry 139:282–286, 1982

Thielman SB, Blazer DG: Depression and dementia, in Dementia in Old Age. Edited by Pitt B. Edinburgh, Churchill Livingstone, 1986, pp 251–264

Thomae H: Personality and adjustment to aging, in The Handbook of Aging and Mental Health. Edited by Birren J, Sloane RB. Englewood Cliffs, NJ, Prentice-Hall, 1980, pp 285–309

Thompson LW, Gallagher D, Steinmetz-Breckenridge J: Comparative effectiveness of psychotherapies for depressed elders. J Consult Clin Psychol 55:385–390, 1987

Tourigny-Rivard M, Raskin DM, Rivard D: The dexamethasone suppression test in an elderly population. Biol Psychiatry 16:1177–1184, 1981

Ulrich RF, Shaw DH, Kupfer DJ: Effects of aging on EEG sleep in depression. Sleep 3:31–40, 1980

Verwoerdt A: Clinical Geropsychiatry. Baltimore, MD, Williams & Wilkins, 1976

Vogel GW, Vogel F, McAbee RS, et al: Improvement of depression by REM sleep deprivation: new findings and a theory. Arch Gen Psychiatry 37:247–253, 1980

Weiner RD: The role of electroconvulsive therapy in the treatment of depression in the elderly. J Am Geriatr Soc 30:710–712, 1982

Weiner RD, Coffey CE: ECT in the medically ill, in Principles of Medical Psychiatry. Edited by Stoudemire A, Fogel B. New York, Grune & Stratton, 1987, pp 113–134

Weissman MM, Prusoff BA, Klerman GC: Personality and the prediction of long-term outcome in depression. Am J Psychiatry 135:797–800, 1978

Weissman MM, Bruce ML, Leaf PJ, et al: Affective disorders, in Psychiatric Disorders in America: The Epidemiologic Catchment Area Study. Edited by Robins LN, Regier DA. New York, Free Press, 1991, p 53

Wells CE: Pseudodementia. Am J Psychiatry 136:895–900, 1979

Wesner RB, Winokur G: The influence of age on the natural history of unipolar depression when treated with ECT. European Archives of Psychiatry and Neurological Sciences 238:149–154, 1989

Whitlock FA, Siskind M: Depression and cancer: a follow-up study. Psychol Med 9:747–752, 1979

Wigdor BT: Drives and motivations with aging, in The Handbook of Aging and Mental Health. Edited by Birren JE, Sloane RB. Englewood Cliffs, NJ, Prentice-Hall, 1980, pp 245–261

Winokur G: The Iowa 500: heterogeneity and course in manic-depressive illness (bipolar). Compr Psychiatry 16:125–131, 1975

Yesavage JA, Brink TL, Rose TL, et al: Development and validation of a geriatric depression screening scale: a preliminary report. J Psychiatr Res 17:37–49, 1983

Young RC, Falk JR: Age, manic psychopathology, and treatment response. International Journal of Geriatric Psychiatry 4:73–78, 1989

Zimmerman M, Coryell W, Pfohl B: Prognostic validity of the dexamethasone suppression test: results of a six-month prospective follow-up. Am J Psychiatry 144:212–214, 1987

Zung WWK: A self-rating depression scale. Arch Gen Psychiatry 12:63–70, 1965

Zung WWK, Green RL: Detection of affective disorders in the aged, in Psychopharmacology in Aging. Edited by Eisdorfer C, Fann WE. New York, Plenum, 1972, pp 213–224

CHAPTER 14

Schizophrenia and Paranoid Disorders

Harold G. Koenig, M.D., M.H.Sc.
Caron Christison, M.D.
George Christison, M.D.
Dan G. Blazer, M.D., Ph.D.

Suspiciousness, persecutory ideation, and paranoid delusions are common psychiatric symptoms seen by the clinician working with cognitively impaired or emotionally disturbed older adults. In a study of older persons in the San Francisco community, Lowenthal (1964) found that 17% of those rated psychiatrically impaired had symptoms of suspiciousness and 13% had delusions. Heston (1987) reported that whereas only about 2% of psychiatric patients fulfilled syndromal criteria for paranoid disorder, 13% had paranoid ideation. In other community studies, Lowenthal (1964) observed suspiciousness in 2.5% and paranoid delusions in 2% of unselected older adults. Likewise, Christenson and Blazer (1984) found that 4% of an elderly community sample suffered from generalized persecutory ideation.

Unlike these earlier studies, the Epidemiologic Catchment Area (ECA) community surveys, which included more than 5,700 adults over age 60, showed rates of less than 0.1% for schizophrenia (Myers et al. 1984). An examination of the ECA studies, however, reveals that a primary reason for so few cases of schizophrenia is that diagnostic criteria specified by DSM-III (American Psychiatric Association 1980) required onset before age 45. Many impaired older adults may not remember when symptoms first began, and collateral information from significant others may not be available. Furthermore, elderly individuals with schizophrenic symptoms may have these attributed to organic mental syndromes, mood disorders, or sensory deficits. For more than 1,600 individuals 60 years of age and older in the ECA study at Duke University (a survey of urban and rural North Carolina), the unweighted prevalence of schizophrenia or schizophreniform disorder was 0.2% (Blazer et al. 1988). Nearly 8% of the sample, however, reported at least one current symptom of schizophrenia, with 4.3% reporting delusions and 5.4%, hallucinations.

The confusion and controversy surrounding the diagnosis of schizophrenia in the elderly center on at least two factors: 1) the definition of a case of schizophrenia (can a case of schizophrenia develop after the age of 45?), and 2) the range of clinical conditions that may manifest as schizophrenia-like symptomatology. A number of authors have reported that a symptom picture virtually identical to that of schizophrenia as defined by DSM-III could have an onset after the age of 45 (Gold 1984; Rabins et al. 1984; Volavka 1985). The argument was straightforward: symptom profiles did not vary except for the criterion requiring onset before age 45. Many patients who suffer from paranoid delusions of late onset respond well to traditional therapies for schizophrenia. The European literature (in which an age criterion has not been used) is often cited to support abolishment of an age criterion. The argument for limiting the onset of schizophrenia to before the age of 45 was that the vast majority of cases of schizophrenia develop before the age of 45. Responding to the former arguments, the authors of DSM-III-R (American Psychiatric Association 1987) allowed an onset of schizophrenic symptoms after age 44, labeling such individuals as having "late-onset" schizophrenia.

Nevertheless, vigorous debate continues on the utility of making distinctions between early-onset and late-onset schizophrenia, with a number of authors challenging results from outcome studies that claim predictive validity (Hassett et al. 1992). In fact, DSM-IV (American Psychiatric Association 1994) is strictly phenomenological in its categorization of schizophrenia, removing the age criterion entirely and deleting late onset as a separate category. Field trials, however, continue (Jeste et al. 1995).

Historical Perspectives

The controversy regarding schizophrenia-like illnesses in late life derives in part from the historical evolution of the term *late paraphrenia*. In 1919, Kraepelin (1919/1971) used *paraphrenia* to describe a disorder characterized by the onset of predominantly paranoid delusions, with or without hallucinations, in a comparatively small group of patients. Although these patients had many characteristics in common with patients who had dementia praecox, Kraepelin, distinguished between the two groups

by stating that the paraphrenic patients exhibited "far slighter development of the disorder of emotion and volition," and that the "dullness and indifference which so frequently form the first symptoms of dementia praecox" were not seen in paraphrenia until, perhaps, "the latest periods of the malady." As a diagnostic entity, paraphrenia subsequently fell into disuse because follow-up of Kraepelin's paraphrenic group revealed that the diagnosis was changed to schizophrenia in more than half the cases (Kolle 1931; Mayer-Gross 1932).

Roth (1955) reintroduced the term paraphrenia, defining it as a syndrome characterized by

> a well-organized system of paranoid delusions with or without auditory hallucinations existing in the setting of a well-preserved personality and affective response. . . . In the great majority of these patients, the illness commences after the age of 60. (p. 281)

He used the term descriptively, and in an empirical follow-up study demonstrated that the outcome in elderly patients suffering from paraphrenia differed from the outcome in those with a diagnosis of affective disorder or dementia. Because the syndrome of paraphrenia did not appear to be the same as schizophrenia (though it resembled schizophrenia), and because the syndrome was frequently found among the elderly, the term *late paraphrenia* emerged.

The existence of a group of patients with schizophrenia-like symptoms that begin in late life and are not due to affective or dementing illnesses has been evaluated in several studies. Baron et al. (1983) found that among 93 chronic schizophrenic patients, none became ill after the age of 40 (although the oldest subject in the study was only 48 years old). Studies such as this can be used to support the DSM-III age criterion for schizophrenia. In contrast, Fish (1960), Essa (1982), and Marneros and Deister (1984) each found a substantial number of subjects who experienced the onset of schizophrenia-like symptoms after the age of 50, with many having demonstrated the first onset of these symptoms after the age of 65. Analyzing data on hospitalized patients with schizophrenia, Harris and Jeste (1988) found that 13% had an onset of psychotic symptoms in their 50s, 7% in their 60s, and 3% in their 70s and 80s.

Post (1966) identified three patterns of symptom presentation among paraphrenic patients in later life. The first was characterized by auditory hallucinations and false beliefs of persecution; the second, by understandable delusions (such as feelings of being observed or having one's conversation taped); and the third, by evidence of the so-called first-rank symptoms of schizophrenia as elucidated by Schneider (1959). Post believed that the etiology of the paranoid state—whether it was due to organic causes, social isolation, or sensory loss—was not related to the symptom pattern. Like others, Post recognized that a poor premorbid history among some patients suggested that they were borderline schizophrenic before the onset of the overt disorder in late life. Nevertheless, he emphasized that the overt symptoms of the disorder did manifest for the first time in late life.

Differential Diagnosis of Schizophrenia-Like Symptoms in Late Life

Eisdorfer (1980) has suggested some useful constructs for the differential diagnosis of schizophrenia-like symptoms with an onset in late life: 1) suspiciousness, 2) transitional paranoid reactions, and 3) paraphrenia—late-onset paranoia as suggested by Roth (1955) or paranoia associated with schizophrenia of late onset. In this section we review these as well as other causes for late-life psychosis, including early-onset schizophrenia, psychoses induced by organic causes, major affective disorders, and late-life delusional disorder (previously called paranoid disorder).

Suspiciousness

Most older adults who demonstrate heightened suspiciousness, such as those who have been identified in community surveys (Christenson and Blazer 1984; Lowenthal 1964), never come into contact with a mental health professional. Such individuals offer vague complaints of external forces controlling their lives. On occasion, such beliefs can become focal, often addressed toward children. Feelings of being deserted by their children or that their children have plotted against them may become so severe that they force the children to seek counsel, yet these older adults continue daily activities with little difficulty. A sense of loss of control, coupled with an inability to evaluate the social milieu properly, provides adequate grounds for the development of mild suspiciousness.

The clinician is more likely to encounter suspiciousness associated with loss of memory and attention, particularly when these losses are associated with hearing or visual deficits. Frequently a problem among patients in long-term care facilities who are suffering from a dementing illness, accusations can plague both family and staff. Such suspiciousness is usually disjointed, not focused, and not accompanied by emotional distress, except for brief episodes. Complaints of objects being stolen, medicines being swapped, misbehavior of attendants in other parts of the facility, and so forth are common symptoms. Inability to organize environmental stimuli and comprehend the frequently confusing activities of a hospital or long-term care facility may contribute to the onset such symptoms. To what extent an underlying hostile and paranoid personality style contributes to such suspiciousness is not known.

Transitional Paranoid Reaction

Eisdorfer's second variety of paranoid disorder derives from the work of Post (1973), who describes focal, narrow, and situational paranoid hallucinations. Again, commonly, individuals who exhibit such symptoms are women who live alone and who believe a plot exists against them. The focus of these hallucinations and delusional thinking usually begins outside the person's house and moves gradually inward, to complaints of noises in the basement and attic and progressing even to physical abuse or molestation—hence, the transition from without to within. Factors that may contribute to this transitional paranoia include social isolation and perceptual difficulties (Eisdorfer 1980; Post 1965).

These transitional paranoid reactions may also accompany moderate to severe dementia, either primary degenerative dementia or multi-infarct dementia. Not infrequently, patients in long-term care facilities complain of fragmented yet elaborately constructed plots against them. For example, if their room is overheated, they imagine personnel have contrived to incinerate the facility. Others protest plots by family members to dispossess them of their possessions, often the family home from which they have been moved to the institution. As the plot evolves in the elder's imagination, the threat moves closer to the individual. Similar to the suspiciousness associated with dementia, the emotions associated with these fragmented paranoid reactions may be strong at times but are not sustained. Clinicians must continually remember, however, that there may be justification for what appear to be paranoid accusations, given the vulnerability of many frail elderly persons to being taken advantage of by others, including family members.

Paraphrenia

Eisdorfer's final category is paraphrenia and paranoia associated with schizophrenia-like illness. Although Roth (1955) distinguished late-onset paraphrenia from paranoid schizophrenia, others would not make this distinction. Investigators who distinguish a syndrome of late-onset paraphrenia emphasize that this is a primary disorder—that is, it is not due to affective illness or an organic mental disorder. Paranoid delusions and hallucinations are almost always apparent, yet the gross disturbances of affect, volition, or function seen in patients with schizophrenia are not prominent. The course may be chronic, but deterioration to the extent observed in the course of schizophrenia or Alzheimer's disease is not characteristic. As can be seen, the distinction between transitional paranoid states and late paraphrenia is unclear, as is the distinction between late paraphrenia and classic paranoid schizophrenia.

Late-Onset Schizophrenia

DSM-III-R dropped the old term *paraphrenia* and created a new diagnostic category, *late-onset schizophrenia*. Although DSM-IV has removed the late-onset specifier, the term *late-onset schizophrenia* continues as a commonly used diagnostic category and the research remains inconclusive. Many elders previously labeled as having paraphrenia now fall into this group. Late-onset schizophrenia is distinguished from mere suspiciousness or transitional paranoid reactions by the presence of bizarre delusions (often of a persecutory nature) and, often, of hallucinations. Delusions are systematized in a high proportion of patients and frequently involve mental or physical influence by others. Somatic, erotic, and grandiose delusions may also be encountered. At times such patients may be difficult to distinguish from those with somatization disorder or obsessive ruminations, although the bizarre nature of the de-

lusions provides an essential clue. Auditory hallucinations are the second most common symptom encountered in patients with this disorder. Schneiderian first-rank symptoms such as thought broadcasting or insertion, although less common than in younger patients with schizophrenia, may also occur. According to Jeste and colleagues (1988), inappropriate affect and loose associations are less common in late-onset than in early-onset schizophrenia. In general, late-onset schizophrenia is felt to have a more benign course than the early-onset variety, a feature noted by many earlier investigators and by authors of more recent work (Rzewuska and Wronska 1992).

To receive the DSM-III-R diagnosis of late-onset schizophrenia, older adults had to meet DSM-III-R criteria for schizophrenia, fulfill the 6-month duration requirement, and experience symptoms that began after age 45—including any prodromal symptoms involving a deterioration in social and occupational functioning, social isolation, changes in affect, or problems with personal hygiene. A number of recent epidemiological studies have provided further information on symptom presentation in late-onset schizophrenia. Yassa and colleagues (1993) reported that 2.4% of 288 admissions to a Canadian geropsychiatry unit were of patients who fulfilled criteria for late-onset schizophrenia (all women). Bizarre delusions (typically paranoid) and auditory hallucinations were common; negative symptoms were rare. In a study of 83 patients with "late paraphrenia," Howard and colleagues (1993) reported persecutory delusions in 87%, nonverbal auditory hallucinations in 64%, verbal third-person hallucinations in 51%, and visual hallucinations in 30%; they also found thought insertion in 16% and thought withdrawal in 6%, despite claims by earlier investigators of the rarity of these symptoms.

Chronic Early-Onset Schizophrenia

Schizophrenic patients with onset of symptoms before age 45 and a chronic course may have an exacerbation of symptoms in later life. Part of the difficulty in distinguishing the spectrum of paranoid symptomatology in late life derives from a poor understanding of the natural course of schizophrenia. Chronic institutionalization of schizophrenic patients in the past, coupled with increased mortality among this population, has rendered community follow-up studies inadequate. Tsuang and Dempsey (1979) found that 200 persons who developed schizophrenia before the age of 40 were four times more likely to die during the first 9 years after onset; this finding was confirmed by Black and Fisher (1992), who reported a suicide rate in this group 23 times higher than that expected in the general population. Talbott (1981) documented that almost one-half of the patients who have been deinstitutionalized over the last 30 years—about 750,000 persons—are now in nursing homes. At follow-up, Tsuang and Dempsey (1979) also found that among those survivors to late life who were diagnosed as schizophrenic early in life, 18% were hospitalized in mental institutions and 48% were in nursing homes. Other studies have indicated that, on average, approximately one-third of schizophrenic patients either experience full remission or have mild symptoms over the long run, although the range is from 6% to 50% (McGlashan 1986).

Psychoses Induced by Organic Causes

First and foremost, organic factors must be ruled out when an older adult demonstrates paranoid or schizophrenia-like symptoms for the first time in late life. Medical disorders that are associated with psychotic symptoms in late life include endocrinopathies (thyroid, parathyroid, adrenal, and pancreatic dysfunction); neurological disorders (all varieties of dementia, seizure disorders, hydrocephalus, multiple sclerosis, brain tumors, encephalopathy, encephalitis, neurosyphilis); vitamin deficiencies (B_{12}, thiamine, niacin, folate); and other disorders (systemic lupus erythematosus, temporal arteritis, electrolyte abnormalities) (Jeste et al. 1991). Many medications can produce hallucinations at toxic, therapeutic, or subtherapeutic doses, and frail elderly persons are frequently at higher risk for such side effects. Alcohol or drug withdrawal states must also be considered, because these can produce psychotic symptoms.

Older persons with Alzheimer's, multi-infarct, or alcoholic dementia frequently experience disruptive paranoid or psychotic symptoms. Wragg and Jeste (1989) reported delusions (mostly persecutory) in 30% (range: 10%–73%) of patients with Alzheimer's disease. As noted earlier, complex or systematized delusions are rarely seen in patients with dementia. Hallucinations (visual slightly more than

auditory) have been reported in 21%–49% of patients with Alzheimer's disease (Wragg and Jeste 1989). As the severity of dementia progresses, however, delusions and hallucinations tend to lessen (Cummings et al. 1987), because a certain degree of cognitive function is necessary for psychotic symptoms to be manifested.

On the other hand, severe cognitive impairment is often seen in elderly persons with early-onset schizophrenia; the cause for such impairment has been a source of speculation (Charlesworth et al. 1993). Purohit and colleagues (1993) performed postmortem examinations on the brains of 12 severely demented elderly schizophrenic patients, comparing them with the brains of a similar number of age-matched control subjects and patients with Alzheimer's disease. In none of the schizophrenic cases were the neuropathological changes characteristic of Alzheimer's disease demonstrated. The relationship between cognitive disorders and paranoid and schizophrenia-like symptoms is further discussed below.

Affective Disorders With Psychotic Features

Older patients with psychotic depression or mania may demonstrate paranoia and schizophrenia-like symptoms. Because paranoid symptoms can be so dramatic in late-onset major depression, Meyers and Greenberg (1986) have suggested that depressed, delusional older adults should be distinguished and treated differently from their depressed but nondelusional counterparts. Mood symptoms usually predominate in these individuals, and there may be either a personal or family history of depression or mania. Careful history taking may determine that mood symptoms preceded the development of psychotic symptoms, may uncover a precipitating stressful event (a financial catastrophe or the death of a spouse, for example), or may reveal a periodicity to the patient's symptoms suggestive of affective disorder.

Late-Life Delusional Disorder

The term *delusional disorder* used in DSM-III-R replaced *paranoid disorder* as used in DSM-III. Delusional disorder often resembles late-onset schizophrenia, although the former is less likely to be associated with bizarre delusions, auditory hallucinations, Schneiderian first-rank symptoms, deteriorating social and occupational functioning, or changes in affect. In addition to including delusions of persecution or jealousy, the category of delusional disorder has been broadened to include erotomanic, somatic, grandiose, and other unspecified delusions. These delusions are characterized as nonbizarre and involve situations that may conceivably occur in real life (being watched, stolen from, or poisoned, for example). They are typically chronic and well systematized, and—in contrast to delirium or dementia—are associated with little or no impairment of memory, orientation, or intellectual functions. Hallucinations, if present, are not prominent. DSM-IV requires that symptoms be present for at least 1 month. Premorbid personality disorders (avoidant, paranoid, schizoid) may be more prevalent in persons who eventually develop delusional disorder. Onset of symptoms must be on or after age 45 to be considered "late onset" (DSM-III-R). The average age at onset for delusional disorder in the general population is 40–49 in men and 60–69 in women. Therefore, this disorder usually first appears in middle or late life.

Other DSM-IV Psychotic Disorders

Other psychotic disorders listed in DSM-IV are brief psychotic disorder, schizophreniform disorder, and schizoaffective disorder. With *brief psychotic disorder,* an elderly person experiences a sudden onset of psychotic symptoms that endure for a total duration of less than 1 month, are often precipitated by a stressful life event (such as bereavement), and result in a complete resolution of symptoms without impact on level of functioning. Older patients who have schizophrenia-like symptoms lasting more than 1 month but less than 6 months are diagnosed as having *schizophreniform disorder.* elderly persons who have schizophrenia-like symptoms but do not fulfill criteria for schizophrenia, have a history of major affective disorder, and have a history of psychotic symptoms in the absence of mood symptoms for 2 weeks or longer are diagnosed as having *schizoaffective disorder.*

Diagnostic Evaluation

A detailed history must be obtained from the patient and corroborated by a spouse, children, other relatives, neighbors, or an employer. Collateral sources of information may reveal that prodromal symptoms were present for some time before the patient's awareness. If hospitalizations or other psychiatric evaluations have occurred, records should be obtained and examined. All medications must be reviewed carefully, particularly those with anticholinergic effects that may induce delirium. All patients require a careful physical and neurological examination, along with laboratory tests such as a chemistry panel, thyroid studies, serologic tests for syphilis, and vitamin B_{12} and folate levels. Magnetic resonance imaging (MRI) is indicated in patients with a positive neurological exam or in cases in which the clinician suspects that structural abnormalities underlie or coexist with paranoid or schizophrenic symptoms (Miller et al. 1989). In summary, it is imperative to rule out reversible medical or surgical illness that may represent psychoses from organic causes.

Factors Associated With Late-Onset Paranoid and Schizophrenic Disorders

Cognitive Disorders

Transient cognitive disturbances, such as delirium, are probably the most important and frequent causes of paranoid symptoms in elderly persons (Lipowski 1983). Confusion is one of the more common causes for referral of a patient to the geropsychiatrist. In a multicenter study in Great Britain, 35% of the patients aged 65 and older exhibited delirium on admission or developed it during the hospital stay under study (Hodkinson 1976). Transient cognitive disorders can result in a number of symptoms, including disordered perception, disordered thinking, impaired memory, decreased alertness, and psychomotor agitation or retardation. Problems with perception often are manifested by a reduced capability to distinguish actual environmental stimuli from imagery, dreams, and even hallucinations (Lipowski 1980). Patients report visits from relatives or friends who are deceased, travels to areas they remember in the past, and conversations in which reality is intermixed with fantasy. Acute delirium often precipitates a dramatic affective response to these perceptual abnormalities; the patient with chronic dementia, however, can report illusions and hallucinations with little affect.

Cognitive dysfunction also contributes to disorganized and fragmented thinking. In the midst of an acute brain syndrome, paranoid ideation and delusions of persecution (unsystematized and transient) have been reported to occur in 40%–55% of older adults (Simon and Cahan 1963). As described by Lipowski (1983), the elderly delirious patient, in contrast to the younger patient with delirium, is less likely to combine florid reports of hallucinations associated with delusional thinking. In an elderly individual with delirium, an impoverished and incoherent thought process is accompanied by impaired reasoning and judgment associated with general suspiciousness and isolated reports that are clearly delusional.

Gender

Female gender is another factor reported by most investigators to be associated with late paraphrenia. Women predominate over men by a ratio of 5:1 or higher. The increased propensity for women to suffer from paranoid symptoms in late life, as demonstrated even in age-adjusted studies, is in contrast to the 1:1 sex ratio found in early-onset schizophrenia. In a study from Graylingwell Hospital of 42 patients with late paraphrenia, Kay and Roth (1961) found 39 women with the disorder, but only 3 men. Marneros and Deister (1984) found that among 1,208 first psychiatric admissions with schizophrenia, 85% were women among the group over the age of 50. Rabins et al. (1984) found an 11:1 ratio of women to men in a study of 35 patients over the age of 44.

A number of factors have been posited to explain the increased risk for women to develop paranoid disorders and late-onset schizophrenia. Some ascribe this to women's greater longevity and exposure to neuropsychosocial stressors. Others have suggested that women tend to develop schizophrenic symptoms later than men do, and therefore women have a later "peak" of symptom manifestation. For example, Zigler and Levine (1981) found that men with schizophrenia are hospitalized about 5 years earlier than women with schizophrenia. Seeman (1981) speculated that dropping estrogen levels in women may contribute to their increased vulnerability. As evidence, she points out that hormonal instability during the postpartum period has been associated with high vulnerability to behavioral decompensation. Another suggestion is that older women with schizophrenic symptoms are more likely to come to the attention of health care providers. A review of the evidence, however, does not provide a satisfactory explanation of the preponderance of women with this disorder.

Social and Occupational Functioning

Another factor associated with schizophrenia-like symptoms in late life is poor social and occupational adjustment. The majority of patients suffering from paraphrenia, according to most investigators, were capable of supporting themselves until retirement or the onset of their illness (Kay 1963). According to clinical experience, however, these individuals were likely in earlier life to be isolated, to work in occupations that required little social interaction, and to be marginal in their social relations outside of work. This caused a number of early investigators (Kay and Roth 1961; Herbert and Jacobson 1967; Odegaard 1953) to hypothesize that the prepsychotic personalities of patients suffering from late-onset schizophrenia tended to be schizoid or paranoid. Prepsychotic behavior was characterized by explosive tempers, adherence to minority religious sects, and—among men—antisocial behavior. Marriages tended to be fragile, with a high incidence of divorce, and the patients were described by their children and neighbors as cold, unloving, and eccentric. When compared with persons with early-onset schizophrenia, however, those with late-onset schizophrenia were more likely to have been married, held employment, and had children (Jeste et al. 1988).

Social isolation may be another contributory factor in the development of schizophrenia-like symptoms. The suspicious or paranoid older adult is often a loner. This condition can be due to loss of family and friends, coupled with a relatively isolated lifestyle. Prolonged social isolation is a fertile breeding ground for the gradual development of distorted thoughts that eventually progress to delusions regarding neighbors, the neighborhood, or the state of the world. To be isolated is to be uninformed, which encourages suspicion and can lead to fabrication of explanations of the unknown.

Sensory Impairment

A number of investigators have reported the association of schizophrenia-like symptoms in late life with sensory impairment. In a community study of older adults (Christenson and Blazer 1984), nearly 78% of subjects with persecutory ideations had impaired vision, compared with 51% without persecutory beliefs. Hearing was impaired in 58% of the symptomatic subjects, but in only 36% of the nonsymptomatic subjects. Post (1966) found "deafness" in 30% of older adults with persistent paranoid symptoms, compared with 11% who were depressed and 7% of the normal community subjects. In a more detailed study, Cooper et al. (1974, 1976) found that, when tested with audiometric devices, patients with paranoid psychosis had hearing losses of significantly greater magnitude than did patients with depressive disorders. Leuchter and Spar (1985) compared elderly psychotic inpatients with elderly nonpsychotic inpatients. Auditory impairment was more prevalent among the psychotic patients than among the control subjects (21% vs. 12%), and visual impairment was more common as well (34% vs. 18%). Cooper and Porter (1976) found an increased prevalence of cataracts among paranoid patients compared with patients who were depressed.

For the patient with sensory impairment, psychotic symptoms, such as hallucinations, may fill in for stimuli that are absent; auditory or visual hallucinations resulting from sensory deprivation have been called "Charles Binet hallucinations." With respect to the development of paranoid ideation, if isolated elderly individuals do not hear speech clearly—especially when in a group situation—they may conclude that others are talking about them, or they may refer to themselves the fragments of speech that are partially heard (Zarit 1980).

Marital Status

As noted earlier, the results of most studies suggest that the patient with late-onset paranoia or schizophrenia is more likely to have been married than is the patient with early-onset schizophrenia (Bridge and Wyatt 1980; Marneros and Deister 1984). However, this finding is confounded by functional impairment in the earlier-onset group during the years when these individuals are most likely to be married.

Family Psychiatric History

If individuals with late-onset schizophrenia represent a subset of patients with true schizophrenia, one would expect the prevalence of schizophrenia among family members to be comparable for early- and late-onset cases. In a study of 148 patients with onset of paranoia after the age of 50, Funding (1961) found the expectancy rate for schizophrenia among siblings to be 2.5%. This is greater than the approximately 1% reported for the general population, but less than the prevalence of nearly 10% reported among siblings for younger schizophrenic patients. In a study of 57 patients with late-onset paranoid symptoms, Kay (1963) discovered that 19% of the probands had at least one relative with schizophrenia. The risk among siblings was 4.9%, and the risk for children, 7.3%. Onset of schizophrenia among these relatives was before age 40 in the large majority of cases. Rabins et al. (1984) also found a higher likelihood of schizophrenia among family members of patients with paraphrenia than among age- and sex-matched controls with affective disorder.

In the majority of these investigations, the rate of schizophrenia in relatives of paraphrenic (or late-onset schizophrenic) probands falls between that of the general population and that of relatives of early-onset schizophrenic probands. Conclusions about these observations, however, remain tentative due to methodological problems encountered in these studies. For instance, not all family members could be followed into old age to ensure that all cases of both early- and late-onset schizophrenia were detected; physical illness and relocation also cause problems in such studies. Certainly, in terms of family history, late-onset paranoid disorders are more closely related to schizophrenia than to the affective disorders, but the genetic loading appears less prominent than for the early-onset illness.

Intrapsychic Factors

A potential psychological risk factor for late-onset paranoid symptoms is having primitive defense mechanisms for dealing with loss (Eisdorfer 1960, 1980). The older person with a long-standing propensity to use projection as a defense may expel grief and may adjust to loss by blaming others rather than working through grief internally. A tendency to see losses as being due to external factors can contribute to suspiciousness and paranoia. Potential areas of loss include employment, role in society, and functional capacity. Of particular importance, as described above, is the loss of perceptual ability and poorer cognitive capacity with associated attentional and mnemonic deficits. The characteristic of many of these losses is that they are not under the control of the older adult and may be almost imperceptible to the patient. Nevertheless, they challenge the elder's mastery of the world, leading to a search for an explanation to account for the losses.

Treatment of Paranoid or Schizophrenic Symptoms in Late Life

The core of effective management of the patient with late-onset schizophrenia-like symptoms is treatment with antipsychotic medications. Post (1966) reported that those patients who improved most were those who received adequate treatment and maintenance with neuroleptic medications. Leuchter and Spar (1985) followed 15 patients who suffered from late-onset primary psychotic symptoms and found that the 10 patients treated with phenothiazines had a significantly better outcome than those who were not treated. Late-onset schizophrenia tends to be a chronic illness, and spontaneous remissions are uncommon (Herbert and Jacobson 1967; Kay and Roth 1961). Discontinuation of neuroleptics generally causes an exacerbation of symptoms (Yassa et al. 1993). The patients who have been followed in treatment studies (when organic problems were not present) have an outcome as good as, if not better than, that of patients who demonstrate schizophrenic symptoms earlier in life. For example, Post (1966) found that of 75 patients treated with either trifluoperazine (10–60 mg/day) or thioridazine (75–600 mg/day), 43 experienced a complete remission, whereas only 8 showed no response. With follow-up over several months to 3 years, the majority of these patients stayed symptom free when they received adequate initial phenothiazine treatment and maintenance.

Unfortunately, the clinician treating the paranoid older adult with neuroleptic medication faces the fact that tardive dyskinesia (TD) due to long-term (and even short-term) treatment with antipsychotic medications is more prevalent in late life.

Mukherjee et al. (1982) found age to be significantly correlated with TD in 153 psychiatric outpatients. After reviewing 76 selected studies on the prevalence of TD, Yassa and Jeste (1992) reported that rates reached a peak in men between 50 and 70 years old, but continued to rise after age 70 in women; the women also had more severe symptoms. In a 5-year study of 99 elderly psychiatric patients without prior exposure to neuroleptics, Yassa and colleagues (1992) found that 35% of treated patients developed TD; interestingly, those with major depression were significantly more likely to develop TD than were elders with organic brain syndromes or delusional psychoses. Therefore, age, gender, length of neuroleptic treatment, cumulative dose of neuroleptics, and the presence of affective symptoms all must be included as factors that increase the likelihood of development of TD (DeVeaugh-Geiss 1982; Yassa et al. 1992). Despite the most cautious approach, however, TD will develop in some patients; in that event, some data suggest that discontinuing the neuroleptic may cause improvement in some cases (Yassa 1991).

In general, low doses of neuroleptics are adequate for controlling psychotic symptoms in most older adults. The clinician must monitor response carefully and inform both patient and close family members about potential side effects such as orthostatic hypotension, anticholinergic effects, oversedation, parkinsonism, neuroleptic malignant syndrome, tardive dyskinesia, and tardive dystonia. Although a higher dose of medication is required for patients with more severe symptoms, initial starting dosages—especially for outpatients with paranoid symptoms—range from 10 to 25 mg daily for thioridazine, from 2 to 4 mg daily for thiothixene, and from 0.5 to 3 mg daily for haloperidol.

The choice of medication usually depends on what side effects the clinician wishes to avoid. Because of its orthostatic and anticholinergic side effects, thioridazine may be troublesome for the frail elderly person who is prone to falling or for the elderly man with prostatic hypertrophy who is at risk for outflow obstruction. These adverse effects can be minimized by keeping the total daily dosage below 80 mg. The sedative effects of thioridazine may be particularly useful in agitated, psychotic patients, although dosages higher than 80 mg/day may be required for a therapeutic response. Haloperidol is a useful drug when sedation is less important, a stronger neuroleptic is needed, and/or the clinician wishes to avoid the orthostatic or anticholinergic effects associated with low-potency neuroleptics. On the other hand, haloperidol presents significant problems for the older person with preexisting rigidity or tremor who is inclined to develop parkinsonian side effects; furthermore, the onset of akathisia in the already delusional patient may undermine initial efforts to encourage compliance with medication. In a small study of 18 psychogeriatric patients, Oberholzer and colleagues (1992) have demonstrated the safety and effectiveness of low-dose clozapine for elderly patients who develop severe neurological side effects.

Most older persons are willing to use a medication if it is explained that the medication will be of value in improving sleep and decreasing anxiety. Medication compliance is usually less of a problem for the paranoid older adult than it is for paranoid patients at earlier stages of the life cycle. Most elders trust their clinicians and are willing to adhere to the suggestions made for optimal therapy. When objections to medications occur, alliance with a family member is beneficial. Parenteral depot neuroleptics may have advantages over oral medications in cases of noncompliance (Raskind et al. 1979). Strong objection to medication or any intervention, however, may indicate the need for hospitalization.

Drug therapy is not the sole intervention available for the paranoid older adult. Clinicians must work to establish a trusting, supportive relationship with the patient. Some delusional patients require a somewhat distant, "medical-type" of approach, which is viewed as less threatening. Nevertheless, respect for the patient, a willingness to listen to whatever complaints and fears the patient experiences, and availability by telephone when crises occur contribute to an improved therapeutic alliance. A professional, matter-of-fact posture is valued by the distressed paranoid elder. He or she wants the attention of the clinician at the time concerns occur. Most elders do not abuse the telephone, and if a patient calls, a return phone call is important.

Of equal importance in treating the paranoid older adult is the development of relationships with persons in the patient's social environment. The value of family relations is obvious: family members are often the first to notice a deterioration in the patient's condition and are therefore the first to contact the physician regarding the problem. In addition, police officers, neighbors, pharmacists, and so forth,

can serve as valuable allies. Older persons with paranoia living in relatively contained communities are well known in these communities. Neighbors and contacts who have known the individual for years not only will recognize a change in behavior but also can serve as valuable allies for limiting the destructiveness of this behavior. Paranoid symptoms can be tolerated by communities—more than many clinicians expect—when they are understood. The clinician and social worker must help to facilitate a network among these various contacts in the community. Needless phone calls to the police, investigations, neighborhood rifts, and so forth can be avoided if a network for supporting and caring for the paranoid older adult is allowed to become established around that elder. Fragmented neighborhoods and a fast-paced lifestyle, common in the latter part of the 20th century, make the development of such a network less likely. Nevertheless, the possibility exists for even transient participants in the patient's life to form a network.

Many inexperienced clinicians try to confront the older paranoid patient with the lack of reason and false assumptions inherent in paranoid ideation. By definition, a delusion is a fixed, false belief that does not yield to persuasion or logic. Frontal attacks are of no value in managing the paranoid older adult, and frequently result in severance of the therapeutic relationship. On the other hand, clinicians must not be deceitful by pretending to agree with paranoid ideation when in fact they do not agree. Rather, the therapeutic alliance can be facilitated if the clinician makes statements such as, "I don't see the situation as you do, but I can understand how you might view it the way you do and I wish to help you nevertheless." Neuroleptic medications often do not cause delusions to disappear; instead, they simply make the delusions less distressing and more tolerable to the patient. Even if paranoid or delusional symptoms remit with treatment, the older adult may not relinquish the belief that these symptoms were reasonable and real.

If behavior resulting from paranoid ideation becomes dysfunctional or dangerous, behavioral approaches may be required to constrain that behavior. For the outpatient, these techniques are usually best implemented by family and friends. Limiting the distance that the elder drives, limiting the use of the telephone, and obtaining guardianship—and therefore the ability to manage the elder's finances—are some of the constraints that can be applied in managing the paranoid older adult.

Finally, if physical health can be improved or if sensory deficits and social isolation can be alleviated, paranoid symptoms may sometimes correct themselves. The "hard core" paranoid person will have more difficulty in social interactions, but the individual with transitional paranoid ideation or suspiciousness will do better with frequent social contacts. When hearing problems are corrected or vision is improves, increased function often follows.

References

American Psychiatric Association: Diagnostic and Statistical Manual of Mental Disorders, 3rd Edition. Washington, DC, American Psychiatric Association, 1980

American Psychiatric Association: Diagnostic and Statistical Manual of Mental Disorders, 3rd Edition, Revised. Washington, DC, American Psychiatric Association, 1987

American Psychiatric Association: Diagnostic and Statistical Manual of Mental Disorders, 4th Edition. Washington, DC, American Psychiatric Association, 1994

Baron M, Gruen R, Asnis L, et al: Age-of-onset in schizophrenia and schizotypal disorders: clinical and genetic implications. Neuropsychobiology 10:199–204, 1983

Black DW, Fisher R: Mortality in DSM-III-R schizophrenia. Schizophr Res 7:109–116, 1992

Blazer DG, George LK, Hughes D: Schizophrenic symptoms in an elderly community population, in Epidemiology of Aging. Edited by Brody J, Maddox GL. New York, Springer, 1988, pp 134–149

Bridge TP, Wyatt RJ: Paraphrenia: paranoid states of late life, I: European research. J Am Geriatr Soc 28:193–200, 1980

Charlesworth GM, Hymas N, Wischik CM, et al: Case conference report: late paraphrenia, advanced schizophrenic deterioration and dementia. International Journal of Geriatric Psychiatry 8:765–773, 1993

Christenson R, Blazer DG: Epidemiology of persecutory ideation in an elderly population in the community. Am J Psychiatry 141:1088–1091, 1984

Cooper AF, Porter R: Visual acuity and ocular pathology in the paranoid and affective psychoses of later life. J Psychosom Res 20:97–105, 1976

Cooper AF, Kay DWK, Curry AR, et al: Hearing loss in paranoid and affective psychoses of the elderly. Lancet 2:851–854, 1974

Cooper AF, Garside RF, Kay DWK: A comparison of deaf and nondeaf patients with paranoid and affective psychoses. Br J Psychiatry 129:532–538, 1976

Cummings JL, Miller B, Hill MA, et al: Neuropsychiatric aspects of multi-infarct dementia and dementia of the Alzheimer type. Arch Neurol 44:389–393, 1987

DeVeaugh-Geiss J (ed): Tardive Dyskinesia and Related Involuntary Movement Disorders: The Long-Term Effects of Antipsychotic Drugs. Boston, MA, John Wright, 1982

Eisdorfer C: Rorschach rigidity and sensory decrement in a senescent population. J Gerontol 15:188–190, 1960

Eisdorfer C: Paranoia and schizophrenic disorders in later life, in Handbook of Geriatric Psychiatry. Edited by Busse EW, Blazer DG. New York, Van Nostrand Reinhold, 1980, pp 329–337

Essa M: Late-onset schizophrenia (letter). Am J Psychiatry 139:1528, 1982

Fish F: Senile schizophrenia. Journal of Mental Science 106:938–946, 1960

Funding T: Genetics of paranoid psychoses in later life. Acta Psychiatr Scand 37:267–282, 1961

Gold DD: Late age of onset schizophrenia: present but unaccounted for. Compr Psychiatry 25:225–237, 1984

Harris MJ, Jeste DV: Late-onset schizophrenia: an overview. Schizophr Bull 14:39–55, 1988

Hassett AM, Keks NA, Jackson HJ, et al: The diagnostic validity of paraphrenia. Aust N Z J Psychiatry 26:18–29, 1992

Herbert ME, Jacobson S: Late paraphrenia. Br J Psychiatry 113:461–469, 1967

Heston LL: The paranoid syndrome after midlife, in Schizophrenia and Aging. Edited by Miller NE, Cohen GD. New York: Guilford, 1987, pp 249–257

Hodkinson HM: Common Symptoms of Disease in the Elderly. Oxford, Blackwell, 1976

Howard R, Almeida D, Levy R: Schizophrenic symptoms in late paraphrenia. Psychopathology 26:95–101, 1993

Jeste DV, Harris MJ, Pearlson GD, et al: Late-onset schizophrenia: studying clinical validity. Psychiatr Clin North Am 11:1–14, 1988

Jeste DV, Manley M, Harris MJ: Psychoses, in Comprehensive Review of Geriatric Psychiatry. Edited by

Sadavoy J, Lazarus L, Jarvik L. Washington, DC, American Psychiatric Press, 1991, pp 353–369

Jeste DV, Harris MJ, Drull A, et al: Clinical and neuropsychological characteristics of patients with late-onset schizophrenia. Am J Psychiatry 152:722–730, 1995

Kay DWK: Late paraphrenia and its bearing on the aetiology of schizophrenia. Acta Psychiatr Scand 39:159–169, 1963

Kay DWK, Roth M: Environmental and hereditary factors in the schizophrenias of old age ("late paraphrenia") and their bearing on the general problem of causation in schizophrenia. Journal of Mental Science 107:649–686, 1961

Kolle K: Die Primare Verrucktheit. Leipzig, Germany, Thieme, 1931

Kraepelin E: Dementia Praecox and Paraphrenia (1919). Translated by Barclay RM. Edited by Robertson GM. Huntington, NY, Robert E. Krieger, 1971

Leuchter AF, Spar JE: The late-onset psychoses: clinical and diagnostic features. J Nerv Ment Dis 173:488–494, 1985

Lipowski ZJ: Delirium update. Compr Psychiatry 21:190–196, 1980

Lipowski ZJ: Transient cognitive disorders (delirium, acute confusional states) in the elderly. Am J Psychiatry 140:1426–1436, 1983

Lowenthal MF: Lives in Distress. New York, Basic Books, 1964

Marneros A, Deister A: The psychopathology of "late schizophrenia." Psychopathology 17:264–274, 1984

Mayer-Gross W: Die Schizophrenie. Berlin, Germany, Springer, 1932

McGlashan TH: Predictors of shorter-medium and longer-term outcome in schizophrenia. Am J Psychiatry 143:50–55, 1986

Meyers BS, Greenberg R: Late-life delusional depression. J Affect Disord 11:133–137, 1986

Miller BL, Lesser IM, Boone K, et al: Brain white-matter lesions and psychosis. Br J Psychiatry 155:73–78, 1989

Mukherjee S, Rosen AM, Cardenas C, et al: Tardive dyskinesia in psychiatric outpatients. Arch Gen Psychiatry 39:466–472, 1982

Myers JK, Weissman MM, Tischler GL, et al: Six-month prevalence of psychiatric disorders in three communities: 1980 to 1982. Arch Gen Psychiatry 41:959–967, 1984

Oberholzer AF, Hendriksen C, Monsch AU, et al: Safety and effectiveness of low-dose clozapine in psychogeriatric patients: a preliminary study. Intl Psychogeriatr 4:187–195, 1992

Odegaard O: New data on marriage and mental disease: the incidence of psychoses in the widowed and the divorced. Journal of Mental Science 99:778–785, 1953

Post F: The Clinical Psychiatry of Late Life. Oxford, UK, Pergamon, 1965

Post F: Persistent Persecutory States of the Elderly. Oxford, UK, Pergamon, 1966

Post F: Paranoid disorders in the elderly. Postgrad Med 53:52–56, 1973

Purohit DP, Davidson M, Perl DP, et al: Severe cognitive impairment in elderly schizophrenic patients: a clinicopathological study. Biol Psychiatry 33:255–260, 1993

Rabins P, Pauker S, Thomas J: Can schizophrenia begin after age 44? Compr Psychiatry 25:290–293, 1984

Raskind M, Alvarez C, Merlin S: Fluphenazine enanthate in outpatient treatment of late paraphrenia. J Am Geriatr Soc 27:459–463, 1979

Roth M: The natural history of mental disorder in old age. Journal of Mental Science 101:281–301, 1955

Rzewuska M, Wronska A: Characteristics of early and late onset of schizophrenia. Psychiatr Pol 26:337–345, 1992

Schneider K: Clinical Psychopathology. Translated by Hamilton MW. New York, Grune & Stratton, 1959

Seeman MV: Gender and the onset of schizophrenia: neurohumoral influences. Psychiatric Journal of the University of Ottawa 6:136–138, 1981

Simon A, Cahan RB: The acute brain syndrome in geriatric patients. Psychiatric Research Reports 16:8–21, 1963

Talbott JA: The National Plan for the Chronically Mentally Ill: a programmatic analysis. Hosp Community Psychiatry 32:699–704, 1981

Tsuang MT, Dempsey GM: Long-term outcome of major psychoses, II: schizoaffective disorder compared with schizophrenia, affective disorders, and a surgical control group. Arch Gen Psychiatry 39:1302–1304, 1979

Volavka J: Late-onset schizophrenia: a review. Compr Psychiatry 26:148–156, 1985

Wragg R, Jeste DV: An overview of depression and psychosis in Alzheimer's disease. Am J Psychiatry 146:577–587, 1989

Yassa R: The course of tardive dyskinesia in newly treated psychogeriatric patients. Acta Psychiatr Scand 83:347–349, 1991

Yassa R, Jeste DV: Gender differences in tardive dyskinesia: a critical review of the literature. Schizophr Bull 18:701–715, 1992

Yassa R, Nastase C, Dupont D, et al: Tardive dyskinesia in elderly psychiatric patients: a 5-year study. Am J Psychiatry 149:1206–1211, 1992

Yassa R, Dastoor D, Nastase C, et al: The prevalence of late-onset schizophrenia in a psychogeriatric population. J Geriatr Psychiatry Neurol 6:120–125, 1993

Zarit SH: Aging and Mental Disorders: Psychological Approaches to Assessment and Treatment. New York, Free Press, 1980

Zigler E, Levine J: Age on first hospitalization of schizophrenics: a developmental approach. J Abnorm Psychol 90:458–467, 1981

CHAPTER 15

Anxiety and Panic Disorders

Javaid I. Sheikh, M.D.

Anxiety is a normal and ubiquitous emotion with adaptive value, in that it acts as a warning system alerting a person of noxious events or impending danger. This system can be considered maladaptive, however, when anxiety becomes unjustifiably excessive and, thus, morbid. This morbid anxiety usually manifests in the form of a multitude of cognitive (worry, fearfulness), behavioral (hyperkinesis, phobias), and physiological (palpitations, hyperventilation) symptoms. The severity of such anxiety may range from excessive worrying about everyday concerns regarding job and relationships to episodes of intense anxiety and fear (panic attacks). Anxiety disorders are diagnostic entities comprising various combinations of signs and symptoms of morbid anxiety with criteria regarding their intensity and duration, as described in DSM-IV (American Psychiatric Association 1994). Although anxiety disorders in elderly persons are among the most frequently encountered psychiatric conditions, they remain among the least studied (Sheikh 1992). In this chapter I begin with a diagnostic classification of anxiety disorders based on DSM-IV, discuss the phenomenology of anxiety disorders in elderly persons, summarize epidemiological data in the literature, present a systematic way of completing a diagnostic workup, and describe various treatment strategies for managing elderly patients with anxiety disorders.

Diagnostic Classification and Phenomenology

DSM-IV describes operationally defined, phenomenologically oriented diagnostic criteria for various anxiety disorders. A list of various anxiety disorders based on DSM-IV classification appears in Table 15–1. Following in this section are brief descriptions of the symptomatology associated with various anxiety disorders, along with additional features that are specific to the elderly population.

Dr. Sheikh's work is supported in part by Grant MH-49226-02 from the National Institutes of Health, United States Department of Health and Human Services. This chapter is adapted from a review written for the *Comprehensive Review of Geriatric Psychiatry—2*, 2nd Edition. Edited by Sadavoy J, Lazarus LW, Jarvik LF, et al. Washington, DC, American Psychiatric Press, 1996.

Table 15–1.   DSM-IV anxiety disorders

→ Panic disorder
  with agoraphobia
  without agoraphobia
→ Agoraphobia without history of panic disorder
→ Social phobia
→ Specific phobia
→ Generalized anxiety disorder
→ Obsessive-compulsive disorder
→ Acute stress disorder
→ Posttraumatic stress disorder
→ Anxiety disorder due to a general medical condition and substance-induced anxiety disorder
→ Anxiety disorder not otherwise specified (NOS)

Source.   American Psychiatric Association 1994.

Panic Disorder

Panic disorder is manifested by recurrent episodes of severe anxiety or fear—panic attacks—that are accompanied by multiple somatic and cognitive symptoms. For example, during a panic attack one may experience palpitations, shortness of breath, chest pain or discomfort, sweating, hot and cold flashes, tingling in hands or feet, fear of dying, and fear of losing control. Panic attacks can either occur unexpectedly (uncued) or be situationally bound (cued)—that is, occurring in specific feared situations. Many patients with recurrent panic attacks go on to develop fear of being in places from where escape might be difficult in case incapacitating panic attacks should occur. Such a fear of panic may lead, over time, to multiple avoidance responses (agoraphobia). Thus, panic disorder can be present with or without agoraphobia. Panic disorder is typically chronic in its course, with frequent recurrences and remissions.

Preliminary investigations suggest that many older patients with onset of panic attacks in early life seem to continue with such symptoms in later life, having received inadequate or no treatment over the intervening years (Sheikh et al. 1991). It also appears that although it may not be very common for panic disorder to appear de novo in old age, it does occur (Luchins and Rose 1989; Sheikh et al. 1988). Data from ongoing studies in our program suggest that late-onset panic disorder (LOPD) may be characterized by fewer panic symptoms, less avoidance, and lower scores on somatization mea-

sures compared with early-onset panic disorder (EOPD) in older populations (Sheikh 1991, 1993).

Agoraphobia Without History of Panic Disorder

Agoraphobia, the central feature of which is a fear of being in public places or situations from which escape might be difficult, is rare in the absence of a history of panic attacks. It is not clear whether some patients with agoraphobia without history of panic disorder have a variant of panic disorder. Agoraphobia without history of panic disorder has not been studied in the elderly.

Social Phobia

Social phobia is diagnosed in the presence of a persistent fear of one or more social situations. Common examples include fear of public speaking or the inability to eat food or write in the presence of others. Attempts to enter the phobic situation are typically accompanied by marked anticipatory anxiety. Epidemiological evidence (Blazer et al. 1991) suggests that this disorder is chronic and persists in old age. Although systematic studies of social phobia in the elderly are lacking, our clinical experience suggests that eating or writing in public, due to the presence of dentures and tremors, respectively, may be more bothersome to the elderly than is public speaking.

Specific Phobia

The diagnostic characteristic of a specific phobia is a marked excessive or unreasonable, persistent fear of an object or situation. Examples include fear of flying, animals, receiving a medication through injection, and seeing blood. The diagnosis is made only if avoidance or anxious anticipation causes significant distress or dysfunction. Systematic studies of specific phobias in the elderly are lacking, in general. However, it does appear that in urban settings, fear of crime is particularly prevalent in the elderly population (Clarke and Lewis 1982), leading to nocturnal neurosis in some cases (Cohen 1976).

Generalized Anxiety Disorder

Generalized anxiety disorder is manifested by excessive anxiety or worry (apprehensive expectations) on most days for 6 months or longer. The worry is pervasive in that it focuses on many life circumstances, and the person finds it difficult to control the worry and to focus attention on tasks at hand. The worry is associated with six of the following symptoms of autonomic hyperactivity, motor tension, or hyperarousal:

1. Motor tension—trembling, muscle tension, restlessness, fatigability
2. Autonomic hyperactivity—shortness of breath, rapid heart rate, sweating or cold clammy hands, dry mouth, dizziness, digestive disturbances, hot flashes or chills, frequent urination, and trouble swallowing or "lump in throat"
3. Hyperarousal—feeling "on edge," exaggerated startle response, difficulty concentrating, insomnia, and irritability

Many elderly patients with this syndrome may also present with features of depression, thus making the diagnosis and therapeutic decisions difficult at times.

Acute Stress Disorder

Acute stress disorder, a new category in DSM-IV, describes acute reactions—lasting no longer than 1 month—that are manifested by anxiety as a response to extreme stress. Little information is available about this disorder at this time, although it is not unreasonable to assume that in some patients it may be a harbinger of the development of posttraumatic stress disorder.

Posttraumatic Stress Disorder

The central criterion for posttraumatic stress disorder (PTSD) is the development of characteristic symptoms after a person has experienced, witnessed, or been confronted with an event or events that involve actual or threatened death or serious injury, or a threat to the physical integrity of oneself or others. The person's response to the stressor must involve intense fear, helplessness, or horror. The symptoms experienced are usually a combination of three categories: 1) reexperiencing of the traumatic event (in the form of images, thoughts, perceptions, dreams, illusions, hallucinations, or flashbacks); 2) avoidance of stimuli associated with the trauma

or numbing of general responsiveness (depression-like symptoms); and 3) experiencing symptoms of increased arousal (anxiety-like symptoms). The symptoms usually begin soon after the trauma but can be delayed for a number of months or years. The disorder itself can be acute (less than 3 months in duration) or chronic (lasting for longer than 3 months). Reports of PTSD in elderly survivors of the Holocaust (Kuch and Cox 1992) and among elders who were prisoners of war during World War II (Speed et al. 1989) indicate that PTSD can be a chronic disorder continuing into old age. A recent report also documents development of PTSD for the first time in old age among survivors of the 1988 Armenian earthquake (Goenjian et al. 1994). It appears that although the overall severity of PTSD seemed similar among young and elderly survivors of the earthquake, the elderly reported less reexperiencing but more symptoms of hyperarousal compared with the younger people. It may be premature to assign any significance to these differences before additional studies replicate these findings.

Obsessive-Compulsive Disorder

Obsessive-compulsive disorder is characterized by recurrent obsessions or compulsions that are sufficiently severe to cause marked distress or dysfunction in occupational or personal matters. *Obsessions* are thoughts, impulses, or images that are experienced as intrusive and ego-dystonic and that cause marked anxiety or distress. Obsessions are not simply worries about real-life problems; common examples include repetitive thoughts of violence toward a loved one, or of contamination by germs or dirt, and repetitive doubts about having injured or offended someone. *Compulsions* are ritualistic behaviors (for example, handwashing, ordering, checking) or mental acts (such as praying, counting, or repeating words silently) that are performed in response to an obsession or according to certain rules that must be applied rigidly. Usually the compulsive behavior or mental act is designed to prevent discomfort or some dreaded situation and is often recognized by the individual as being either excessive or unrealistic. Attempting to resist a compulsion produces tension that can be relieved by yielding to the compulsion. Epidemiological data regarding this disorder suggest a 6-month prevalence of about 1.5% in the elderly (Blazer et al. 1991), although relatively little is known about any special manifestations in the elderly.

Anxiety Disorder Due to a General Medical Condition and Substance-Induced Anxiety Disorder

Anxiety disorder due to a general medical condition and substance-induced anxiety disorder, two anxiety disorders that are new categories in DSM-IV, are defined by etiology.

Anxiety Disorder Not Otherwise Specified

The category of anxiety disorder not otherwise specified includes disorders with prominent anxiety symptoms that are not classifiable as specific anxiety disorders. Examples include clinically significant symptoms of anxiety and depression when criteria are not met for either a specific mood or anxiety disorder, or situations in which a clinician is unable to determine whether an anxiety disorder is primary, secondary, or substance-induced.

Epidemiology

Very few epidemiological studies of anxiety disorders in the elderly have been done. Studies belonging to the era before the introduction of DSM-III (American Psychiatric Association 1980) tended to categorize anxiety and depression into a mixed, anxious-depressive neurosis following the tradition at that time (Bergman 1971; Post 1972). It is thus difficult to discern the prevalence of different anxiety disorders based on those studies.

More recently, in a comparison of the Epidemiologic Catchment Area (ECA) data of a middle-aged group (45–64 years) with an older aged group (65+ years), Blazer et al. (1991) documented the 6-month and lifetime prevalence in the Duke ECA community sample for all anxiety disorders excluding PTSD. Their analysis shows that both 6-month and lifetime prevalence of all anxiety disorders decline somewhat from the middle-aged to the older aged group, though the prevalence figures for the older aged still stand at a formidable combined (all anxiety disorders) 19.7% for the 6-month period and 34.05% for the lifetime (see Table 15–2). These data indicate that anxiety disorders as a group are the most common psychiatric conditions in the elderly,

Table 15–2. Six-month and lifetime prevalence of anxiety disorders by age for the Duke ECA community sample

Diagnosis	6-month prevalence		Lifetime prevalence	
	Age groups (years)			
	45–64	65+	45–64	65+
Simple phobia	13.29	9.63	18.11	16.10
Social phobia	2.04	1.37	3.18	2.64
Agoraphobia	7.30	5.22	9.40	8.44
Panic disorder	1.10	0.04	2.04	0.29
OCD	2.01	1.54	3.33	1.98
GAD	3.10	1.90	6.70	4.60

Note. ECA = Epidemiologic Catchment Area; GAD = generalized anxiety disorder; OCD = obsessive-compulsive disorder. *Source.* Reproduced from Blazer D, George LK, Hughes D: "The Epidemiology of Anxiety Disorders: An Age Comparison," in *Anxiety in the Elderly.* Edited by Salzman C, Lebowitz BD. New York, Springer, 1991, p. 21. Used with permission.

just as they are in younger populations. There is also the suggestion that anxiety disorders may result in higher medical and psychiatric comorbidity. For example, in a study from the United Kingdom, Lindesay (1991) indicated that when elderly individuals with phobic disorders are matched by age and gender to control subjects without a history of phobic disorders, phobic disorders are associated with considerably higher psychiatric and medical morbidity. It also appears that despite higher rates of contact with general practitioners among phobic elderly individuals compared with control subjects, only one of the phobic elderly persons in this study was receiving psychiatric help.

In conclusion, it appears that anxiety disorders are among the most common psychiatric ailments experienced by older adults and among the least studied in that age group.

Diagnostic Workup and Differential Diagnosis

Several factors can confound proper assessment of anxiety in the elderly. First, many medical conditions can masquerade as somatic manifestations of anxiety. These may include cardiovascular problems (such as angina pectoris or cardiac arrhythmias), endocrine disorders (for example, hyperthyroidism or hypoglycemia), pulmonary disorders (including pulmonary embolism and chronic obstructive pulmonary disease), and neurological illnesses (such as temporal lobe epilepsy or movement disorders). Second, any major medical illness can produce anxiety as an expected response to a physical stressor. Third, many medications can produce symptoms of anxiety. Examples of such medications include sympathomimetic compounds such as pseudoephedrine hydrochloride in over-the-counter drugs, thyroid replacement therapies, neuroleptics, antidepressants, and steroids, among others. In addition, withdrawal from sedatives, hypnotics, or alcohol must be considered in the differential diagnosis. Fourth and last, but not the least, depression can be the possible principle disorder with concomitant anxiety as a comorbid condition. With these caveats in mind, evaluation of geriatric anxiety is usually accomplished in three major ways: clinical evaluation, assessment by rating scales, and laboratory investigations.

Clinical Evaluation

The clinical evaluation includes a history of present and past illness (for example, panic disorder usually has remissions and relapses); the use of prescription and over-the-counter medications (including cold remedies, anticholinergic drugs, and over-the-counter hypnotics or stimulants); alcohol use; and family history (such as panic disorder). A mental status examination may reveal some of the cognitive and behavioral signs and symptoms of anxiety, including apprehension, distractibility, hyperkinesis, and startle response. Physiological signs and symptoms detected during the physical examination—including increased heart rate, rapid breathing, sweating, and trembling—can provide additional clues.

Psychometric Assessment

Clinical evaluation of anxiety in the elderly can be aided by the use of anxiety rating scales. These can also serve as instruments to document the effectiveness of various psychological and pharmacological therapeutic interventions. These scales are primarily of two kinds: observer rated and self-rated. The most commonly used observer-rated scale is the Hamilton Anxiety Scale (HAS; Hamilton 1959). It has 14 items listing 89 symptoms that measure psychic and somatic components of anxiety, with each item rated on five levels of severity from "none" (0) to "very severe" (4). A rating of 18 or above is generally considered to be suggestive of clinically significant anxiety. The HAS should be used selectively, however, as it may be cumbersome for many elders to go through the list of 89 symptoms without becoming very fatigued. In addition, when interpreting the score, it is worth considering that elderly persons tend to overendorse the somatic items.

Several of the self-rated anxiety scales can be quite useful as adjuncts to clinical evaluation. These include the State-Trait Anxiety Inventory (Speilberger et al. 1970), the Beck Anxiety Inventory (Beck et al. 1988), and the Symptom Checklist 90—Revised (SCL-90-R; Derogatis 1975). A more detailed discussion of the advantages and disadvantages of various anxiety rating scales in the elderly is available elsewhere (Sheikh 1991).

Laboratory Tests

Laboratory tests can aid in diagnosing anxiety disorders induced by underlying medical conditions and substance abuse. A complete blood count, an electrocardiogram, vitamin B_{12} and folate levels, thyroid function tests, blood glucose levels, and a drug/alcohol screening can be helpful when used appropriately to rule out medical causes of anxiety.

Management

Safe and effective management of anxiety in the elderly can be accomplished by using pharmacological and/or psychological treatments.

Pharmacological Management

Controlled clinical trials of anxiolytics in the elderly are scarce, and so the standard practice is to use anxiolytics based on effectiveness data from younger populations. Numerous compounds belonging to several different classes of drugs have been used as anxiolytics over the past few decades. These include alcohol, barbiturates, antihistamines, antidepressants, neuroleptics, beta-blockers, benzodiazepines, and azapirones. In prescribing any medications to the elderly, one needs to consider age-related physiological changes in absorption, distribution, protein binding, metabolism, and excretion of drugs. In addition to significantly altering plasma levels of drugs, these changes can lead to excessive accumulation of medications in various body tissues and make elderly patients particularly prone to experiencing toxic side effects, even at dose ranges that are average for the general population. These factors are the basis for the adage, "Start low and go slow." Presented below is a brief description of the various drugs and classes of compounds that are currently in common use as anxiolytics.

Benzodiazepines. Over the last three decades, benzodiazepines have been the most frequently prescribed anxiolytics for both young and older patients. Several researchers have demonstrated—again, generally in younger populations—the efficacy of benzodiazepines in treating patients with generalized anxiety disorder (Hoehn-Saric et al. 1988; Rickels 1978), panic disorder (Ballenger et al. 1988; Tesar et al. 1987), and obsessive-compulsive disorder (Bacher 1990; Hewlett et al. 1990). For treating elderly persons, the short-half-life benzodiazepines such as lorazepam, oxazepam, and temazepam may be preferable in that they are inactivated by direct conjugation in the liver, a mechanism that does not seem to be affected by aging (Moran et al. 1988). Most other benzodiazepines—such as diazepam, chlordiazepoxide, chlorazepate, and flurazepam—tend to be metabolized via oxidative pathways into active metabolites, which, in turn, clear much more slowly in older persons.

Alprazolam, a medication with an intermediate half-life that is commonly used to treat patients with panic disorders, has also been shown to have a half-life of more than 21 hours in elderly persons compared with 11 hours in younger people (Kroboth et al. 1990). In a preliminary analysis of an 8-week study of panic disorder in older patients (age 55 and above) in our program, we have found alprazolam to be more effective than placebo in blocking panic attacks. However, data on long-term effectiveness or safety of this medication in older patients with panic disorder are lacking. Given the probability that long-term use of even short-acting benzodiazepines in older people will result in the accumulation of the drug, any use of benzodiazepines in this population should be for specific indications and time limited, preferably to less than 6 months.

Buspirone. This anxiolytic medication with serotonin-1A agonist properties has demonstrated effi-

cacy in younger patients with generalized anxiety disorder (Rickels et al. 1982; Rickels and Schweizer 1987). Studies of buspirone in geriatric populations have shown the following: 1) the pharmacokinetics are very similar in both the elderly and in younger people; 2) the drug is well tolerated and does not cause sedation or cognitive or psychomotor impairment; 3) it does not produce adverse interactions when co-prescribed with a variety of other medications (including antihypertensives, cardiac glycosides, and bronchodilators); and 4) it is effective for the treatment of patients with chronic anxiety symptoms (Gammans et al. 1989; Napoliello 1986; Robinson et al. 1988). Buspirone also appears to be effective in mixed anxiety-depression syndromes (Robinson et al. 1990). Finally, there is some evidence that this drug may be effective in treating patients with agitated dementia (Colenda 1988; Sakauye et al. 1993). It must be noted, however, that in contrast to research results, clinical experience with this medication suggests that a therapeutic response is somewhat inconsistent.

Antidepressants. Several reports over the last three decades have documented the effectiveness of various antidepressants in younger patients with anxiety disorders. For example, the tricyclic antidepressant (TCA) imipramine and the monoamine oxidase inhibitor (MAOI) phenelzine have proven effective in panic disorder and agoraphobia (Mavissakalian and Michelson 1986; Sheehan et al. 1980; Zitrin et al. 1983). More recently, several researchers have demonstrated the efficacy of the selective serotonin reuptake inhibitors (SSRIs) such as fluoxetine, paroxetine, and sertraline in panic disorder (Ohrstrom et al. 1992; Schneier et al. 1990). In the same vein, the TCA clomipramine (Insel et al. 1983; Thorén et al. 1980; Volavka et al. 1985), and the SSRIs fluoxetine and sertraline (Chouinard et al. 1990; Greist et al. 1992) have been shown to be effective for alleviating symptoms of obsessive-compulsive disorder.

Because controlled studies in patients with various anxiety disorders are lacking, evidence is at best inconclusive for the efficacy of secondary amine TCAs like desipramine or nortriptyline, or of atypical antidepressants (like bupropion or trazodone)—agents that would otherwise be preferable in the elderly because they are less anticholinergic than imipramine or clomipramine (Ballenger 1994). Our practice, therefore, is to use one of the SSRIs as the first line of treatment in older patients with panic disorder or obsessive-compulsive disorder, as these drugs seem to be much better tolerated than imipramine or clomipramine by elderly persons. Finally, there are several case reports suggesting that trazodone, a serotonergic antidepressant, may be quite useful in managing severe anxiety and agitation associated with dementia (Pinner and Rich 1988; Simpson and Foster 1986).

Beta-blockers, antihistamines, and neuroleptics. Although beta-blockers have been used for the treatment of various anxiety disorders for about three decades, their effectiveness remains controversial. One area in which they appear to be consistently useful is the management of somatic anxiety, due to the fact that these agents block autonomic reactions commonly associated with anxiety conditions (Lader 1976; Noyes 1985; Tyrer and Lader 1974). Some reports suggest that beta-blockers like propranolol and oxprenolol may be quite suitable for the treatment of some geriatric patients with anxiety and agitation (Petrie 1983; Petrie and Ban 1981). There is also some suggestion for their usefulness in extremely agitated, demented individuals in very high doses—up to 520 mg/day (Greendyke et al. 1986). A 10-mg dose of propranolol twice a day, to be gradually increased to 20–30 mg twice a day if no response occurs, may be sufficient in some of these cases. Caution should be exercised, however, in using nonselective beta-blockers (β_1 and β_2 blockade) such as propranolol or pindolol in the medically ill elderly. These are generally contraindicated in patients with chronic obstructive pulmonary disease, diabetes mellitus, and congestive cardiac failure. Cardioselective β_1 agents such as atenolol and metoprolol may be used with caution in some of these patients.

To manage mild anxiety, short-term treatment with antihistamines such as hydroxyzine and diphenhydramine has sometimes been used (with monitoring for anticholinergic side effects) with varying degrees of success.

Finally, our clinical experience suggests that low-dose, high-potency neuroleptics like haloperidol (for example, 0.25–0.5 mg twice a day) and fluphenazine can be quite effective in managing severe anxiety and agitation associated with dementia.

In conclusion, a variety of compounds—including benzodiazepines, buspirone, antidepressants, and beta-blockers—seem to show effectiveness for the treatment of various anxiety disorders of the elderly.

Psychological Treatments

Psychological treatments can be quite useful for the management of anxiety disorders in the elderly, either in combination with pharmacological treatments or as alternatives to them. Studies in younger populations suggest that dynamic psychotherapy is of limited therapeutic usefulness as a primary treatment for various anxiety disorders (Sheehan et al. 1980; Weiss 1964; Zitrin et al. 1978). No such studies of dynamic psychotherapy in the elderly exist. Many psychiatrists believe, however, that a psychodynamically oriented, supportive therapy can be a valuable adjunct to medication treatment by enabling the patient to view the therapist as understanding and empathic, thus improving patient compliance with the prescribed medication.

Numerous reports have been published over the years describing the efficacy of cognitive-behavior therapy in anxiety disorders of younger patients. For example, a number of cognitive and behavioral interventions are effective for the treatment of generalized anxiety (Barlow 1988; Beck 1988), panic disorder (Clark 1989; Clark et al. 1985), phobias (Marks 1981, 1987), and obsessive-compulsive disorder (Marks 1981; Rachman and Hodgson 1980) in the general population. In general, systematic studies of the effectiveness of cognitive-behavior therapy in the anxious elderly are lacking. One has to settle for inference based on studies in younger patients, and hope that the methods in these studies will be similarly effective in the geriatric population.

Preliminary data from our ongoing studies indicate that cognitive-behavior therapy can be quite effective in older patients with panic disorder (Swales and Sheikh 1993). Cognitive-behavioral treatment should therefore be considered as an alternative to pharmacological treatment in patients in whom the possibility of side effects and drug interactions is high due to intercurrent medical problems and polypharmacy, or in those for whom compliance with a medication regimen is an issue. It can also be considered as a valuable adjunct to pharmacological treatments in patients who have behavioral symptoms that can be targeted—for ex-

Table 15–3. Strategies for effective management of anxiety disorders in the elderly

Disorder	Treatment of choice	Alternative treatments
Panic disorder with or without agoraphobia	Serotonin reuptake inhibitors (e.g., fluoxetine, paroxetine, sertraline)	Alprazolam, imipramine, phenelzine; cognitive-behavior therapy
Generalized anxiety disorder	Benzodiazepines or buspirone	Cognitive-behavior therapy
Obsessive-compulsive disorder	Serotonin reuptake inhibitors	Clomipramine; cognitive-behavior therapy
Social phobia:		
Generalized	Phenelzine + cognitive-behavior therapy	Benzodiazepines
Specific	Beta-blockers + cognitive-behavior therapy	Buspirone
Specific phobia	Cognitive-behavior therapy or benzodiazepines	Beta-blockers
Acute and posttraumatic stress disorders	As indicated	—

Source. Adapted from Sheikh JI: "Anxiety Disorders," in *Textbook of Geriatric Neuropsychiatry.* Edited by Coffey CE, Cummings JL. Washington, DC, American Psychiatric Press, 1994, p. 292. Used with permission.

ample, a moderate to severe degree of agoraphobia in patients with panic disorder. Table 15–3 summarizes strategies for effective management of anxiety disorders in elderly persons.

Conclusions

Despite increasing research interest in the area of anxiety in younger age groups, few systematic studies of the phenomenology and treatment of anxiety disorders in the elderly have been performed. Data from ECA studies suggest that anxiety disorders remain among the most prevalent of all psychiatric disorders in this age group. Several reports suggest that panic disorder can have its onset in late life, and that this may be a distinct subtype with differences in vulnerability factors, phenomenology, treatment, course, and prognosis. Any evaluation of anxiety in elderly persons should take into account that multiple medical illnesses and medications can produce a similar symptom picture. Anxiety disorders tend to be chronic, interspersed with remissions and relapses of varying degrees. Proper education of the patient, leading to better compliance with the treatment regimen, and recent advances in treatment will almost certainly improve the outlook for these patients for better functioning and a more optimistic prognosis.

References

American Psychiatric Association: Diagnostic and Statistical Manual of Mental Disorders, 3rd Edition. Washington, DC, American Psychiatric Association, 1980

American Psychiatric Association: Diagnostic and Statistical Manual of Mental Disorders, 4th Edition. Washington, DC, American Psychiatric Association, 1994

Bacher NM: Clonazepam treatment of obsessive compulsive disorder (letter). J Clin Psychiatry 51:168–169, 1990

Ballenger JC: Pharmacological treatment of panic disorder, in Handbook of Depression and Anxiety: A Biological Approach. Edited by den Boer JA, Ad Sitsen JM. New York, Marcel Dekker, 1994, pp 275–289

Ballenger JC, Burrows GD, DuPont RL, et al: Alprazolam in panic disorder and agoraphobia: results from a multicenter trial, I: efficacy in short-term treatment. Arch Gen Psychiatry 45:413–422, 1988

Barlow DH: Anxiety and Its Disorders: The Nature and Treatment of Anxiety and Panic. New York, Guilford, 1988

Beck AT: Cognitive approaches to panic disorder: theory and therapy, in Panic: Psychological Perspectives. Edited by Rachman S, Maser JD. Hillsdale, NJ, Lawrence Erlbaum, 1988, pp 91–110

Beck AT, Epstein N, Brown G, et al: An inventory for measuring clinical anxiety: psychometric properties. J Consult Clin Psychol 56:893–897, 1988

Bergman K: The neuroses of old age, in Recent Developments in Psychogeriatrics: A Symposium (British Journal of Psychiatry Special Publ No. 6). Edited by Kay DWK, Walk A. Ashford, England, Headley Brothers, 1971, pp 39–50

Blazer D, George LK, Hughes D: The epidemiology of anxiety disorders: an age comparison, in Anxiety in the Elderly. Edited by Salzman C, Lebowitz BD. New York, Springer, 1991, pp 17–30

Chouinard G, Goodman W, Greist J, et al: Results of a double-blind placebo controlled trial of a new serotonin uptake inhibitor, sertraline, in the treatment of obsessive-compulsive disorder. Psychopharmacol Bull 26:279–284, 1990

Clark DM: Anxiety states: panic and generalized anxiety, in Cognitive Behaviour Therapy for Psychiatric Problems: A Practical Guide. Edited by Hawton K, Salkovskis PM, Kirk J, et al. New York, Oxford University Press, 1989, pp 52–96

Clark DM, Salkovskis PM, Chalkley AJ: Respiratory control as a treatment for panic attacks. J Behav Ther Exp Psychiatry 16:23–30, 1985

Clarke AH, Lewis MJ: Fear of crime among the elderly. British Journal of Criminology 22:49–62, 1982

Cohen CI: Nocturnal neurosis of the elderly: failure of agencies to cope with the problem. J Am Geriatr Soc 24:86–88, 1976

Colenda CC: Buspirone in treatment of agitated demented patient (letter). Lancet 1:1169, 1988

Derogatis LR: The SCL-90-R. Baltimore, MD, Clinical Psychometric Research, 1975

Gammans RE, Westrick ML, Shea JP, et al: Pharmacokinetics of buspirone in elderly subjects. J Clin Pharmacol 29:72–78, 1989

Goenjian AK, Najarian LM, Pynoos RS, et al: Posttraumatic stress disorder in elderly and younger adults after the 1988 earthquake in Armenia. Am J Psychiatry 151:895–901, 1994

Greendyke RM, Kanter DR, Schuster DB, et al: Propranolol treatment of assaultive patients with organic brain disease: a double-blind crossover, placebo-controlled study. J Nerv Ment Dis 174:290–294, 1986

Greist J, Chouinard G, DuBoff E, et al: Double-blind comparison of three doses of sertraline and placebo in the treatment of outpatients with obsessive-compulsive disorder. Poster presented at the Collegium Internationale Neuro-Psychopharmacologium 18th Congress, Nice, France, June 1992

Hamilton M: The assessment of anxiety states by rating. Br J Med Psychol 32:50–55, 1959

Hewlett WA, Vinogradov S, Agras WS: Clonazepam treatment of obsessions and compulsions. J Clin Psychiatry 51:158–161, 1990

Hoehn-Saric R, McLeod DR, Zimmerli WD: Differential effects of alprazolam and imipramine in generalized anxiety disorder: somatic vs. psychic symptoms. J Clin Psychiatry 49:293–301, 1988

Insel TR, Murphy DL, Cohen RM, et al: Obsessive-compulsive disorder: a double-blind trial of clomipramine and clorgyline. Arch Gen Psychiatry 40:605–612, 1983

Kroboth PD, McAuley JW, Smith RB: Alprazolam in the elderly: pharmacokinetics and pharmacodynamics during multiple dosing. Psychopharmacology 100:477–484, 1990

Kuch K, Cox BJ: Symptoms of PTSD in 124 survivors of the Holocaust. Am J Psychiatry 149:3337–3340, 1992

Lader M: Somatic and psychic symptoms in anxiety, in Neuro-psychiatric Effects of Adrenergic Beta-Receptor Blocking Agents, Vol 12: Advances in Clinical Pharmacology. Edited by Carlsson C, Engel J, Hansson L. Munich-Berlin-Vienna, Urban & Schwarzenberg, 1976, pp 21–28

Lindesay J: Phobic disorders in the elderly. Br J Psychiatry 159:531–541, 1991

Luchins DJ, Rose RP: Late-life onset of panic disorder with agoraphobia in three patients. Am J Psychiatry 146:920–921, 1989

Marks IM: Cure and Care of Neuroses: Theory and Practice of Behavioral Psychotherapy. New York, Wiley, 1981

Marks IM: Fears, Phobias, and Rituals: Panic, Anxiety, and Their Disorders. New York, Oxford University Press, 1987

Mavissakalian M, Michelson L: Agoraphobia: relative and combined effectiveness of therapist-assisted in vivo exposure and imipramine. J Clin Psychiatry 47:117–122, 1986

Moran MG, Thompson TL II, Nies AS: Sleep disorders in the elderly. Am J Psychiatry 145:1369–1378, 1988

Napoliello MJ: An interim multicentre report on 677 anxious geriatric out-patients treated with buspirone. Br J Clin Pract 40:71–73, 1986

Noyes R: Beta-adrenergic blocking drugs in anxiety and stress. Psychiatr Clin North Am 8:119–132, 1985

Ohrstrom JK, Judge R, Manniche PM, et al: Paroxetine in the treatment of panic disorder. Proceedings of the annual meeting of the American College of Neuropsychopharmacology, San Juan, Puerto Rico, December 1992

Petrie WM: Drug treatment of anxiety and agitation in the aged. Psychopharmacol Bull 19:238–246, 1983

Petrie WM, Ban TA: Propranolol in organic agitation (letter). Lancet 1:324, 1981

Pinner AE, Rich C: Effects of trazodone on aggressive behavior in seven patients with organic mental disorders. Am J Psychiatry 145:1295–1296, 1988

Post F: The management and nature of depressive illnesses in late life: a follow-through study. Br J Psychiatry 121:393–404, 1972

Rachman SJ, Hodgson RJ: Obsessions and Compulsions. Englewood Cliffs, NJ, Prentice-Hall, 1980

Rickels K: Use of antianxiety agents in anxious outpatients. Psychopharmacology 58:1–17, 1978

Rickels K, Schweizer EE: Current pharmacotherapy of anxiety and panic, in Psychopharmacology: The Third Generation of Progress. Edited by Meltzer HY. New York, Raven, 1987, pp 1193–1203

Rickels K, Weisman K, Norstad N, et al: Buspirone and diazepam in anxiety: a controlled study. J Clin Psychiatry 43 (12, sec 2):81–86, 1982

Robinson D, Napoliello MJ, Schenk J: The safety and usefulness of buspirone as an anxiolytic drug in elderly versus young patients. Clin Ther 10:740–746, 1988

Robinson DS, Rickels K, Feighner J, et al: Clinical effects of the 5-HT$_{1A}$ partial agonists in depression: a composite analysis of buspirone in the treatment of depression. J Clin Psychopharmacol 10 (suppl 3):67S–76S, 1990

Sakauye KM, Camp CJ, Ford PA: Effects of buspirone on agitation associated with dementia. Am J Geriatr Psychiatry 1:82–84, 1993

Schneier FR, Liebowitz MR, Davies SO, et al: Fluoxetine in panic disorder. J Clin Psychopharmacol 10:119–121, 1990

Sheehan DV, Ballenger J, Jacobsen G: Treatment of endogenous anxiety with phobic, hysterical, and hypochondriacal symptoms. Arch Gen Psychiatry 37:51–59, 1980

Sheikh JI: Anxiety rating scales for the elderly, in Anxiety in the Elderly. Edited by Salzman C, Lebowitz BD. New York, Springer, 1991, pp 251–265

Sheikh JI: Anxiety disorders and their treatment, in Clinics in Geriatric Medicine: Psychiatric Disorders in Late Life, Vol 8, No 2. Edited by Alexopoulos GS. Philadelphia, PA, WB Saunders, 1992, pp 411–426

Sheikh JI: Is late-onset panic disorder a distinct syndrome? Proceedings of the 146th annual meeting of the American Psychiatric Association, San Francisco, CA, May 1993

Sheikh JI: Anxiety disorders, in Textbook of Geriatric Neuropsychiatry. Edited by Coffey CE, Cummings JL. Washington, DC, American Psychiatric Press, 1994, pp 279–296

Sheikh JI, Taylor CB, King RJ, et al: Panic attacks and avoidance behavior in the elderly. Proceedings of the 141st annual meeting of the American Psychiatric Association, Montreal, Canada, May 1988

Sheikh JI, King RJ, Taylor CB: Comparative phenomenology of early-onset versus late-onset panic attacks: a pilot survey. Am J Psychiatry 148:1231–1233, 1991

Simpson DM, Foster D: Improvement in organically disturbed behavior with trazodone treatment. J Clin Psychiatry 47:191–193, 1986

Speed N, Engdahl B, Schwartz J, et al: Posttraumatic stress disorder as a consequence of the POW experience. J Nerv Ment Dis 177:147–153, 1989

Spielberger C, Gorsuch RL, Lushene R: Manual for the State-Trait Anxiety Inventory. Palo Alto, CA, Consulting Psychologists Press, 1970

Swales PJ, Sheikh JI: Clinical and research perspectives on anxiety in the elderly. Paper presented at the 146th annual meeting of the American Psychiatric Association, San Francisco, CA, May 1993

Tesar GE, Rosenbaum JF, Pollack MH, et al: Clonazepam vs. alprazolam in the treatment of panic disorder: interim analysis of data from a prospective double-blind, placebo-controlled trial. J Clin Psychiatry 48 (suppl 10):16–21, 1987

Thorén P, Åsberg M, Cronholm B, et al: Clomipramine treatment of obsessive-compulsive disorder, I: a controlled clinical trial. Arch Gen Psychiatry 37:1281–1285, 1980

Tyrer PJ, Lader MH: Response to propranolol and diazepam in somatic and psychic anxiety. BMJ 2:14–16, 1974

Volavka J, Neziroglu F, Yaryura-Tobias JA: Clomipramine and imipramine in obsessive-compulsive disorder. Psychiatry Res 14:85–93, 1985

Weiss E: Agoraphobia in the Light of Ego Psychology. New York, Grune & Stratton, 1964

Zitrin CM, Klein DF, Woerner MG: Behavior therapy, supportive psychotherapy, imipramine, and phobias. Arch Gen Psychiatry 35:307–316, 1978

Zitrin CM, Klein DF, Woerner MG, et al: Treatment of phobias, I: comparison of imipramine hydrochloride and placebo. Arch Gen Psychiatry 40:125–138, 1983

CHAPTER 16

Somatoform and Psychosexual Disorders

Ewald W. Busse, M.D.

Somatoform Disorders

Seven somatoform disorders are included in DSM-III-R and DSM-IV (American Psychiatric Association 1987, 1994) and in the International Classification of Diseases, Tenth Revision (ICD-10) Classification of Mental and Behavioural Disorders (World Health Organization 1992). However, when one compares these three diagnostic systems, it is obvious that there are variations that may result in serious inconsistencies. Consequently, although the clinician will probably want to adhere to a single method, he or she must be aware that such variations exist. Hypochondriasis will be a major focus of this discussion.

Hypochondriasis

The term *hypochondriasis* has its origin in the ancient Greek language. Anatomically, the hypochondrium, from which the name of the psychiatric disorder derives, refers to that part of the body between the ribs and the xiphoid cartilage. The ancient Greeks believed that this part of the body, which includes the spleen, was the seat of morbid anxiety

associated with oneself, depression, bad mood, or simulated disease (Allen and Busse 1994). Although the "spleen theory" of anxiety has not withstood the passage of time, the term hypochondriasis has survived and is, obviously, a part of our modern diagnostic nomenclature.

As a diagnostic term, hypochondriasis is not unlike some other psychiatric diagnostic terms in that it has been frequently redefined and has been omitted from and restored to official classifications of mental diseases. Hypochondriacal *neurosis* was included in DSM-III-R but has been omitted in DSM-IV.

Hypochondriasis disorder is the term used in the ICD-10, which describes this disorder as "a persistent preoccupation with the possibility of having one or more serious and progressive physical disorders" (World Health Organization 1992, p. 164). Further, "attention is usually focused on only one or two organs or systems of the body" (p. 164). Marked depression and anxiety are commonly observed. This disorder rarely develops "after the age of 50 years" (p. 165). The syndrome occurs in both men and women, and there are no special familial characteristics. The diagnostic guidelines further state that the disorder is marked by "persistent refusal to accept the advice and reassurance of several different doctors that there is no physical illness or abnormality underlying the symptoms" (p. 165).

Regardless of this uncertainty about the definition and accuracy of the diagnosis, clinicians are aware that hypochondriasis is a common and often frustrating clinical problem. The certainty of diagnosis in an elderly person is complicated by the existence of physical disabilities and diseases and the increase in socioeconomic stress factors that frequently accompany the aging process.

Diagnostic criteria. The DSM-IV diagnostic criteria for hypochondriasis are listed in Table 16–1. As regards age at onset, "the disorder can begin at any age" (American Psychiatric Association 1994, p. 464). (This criterion is different from what appears in ICD-10, which indicates rare onset after age 50.) In DSM-IV, it is acknowledged that hypochondriasis is commonly associated with a depressive mood; however, these depressive symptoms rarely are severe enough to make antidepressant medication necessary (Gallagher and Thompson 1983).

Table 16–1.   DSM-IV diagnostic criteria for hypochondriasis

A. Preoccupation with fears of having, or the idea that one has, a serious disease based on the person's misinterpretation of bodily symptoms.

B. The preoccupation persists despite appropriate medical evaluation and reassurance.

C. The belief in criterion A is not of delusional intensity (as in delusional disorder, somatic type) and is not restricted to a circumscribed concern about appearance (as in body dysmorphic disorder).

D. The preoccupation causes clinically significant distress or impairment in social, occupational, or other important areas of functioning.

E. The duration of the disturbance is at least 6 months.

F. The preoccupation is not better accounted for by generalized anxiety disorder, obsessive-compulsive disorder, panic disorder, a major depressive episode, separation anxiety, or another somatoform disorder.

Specify if:

> **With Poor Insight:** if, for most of the time during the current episode, the person does not recognize that the concern about having a serious illness is excessive or unreasonable

---

Source. American Psychiatric Association 1994, p. 465.

Hypochondriasis—high bodily concern. In this discussion, the disorder of hypochondriasis is considered to be an anxious preoccupation with the body or a portion of the body that is believed to be diseased or functioning improperly. The complaint can lack a discernible organic explanation or it may be an exaggeration of existing pathology. Investigators in the Duke Longitudinal Studies of Aging used a consistent and sensitive measure that identified subjects with "high bodily concern" (Busse 1993). Observations made over a span of 20 years revealed that more than 33% of subjects experienced an episode of "high bodily concern"—usually mild to moderate. Barsky et al. (1990) noted that transient hypochondriasis is common in a general medical clinic. Subjects in the Duke Longitudinal Studies who initially presented with or who developed high bodily concern were found to have a history of other psychoneurotic reactions, a much lower evaluation of life satisfactions, fewer friends, and fewer wholesome attitudes toward their friends. It is important to note that the subjects considered to have high bodily concern differed from the typical hypochondriacal individual seen in a special clinic. The major difference between the medical clinic hypochondriasis patients and subjects in the Duke Longitudinal Studies was that the clinic patients in Barsky et al.'s study did not persist in seeking medical help, and often the fortuitous disappearance of the source of a stress resulted in an improvement of the high bodily concern. This longitudinal study contributed greatly to the understanding of hypochondriasis, resulted in an identification of the importance of certain psychodynamics in the development of hypochondriasis or high bodily concern (Busse 1982), and contributed to an effective treatment program for those patients in a special clinic (Busse 1986).

The etiology of hypochondriasis and the indicated therapeutic intervention are based on the conviction that hypochondriasis in the elderly is frequently a biological/psychosocial phenomenon. The psychotherapeutic rationale and techniques can be understood and used by any interested and motivated physician. The primary care physician carries a major burden for the care of the elderly, including those with hypochondriasis, and it has been observed that many elderly hypochondriacal patients respond favorably to a combined medical-psychotherapeutic approach. However, treatment of such patients is best accomplished by a psychiatrist working in a general medical clinic or by an adequately trained primary care physician.

Comorbidity in hypochondriasis. With older hypochondriacal patients, physicians must remain alert to the possibility that true organic illness can coexist or develop. Included in the high cost to the patient of being neurotic is the distinct possibility that physical illness can be overlooked because the multiple symptoms make it difficult to separate functional from organic signs or symptoms.

Depression in hypochondriasis. A number of observers have reported that in the Far East, particularly in the People's Republic of China, depression as we now define it is relatively rare. However, the conflicts that might otherwise precipitate depression are expressed in that culture in terms of somatic equivalents. This is explained in a number of ways, including the observation that guilt feelings and depressive affect are rarely or poorly verbalized (Grauer 1984). It is also reported that the diagnosis of neurasthenia is popular in China, and often this diagnosis represents the somatization of a depressive status; the existence of depression is denied by the patients (Kleinman 1982).

Affective disorders in late life may be manifested by exaggerated fears and worries about the body. Depression is the most common affective condition to be masked by physical symptoms. Because depression is more common in the elderly, one might expect to see an increased prevalence of hypochondriacal symptoms in this group. An "advantage" of such symptoms for the depressed patient is that he or she may receive secondary gain in the form of the attention, comfort, touching, and interest associated with interactions with physicians and family members regarding the patient's pain (Busse and Blazer 1980).

Most studies indicate that the prevalence of hypochondriasis is quite high among the depressed elderly. In one study (Alarcon 1964), hypochondriacal symptoms were found in 65.7% of men and 62% of women among a group of 152 depressed patients over the age of 60. The most common presenting symptom was constipation. Hypochondriacal symptoms may be associated with overt symptoms of anxiety or depression. Of those individuals with hypochondriacal symptoms, 24.8% attempted suicide; among those free of such symptoms, only 7.3% attempted suicide. Thus, presence of hypochondria-

cal symptoms in the older patient who also has significant depression may present a potentially critical situation to the clinician.

Lyness (1993) devised a study to examine the relationship of "somatic worry" to age, actual medical illness, and depressed severity. Observations apparently confirm the notion that "somatic worry" is indeed hypochondriasis and is relatively independent of the depression and the medical illness. Further studies are needed to clarify the relationship between age, depression, and medical illness in the production of "somatic worry."

Barsky and colleagues (1992) reported their work with a sample of patients with hypochondriasis (as described by DSM-III-R criteria), whom they compared with a random sample of outpatients in a general medical setting. Careful examination of the subjects' histories as well as their current situations revealed that, in contrast to what was found in the control group, a considerable overlap existed between symptoms of hypochondriasis and the manifestation of depression and anxiety disorders in the sample of hypochondriacal patients. An overlap also occurred between hypochondriasis and other somatoform disorders, particularly somatization disorder, and the investigators concluded that these two diagnostic groupings represent two different ways of describing the same clinical entity. Some of the other data collected by Barsky and colleagues (1990) are also interesting: the mean age of hypochondriac patients was 57.1 years; 76% were women; and 51% were married; and the sample was distributed over a range of social classes.

Epidemiology. A community survey in Durham, North Carolina (Maddox 1964) revealed that approximately 10% of elderly patients who were questioned assessed their physical health to be poorer than it actually was (when health status was rated on an objective basis). These individuals were more depressed and had decreased life satisfaction. Though their physical health status was normal, their activities of daily living were decreased, and they visited their physicians more frequently compared with subjects in a control group. One surprising finding was that these individuals were actually more willing to see a mental health counselor (if they demonstrated some impairment in their mental health) than were the control population. This finding is in contrast to the general belief that the hypochondriacal patient avoids mental health services and gravitates to individuals who they feel will take interest in their physical health only. A separate study found that 53.6% of the elderly surveyed felt themselves to be in better health than others. Thirty-one percent reported that their own health was about the same as that of others, and 9.8% considered their health to be poorer than that of other persons their age (U.S. Department of Health, Education and Welfare 1977).

In a report from another study of the elderly in Durham County, Maddox and Douglass (1973) noted that two of three elderly subjects displayed a reality orientation in their subjective evaluation of health status. Of the one-third of subjects who did not display such a reality orientation, 17% subjectively assessed their health as poor when it was good according to objective evaluation, and 13% assessed their health as good when it was objectively rated as poor.

Together, these studies indicate that between 10% and 20% of community-dwelling elderly persons consider their own health to be poor compared with the health of other persons their own age, and subjectively view their health to be worse than it actually is, as demonstrated on objective examination. These individuals may not all deserve the label "hypochondriacal," but the factors contributing to the development of this negative assessment of health status may form a predictable pattern. This turning attention to the body may 1) facilitate communication and interaction with others (via symptom communication), 2) displace anxiety, 3) be used to form an identification with a deceased or absent loved one, 4) provide self-punishment for unresolved guilt feelings, and 5) be used to control the behavior of individuals within the immediate environment. Regardless of the etiology, these individuals represent a difficult challenge for the treating physician.

Genesis of hypochondriasis. In his review article on the subject, Lipowski (1987) noted that predisposing factors such as genetics, developmental learning, personality, and sociocultural environment play a role in somatization. Swedish investigators have gathered data from adoption studies in regard to familial somatization patterns. Sigvardsson et al. (1984) suggested that somatization is more common in adopted women than in nonadopted women. This raises the issue of genetic predisposition to so-

matization, as adoptees are known to have a higher percentage of biological parents with alcoholism and criminality compared with nonadoptees. There may be a complex interaction between the type of somatizers, alcoholism and antisocial behavior, and sex differences. The interaction between biological predisposition and environmental influences requires additional attention.

Theories that conceptualize the genesis of hypochondriasis as learned behavior from childhood are especially appealing because, intuitively, they make sense. Children suffering from "physical" disorders may get anxious attention from parents (Parker and Lipscombe 1990). They may also learn that one aspect of being sick is that unpleasant duties can be avoided. Somatization may thus become a way to deal with adverse social situations and to maintain self-esteem.

More than 50 years ago, Kanner wrote of his belief that hypochondriacal attitudes in children often reflected school problems or "unhappiness at home" (Kanner 1935). He observed that some mothers focused on their children's somatic functioning rather than on their own, thus teaching the child somatization. This improper maladaptive coping pattern may well continue into adulthood. However, although it is possible that these early childhood influences can shape the child into a hypochondriacal character, it may not necessarily follow, and innate personality characteristics may exist that predispose only some to somatization. Barsky and Klerman (1983) suggested the existence of a "somatic style" and pointed out that there are individuals who "amplify body sensations," focus on and misinterpret them, and reach the conclusion that these sensations may indicate disease. Costa and McCrae (1985) observed that persons who somatize tend to score highly on measures of neuroticism.

Predisposing factors appear by no means to be limited to stressful life events that occur in childhood. Studies on elderly hypochondriacal patients demonstrate that contributing factors can include recurrent exposure to criticism in a situation that provides no possibility of escape, reduction in economic status, loss of spouse and friends, isolation due to socioeconomic factors, and deterioration in marital satisfaction (Busse 1986).

Psychodynamics. Although each individual has different psychosocial stresses and responses, there are four psychological defense mechanisms that often—although not exclusively—play an important role in the dynamics of hypochondriasis in the elderly (Busse 1986):

1. The symptoms may be used as an explanation for failure to meet personal and social expectations and to avoid or excuse recurrent failure.
2. The patient may be experiencing increasing isolation and therefore may be withdrawing psychic interests from other persons or objects and redirecting interests toward the self, the body, and its functions.
3. The patient may be shifting anxiety from a specific psychiatric conflict to a less threatening bodily function.
4. The symptoms may be a means of self-punishment and atonement for unacceptable hostile feelings toward persons close to the individual.

The primary mental mechanisms are reinforced by secondary gain. Secondary gain is the increased attention and sympathy from friends and health care providers that is originally generated by the symptoms. It is important that the clinician keep these mechanisms in mind, since doing so will make the patient's complaints more understandable and provide a logical basis for the therapeutic approach.

Risk factors. Stressful life events are often precipitating factors of hypochondriacal reactions in later mid-life and early late-life years. These events often include exposure to a work or social situation in which the individual suffers prolonged criticism and lacks escape opportunities (Busse 1982). The older person is likely to experience other stresses, such as a reduction in economic status and/or loss of spouse and friends, both of which contribute to social isolation. A deterioration in marital satisfaction can result from chronic disability affecting one of the marital partners.

Remission and course. The longitudinal studies of "normal" aging people conducted at Duke University Center for the Study of Aging and Human Development have yielded some important observations relevant to the problem of hypochondriasis (Busse 1986). Observation of subjects over time revealed that hypochondriacal reactions are often transient, lasting from a few months to several years.

It is not unusual for depressive signs and symptoms to occur concomitantly with hypochondriasis. The hypochondriacal reaction is often an adaptive response to an unfamiliar, serious social stress; hence, improvement is related to the fortuitous disappearance of the stress, such as the moving away of an adult child who has been a persistent critic of the older person.

The subjects observed in the Duke Longitudinal Study I that were classified as having "high bodily concern,"—that is, hypochondriasis—frequently did not seek medical attention but, in fact, resisted the urging of family or friends to seek medical relief for their multiple symptoms. Many of the hypochondriacal subjects used home remedies and excessively used over-the-counter medication. Based on their observations of these subjects, the investigators suggested that if such hypochondriacal persons are forced to see a physician—particularly at the insistence of family or friends—their pattern of maintaining social adjustment and self-esteem is threatened and the hypochondriacal pattern may become solidified.

These longitudinal observations are consistent with those of Barsky and Klerman (1983), who maintain that hypochondriasis is a learned social behavior. It is a type of social communication that is an appeal for sympathy and support. The hypochondriacal person has learned that the illness behavior is a way to obtain support and attention. Furthermore, chronic illness behavior is also reinforced by the successful avoidance of adverse consequences, such as unpleasant duties and obligations. Similar observations were made in the longitudinal studies: the individuals were using somatization as a way to deal with an adverse social situation and as a way of maintaining their self-esteem.

A particular caution is appropriate here concerning diagnostic or exploratory surgical procedures in hypochondriacal patients. It never helps the patient to have a surgical scar that testifies to the fact that a competent physician believed that the patient had something wrong with his or her body. In addition, the operative scar can become a focus of new symptoms that are then attributed to "complications" or "adhesions" following the surgical procedure.

Forms of brief psychotherapy. There are at least 250 "brands of therapy that are advocated for the treatment of mental, emotional, and behavioral problems" (Meredith 1986, p. 30). Each brand of therapy is said by its proponents to have special features that make it more effective, and often certain brands are said to be particularly useful in certain disorders. A number of brief psychotherapies have been described for the treatment of depression (not hypochondriasis) in the elderly. Some of the better-known types are cognitive therapy (Beck et al. 1979; Emery 1981), behavioral therapy (Gallagher et al. 1981; Lewinsohn et al. 1976), interpersonal therapy (Klerman and Weissman 1982), and brief psychodynamic psychotherapy (Bellak and Small 1965). These brief forms of psychotherapy (up to 20 visits) are useful, but are designed for those patients who are actively seeking psychiatric help. In contrast, the therapeutic approach described in this chapter applies to patients who are resistant or unwilling to be referred for psychiatric help.

Brown and Vaillant (1981) described a study involving patients who were severely hypochondriacal—patients who, according to current criteria, would probably be considered to have somatization disorder. Brown and Vaillant reached the conclusion that this type of hypochondriasis can best be defined as "the transformation of reproach toward others arising from bereavement, loneliness, or unacceptable aggressive impulses into self reproach initially and then into complaints of other pain or somatic illness" (p. 725). These investigators noted that encounters with this type of hypochondriacal patient tend to elicit five responses that adversely influence therapeutic approaches: 1) the ignoring of the patient's social history, 2) the covert anger of the patient that may escape the physician's awareness (specifically, the hidden anger of the patient toward the physician), 3) the physician's frustration and resentment that disrupt the doctor-patient relationship, 4) the attempts to offer care that are misdirected and malfunction, and 5) unexpected shifts in the patient's behavior that surprise and distract the physician. Brown and Vaillant concluded that to treat hypochondriacal patients successfully, the physician needs to combine both an intellectual and an emotional understanding of the patient's predicament. The physician must appreciate the traumatic psychosocial history of the patient.

Therapeutic techniques.   The therapeutic techniques described below are designed to assist the primary care physician and the psychiatrist practicing in a general medical setting in dealing on an outpatient basis with the hypochondriacal patient whose symptoms are of relatively recent onset (less than 2 years) (Busse and Blazer 1980). The techniques are basic to, but not sufficient for, the handling of the other six somatoform disorders described in DSM-III-R and for hospitalized patients. Furthermore, these techniques may be of limited usefulness in dealing with multiple physical complaints or when hypochondriasis is associated with an early-onset somatization disorder, schizophrenia, or severe depression. This review of a therapeutic approach contains "basic" information. Additional relevant material can be found in numerous sources, including Busse and Blazer (1980) and Busse (1982, 1986).

Ineffective Treatment Techniques

Limits of revelations.   It seems logical that if the patient is given a full explanation of his or her medical condition—that is, if the patient is informed of the absence of any organic explanation for his or her complaints—this would serve as reassurance. Furthermore, consistent with the patient's "right to know" and with "normal" thinking, the patient should be informed of physical and laboratory studies that are negative. However, if the physician says, "The results of my careful workup indicate that you are physically in good health," many hypochondriacal patients will react poorly. Such an abrupt revelation implies that the person's symptom profile must be of mental origin. The failure of the physician to find an organic explanation for the complaints seems to rob the patient of an unconscious defense mechanism, the disrupting of which further reduces self-esteem. Often after such an abrupt revelation, the patient's complaints will increase and the patient may terminate contact with the physician. Such hypochondriacal patients become medical "shoppers," pursuing a doctor-patient relationship that meets their needs.

Even less-specific explanations of how emotional upsets can sometimes cause physical symptoms are likely to be unsuccessful. Patients may agree that this can happen to some people, but they are sure that a mental or emotional explanation is not applicable in their own case.

To balance the right to know with a measure of

reassurance, it is suggested that the physician include in his or her remarks a supportive statement and manner. For example, "The results of this workup indicate that there is no adequate explanation for your symptoms. It is obvious that you are having problems and I will be pleased to work with you to improve your situation."

Specific diagnosis. Another technique that is unlikely to be successful is to respond to the patient's demand to know "what's wrong with me?" by giving him or her a specific, but false, diagnosis. Often these patients respond by saying they are relieved to know what is wrong with them, but since their symptoms persist and may even increase, they will question the diagnosis and disrupt the relationship with the physician. Instead, the physician should say, "I'm sure it would be reassuring if I had a specific diagnosis, but I don't. However, I am willing to follow your case carefully and I'll try to find some way to improve your health and well-being."

The examples of statements that can be used in response to patients are, of course, only suggestions; a physician must respond in a way that is consistent with his or her personal style. However, it is important to keep in mind the two essential elements of such statements: 1) inclusion of supportive remarks, indicating a commitment to helping the patient, and 2) avoidance of statements that may threaten the patient's need to maintain a hypochondriacal defense.

Effective Treatment Techniques

For hypochondriacal persons to continue to live comfortably with their families and in society, their psychological defense of hypochondriasis must be maintained until adequate coping mechanisms are developed as a replacement. The physician must understand this need, must listen to the patient's "organ recital" until a positive doctor-patient relationship has been established, should use this relationship to provide the basis for a discussion of areas of emotional conflict, and must help the patient to seek new methods of coping. The physician should make it clear that he or she is aware that the patient is experiencing discomfort and unhappiness and is willing to help.

Use and limitation of medication. A patient-physician relationship is assisted by the use of prescribed medication or a placebo. The physician must be careful to avoid prescribing any medication that is likely to produce side effects, the occurrence of which only complicate an already confused clinical picture. Addictive drugs should be avoided, and medications that the patient has already used without success should not be used. Although only 2.4% of physicians who care for hypochondriacal patients use placebos, such agents have value in practice and research (Busse and Maddox 1985; Poe and Holloway 1980).

The use of prescribed "medication" may be criticized because it implies to the hypochondriacal patient that he or she actually has an organic illness. This criticism is not without merit, but, on the other hand, many hypochondriacal elderly patients actually do experience improvement in their physiological functioning as a result of such "treatment." For example, hypochondriacal elderly patients who suffer from sleep disturbances often respond positively to the improved medical surveillance (and, in fact, such a positive response may allow elimination of the use of hypnotic drugs). Again, the physician must remember that medications and placebos do have symbolic value. A hypochondriacal complaint is a distress signal, and patients' anxiety may be reduced and self-esteem increased by knowing that a reputable, professional person is "taking care" of them.

The roles of relatives. The handling of relatives is an important part of the treatment process. Relatives or friends, particularly those who begin to suspect that the patient's symptoms are of emotional rather than physical origin, may request an interview with the physician to confirm their suspicions. Under these circumstances, the physician should avoid saying that the patient's symptoms are of psychological origin. Rather, physicians should communicate that they consider the patient to be ill and worried, that the patient needs help, and that they will do whatever they can to be of value. One of the surest ways for a patient to lose confidence in the physician is to learn from a relative or friend that the physician confirmed another's belief that the patient's complaints are imaginary.

Frequency of visits. It is generally wise to see a hypochondriacal patient once a week for at least 8–10 weeks. After that point, the time between appointments can be lengthened. Appointments should be made for a definite time. (It is interesting to note how many hypochondriacal patients will respond by saying that the time suggested is inconvenient and will ask for another time to be arranged. The frequency with which this pattern occurs in this population leads to the conclusion that it is a way of testing physicians to determine the extent of their interest in the patient.) Generally, the physician should insist that the patient adhere to a selected time for appointments and adhere to the therapeutic regimen. Firmness gives the patient new confidence that the physician is making a determined effort to be of help.

Length of interview. It is desirable to adhere to an appointment schedule. Although the first contact may require considerable time, return visits can be reduced to between 15 and 20 minutes. The patient should be told when and how long the next appointment will be. This will discourage hypochondriacal patients from making bids for additional time. When the duration of the interview has not been specified, the patient—sensing that the interview is about to be concluded—may "suddenly" remember something very important, thereby seeking to extend the period of contact with the physician. One way to handle such a situation, should it occur, is to suggest to the patient that because the suddenly remembered topic is so important, it should be given more time and should be taken up at the next visit.

Hostility. In the second or third interviews, it is not unusual for the patient to express hostility toward a previous physician. The treating physician must refrain from defending the colleague and must confine remarks to recognition that the patient's experiences have been both upsetting and disappointing. It might be helpful, occasionally, to mention that perhaps the patient is concerned whether the physician will maintain an interest in the patient and continue to seek ways of helping. Such a demonstration of understanding and acceptance of the patient's views can be very constructive.

Resistance. Psychiatrists who work with elderly hypochondriacal persons must recognize that it is highly likely that they will encounter more resistance and more expressions of hostility from these patients than would ordinarily be directed toward physicians in other specialties. Many patients believe that the role of the psychiatrist is to determine or demonstrate that their physical symptoms are of mental origin. It is not unusual for patients to confront the psychiatrist by asserting that imagination or nervousness plays no role in their symptoms. One way of dealing with such resistances is for the psychiatrist to state that he or she recognizes that other individuals may have indicated that the symptoms were of mental or emotional origin, and that this is understandably upsetting to the patient. It may also be helpful to point out to the patient that the psychiatrist's therapeutic role is not limited to psychiatry, but involves the total health and well-being of the individual.

Content of Follow-Up Visits

Interpersonal events. As return visits continue, the physician encourages the patient to give details regarding the interpersonal events that occurred between interviews. Gradually the patient shifts away from physical complaints to placing a greater emphasis on psychosocial conflicts related to the family, work, and friends. When this change develops, treatment can follow two paths. First, patients may gradually lose the intensity of their preoccupation with their imaginary illness as a result of confidence and improved self-esteem gained in the physician-patient relationship. Second, patients may become aware that exacerbations of symptoms occur as the result of certain events, but in the intervening period they can return to a more active and more efficient participation in their interpersonal relationships.

Insight. A still brighter outlook can be anticipated if the patient begins to develop some insight into the situation. The patient may notice that the symptoms become worse after an argument or after being criticized and, as a result, will begin to discuss ways of handling such stressful situations. As defense mechanisms become more effective, the patient will often begin to abandon the physical complaints.

Somatoform Pain Disorder (DSM-III-R)—Pain Disorder (DSM-IV)

Table 16–2 lists the DSM-III-R diagnostic criteria for *somatoform pain disorder*. A comparison of the definitions of pain disorder and hypochondriasis does not reveal a clear distinction between the two disorders.

Table 16–2.	DSM-III-R diagnostic criteria for somato-form pain disorder

A. Preoccupation with pain for at least 6 months.
B. Either (1) or (2):
   (1) appropriate evaluation uncovers no organic pathology or pathophysiologic mechanism (e.g., a physical disorder or the effects of injury) to account for the pain
   (2) when there is related organic pathology, the complaint of pain or resulting social or occupational impairment is grossly in excess of what would be expected from the physical findings.

Source. American Psychiatric Association 1987, p. 266.

The existence of pain is the predominant symptom in a pain disorder, whereas hypochondriasis is based on "physical signs and sensations" (p. 266).

DSM-IV includes two subgroups under the diagnosis of "pain disorder": *pain disorder associated with psychological factors* and *pain disorder associated with both psychological factors and a general medical condition* (see Table 16–3). The first subgroup should not be diagnosed "if criteria are also met for somatization disorder" (American Psychiatric Association 1994, p. 462). For both subgroups, it should be specified whether the condition is acute (less than 6 months' duration) or chronic (lasting 6 months or longer).

In contrast, ICD-10 uses a single category—*persistent somatoform pain disorder.* Further, it specifies that the persistent pain "occurs in association with emotional conflict or psychosocial problems that are sufficient to allow the conclusion that they are the main causative influences" (World Health Organization 1992, p. 168).

The psychophysiology of pain is discussed in Chapter 3. For additional information, see Jessel and Kelly 1993 and Brose and Spiegel 1992.

Periodic pain is experienced by all individuals throughout their lives. However, persistent pain is a problem that is seen more frequently in late and older middle life, and is estimated to afflict 25%–50% of the elderly living in the community (Tait 1993). Pain in elderly individuals is usually associated with degenerative conditions, with pathological conditions (particularly cancer), and with trauma to the body and to the brain. The problem with pain is quite prevalent in nursing homes, affecting approximately 80% of residents.

Table 16–3.	DSM-IV diagnostic criteria for pain disorder

A. Pain in one or more anatomical sites is the predominant focus of the clinical presentation and is of sufficient severity to warrant clinical attention.
B. The pain causes clinically significant distress or impairment in social, occupational, or other important areas of functioning.
C. Psychological factors are judged to have an important role in the onset, severity, exacerbation, or maintenance of the pain.
D. The symptom or deficit is not intentionally produced or feigned (as in factitious disorder or malingering).
E. The pain is not better accounted for by a mood, anxiety, or psychotic disorder and does not meet criteria for dyspareunia.

Code as follows:

307.80   Pain Disorder Associated With Psychological Factors: psychological factors are judged to have the major role in the onset, severity, exacerbation, or maintenance of the pain. (If a general medical condition is present, it does not have a major role in the onset, severity, exacerbation, or maintenance of the pain.) This type of pain disorder is not diagnosed if criteria are also met for somatization disorder.

Specify if:

Acute: duration of less than 6 months

Chronic: duration of 6 months or longer

307.89   Pain Disorder Associated With Both Psychological Factors and a General Medical Condition: both psychological factors and a general medical condition are judged to have important roles in the onset, severity, exacerbation, or maintenance of the pain. The associated general medical condition or anatomical site of the pain (see below) is coded on Axis III.

Specify if:

Acute: duration of less than 6 months

Chronic: duration of 6 months or longer

Note: The following is not considered to be a mental disorder and is included here to facilitate differential diagnosis.

Pain Disorder Associated With a General Medical Condition: a general medical condition has a major role in the onset, severity, exacerbation, or maintenance of the pain. (If psychological factors are present, they are not judged to have a major role in the onset, severity, exacerbation, or maintenance of the pain.) The diagnostic code for the pain is selected based on the associated general medical condition if one has been established (see Appendix G) or on the anatomical location of the pain if the underlying general medical condition is not yet clearly established—for example, low back (724.2), sciatic (724.3), pelvic (625.9), headache (784.0), facial (784.0), chest (786.50), joint (719.4), bone (733.90), abdominal (789.0), breast (611.71), renal (788.0), ear (388.70), eye (379.91), throat (784.1), tooth (525.9), and urinary (788.0).

Source. American Psychiatric Association 1994, pp. 461–462.

Clinical implications of pain. Although age affects many perceptions—including vision, hearing, taste, and smell—it is not clear what changes in pain, if any, are associated with aging. Age does not influence pain thresholds for such diverse stimuli as tooth shock or forearm heat (Harkins et al. 1986). When psychophysiological procedures are designed to measure response to a noxious stimulus, changes may be detected; however, these changes may be attributed to differences in response (e.g., speed of response) rather than to differences in pain perception (i.e., to nociceptive differences).

The pain experienced with myocardial infarction varies in type and severity. The clinician is justified in being concerned that age-associated pain changes may influence the diagnostic criteria that are customarily used. One survey of patients who suffered a myocardial infarction showed that 30% of those over age 70 did not experience pain as a major presenting symptom, and an almost comparable percentage (23%) of younger persons had the same painless experience (MacDonald et al. 1983). It is debatable whether age-associated biological changes actually affect pain perception, but this disputability is not mentioned in the major medical textbooks.

The presentation of pain associated with appendicitis is similar among patients, regardless of age: generalized abdominal pain localized to the right lower quadrant and associated with nausea and vomiting. What may be lacking in the elderly individual are the elevation of temperature and the leukocytosis that often round out the symptom profile in younger patients. The absence of these latter manifestations may account for the diagnostic difficulties that are sometimes encountered in elderly individuals with appendicitis (Albano et al. 1975; Glenn 1978).

It is clear that persistent or frequently recurring pain is associated with physical disorders that are common in late life. These include osteoarthritis, rheumatic arthritis, angina of effort, herpes zoster, and gout. There are other conditions that more likely produce chronic pain in younger adults. These include arthralgia, pleuritic pain, headaches, and backaches. It is highly likely that the presence of persistent pain does have significant effect on psychological functioning, but this is true for both middle-aged and elderly persons (Harkins and Nowlin 1985).

Pain and depression. The symptom overlap between pain and depression is of great clinical importance. Lindsay and Wycoff (1981) observed that 59% of patients who request treatment for depression also have recurrent benign pain. In contrast, 87% of patients in chronic pain clinics are depressed. Patients with chronic pain often report insomnia, eating disturbances, and loss of interest in social activities and in sex (Lindsay and Wycoff 1981). Patients with chronic pain complaints often deny feeling depressed, but their other symptoms suggest the existence of a depression; these include loss of energy, poor concentration, and inappropriate guilt, as well as symptoms such as sleep disturbances, early morning awakening, and psychomotor retardation. The degree of frequency of comorbidity of chronic pain and depression has resulted in the speculation that the two achieve expression through common pathways. Many clinicians believe that the existence of the chronic pain syndrome in some patients results in a secondary depression. In other cases, pain is a masking symptom of depression (Blazer 1993). As previously noted, physical illnesses—particularly degenerative diseases—are the source of chronic pain. Such pain is not related to aging.

Because of the overlap of depression and chronic pain, the use of antidepressants in the management of patients with chronic pain has proved to be of value in many cases. Interestingly, the antidepressant medication may act more rapidly on pain than it does on the other manifestations of the depression. Therefore, it is important for the patient to keep taking the medication despite the reduction in pain. Kwentus and colleagues (1985) reported that some elderly patients who complain of chronic pain have long-standing personality disorders. The pain behaviors that such individuals display may be particularly troublesome. Pain complaints may serve to manipulate friends, relatives, and physicians. In many respects, this is not unlike the secondary gain found in hypochondriasis.

Obviously the psychiatrist must assist in a therapeutic approach by designing a multidisciplinary effort that discourages pain-intensifying, reinforcing behaviors. Some helpful techniques include using set-dose analgesic drug therapy rather than prescribing pain medications for as-needed administration; reinforcing involvement in activities unrelated to pain; according selective inattention to pain complaints; and avoiding prolonged discussion of pain

(Tait 1993). Clinicians must remember a particular caveat in the management of pain in elderly patients: many elderly people are receiving multiple medications for a variety of physical disorders, and drug interactions may seriously complicate the clinical picture.

Relief of pain.   For several thousand years before the birth of Christ, the Egyptians knew that extracts from the white poppy would relieve pain. Furthermore, we know from stone carvings in tombs from the fifth dynasty—about 2500 B.C.—that the Egyptians used an electric fish found in the Nile River to treat a variety of pain conditions.

Acupuncture has been used in the Orient, particularly in China, for thousands of years (Beardsley 1993). The classical textbook of Oriental medicine, *Nei Ching,* refers to the relief of pain by techniques of stimulation of tissue at special sites with sharp objects such as fish bones, stones, or bamboo sticks. An alternative method was to warm these points by pouring small urnsful of burning moxa (herbs) on the skin. Although acupuncture was used for relief of pain, it was not until 1955 that the technique of acupuncture anesthesia was developed in China. In the late 1950s, Chinese medical workers became aware that acupuncture reduced the pain of toothache, sore throat, tooth extraction, and tonsillectomy. This observation formed a basis for expanding the technique for use in more extensive surgical procedures. Initially, practitioners of acupuncture as surgical anesthesia used many needles, but over the years the number has been reduced; currently, only one to four needles are used for many important procedures. In addition, many of today's practitioners supplement their technique with electrical stimulation, eliminating the old procedure of rotating the needles by hand to maintain an input of sensation (Busse and Busse 1979). Acupuncture is usually employed as anesthesia for surgical procedures after several days of trial and education of the patient. As the technique is practiced in China, supplementary drugs are used occasionally, but they are usually of relatively low dosage.

Although most patients insist that they feel no pain when the needle is inserted, effective anesthesia with acupuncture requires that the patient feel sore, distended, heavy, and numb over the site of the needle placement. The needle is usually inserted to a depth of ¼ inch to 1 inch, depending on the patient's body build, location of needle, and so forth. Needle insertion is carried out with care to avoid puncturing blood vessels or disrupting vital organs. Ear points are frequently used. With ear points, some patients do report experiencing pain upon needle insertion.

The most plausible explanation for the effectiveness of acupuncture is consistent with the Melzack and Wall (1965) theory of gate control of pain. This theory holds that certain types of stimuli will flood gates in the nervous system and prevent other types of stimuli from going through these gates. It is also very likely that there is considerable individual variation as to those who respond to acupuncture.

Transcutaneous electrical nerve stimulation (TENS) is a technique for pain control derived from acupuncture that is widely advocated in Sweden (Sjolund and Eriksson 1985). Other methods have been developed to stimulate nervous tissue with devices implanted in the body. Two that have come into clinical use are spinal cord stimulation and dorsal column stimulation. These techniques are used after other measures, such as TENS, have failed.

Treatment of chronic pain.   Chronic pain, by definition, is pain that has persisted for some time; the underlying cause may or may not be identified with a disease process. As noted in Chapter 3, chronic pain serves no useful biological function. Further, the recognized pain pathways may not be involved in the perception of chronic pain, and interruption of these pathways ordinarily results in only transient relief. Furthermore, Gildenberg and DeVaul (1985) believe that cutting pain pathways and the commonly used analgesics not only are ineffective against chronic pain but may actually potentiate it. These authors observe that although there are similarities among patients with chronic pain, each must be considered as an individual, and the physician must be alert to the possibility that a patient's pain has been overevaluated. In such cases, pain plays a central role in how the patients relate to themselves and to others. Social factors may be present that reinforce the pain behavior, and the physician must be careful because such patients often have succeeded in maneuvering physicians into attempting ill-advised medical or surgical procedures. Gildenberg and DeVaul concluded, "Little in the way of pain management can be accomplished unless and until both patient and treating physician exchange the goal of pain relief for that of rehabilitation" (p. 89). In the case of cancer, however, caution must be exercised; these authors noted that pain from malignancies is unusual in that it contains features of both chronic and acute pain (i.e., chronic pain with acute exacerbations). Chronic cancer pain can often be alleviated by interrupting pain pathways.

Medications are used to reduce peripheral pain. The analgesic action of acetylsalicylic acid (aspirin) can be explained by the inhibition of cyclooxygenase. This enzyme controls the synthesis from arachidonic acid of prostaglandins, prostacyclins, and thromboxanes, all of which appear to be associated with pain generation. Many other drugs also inhibit cyclooxygenase. Ibuprofen, which is now commonly used, seems to have both an analgesic and an antiinflammatory effect. The corticosteroids have somewhat similar antiinflammatory/analgesic effects.

Pain clinics. Pain clinics, which currently exist in many medical centers, are usually staffed by a multidisciplinary team. Often a psychiatrist plays a critical role in evaluating and devising a therapeutic plan. The therapeutic plan must take into account the estimate of the degree to which the patient may be aggravating or exaggerating the persistent pain, the patient's personal characteristics, and the environment in which the patient exists.

Although elderly individuals frequently report recurrent or persistent pain, they are underrepresented in the patient population of a multidisciplinary pain clinic. This suggests either that the elderly person tolerates chronic pain as an accepted part of the aging process, or that the referring physician is pessimistic as to what the clinic may offer an older person.

The pain experiences of residents in nursing homes are undoubtedly complicated by physical, emotional, and environmental factors. Added to this already complex picture are the communication difficulties that some residents have. A successful pain treatment plan must be individually constructed so that it adequately deals with the numerous factors that are inherent in a chronic pain syndrome. Unfortunately, chronic pain in elderly individuals can rarely be eliminated completely. It is more realistic to expect to reduce the intensity and frequency of pain exacerbations. Restoring functional capacity improves the mood and the quality of life.

In prescribing medications, it is important for clinicians to remember that drug use in the elderly differs considerably from that in younger adults. Side effects may be particularly troublesome for older persons. A paper published by Brose and Spiegel (1992) includes an excellent detailed table elucidating the 15 common opiates, giving various pharmacokinetic parameters; I recommend this as an important resource for the geriatric psychiatrist.

Patient-controlled analgesia (PCA) has become widely used in hospital settings. This allows the patient to self-administer analgesics as needed, but without exceeding a predetermined limit. Various types of PCA systems are in use, but regardless of the specific system used, the results have been favorable. Patients generally express satisfaction with PCA; they report fewer pain complaints and rarely need to exceed the predicted dose and time limits that are built into the system.

Sexual Behavior and Disorders

Under the category of sexual disorders, DSM-III-R lists two subclasses and defines 9 paraphilias and 10 sexual dysfunctions. The psychopathology of paraphilias is primarily that of a distorted sex object and an aberration of sexual expression and enjoyment. Sexual dysfunctions are manifested by physiological disturbances that are linked etiologically to mental and emotional disorders. Although not classified as somatoform disorders, these dysfunctions not only are held to be physical manifestations of presumed psychological factors but also are without satisfactory explanation based on organic pathology or pathophysiology. Only a few of the sexual disorders are of major concern to the geriatric psychiatrist. DSM-IV contains a number of diagnostic changes. Under the "Sexual and Gender Identity Disorders" heading are 4 subcategories and 30 diagnostic entities. Those listed under *sexual dysfunction due to a general medical condition* are all encountered in the practice of geriatrics.

Sexual Activity in Late Life

Over the last 30 years, sexuality in late life has been given increasing attention by investigators and has gained gradual acceptance in society. Researchers in this area have done much to dispel a variety of myths that once existed surrounding the topic of sexuality in late adulthood.

Although young and middle-aged adults have clearly become sexually more permissive in regard to their own generations, many adult children have difficulty accepting elderly parents who, by their behavior, indicate a continuing sexual interest. An adult child, observing the flirtatious behavior of an elderly parent, often becomes disturbed and questions the mental and emotional soundness of the parent. In turn, many elderly persons are aware that this type of behavior bothers their adult children and deliberately avoid such anxiety-producing behavior when in their presence.

Butler and Lewis (1976) observed that sexual activity in an elderly man is more likely to be sanctioned than that in a woman of comparable age. Furthermore, it is generally considered acceptable for the elderly man to marry a younger woman. In contrast, women who show an interest in sexuality are seen as depraved or "grasping for lost youth." Sexual interest by an older woman involving a younger man is unlikely to be socially embraced.

Contributing to these differences in the attitudes toward men and women is the discrepancy of the male-to-female ratio in the general population. Since older women outnumber older men, it is obvious that the surviving man has the opportunity to expand his sexual choices, whereas the elderly woman is restricted by the reality of the male/female imbalance within the population (Taeuber 1993).

Physiological Changes Affecting Sexuality

The aging man and woman undergo important anatomic and physiological sex changes, as the work of several researchers demonstrates. The pioneer investigations of Masters and Johnson (1979) can be divided into two categories. The first category consisted of laboratory observations related to the anatomic and physiological changes in old age; the second category was composed of data derived from interviews with a larger but self-selected group of older subjects. Laboratory investigations were conducted on 35 men whose ages ranged from 51 to 89 years. Sociosexual interviews were carried out with 212 men over the age of 50 years. The women involved in these studies included 61 menopausal and postmenopausal subjects. In this grouping, the youngest was 41 and the oldest, 78. Thirty-four of the participants were considered to be postmenopausal.

Men. In aging men, the nipple erection that usually accompanies the act of ejaculation declines over time so that the majority of men (if not all men) over age 60 do not demonstrate nipple erection at the time of ejaculation. The correlation of these two events is expected in men under the age of 60.

It is evident that most, if not all, physiological processes are slowed with the passing of time. Consequently, it takes an aging man longer to achieve erection. The slowing of the sexual arousal process is inevitable, and this slowing should be recognized as normal by both the man and his partner. For men aged 60 or older, full penile erection is frequently not attained until just before ejaculation. However, the maintenance of penile erection over long periods of time without ejaculation is often an achievement of old age.

Probably the most important change in male sexual function associated with the aging process is the reduction in both the frequency of ejaculation and the need to ejaculate. A man in his middle or late 60s often finds that his demand for ejaculatory release of sexual tension levels out to about once a week, although he may enjoy sexual intercourse two or more times a week. Again, the reduced demand for ejaculatory release should be accepted without reservation by both partners.

The majority of aging men experience a decreased ability to become erect at the sight of a person whom they consider attractive, or as a result of a sexual thought or fantasy. Because of this psychological change, men often are fearful that they are losing their potency. The change is really based on tactile stimulation since this becomes the most important means of obtaining an erection. Auditory stimulation—including speech—also plays a role.

The existence or absence of the male climacteric (similar to the female menopause) continues to be a subject of debate. The testes of the aging male show little change in normal structure. The clinician who elects a trial of hormone replacement for the elderly man must exercise considerable caution, because testosterone frequently exacerbates benign prostatic hypertrophy (BPH), a condition that is quite common in elderly men. Furthermore, testosterone is definitely contraindicated if a neoplasm of the prostate is suspected, because this hormone accelerates the development of carcinoma. Another potential complication is polycythemia. Therefore, if testosterone is given to a man, regular hemoglobin and red cell determinations are important, and attention must be paid to the possibility of prostatic changes. Hormone replacement therapy is very controversial, and there exists a need for carefully designed long-term research projects to provide more information on its risks and benefits.

Women. The aging process has obvious physiological influences on the sexual response cycle of women. Production of vaginal lubrication is the exact physiological counterpart of the male erection: the onset of lubrication may be delayed, and the degree of lubrication that a woman once experienced may not be achieved. These changes develop relatively rapidly as a result of reduced estrogen production during the years leading up to and following cessation of menses. The postmenopausal woman may report that she is more easily distracted during the sexual response cycle, and that she is more likely to be distracted by stimuli that had never interfered previously.

Unless estrogen is replaced by exogenous sources, the mucosal lining of the vagina becomes very thin and atrophic after menopause. Hence, the vaginal wall is vulnerable to the trauma associated with intercourse, and local irritation and bleeding may occur. In addition, aging usually brings a loss of some of the fatty integument of the external genitalia, and constriction of the vaginal introitus; thus, several factors may contribute to distress or pain during intercourse (National Institute on Aging 1992).

Although it is rare, some postmenopausal women experience painful tonic contractions of the uterus with orgasm. In younger women, the uterus contracts rhythmically with orgasm, in a pattern not dissimilar to the contractions observed during the first stage of labor. However, in advanced years, the rhythm of the contractions may be lost, and a spasm can occur that is experienced as a severe lower abdominal pain. This type of spastic uterine response accompanying orgasm reflects a state of sex steroid starvation. Consequently, hormone replacement therapy is particularly useful in such cases.

Sexual Behavior and Attitudes
Several reports related to sexual behavior and attitudes that are based on data derived from the Duke Longitudinal Studies have appeared in journals (Pfeiffer and Davis 1972; Verwoerdt et al. 1969). The data concerned with the frequency of sexual activity

have remained relatively consistent over two decades. The sexual changes that occur provide useful information to clinicians, but may reflect cohort differences rather than age changes. An actual cross-sectional analysis published in the 1950s (Busse et al. 1954) showed that the amount of sexual activity among older persons was correlated with socioeconomic status—the better the socioeconomic status, the more likely the continuation of sexual activity. Since then it has become evident that the important variable of physical health must be given primary attention, because physical health is a critical determinant regardless of socioeconomic status. Individuals who live in poverty or near poverty are not as likely to be in good health as those who are economically better off. Consequently, it is clear that there are several interacting factors that influence the continuation or termination of sexual activity.

Sexual activity between marital partners tends to be maintained until after the age of 75. Approximately 60% of married couples between the ages of 60 and 74 remain sexually active. After the age of 75, coitus is practiced by less than 30% of married couples. The continuation of sexual activity depends on several interrelated factors, including the availability of a sexual partner. Among married persons, the physical and mental health of the partners is important, as are the patterns of sexual interest and activity that were established in early adulthood. Only 7% of the elderly subjects without a wife or husband continued to have sexual relations in old age. This small percentage drops rapidly with advancing age. Compared with healthy women, a larger number of men in good health—four out of five—expressed a continuing interest in sexual activity. Verbalized interest in sex is reported by only about one-third of elderly women. This difference may be the direct result of the lack of stimuli for women, because older woman live in a predominantly female world.

The accuracy of the incidence of sexual activity in middle and late life is enhanced by distinguishing cohort effects as well as age and gender. George and Weiler (1981) indicated that cross-sectional studies can be misleading and that longitudinal studies of multiple cohorts (ranging in age from 46 to 71 years) have shown that the pattern of sexual intercourse remains relatively stable over a span of 6 years. These investigators identified several patterns of sexual activity within the sample they studied. Over a 6-year span that included four test dates, they found that 58.27% of the subjects reported exactly the same level of sexual activity; 7.9% reported no sexual activity at all at each of the four test dates. About 5% of the sample reported an increase in sexual activity; approximately one-half of this group resumed sexual activity after a period of cessation. About 20% reported a decrease in sexual activity. The remaining 10+% showed fluctuation in patterns of sexual activity. Consistent with other reports, men reported higher levels of sexual interest and activity than did women. Both men and women attributed the responsibility for cessation of sexual activity to the male partner. The findings of George and Weiler suggest that as the number of intact couples surviving to old age increases (as is currently the case), there will be a concomitant increase in the number of older people reporting continuity in sexual behavior.

Marriage Trends

Taeuber (1993) reported that two-thirds of men aged 65 and older live with wives, but only one-third of women over 65 have husbands. Most older men are married, whereas most older women are widows; there are almost four times as many widows as widowers. It should be noted that about two-fifths of the older married men have wives under 65 years old. At least 45,000 marriages are performed each year in which the groom and/or the bride is 65 years of age or over. The number of marriages among elderly people has been steadily increasing.

Gavzer (1987) claimed that in recent years there has appeared a trend for older women to marry younger men. In 1983 there were 151,000 marriages in which the bride was at least 5 years older than the bridegroom. This represented 6.2% of all marriages in 1983. By comparison, only 3.7% of brides in 1970 were 5 or more years older than their husbands. This trend toward older women marrying younger men is believed to be widespread, but is led by celebrities who turn the tables on convention. Wilson (1983) presented data suggesting that 37.1% of brides aged 65 and older are marrying younger men. This trend is compatible with the variation of life expectancy at age 65: for men, approximately 14+ years, and for women, 18+ years.

The marital status of the "aged" group—that is, those age 75 or older—reflects the social tradition for many men to marry younger women. Twice as many aged men as women are married, and only one-third of them have wives over age 75. About one-half have wives between 65 and 74 years of age, and one-fifth have wives under 65 years of age. Of men age 75 years or older, 33.9% are living with their wives. In contrast, only 17.8% of women 75 years of age or older are living with their husbands. Of these women, about 3% have husbands under 65 years of age, roughly 20% have husbands between the ages of 65 and 74, and the remainder have husbands their own age or older. Each year, about 2,000 women 75 years of age or older marry, and about 6,000 men 75 years of age or older marry. Both of these groups are usually moving out of widowhood. Of these 8,000 marriages, more than 4,000 involve one partner under age 75.

Sexual Problems in Late Life

Men

Episodic impotence—or *erectile dysfunction*, the preferred term (National Institutes of Health 1992)—occurs in most men, and although the men who experience it are concerned, it does not have the same devastating impact as persistent impotence. The masculine component of self-image is largely attributable to sexual potency. Although organic impotence is rarely life threatening, it has far-reaching consequences, often producing serious anxiety and depression. Estimates of the incidence of biological causes of impotence fluctuate from 10% to 70%. The incidence of impotence from biological causes is age related. One estimate is that 70% of cases of impotence that occur in men over the age of 70 years are attributable to organic etiologies (Crenshaw 1985).

Nocturnal penile tumescence is regularly associated with rapid eye movement (REM) during sleep. The total tumescence time occurring during a stage of REM sleep decreases from age 13 through late life (age 79). Non–REM-related penile tumescence also occurs, but it is not a dominant feature of nocturnal penile tumescence. A procedure can easily be conducted at home to determine the absence or presence of erections and their quality during sleep. Such tests can make a significant contribution in the evaluation of any organic factors, including drug-induced impotence (Karacani et al. 1975).

Reports have shown that intracavernous injection of papaverine or a papaverine-phentolamine mixture can produce penile erection of satisfactory quality for sexual intercourse (Trapp 1987). Unfortunately, this report did not provide the age distribution of the 700+ patients who were evaluated for sexual dysfunction; impotence was the primary complaint of 700 of these patients. In a study reported by Trapp (1987), a series of 136 patients were treated for their impotence by pharmacological erection techniques. Of this group, 61% were believed to have vascular pathology, 18% were diabetic, less than 1% of the cases were neurological in origin, and 15% were considered to be of psychological origin. The age range in this particular sample was 27–74 years. The only complication that has been identified is the appearance of an erection lasting for 8 hours and requiring reversal; this occurred in 2.3% of the patients. However, it is anticipated that some long-term side effects might develop, probably due to sclerosis or scarring. Although Trapp (1987) presents no clear outcome evaluations, the results of such pharmacological intervention are sufficiently encouraging to warrant very careful further research.

Morley and Kaiser (1992) confirmed that vascular disease involving the penile arteries is the most common cause of impotence in older males and adds that this is "a harbinger of atherosclerosis in other parts of the body" (p. 159).

With aging there is a diminished volume of ejaculate as well as the force with which the ejaculate is expelled. In addition, ejaculation may not occur; the absence of an ejaculation does not preclude a satisfactory, orgasm-like experience. Moreover, men are capable of ejaculating with a completely flaccid penis. Consequently, they can experience an orgasm without having an erection. This particular condition is usually the result of anxiety. Thus, a problem in one area need not affect another mechanism. This phenomenon can be explained by the existence of different neuronal mechanisms controlling erection, arousal, and ejaculation.

Drugs such as thioridazine can both inhibit ejaculation and produce impotence. Because individuals respond differently to a wide spectrum of medications, no physician should dismiss without further consideration a patient's claim that his impotence is a side effect of a medication. Furthermore, it is important to remember that some medications have a long half-life, and the withdrawal of medication often will not have a prompt positive response.

Women

As a woman ages, very little change occurs in orgasmic capacity. There is some decreasing intensity of orgasmic response, and the woman is slower to achieve orgasm, but many elderly women discover for the first time that they are capable of multiple orgasms.

Because the vaginal walls may have thinned and because vaginal lubrication may occur more slowly and in decreased volume, use of a water-soluble lubricant during sexual activity is advisable. Furthermore, if a woman has been sexually inactive for a long period, her vagina may show signs of atrophy and adhesions. A sexually inactive woman in her late 60s or 70s should not resume intercourse without adequate preparation. If such physical changes have occurred, mechanical dilatation supplemented with hormone replacement therapy will permit the elderly woman to return to sexual functioning without discomfort or injury.

Painful sexual intercourse in older women can usually be traced to an estrogen deficiency. However, a retroverted uterus that is diseased can also be a source of pain (Leiblums et al. 1983).

Illness and Disability

Cardiovascular disease, especially if a person has had a myocardial infarction, has led many older people to give up sex completely for fear of causing another heart attack; this problem is especially prevalent among men. Actually, the risk of death during sexual intercourse is very low. Although a person who has suffered a heart attack should seek medical advice, sex usually can and should be resumed after a period of 12–16 weeks. A rehabilitation program of activity including sexual experiences may decrease the risk of a future attack (National Institute on Aging 1985).

Diabetes in late life is not infrequently associated with impotence. However, if the diabetes is under adequate control—particularly by means of diet and exercise—improvement can occur. Unfortunately, even in some cases of well-controlled diabetes, impotence persists.

Stroke rarely damages areas in the brain that affect the physical aspects of sexual function, but residual incapacities may require that different positions be used; in some cases, physical support systems may be necessary to complete the sexual act.

Arthritis is a very common problem in late life, and the pain that results from physical activity may limit sexual responses. The painful experience can be reduced by the use of medication, exercise, and attention to position and the timing of sexual activity.

Although hysterectomy or a mastectomy does not alter a woman's capability for sexual responsiveness, psychological and emotional factors may impair sexual activity. In recent years, prompt reconstructive surgery after breast removal seems to have had a positive effect on some women who undergo mastectomy.

Prostatectomy for benign conditions rarely affects potency of the male. Seminal fluid may be absent or reduced postsurgically, but sexual capacity and enjoyment after prostatectomy should return to the presurgical level. Men who have cancer and require a perineal surgical approach are likely to become impotent.

Excessive use of alcohol reduces potency in men and delays orgasm in women. Many elderly persons carefully control their alcoholic intake, having observed that a small amount may produce a positive effect, whereas a larger amount may eliminate the pleasurable response.

Aging and Homosexuality

A Consumers Union report published in 1984 reported on an in-depth survey of 4,246 individuals (2,402 men and 1,844 women) between 50 and 93 years old (Brecher 1984). The study included 324 women aged 70 years or older and 498 men aged 70 years or older. In accord with the general population, the men were much more likely to be married than the women. Of this large sample, only 56 of the men considered themselves to be homosexuals and only 9 of the women considered themselves to be lesbians. However, Brecher noted that many of those in the sample reported having had casual homosexual experiences, usually during adolescence or earlier. Casual homosexual experiences do occur in the lives of older men and women, even though they have usually considered themselves to be heterosexual; a few consider themselves to be bisexual. Although the title of this report was "Love, Sex, and Aging," no data were presented regarding homosexuality and coping with aging. The attitudes and reactions of a few subjects were reported, and it was noted that as these homosexual men grew older,

they became aware that fewer persons were interested in having sex with them.

Corby and Solnick (1980) presented a detailed review of homosexuality and aging. Their data indicated that some women who reported homosexual activity experienced all such relationships before the age of 30, thereafter living a heterosexual lifestyle. Other women engaged in satisfactory heterosexual relationships and then lived a lesbian lifestyle in later years. Corby and Solnick postulated that changes between heterosexual and lesbian lifestyles are influenced by the social situation, which affects partner-gender choice. They also suggested that homosexual activity in women was likely to be discontinued in most subjects by the age of 50.

Corby and Solnick (1980) observed that older gay men were much more youth oriented than heterosexual males and, consequently, tended to view aging more negatively and to consider themselves "old" at earlier ages than did straight men.

Intimacy in Late Life

Intimacy is a term that is accepted by most behavioral scientists as a word for a somewhat vague but definite human need. According to Weg (1987), intimacy may remain present throughout the life span, although it can wax and wane. It is often suggested that intimacy in the latter part of the life span increases in importance as other sources of self-esteem are diminished. The decline in sexual capacity may be one of those alterations that is compensated for by increased intimacy. In a discussion of sex and aging, Calderone and Johnson (1981) say that intimacy occurs "when people delight each other and delight in each other in an atmosphere of security based upon mutuality, reciprocity, and total trust in each other" and that "this is surely the kind of relationship that every human being seeks, even if it does not involve physical sex" (p. 62). Although sexual behavior is considered to be a type of intimacy, it is not a totally favorable experience when it is devoid of mutual caring, responsibility, and open communication. The need for physical intimacy clearly occurs in older people, and many older persons appear to be "touch hungry" (Renshaw 1984). This need can be satisfied by physical contact with other adults, but particularly by grandchildren and pets. Intimacy includes various components such as physical, social, intellectual, spiritual, and emotional characteristics. Each may occur relatively independently and have a cyclical aspect.

Intimacy in late life is particularly important because it can effectively serve as an intervening, mediating, or buffering factor in adaptation to stress (Weiss 1983). Moreover, marital success in late life seems to be tied to intimacy. According to Weg (1987), older men and women have described the most rewarding aspects of marriage as companionship and being able to express true feelings to each other. Marriages get into trouble when it is apparent that there are different values and that there is a lack of mutual interest. All older couples do not improve their intimacy, and the realization of the lack of intimacy may become very apparent early in the retirement years. The continuation of physical sexual activity is linked to general intimacy. In late life it is unlikely that one will occur without the other.

Passion and romance continue into old age. Observers of the behavior of older people in social situations, such as senior centers, often note the festive dress and flirtatious behavior that emerge during certain social activities, especially dancing and singing. Playing games also provides this opportunity. The flirtatious behavior includes verbal remarks, changes in facial behavior, body movements, and touching. Such behavior rarely becomes objectionable and it is obviously important in providing an opportunity to pursue one form of increasing intimacy (Bulcroft and O'Conner-Roden 1986).

Sexuality and Institutionalized Elderly Persons

Of all behavioral problems encountered in skilled nursing facilities, those that are of a sexual nature are considered to be among the most disturbing. Too frequently, the facility staff members do not seem to take into account the realization that sexuality has been an important part of the patients' self-image and that it remains important. Staff attitudes and beliefs may contribute to the problems encountered with sexual behavior.

A variety of behavioral disturbances occur among the elderly persons in nursing homes. In a survey of a large number of patients in 42 skilled nursing facilities (Zimmer et al. 1984), 64.2% of the patients were reported to have significant behavioral problems. Of these, 23.6% had "serious problems." These highly disturbing problems included

exposure of genitalia and masturbation. The staffs of these facilities were obviously horrified by such acts. Wasow and Loeb (1979) reported the results of another survey in which residents were asked if *patients* should have sex; 39% of the men and 53% of the women said no. When asked if *old people* should be allowed to have sex, 81% of the men and 75% of the women said "yes" (Wasow and Loeb 1979).

Consistent with other studies of sexual behavior in late life, it appears that the concept of sexual activity among institutionalized elderly persons is related to these elders' interests and attitudes toward sexuality in the past and to their prior level of sexual activity. If physical intimacy has been important in the past, it remains so. Although nursing home residents have physical and/or mental disabilities, some retain a capacity for sexual pleasure.

Sexual problems concerning nursing home residents may involve only one individual (open masturbation), whereas other problems (unwelcome sexual advances) may involve other residents, staff members, and/or family and other visitors. One author reported that sexual behavior between two residents seemed to mobilize "the paternalistic tendencies of the staff" (McCartney et al. 1987, p. 332). A serious staff reaction can be anticipated when a nondemented or mildly demented resident pursues another resident who is more demented. This produces a situation that staff members may perceive as a relationship between a perpetrator and a victim. To resolve such staff/resident conflicts, it is important that there be staff meetings in which staff members can express their discomfort and be helped to understand that a resident's activity is not to be limited by someone else's moral values. Although it is necessary, of course, to prevent sexual abuse of a resident, a regressing adult should not be any more condemned or made to feel any more shame or guilt than should a developing child (McCartney et al. 1987). Morley and Kaiser (1992, p. 163) observed that inappropriate sexual advances by residents in long-term care settings not only are a problem for the staff but also are distressing for the delinquent resident's spouse, who often requires support.

References

Alarcon R: Hypochondriasis and depression in the aged. Gerontologia Clinica 6:266–268, 1964

Albano WA, Zietinstic CM, Organ CH: Is appendicitis in the aged really different? Geriatrics 30:81–88, 1975

Allen A, Busse E: Hypochondriacal disorder, in Principles and Practice of Geriatric Psychiatry. Edited by Copeland J, Abou-Saleb M, Blazer DG. London, Wiley, 1994, pp 757–760

American Psychiatric Association: Diagnostic and Statistical Manual of Mental Disorders, 3rd Edition, Revised. Washington, DC, American Psychiatric Association, 1987

American Psychiatric Association: Diagnostic and Statistical Manual of Mental Disorders, 4th Edition. Washington, DC, American Psychiatric Association, 1994

Barsky AJ, Klerman GL: Overview: hypochondriasis, bodily complaints, and somatic styles. Am J Psychiatry 140:273–283, 1983

Barsky AJ, Wyshak G, Klerman GL: Transient hypochondriasis. Arch Gen Psychiatry 47:746–752, 1990

Barsky AJ, Wyshak G, Klerman GL: Psychiatric comorbidity in DSM-III hypochondriasis. Arch Gen Psychiatry 49:101–108, 1992

Beardsley T: Holistic therapy collides with reductionist science. Sci Am 269:39–44, 1993

Beck AT, Rush AJ, Shaw BF, et al: Cognitive Therapy of Depression. New York, Guilford, 1979

Bellak L, Small L: Emergency Psychotherapy and Brief Psychotherapy. New York, Grune & Stratton, 1965

Blazer DG: Physical illnesses that cause depressive symptoms in late life, in Depression in Late Life, 2nd Edition. Edited by Blazer DG. St. Louis, MO, CV Mosby, 1993, pp 223–234

Brecher EM: Love, Sex, and Aging: A Consumers Union Report. Mount Vernon, NY, Consumers Union, 1984

Brose WG, Spiegel D: Neuropsychiatric aspects of pain management, in The American Psychiatric Press Textbook of Neuropsychiatry, 2nd Edition. Edited by Yudofsky SC, Hales RE. Washington, DC, American Psychiatric Press, 1992, pp 245–276

Brown HN, Vaillant GE: Hypochondriasis. Arch Intern Med 141:723–726, 1981

Bulcroft K, O'Conner-Roden M: Never too late. Psychology Today 20:66–69, 1986

Busse EW: Hypochondriasis in the elderly. Am Fam Physician 25:199–202, 1982

Busse EW: Treating hypochondriasis in the elderly. Generations 10:30–33, 1986

Busse EW: Duke University Longitudinal Studies of Aging. Z Gerontol 26:123–128, 1993

Busse EW, Blazer DG: Disorders related to biological functioning, in Handbook of Geriatric Psychiatry. Edited by Busse EW, Blazer DG. New York, Van Nostrand Reinhold, 1980, pp 390–414

Busse EW, Busse OS: Medical care and education: impressions of China 1979. Center Reports on Advances in Research (Duke University Center for the Study of Aging and Human Development), December 1979, pp 1–6

Busse EW, Maddox GL: Duke Longitudinal Studies of Normal Aging, 1955–1980. New York, Springer, 1985

Busse EW, Barnes RH, Silverman AJ, et al: Studies of processes of aging, VI: factors that influence the psyche of elderly persons. Am J Psychiatry 110:897–903, 1954

Butler RN, Lewis MI: Sex After Sixty. New York, Harper & Row, 1976

Calderone MS, Johnson EW: The human response systems: how they develop and how they work, in The Family Book About Sexuality. Edited by Calderone MS, Johnson EW. New York, Harper & Row, 1981, pp 61–62

Corby N, Solnick RL: Psychosocial and physiological influences on sexuality in the older adult, in Handbook of Mental Health and Aging. Edited by Birren JE, Sloane RB. Englewood Cliffs, NJ, Prentice-Hall, 1980, pp 893–921

Costa PT, McCrae RR: Hypochondriasis, neuroticism, and aging. Am Psychol 40:19–28, 1985

Crenshaw TL: Age-related changes in sexual function. Geriatric Consultant 3:26–29, 1985

Emery G: Cognitive therapy with the elderly, in New Directions in Cognitive Therapy. Edited by Emery G, Hollon S, Bedrosian R. New York, Guilford, 1981, pp 102–116

Gallagher DE, Thompson LW: Depression in the Elderly: A Behavioral Treatment Manual. Los Angeles, CA, University of Southern California Press, 1981

Gallagher DE, Thompson LW: Effectiveness of psychotherapy for both endogenous and nonendogenous depression in older adult outpatients. J Gerontol 38:707–712, 1983

Gavzer B: Why more older women are marrying younger men. Parade Magazine, March 1987, pp 12–13

George LK, Weiler SJ: Sexuality in middle and late life. Arch Gen Psychiatry 38:919–923, 1981

Gildenberg PL, DeVaul RA: The Chronic Pain Patient: Evaluation and Management (Pain and Headache Series, Vol 7). New York, S Karger, 1985

Glenn F: Surgical principles for the aged patient, in Clinical Aspects of Aging. Edited by Reichel W. Baltimore, MD, Williams & Wilkins, 1978, pp 166–170

Grauer H: Geriatric depression in the West and the Far East. Psychiatric Journal of the University of Ottawa 9:118–120, 1984

Harkins SW, Nowlin JB: Persistent pain in the elderly. Paper presented at the annual meeting of the American Psychological Association, Los Angeles, CA, August 1985

Harkins SW, Price DD, Martelli M: Effects of age in pain perception. J Gerontol 41:58–63, 1986

Jessel TM, Kelly DD: Pain and analgesia, in Principles of Neural Science, 3rd Edition. Edited by Kandel ER, Schwartz JH, Jessel TM. Norfolk, CT, Appleton & Lange, 1991, pp 385–399

Kanner L: The minor psychoses, in Clinical Psychiatry. Edited by Kanner L. Springfield, IL, Charles C Thomas, 1935, pp 448–483

Karacani I, Williams R, Thornby J, et al: Nocturnal penile tumescence and REM sleep. Am J Psychiatry 132:932–937, 1975

Kleinman AM: Neurasthenia and depression: a study of somatization and culture in China. Cult Med Psychiatry 6:117–190, 1982

Klerman GL, Weissman MM: Interpersonal psychotherapy: theory and research, in Short-Term Psychotherapies for Depression. Edited by Rush AJ. New York, Guilford, 1982, pp 46–54

Kwentus JA, Harkins SW, Lignon N, et al: Current concepts of geriatric pain and its treatment. Geriatrics 40:48–54, 1985

Leiblums S, Bachmann G, Kemmann E, et al: Vaginal atrophy in the postmenopausal woman: the importance of sexual activity and hormones. JAMA 249:2195–2198, 1983

Lewinsohn PM, Biglan A, Zeiss A: A behavioral treatment of depression, in Behavioral Management of Anxiety, Depression and Pain. Edited by Davidson P. New York, Brunner/Mazel, 1976, pp 71–99

Lindsay PG, Wycoff FM: The depression syndrome and its response to antidepressants. Psychosomatics 22:571–577, 1981

Lipowski ZJ: Somatization: the experience and communication of psychological distress as somatic symptoms. Psychother Psychosom 47:160–167, 1987

Lyness JM, King DA, Conwell Y, et al: Somatic worry and medical illness in depressed inpatients. American Association for Geriatric Psychiatry 1(4):288–295, Fall 1993

MacDonald J, Ballie J, Williams B, et al: Coronary care in the elderly. Age Ageing 12:17–20, 1983

Maddox GL: Self-assessment of health status. Journal of Chronic Diseases 17:449–460, 1964

Maddox GL, Douglass EB: Self-assessment of health: a longitudinal study of elderly subjects. J Health Soc Behav 14:87–93, 1973

Masters W, Johnson V: Geriatric sexuality, in Textbook of Sexual Medicine. Edited by Kolodny R, Masters W, Johnson V. Boston, MA, Little, Brown, 1979, pp 103–116

McCartney JR, Henry I, Rogers D, et al: Sexuality and the institutionalized elderly. J Am Geriatr Soc 35:331–333, 1987

Melzack R, Wall PD: Pain mechanisms: a new theory. Science 150:973–979, 1965

Meredith N, Turner P: Therapy under analysis. Science 86:29–52, 1986

Morley JE, Kaiser FE: Aging and sexuality, in Facts and Research in Gerontology. Edited by Vellas B, Albareda JL. New York, Springer, 1992, pp 157–165

National Institute on Aging: Sexuality in Late Life. Bethesda, MD, National Institute on Aging, 1985

National Institute on Aging: Menopause (ISBN-0-16-038139-8). Washington, DC, U.S. Government Printing Office, December 1992

National Institutes of Health: NIH Consensus Statement: Erectile Dysfunction, Vol 10, No 4 (1–31). Bethesda, MD, National Library of Medicine, December 1992

Parker G, Lipscombe P: The relevance of early parental experiences to adult dependency, hypochondriasis, and utilization of primary physicians. Br J Med Psychol 53:355–363, 1990

Pfeiffer E, Davis GD: Determinants of sexual behavior in middle and old age. J Am Geriatr Soc 20:141–148, 1972

Poe WD, Holloway DA: Drugs and the Aged. New York, McGraw-Hill, 1980

Renshaw DC: Touch hunger—a common marital problem. Medical Aspects of Human Sexuality 18:63–70, 1984

Sigvardsson S, Von Knorring AL, Bohman M, et al: An adoption study of somatoform disorders: the relationship of somatization to psychiatric disability. Arch Gen Psychiatry 41:853–859, 1984

Sjolund B, Eriksson M: Relief of Pain by TENS. Chichester, UK, Wiley, 1985

Taeuber CM: Sixty-Five Plus in America. International Institute on Aging, Malta, Union Print Company, 1993

Tait RC: Management of pain in the elderly, in Problem Behaviors in Long-Term Care. Edited by Szwabo PA, Grossberg GT. New York, Springer, 1993, pp 133–146

Trapp JD: Pharmacologic erection program for the treatment of male impotence. South Med J 80:426–427, 1987

U.S. Department of Health, Education and Welfare: National Institute on Drug Abuse Services Research Report: A Study of Legal Drug Use by Older Americans (Publ No 77-495). Washington, DC, U.S. Department of Health, Education and Welfare, 1977

Verwoerdt AE, Pfeiffer E, Wang HS: Sexual behavior in senescence, II: patterns of sexual activity and interest. Geriatrics 24:137–154, 1969

Wasow M, Loeb M: Sexuality in nursing homes. J Am Geriatr Soc 27:73–79, 1979

Weg RB: Intimacy and the later years, in Handbook of Applied Gerontology. Edited by Lesnoff-Caravaglia G. New York, Human Sciences Press, 1987, pp 127–142

Weiss LJ: Intimacy in adaptation, in Sexuality in the Later Years: Roles and Behavior. Edited by Weg RB. New York, Academic Press, 1983, pp 130–138

Wilson BF: Marriage in the elderly. Hyattsville, MD, National Center for Health Statistics, 1983

World Health Organization: The ICD-10 Classification of Mental and Behavioural Disorders: Clinical Descriptions and Diagnostic Guidelines. Geneva, Switzerland, World Health Organization, 1992

Zimmer JG, Watson N, Treat A: Behavioral problems among patients in skilled nursing homes. Am J Public Health 74:1118–1121, 1984

CHAPTER 17

Bereavement and Adjustment Disorders

Dolores Gallagher-Thompson, Ph.D.
Larry W. Thompson, Ph.D.

In this chapter we cover the topic of late-life bereavement in some depth, as there has been a tremendous increase in the amount of clinical and empirical research done on this topic in the recent past. Much more is known about it, comparatively speaking, than about the second topic to be addressed in this chapter—namely, adjustment disorders in the aged. We present a variety of ways to define and understand the process of "normal grief," along with issues such as what constitutes (and how to assess) "abnormal grief," how grief manifests in older adults, how it changes over time, and some of the risk factors that tend to increase its intensity. Finally, we review a variety of interventions that have been found to be helpful from a treatment perspective, including our own work with cognitive-behavior therapy. In the section on adjustment disorders we review what little research and clinical data are currently available, and conclude with some information about how elderly persons tend to cope with stressful life events that are less threatening than the death of a loved one. We hope that this may encourage future research and clinical investigation regarding this important, but generally overlooked topic in geriatric psychiatry.

Late-Life Bereavement

Who Are the Elderly Bereaved?

The question "Who are the elderly bereaved?" is not simple to answer in terms of epidemiological information because the terms *bereavement* and *grief reaction* have been used to refer to any number of losses experienced by older adults. These losses include, but are not limited to, the death of a spouse, an adult child, another family member, or a close personal

Preparation of this work was supported in part by grants RO1–AGO1959 from the National Institute on Aging and RO1-MH36834 and RO1-MH37196 from the National Institute of Mental Health.

friend, as well as divorce (Cain 1988); prolonged caregiving for a severely impaired relative (Bass et al. 1991); and/or significant decline in one's own health, attractiveness, capabilities, opportunities, and so forth (Kalish 1987). When used in its narrowest sense, bereavement refers to the reaction or process that results after the death of someone close. In terms of prevalence, we have data only on the frequency of occurrence of widowhood. In the United States, the mean age at which this takes place is 69 years for men and 66 years for women. Among persons age 65 and over, 51% of women and 13% of men are widowed. Because women live longer than men, in general, the mean duration of widowed life is approximately 14 years for women versus only 7 years for men (United States Bureau of the Census 1984). These data—plus the fact that widowed men are more likely to remarry after their spouse's death—are often interpreted to mean that widowhood is a women's issue; however, this is a narrow perspective, because many research studies have shown that older men are at a high risk for their own subsequent mortality after a wife's death. These and other gender differences will be discussed below in more detail.

Theories About Adjustment to Permanent Losses

A number of theoretical perspectives have been developed to explain how people (of any age) respond to significant loss. It is beyond the scope of this chapter to review them all in depth; the interested reader is referred to a comprehensive, definitive report issued by the Institute of Medicine (Osterweis et al. 1984) for this information. Here we will briefly note the major positions that have influenced the field, beginning with the classic work of Freud in "Mourning and Melancholia" (1917/1957). His thesis was that the prime task of mourning was the gradual surrender of psychological attachment to the deceased; if this was not done properly, Freud contended, various kinds of psychopathology would result. In contrast, Bowlby (1961), in his attachment theory, emphasized that bereavement, as an involuntary separation from a loved one, gives rise to many forms of attachment behavior (such as separation anxiety and pining), the functions of which are not withdrawal from the lost object, but reunion with it.

Others, such as Parkes (1972) and Horowitz (1976), have proposed models that involve phases or stages of reaction to the death of a loved one. This approach has subsequently been applied to many other types of losses, such as permanent disability, rape, and life-threatening illness (see Wortman and Silver [1987] for a review of these stage models). Despite the differences in the type of trauma, most 20th-century theorists agree on a general course over time, which consists of the following. The first phase begins at the time of the death (or traumatic event) and persists for several weeks. Shock and disbelief, combined with coldness, emotional numbness, emptiness, and cognitive confusion characterize this period, along with frequently intense "free-floating" anxiety and significant mood fluctuations. Specific somatic symptoms include sleeplessness, loss of appetite, and vague muscular aches and pains, leading to increased contact with primary care physicians and, commonly, requests for medication to alleviate some of the distressing symptoms.

The second phase generally begins as the numbness and anxiety start to decrease—usually in about 4–6 weeks—and often lasts for the better part of a year. During this period, family and friends gradually become less available and/or helpful; they often convey the message that the bereaved person should be "getting on with life" and should be "getting over" his or her grief long before the individual is ready to do so. In fact, it is only with increased time that the finality of the loss becomes more apparent to the bereaved person, and more of the sadness, anger, guilt, relief, and other strong emotions begin to surface, causing emotional lability and confusion. Specific symptoms such as frequent crying, chronic sleep disturbance, blue mood, poor appetite, low energy, feelings of fatigue, loss of interest in daily living, and problems with attention and concentration are common. Nevertheless, most do not develop the clinical syndrome of major depression, despite the fact that certain symptoms of grief and depression overlap (for more detail, see "Operational Definitions of 'Normal' and 'Abnormal' Grief," and "Definitional Problems and Issues," below).

Parkes (1972) referred to this second phase as a time of "yearning and protest," characterized by actual searching for the deceased in both behavioral and cognitive ways—for example, actually going to places frequented by the deceased person. Such endeavors bring momentary comfort and also, paradoxically, intensify feelings of grief. The bereaved often wishes that the loved one would come in the door, or be around the corner. Often, someone so similar is seen that for a moment, the survivor is certain it must be the deceased.

Bereaved persons often report auditory or visual hallucinatory-like experiences of the deceased and/or a strong "sense of presence" of the individual. They may see the deceased sitting in his or her favorite chair, or hear their name being called, or receive a reassuring message that all is well. These vivid experiences appear to be a very normal part of the grief process, and have been documented as such in the clinical literature for more than 20 years. Rees (1971) provides an early perspective and Grimby (1993) gives more recent data on these cognitive phenomena, confirming that for most elderly persons, these illusions and/or hallucinations are generally experienced as pleasant and helpful.

Other cognitive components of this time period include frequent searching for the meaning of the death, along with an explanation for why it occurred when it did. This process often has religious and/or philosophical overtones, and generally involves activities such as discussions with clergy, attendance at religious services and events, and reading pertinent material on the subject. In addition, there is frequent review of the memories and scenes associated with the death, as if to reinforce that it occurred and that it cannot be undone. Although it can be difficult for friends and family members, having heard it all many times before, to weather this phase with the bereaved, it is particularly important that emotional and social support continue during this period.

The third and final phase of adaptation to loss involves the gradual disengagement of some or most of the psychic energy that has been bound up with the deceased (or with the traumatic event), and reinvestment of that energy in other persons and activities. Lopata (1975) called this the "identity reconstruction" process, and suggested that it could take a minimum of about one additional year for this to occur, particularly in the case of a major loss, such as the death of a spouse or adult child. The process will be longer or shorter depending on the centrality of roles that were lost as a result of the death or traumatic event, and the amount and kind of new learning that must take place for a new sense of self to develop and become firmly established. During this period, most of the troublesome somatic symptoms described above will abate, along with the unique cognitive and behavioral components noted previously. Loneliness tends to diminish as new social relationships are developed and skills are learned that are needed to function adequately in new roles (although for some, the thrust is to strengthen relationships and roles that were in place before the death or traumatic event, rather than to develop new options). In either case, as Parkes and Weiss (1983) have noted, the bereaved person's model of his or her inner self, and the outer world or environment, must change to match the present, new reality.

It should be noted that although these stage theories of adaptation have been widely accepted by health care professionals—and have been written about in the psychiatric, nursing, social work, and psychological literatures—there is actually little empirical evidence to support them. Also, this position could be problematic if adhered to rigidly while assessing and/or treating bereaved individuals. It is vital to recognize that the bereaved do not proceed from one clearly identifiable phase to another in an orderly fashion. Rather, according to Osterweis et al. (1984) and many other clinicians and researchers since then, people differ considerably in the specific manifestations of grief that they experience and in the order and speed with which they move through the process. In the case of older adults, this is even more true; many experience multiple losses, often without sufficient time in between to complete the grieving for one event before the next one occurs. Kastenbaum (1981) has termed this "bereavement overload" and has suggested that because of multiple losses, the process of grieving is likely to be significantly different and more complex among older compared with younger individuals. Again, however, there are little empirical data on this point at the present time. In brief, one might best view these stages or phases of adaptation to loss in descriptive terms, and use caution in not oversimplifying one's understanding of a very complicated phenomenon. As Shuchter and Zisook (1993) conclude, "grief's duration may be prolonged, at times even indefinite, and its intensity varies over time, from person to person, and from culture to culture. It cannot be understood from a static or linear perspective" (p. 43).

Operational Definitions of "Normal" and "Abnormal" Grief

Given that there is such wide variability in how people proceed through the grief process, how can we determine what is "normal" and what is not? As Shuchter and Zisook (1993) have noted, such a determination is very difficult; they suggest that those who work in the field of bereavement and grief are still trying to validate and operationalize this construct. According to both DSM-III-R (American Psychiatric Association 1987) and DSM-IV (American Psychiatric Association 1994), bereavement is in the V Code section, meaning it is a condition that may be the focus of attention or treatment but is not directly attributable to a mental disorder. Uncomplicated bereavement is defined in DSM-III-R as follows:

> This category is used when the focus of attention or treatment is a normal reaction to the death of a loved one (bereavement). A full depressive syndrome frequently is a normal reaction to such a loss, with feelings of depression and such associated symptoms as poor appetite, weight loss, and insomnia. However, morbid preoccupation with worthlessness, prolonged and marked functional impairment, and marked psychomotor retardation are uncommon and suggest that the bereavement is complicated by the development of a major depression. (American Psychiatric Association 1987, p. 361)

DSM-III-R goes on to point out other features to help distinguish "uncomplicated" from "complicated" bereavement. Uncomplicated bereavement may have such features as guilt (if present, it is chiefly about things done or not done by the survivor at the time of the death); thoughts of death or dying (if present, limited to the survivor thinking he or she should have died with the deceased person); and depressed mood (viewed by the bereaved person as "normal" and not cause for great concern). According to this view, normal grief would be characterized by some but not all of the common symptoms of the clinical syndrome of depression, and there would be differences in intensity as well. The diagnosis of a normal grief reaction would be made when both quantitative and qualitative features of the reported symptoms are taken into account,

whereas a diagnosis of complicated bereavement would be made if a major depressive disorder is present in addition to the features of normal grief.

Because this differentiation has not always been easy to make, DSM-IV is more explicit in delineating several specific symptoms that are not considered to be characteristic of a "normal" grief reaction:

> These include: 1) guilt about things other than actions taken or not taken by the survivor at the time of the death; 2) thoughts of death other than the survivor feeling that he or she would be better off dead or should have died with the deceased person; 3) morbid preoccupation with worthlessness; 4) marked psychomotor retardation; 5) prolonged and marked functional impairment; and 6) hallucinatory experiences other than thinking that he or she hears the voice of, or transiently sees the image of, the deceased person. (American Psychiatric Association 1994, pp. 684–685)

Definitional Problems and Issues

Although these operational definitions have been helpful and have provided guidance for diagnostic decision making, they are at some variance with what has been in the clinical literature for some time and, many would say, are not detailed enough to be really helpful to the practicing clinician. For example, Middleton and colleagues (1993) note that even a modest sampling of the literature highlights the fact that there are many inconsistencies in how normal and abnormal grief are defined. They indicate that the following terms have been used, at various times and by various authors (often using their own idiosyncratic meanings), to denote some variation from normal grief: absent or denied, abnormal, complicated, distorted, morbid, maladaptive, truncated, atypical, intensified and prolonged, unresolved, and neurotic. They raise such questions as: Could grief accentuate preexisting pathology, and if so, how would that be diagnosed? Would a major depression that develops after the loss of a loved one represent a form of "abnormal" grieving, or should it be regarded as an affective disorder in its own right? Wortman and Silver (1987) raise other important questions that should be addressed as one thinks about what constitutes normal versus abnormal grief, such as: Is it really necessary to substantially reduce one's attachment to the deceased in order to "resolve" one's grief? Is it reasonable to expect a bereaved person to recover substantially within the "typical" span of 2 years, which is the duration most often used to demarcate a chronic grief reaction? In fact, in partial response to these issues, Wortman and Silver (1987) present data from several investigations showing that continued attachment to the deceased is often viewed as comforting by the survivor and does not appear to interfere with subsequent healthy adjustment. Also, they point out that even when individuals appear to have recovered from their loss, there is some evidence to suggest that feelings of grief may reemerge for brief periods for many years—for example, anniversary reactions may occur throughout the survivor's lifetime and should present no cause for alarm.

In summary, at present there appears to be more divergence than convergence of opinion about what exactly constitutes a normal versus an abnormal grief reaction, at any age. We suggest, as a starting point, consistent use of the currently available (and evolving) diagnostic criteria, which clearly affirm that normal grief is not equivalent to the clinical syndrome of major depression, and which indicate specific symptoms to be evaluated to determine if their presence and/or severity level would suggest that a differential diagnosis is needed. The results of our own psychometric work in this regard—using some common self-report questionnaires to assess both depression and level of grief—generally support this position (Breckenridge et al. 1986; Gallagher-Thompson and Thompson 1994). Much can also be learned from the results of several empirical studies of how elders have adapted to major losses over time. These studies provide considerable data about what appears to be the normal course of adaptation to spousal bereavement over a 2- to 3-year period; unfortunately, few longer-term studies have been done to assess the impact of this major life event over a period of a decade or more.

What Have We Learned From Longitudinal Studies of Late-Life Bereavement?

In about the past decade, the National Institute on Aging has funded a number of longitudinal investigations of how older adults have adapted to bereavement of various kinds, with an emphasis on death of the spouse. Preliminary results from several

of these studies can be found in the edited book by Lund (1989), containing chapters by Lund, Caserta, and Dimond on their work predominantly with Mormon elders in Utah, along with chapters by Van Zandt and associates on rural bereaved elders, and Faletti and colleagues on predominantly Jewish elders in Miami. More recent reports of the Utah study can be found in the edited book by Stroebe and colleagues (1993). It is a very comprehensive volume on a number of topics pertaining to late-life bereavement, including data-oriented chapters by Lund, Caserta, and Dimond and by our own research group. There we present a comprehensive summary of the University of Southern California longitudinal study of adaptation to spousal bereavement, and include information contrasting the natural-death survivors of that study with survivors of elder suicides (Gallagher-Thompson et al. 1993).

For the most part, data from these studies have been fairly consistent in their findings on the kinds of symptoms that change over time; the rate of change that can be expected to occur; and the presence or absence of gender differences. When standard measures are used to determine outcomes such as depressed mood and related symptoms, anxiety, well-being, and level of grief, it has been found that the most significant differences between bereaved subjects and nonbereaved control subjects (evaluated at the same points in time) occur in the first 2–6 months after the spouse's death, when elevated levels of distress are common across a variety of measures. Typically, bereaved women reported more psychological distress than bereaved men, although this was not found in all studies (cf. Lund et al. 1986). By 12 months postloss, the levels of reported distress were no longer significantly different between bereaved and nonbereaved control subjects, although women's distress generally remained higher (Harlow et al. 1991; Lund et al. 1989; Thompson et al. 1991). This suggests that considerable recovery was evident by the end of 1 year. Also, it should be noted that although the trend was for intensity of distress to be reduced somewhat by 6 months postloss, many unpleasant symptoms were still present; as Harlow and colleagues (1991) state, this means that there is evidence for amelioration of symptoms by 6 months but not for their disappearance.

There is one notable exception to these results regarding psychological distress measures, and that concerns the level of grief reported by the bereaved over time. For example, in the study by Thompson and co-workers (1991), the elderly men and women in that sample obtained mean scores that were higher than the currently published normative scores for experienced grief, using the Texas Revised Inventory of Grief as the measure (Faschingbauer 1981). This was true not only immediately after the spouse's death (2 months postloss) but also at the 12- and 30-month follow-ups. Also, there were no gender differences on this measure, contrary to what was reported for other indices of psychological distress. Thompson et al. (1991) interpreted these findings to mean that the experience of grief remains high over at least a 30-month interval after the spouse's death, and that it is distinct from the experience of depressed mood and related symptoms, which decline significantly over that same interval. In other words, depression and grief can be distinguished using brief self-report questionnaires, and one can anticipate that the former will abate considerably over time, whereas the latter may remain quite high, and yet be considered normal for an older adult. These findings are consistent with those of Zisook and Shuchter (1985, 1986), who also found that the experience of grief (as indexed by a continuing sense of attachment to the deceased) was still strong, at times, even 4 years postloss. Thus, "recovery" may be an unrealistic goal when working with older bereaved patients, particularly if recovery means that experiences such as still missing the deceased and still fondly remembering the past are not to be tolerated.

Risk Factors for Intensifying the Grief Experience

Grief has been characterized by many as not only a highly charged emotional state but also a significant risk factor for the development of a wide range of negative outcomes, including mortality and major physical and mental health disturbances. On the other hand, come other clinicians and researchers have been struck by the apparently remarkable resilience of many older adults to survive and cope quite well, overall, with the profound losses of old age. As McCrae and Costa (1993) have pointed out in their 10-year follow-up study of a national sample of bereaved men and women, the great majority of individuals showed considerable ability to adapt to

this major life stress (although length of "recovery" seemed to vary considerably). Nevertheless, despite this optimism, it seems important to attempt to identify "at risk" elders who may have an increased likelihood for negative outcomes after their spouse's death (Sanders 1993).

Along these lines (although the reader must keep in mind that results of specific studies may conflict and generalizations can be difficult to make), a number of studies have shown that there are several specific variables that, when present, tend to result in a more intense or difficult bereavement. These variables are 1) age of the survivor, 2) gender of the survivor, 3) mode of death, 4) presence of significant depression shortly after the death, 5) self-esteem and perceived coping, 6) prior relationship satisfaction, and 7) social support. Some additional factors, such as strength of religious commitment and involvement, access to appropriate mourning rituals (and participation in them), and how roles are redistributed in the family after the death, can also have an impact on how the grief process is experienced, although the literature is by no means clear on the relative contribution of each of these factors.

Regarding the *age* of the survivor, some studies have shown that older persons adapt better than younger persons to the loss of their spouse. For example, Zisook and colleagues (1993) found that their oldest subjects demonstrated the most consistent improvement in distress levels over time; in contrast, Sable (1991), among others, found that older widows were more distressed throughout the first three years of bereavement than their younger counterparts.

Regarding the survivor's *gender,* considerable research data point to the fact that older bereaved men who have lost their spouses are at high risk for their own death. In their recent review of both cross-sectional and longitudinal studies on this topic, Stroebe and Stroebe (1993) concluded that "the bereaved are indeed at higher risk of dying than are nonbereaved persons. Highest risk occurs in the weeks and months closest to loss, and men appear to be relatively more vulnerable than women" (p. 188).

An empirical study by Bowling (1988–1989) of more than 500 elderly widowed persons followed for 6 years after their bereavement revealed that men age 75 and older had excessive mortality compared with men of the same age in the general population. Bowling also found that certain additional variables predicted mortality, including low social contact. Our own research on this topic provides additional data in support of the notion that it is not just male gender alone that is a risk factor for mortality, but gender in combination with other factors, most notably, social isolation. In this research (described in Gallagher-Thompson et al. 1993), we found that the widowers who had died within the first year of spousal bereavement had reported more often than survivors that their wife was their main confidante; in addition, they had reported minimal involvement in activities with other persons after their wife's death, so after she was gone, their social network virtually disappeared.

Regarding *mode of death,* the results of many studies have demonstrated that adaptation is more difficult when the death is violent (as in a homicide or suicide), stigmatized (as in the case of AIDS), or very unexpected and unanticipated (for more detailed discussion of the clinical impact of these factors, see O'Neil 1989; Osterweis et al. 1984, Parkes and Weiss 1983, and Worden 1991). In our experience comparing older adults whose spouses died of natural causes with older adults whose spouses committed suicide, the impact of the suicide death was considerably more severe on the subsequent bereavement process of the survivor. Although this effect was not very notable at early times of measurement in this longitudinal study—for example, 2 months and 6 months postloss (see Farberow et al. 1987)—it became quite evident over the latter course of the 2½-year measurement period. In contrast to the natural-death survivors, whose feelings of depression and other negative affects were substantially reduced by 1 year postloss, suicide survivors maintained high levels of depression and distress longer—levels in this group generally did not come down significantly until the final follow-up, about 30 months postloss (for complete details, see Farberow et al. 1992a). Farberow and colleagues (1992a) concluded that although over time most of the severe distress subsided, the subjects experienced different courses and had varying remaining levels of distress after 30 months of bereavement. Results also showed that both the suicide and natural-death survivors seemed to manage their new roles and responsibilities adequately by the endpoint, despite the different patterns of emotional distress that they experienced in the interim. Thus, in terms of

whether or not to view a spouse's death by suicide as presenting a significant risk factor for difficult bereavement in the surviving spouse, it appears that this mode of death will make the process more psychologically stressful, particularly during the first year of bereavement. Similar studies have not been carried out for elders whose spouses (or other family members) were homicide victims, nor has much research been done on the impact of stigmatized deaths and/or very sudden deaths. However, Moss and colleagues (1993) did perform a very careful study on the impact of mothers' deaths on middle-aged daughters; these investigators found that relatively sudden deaths were associated with more intense grief than were deaths that occurred in a nursing home, where, presumably, there was time to prepare and say good-bye.

The presence of *clinically significant symptoms of depression* within the first 2 months after a spouse's death is a significant risk factor for poor outcome over time. Lund and co-workers (1993), who found that intense negative emotions at 2 months postloss—such as desire to die and frequent crying—were associated with poor coping 2 years later. Wortman and Silver (1989) reviewed a number of studies indicating that depression confounds successful resolution of grief. In our own work investigating the relationship of depression to later bereavement outcome—summarized in Gilewski et al. (1991)—we found that individuals in the moderate to severe range of self-reported depression were at greatest risk for all other psychopathological symptoms, such as increased anxiety, hostility, interpersonal sensitivity, and other indices of global psychiatric distress. This was true whether or not they were suicide or natural-death survivors. However, the suicide survivors who were moderately to severely depressed at the outset had the highest mean score of any subgroup on the depression measure that was used, maintained higher mean levels of depression over time, and were more likely to score high on other distress measures. These data suggest that, once again, the interaction of one or more risk factors may contribute to the greatest distress.

Regarding the impact of *self-esteem and perceived coping ability,* several papers have suggested that those elderly bereaved with poor self-esteem and/or inadequate coping skills are at greater risk for a difficult bereavement process. Johnson and colleagues (1986) conducted one of the few studies that directly addressed these variables in elders; as expected, individuals who reported themselves to be high in self-esteem and to be effective copers early on in the bereavement process remained high in self-esteem and remained effective copers throughout the first year of bereavement, whereas those who initially reported high stress levels generally continued to be high in stress at subsequent times of measurement.

Regarding the role of *satisfaction with the relationship* and how that might affect the subsequent grief process, this is another variable that has been widely addressed in the clinical literature (cf. Parkes and Weiss 1983; Worden 1991) but with little empirical research to support or refute the clinical lore. Only one recent empirical study could be found that focused on the relationship between the bereaved elders' retrospective assessment of marital adjustment and subsequent levels of self-reported depression, and its results are equivocal. Futterman and co-workers (1990) found that, compared with the non-bereaved, currently married control group in the study, more positive ratings of marital satisfaction were made by the bereaved, and—contrary to expectations—more positive ratings of satisfaction were associated with more severe depression. This pattern of results did not change significantly during the 2-year course of the study, nor was it influenced by gender. The investigators suggested that idealization of the deceased spouse may occur in terms of the satisfaction ratings, thus making it difficult to distinguish the true role of relationship satisfaction to later bereavement outcomes. Clearly, more research is needed on this dimension. Ideally, the quality of the relationship would be measured before and after the spouse's death to more clearly determine how the actual versus the possibly idealized ratings affect the subsequent course of bereavement.

The role of *social support* is less ambiguous, overall. Since the publication of Cobb's classic paper (1976) on the stress-buffering effects of social support, it has been widely recognized as a moderator of many kinds of life stress. A comprehensive review of the role of social support in mitigating the effects of bereavement can be found in Stylianos and Vachon (1993), who make the point that social support should really be viewed as a multidimensional process, including such aspects as size, structure, quality, types of support, and appraisal of support (as satisfactory or not). In this respect, the construct of social support becomes more complex to describe and to measure. In the literature to date, most studies have focused on only one aspect of support, although there is no single aspect that has been most frequently selected for study. Specifically with regard to late-life spousal bereavement, Dimond et al. (1987) found in their longitudinal study that the total size of the reported support network at baseline was positively correlated with perceived coping skills and life satisfaction at later times of measurement. They also found that quality of the network was inversely related to later depression and positively correlated with later measures of life satisfaction. Finally, through a series of multiple regression analyses, they found that several baseline social network factors made independent contributions to the variance accounted for in predicting depression at later times of measurement, suggesting that the role of social support in mitigating severe negative reactions to loss of a spouse has been replicated for older individuals.

Our own research with both natural-death and suicide survivors also confirms and supports this position. In a series of analyses directly comparing these two groups, Farberow and colleagues (1992b) found that the suicide survivors received significantly less emotional and practical support for their feelings of depression and grief than did the natural-death survivors. This was particularly true about 6 months postloss. Also, the suicide survivors did not feel that they could confide in members of their network any more than did the nonbereaved comparison group. Gender differences were also noted, with the bereaved women from both groups reporting that they received more support overall than did either group of bereaved men. The most common sources of support were other family members (particularly adult children), followed by friends, then siblings. Another significant difference concerned how social supports changed over time: the survivors of spouses who had natural deaths reported keeping roughly the same level of feelings for the people in their network, whereas the feelings of the suicide survivors (especially the men) fluctuated considerably over the 30 months. However, by the endpoint—as with the emotional distress measures discussed earlier in this chapter—both practical and emotional supports had increased in the suicide survivor groups and were more comparable to the levels reported by the natural-death survivors.

Taken together, these various studies suggest that certain risk factors, either singly or in combination, do appear to be associated with a more difficult subsequent grief process in elderly individuals. However, it is important to keep in mind that most of this research has been conducted with volunteer subjects, often from relatively advantaged socioeconomic backgrounds, who could see some benefit to themselves from being interviewed. Much remains to be learned about the process of bereavement among those elderly who are economically disadvantaged, or in very poor health, or who have little or no family to rely on. In addition, we need to study more about the interactive effect of several of these risk factors (particularly as they may change over time in their relative intensity or salience to the individual), as well as investigate whether or not the same risk factors would be relevant for bereavement from other causes, such as divorce, death of an adult child or parent, or losses of other kinds.

Interventions to Treat the Elderly Bereaved

Given the fact that the literature is not conclusive on many of the points discussed above, we will nevertheless begin the discussion of interventions to treat the elderly bereaved by asking the reader to think about selecting an intervention on the basis of responses obtained to the following questions: 1) Does the symptom picture fall within the realm of "normal grief" or does it appear to be grief complicated by the presence of a clinical level of depression or some other psychiatric disorder? and 2) What risk factors seem to be present that would suggest that this individual may have a difficult grieving process ahead? By thoughtfully considering responses to these and related questions, one can aim to match the intervention strategy to the needs and profile of the individual patient.

Treatment of complicated bereavement. There is general consensus in the field that if a clinical level of depression (or another significant psychiatric disorder, such as substance abuse or generalized anxiety disorder) is present, then that problem should be treated first, with medication and/or psychotherapy, so that it can resolve sufficiently to permit the grieving process to become the focus of attention when the patient is ready (NIH Consensus Confer-

ence 1992; Parkes and Weiss 1983; Reynolds 1992). As Reynolds (1992) has indicated, "Our clinical practice has been to intervene as early as 2 months, and certainly by 4 months, in the presence of clear syndromal major depression" (p. 50).

Various forms of individual or group psychotherapy have also been used to treat patients with complicated bereavement reactions. Reviews and critiques can be found in several current sources. Raphael and colleagues (1993) briefly describe a variety of methods, including psychodynamic approaches, behavioral therapies, and cognitive therapies for complex grief reactions, along with less intensive counseling techniques that have generally been used in more normal grief situations. They have included a very clear presentation of Horowitz's (1976) time-limited psychodynamic therapy in which separation and loss are regarded as the key issues to work through in a 12-session model. Techniques such as abreaction, catharsis, and interpretation of defenses and affects have been used in order to facilitate realistic appraisals of the implications of the death and to explore the impact of the loss of the relationship on the self-concept of the bereaved person. This model has been empirically studied by Horowitz and colleagues in several reports (see Marmar et al. 1988 for a description of application of this approach to older bereaved women who were also depressed).

The effective use of a relatively brief, intensive, structured behavioral program, called "guided mourning," to facilitate the resolution of chronic grief was reported by Mawson and co-workers (1981), and more recently has been replicated by Sireling and associates (1988). In this approach, 90-minute sessions were held three times weekly for 2 weeks, with subsequent less intense follow-up for 28 weeks; patients were helped to repeatedly confront aspects of their loss so that they could relive painful memories and eventually diminish the negative affects associated with them.

Several forms of cognitive and cognitive-behavior therapy have also been successfully used to treat patients with complex bereavement reactions. The "personal construct" approach of Viney (1990) has focused on the description of core constructs that tend to be disrupted in intense grief, along with methods for reconstructing personal beliefs about oneself, in order to promote adaptation. Treatment of prolonged grief in a 70+-year-old widower using a blend of cognitive and behavioral techniques (such as challenging dysfunctional thoughts and learning to talk about his grief with his adult children) has been described by Florsheim and Gallagher-Thompson (1990). Other examples of the use of cognitive/behavioral methods to treat patients with complicated grief reactions can be found in an excellent conceptual chapter on this topic by Abrahms (1981) and in very detailed case studies by Gantz et al. (1992) and Kaplan and Gallagher-Thompson (1995).

Perhaps one of the most comprehensive and clinically useful books on this topic has been written by Worden (1991). He describes various approaches that he developed for the treatment of grief, while distinguishing between certain methods called "grief counseling" (for normal grief reactions) and "grief therapy" (for inhibited, chronic, or unresolved grief). His methods for grief therapy include reviving memories of the deceased, along with facilitating the experiencing of a broad range of emotions to accompany these memories; helping the patient to acknowledge and deal with ambivalent feelings (in order to eventually achieve a balance); exploring and defusing "linking objects" (those objects a mourner keeps in order to maintain a relationship with the deceased); and helping the bereaved to say a final good-bye as part of therapy. Worden recommends specific modifications of this approach to help patients grieve particularly difficult losses, such as suicides and other forms of sudden death. He also integrates techniques such as psychodrama and role playing in order to intensify the emotional experience and provide the patient with options for working through the painful emotions.

Treatment of normal grief reactions. There are differences of opinion regarding the use of medication to treat the unpleasant symptoms of depression (such as sleep and appetite problems) that typically accompany the first year of bereavement in patients experiencing a normal grief reaction. According to some psychiatrists and other health care providers, medication should be used sparingly, and only briefly, if at all, because it is assumed that in order to recover adequately from grief it is necessary to experience it fully and to live through the experience (cf. Parkes 1972; Worden 1991). Others believe that one should intervene "sooner rather than later,"

given the tendency of depressive symptoms to persist throughout the first year of spousal bereavement (cf. Reynolds 1992). Still others say that there is no empirical evidence that one must suffer through a difficult grieving process in order to be able to resume one's life effectively; therefore, pharmacological (and other) treatments for pain and suffering should be available to those who request them (Wortman and Silver 1987).

Currently there are two well-recognized approaches to facilitate the experience (and expression) of normal grief. As noted above, Worden's work (1991) has specified several methods of "grief counseling" for exactly this purpose, including use of guided imagery to facilitate communication with the deceased, and the use of symbols (such as photos of the deceased) to evoke emotional expression. Worden is also noted for his conceptualization of mourning as consisting of four "tasks" that must be worked through before grief can adequately be resolved: accepting the reality of the loss, experiencing the pain of grief, adjusting to an environment in which the deceased is truly no longer there, and emotionally detaching sufficiently from the deceased to be able to resume a normal life. Bereaved persons are helped to accomplish these tasks through brief individual or group counseling, seen as adjunctive to their own psychological work on these issues.

Because the majority of bereaved persons (particularly elders) do not seek professional assistance for their grief, group counseling is much more widely used—that is, attending a support group specifically for bereaved persons has been the most common intervention recommended, and pursued, by those experiencing an uncomplicated (but painful and lonely) bereavement. A thorough review of the relatively sparse extant literature on bereavement self-help groups has been done by Lieberman (1993). He describes what are thought to be the basic curative factors in such groups, including their "family-like" atmosphere, encouragement of intense emotional expression, and sanction for development of a new self-image that reflects one's current status as an "I" rather than a "we." In contrast to the various forms of psychotherapy reviewed above, which tend to be relatively brief (or at least time-limited in their scope), self-help groups encourage long-term involvement; as Lieberman (1993) pointed out, "membership is indeterminate and may persist far beyond professionally defined recovery" (p. 420). After reviewing the empirical data in support of this approach, Lieberman concluded that self-help groups for grieving persons have been successfully used around the country, often with specific emphases (such as the "Compassionate Friends" self-help network for grieving parents), and that it is reasonable to expect that a large segment of the bereaved population can meet their social and psychological needs through this kind of intervention.

A final intervention that seems to us to hold promise, particularly for older men whose wives have died (and who are at risk for their own subsequent mortality), is one that proposes to help the bereaved develop new affectional bonds to replace the major bond that was severed through death (Stoddard and Henry 1985). This approach is based on the assumption that most older men have only one strong emotional bond (with their wives); when that ends, the ensuing void must be filled with other affectional/emotional relationships, in order to protect against increased vulnerability for negative outcomes. This therapy consists of encouragement and support to develop social friendships into relationships that are emotionally fulfilling and not just socially gratifying. Although there is limited empirical support for this method at present, it is a conceptually appealing approach that warrants further investigation.

As with the other interventions discussed in this chapter, there are, unfortunately, few guidelines to follow in choosing which one (or several) from the available array that might be best to use with a given patient. Clinicians will need to be guided by experience, as well as by future research findings as to the relative efficacy of these methods for patients with specific presenting characteristics.

Adjustment Disorders in Late Life

The diagnostic category of adjustment disorders has been underutilized in the assessment and treatment of older adults. DSM-IV defines adjustment disorder as "clinically significant emotional or behavioral symptoms in response to an identifiable psychosocial stressor or stressors . . . [that] . . . develop within 3 months after the onset of the stressor(s)" (Ameri-

can Psychiatric Association 1994, p. 623). Evidence of impairment in social or occupational functioning should be apparent during the reaction, or there should be symptoms above and beyond what might be expected as a normal reaction to a given stressor. This diagnosis is not applied if the symptom picture meets criteria for another specific disorder or if the reaction appears to be an exacerbation of another mental disorder. If the stressor has a discrete beginning and end, it is assumed that this reaction will subside within a brief time after the stressor disappears. If the stressor is maintained for a long period, it is assumed that the individual will develop a more adaptive pattern of responding over time. By definition, an adjustment disorder must resolve within 6 months after the termination of the stressor. However, symptoms may persist longer if the stressor is chronic or has enduring consequences. The specific type of adjustment disorder is coded according to the predominant symptom pattern (e.g., adjustment disorder with anxious or depressed mood). The new DSM-IV criteria provide for the opportunity to specify whether the adjustment disorder is acute (i.e., if it has persisted for 6 months or less) or chronic (if it has persisted for more than 6 months). This might also lead to an increase in the prevalence of diagnoses of adjustment disorders among the elderly, because in this population stressors are frequently chronic and cumulative, and symptoms often persist longer than 6 months.

DSM-IV reports that adjustment disorders are very common. However, very little attention has been focused on these disturbances in the literature. Out of 10 psychiatry texts we reviewed, only 2 listed adjustment disorder in the index, and it was mentioned within the texts only slightly more often. Virtually no specific data could be found in recent publications concerning prevalence, whether or not there are age or gender differences, or other possible correlates. There has been little interest in this disorder shown in the geropsychiatry literature as well. A literature search covering the past 7 years revealed only one study in geropsychiatry in which the authors reported on the use of this diagnostic category in making consultations on geriatric patients for other medical specialties (Grossberg et al. 1990). This is somewhat surprising, since the increase in stressors experienced by the elderly might lead one to expect a greater proportion of adjustment disorders in this group. In fact, the study referred to above showed that out of 147 geriatric patients seen for psychiatric consultations over a 2-year period, 26% were diagnosed as having an adjustment disorder, second only to affective disorder (27%). One reason for the lack of emphasis in the clinical literature may be that many of the individuals suffering with this disturbance may never have contact with the mental health system. Remedial assistance within the family or from other institutions not connected with the health system may facilitate quick recovery. Age stereotypes regarding emotional illness (Butler and Lewis 1982) may also discourage use of health care resources, or simply delay any help-seeking efforts until the disturbance becomes unbearably severe. This delay in seeking help would in turn increase the likelihood that the arbitrary 6 months may have elapsed, thereby excluding the individual from this diagnostic category.

Blazer (1983) called attention to the possible importance of this diagnostic category in an analysis of the available literature on the epidemiology of depression. He noted that the prevalence of depressive symptoms in community samples ranged from 10% to 45% as reflected in self-report scales, but the actual rate of clinical depression was substantially lower, ranging around 2%–5%, when more stringent interview techniques of assessment were used. He concluded that the discrepancy could be accounted for in part by transient episodes of depressive symptoms accompanying bereavement or an adjustment reaction to other psychosocial stressors. More recent epidemiological studies by Blazer et al. (1987) identified a clinical subtype, referred to as the "symptomatic depression" subgroup, which these investigators suggested may be representative of elderly individuals in the community who are suffering from adjustment disorder. However, Blazer and colleagues acknowledged that a definitive diagnosis could not be made on the basis of their data. The symptomatic depression subgroup constituted 4% of their community sample, but it is likely that even this proportion is an underestimate of the prevalence of the disorder. Further, as mentioned earlier, with the more specific delineation of the time cutoff, which permits a more appropriate use of this diagnosis for chronic stressors, this percentage should increase.

Authors such as Blazer (1983) have provided compelling arguments for the utility of this diagnosis in working with elderly persons. Application of this diagnosis places the focus squarely on the importance of external stressors and the psychological and social resources that the patient has available to cope with whatever unfortunate events might have occurred. Since age-related changes are likely in all of these domains, there are many instances in which this classification could provide a useful working guide for assessment and subsequent treatment efforts in working with elderly patients.

With regard to external stressors, older people experience substantially more serious losses (Chiriboga and Cutler 1980; Lazarus and DeLongis 1983). For example, retirement often leads to loss of the work role; declining health can lead to a host of losses in physical and social functioning; and loss of loved ones and friends can occur not only through death but also by virtue of a move into a new environment, such as a retirement home. Although it is true that some of these losses cannot be avoided, many such losses actually are not unavoidable. In our own work with psychologically distressed elders, for example, we continue to be impressed with how often they have underestimated the importance of their social network when making decisions about moving to a new situation during a time of transition. In many instances, had the significance of old friends and the difficulty of making new ones in a strange setting been given their proper due, the impact of loss of positive life events might have been mitigated. A similar story has been repeated many times for retirement. With proper preparation, individuals can make retirement a transition from one work role to another rather than a loss of role, but all too often the potential hazard of this change is ignored.

The stress of such losses, however, may not be of primary importance; rather, how individuals cope with them may be the critical feature affecting health and well-being in elderly individuals (Billings and Moos 1981; Folkman et al. 1986). Greater acceptance in the field of this position has stimulated considerable interest in possible age differences in coping processes. Some have emphasized increased maturity with age in handling stressful situations (Vaillant 1977). Others have argued that age changes in coping behavior may be minimal, but the kinds and severity of stressors encountered by the elderly are more problematic, thus requiring different types of coping responses (Folkman et al. 1987; McCrae 1982).

Although the explanation for differences in coping behavior is not yet established, there are clear indications that the coping strategies used by older individuals tend to differ from those used by younger individuals. Folkman et al. (1987) reported that in their study, younger persons used proportionately more active, interpersonal, problem-focused forms of coping, whereas the elderly used intrapersonal, emotion-focused forms of coping involving distancing, acceptance of responsibility, and positive reappraisal. McCrae (1982) found that age differences in coping seemed to be due to the different kinds of stressors, but also found that older individuals were generally less hostile in reaction to negative events and less likely to rely on escapist fantasy. Foster and Gallagher (1986) compared elderly depressed patients with nondepressed community volunteers matched for gender, age, and education and found that depressed patients were more likely to use emotional discharge than were those who were not depressed. Although there were no differences between the two groups on appraisal-focused and problem-focused coping, depressed patients rated all of their strategies as significantly less helpful than did the community participants.

The extent to which age-related changes in stressors, social support systems, and coping resources might account for age differences in adjustment reactions is not yet clearly understood. However, the conceptual backdrop emanating from this line of research can provide clear direction for effective treatments of older patients with adjustment disorders. A logical first step would involve a collaborative effort with patients to determine ways of neutralizing the stressful agents. Helping patients to learn how to cope with negative events can also be immensely helpful, particularly with those stressors that are not easily removed, such as chronic physical illness or drastic reductions in income. Such efforts will decrease the likelihood that a prolonged reaction to stress might lead to a more persistent and complicated psychiatric disorder. If stressors are left unchecked, the high frequency of losses and other negative events is likely to render successful adaptation much more difficult, particularly for elderly persons. The end result of this process could be a more severe disorder, requiring hospitalization and the initiation of medical treatment. A frequent endpoint in this reaction to losses and negative events is a depressive episode.

Along these lines, the position advanced by George (1994) is clearly relevant. Recent emphasis on the search for biological factors underlying psychiatric disorders can serve to undermine the importance of external stressors in the development of some types of maladaptive behavior. Increased attention to the diagnostic classification of adjustment disorder, both in the clinical and research setting, may provide a healthy correction to any such trends by keeping the significance of negative events and poor coping behaviors in the foreground. For example, despite recent successes in identifying biological correlates of depression, considerable variance remains unexplained by such markers. This is understandable, given that depression is likely to be the final common pathway of several different causes. However, continued attempts to identify unique symptom patterns that occur in response to external stressors, in the final analysis, should aid in improving the precision of differential diagnostic categories that emphasize specific etiological agents and treatment programs.

References

Abrahms JL: Depression versus normal grief following the death of a significant other, in New Directions in Cognitive Therapy. Edited by Emery G, Hollon S, Bedrosian RC. New York, Guilford, 1981, pp 255–270

American Psychiatric Association: Diagnostic and Statistical Manual of Mental Disorders, 3rd Edition, Revised. Washington, DC, American Psychiatric Association, 1987

American Psychiatric Association: Diagnostic and Statistical Manual of Mental Disorders, 4th Edition. Washington, DC, American Psychiatric Association, 1994

Bass DM, Bowman K, Noelker LS: The influence of caregiving and bereavement support on adjusting to an older relatives' death. Gerontologist 31:32–42, 1991

Billings AG, Moos RH: The role of coping responses and social resources in attenuating the impact of stressful life events. J Behav Med 4:139–157, 1981

Blazer DG: The epidemiology of depression in late life, in Depression and Aging: Causes, Care and Consequences. Edited by Breslau L, Haug MR. New York, Springer, 1983, pp 30–50

Blazer DG, Hughes DC, George LK: The epidemiology of depression in an elderly community population. Gerontologist 27:281–287, 1987

Bowlby J: Processes of mourning. Int J Psychoanal 42:317–340, 1961

Bowling A: Who dies after widow(er)hood? A discriminant analysis. Omega: Journal of Death and Dying 19:135–153, 1988–1989

Breckenridge J, Gallagher D, Thompson LW, et al: Characteristic depressive symptoms of bereaved elders. J Gerontol 41:163–168, 1986

Butler RN, Lewis MI: Aging and Mental Health, 3rd Edition. St. Louis, MO, CV Mosby, 1982

Cain BS: Divorce among elderly women: a growing social phenomenon. Social Casework 69:563–568, 1988

Chiriboga DA, Cutler L: Stress and adaptation: life span perspectives, in Aging in the 1980s. Edited by Poon L. Washington, DC, American Psychological Association, 1980, pp 347–362

Cobb S: Social support as a moderator of life stress. Psychosom Med 3:300–314, 1976

Dimond M, Lund DA, Caserta MS: The role of social support in the first two years of bereavement in an elderly sample. Gerontologist 27:599–604, 1987

Farberow N, Gallagher D, Gilewski M, et al: An examination of the early impact of bereavement on psychological distress in survivors of suicide. Gerontologist 27:592–598, 1987

Farberow N, Gallagher D, Gilewski M, et al: Changes in grief and mental health of bereaved spouses of older suicides. J Gerontol 47:P357–P366, 1992a

Farberow N, Gallagher D, Gilewski M, et al: The role of social supports in the bereavement process of surviving spouses of suicide and natural deaths. Suicide Life Threat Behav 22:107–124, 1992b

Faschingbauer TR: Texas Inventory of Grief—Revised Manual. Houston, TX, Honeycomb Publishing, 1981

Florsheim M, Gallagher-Thompson D: Cognitive/behavioral treatment of atypical bereavement: a case study. Clinical Gerontologist 10:73–76, 1990

Folkman S, Lazarus RS, Gruen R, et al: Appraisal, coping, health status, and psychological symptoms. J Pers Soc Psychol 50:571–579, 1986

Folkman S, Lazarus RS, Pimley S, et al: Age differences in stress and coping processes. Psychol Aging 2:171–184, 1987

Foster J, Gallagher D: An exploratory study comparing depressed and nondepressed elders' coping strategies. J Gerontol 41:91–93, 1986

Freud S: Mourning and melancholia (1917), in The Standard Edition of the Complete Psychological Works of Sigmund Freud, Vol 14. Translated and edited by Strachey J. London, Hogarth Press, 1957, pp 237–258

Futterman A, Gallagher D, Thompson LW, et al: Retrospective assessment of marital adjustment and depression during the first two years of spousal bereavement. Psychol Aging 5:277–283, 1990

Gallagher-Thompson D, Thompson LW: Depression versus normal grief: similarities and differences in assessment and treatment. Paper presented at the annual meeting of the American Society on Aging, San Francisco, CA, March 19, 1994

Gallagher-Thompson D, Futterman A, Farberow N, et al: The impact of spousal bereavement on older widows and widowers, in Handbook of Bereavement. Edited by Stroebe MS, Stroebe W, Hansson R. Cambridge, UK, Cambridge University Press, 1993, pp 227–239

Gantz F, Gallagher D, Rodman J: Cognitive/behavioral facilitation of inhibited grief, in Comprehensive Casebook of Cognitive-Behavior Therapy. Edited by Freeman A, Dattilio F. New York, Plenum, 1992, pp 201–207

George LK: Social factors and depression in late life, in Diagnosis and Treatment of Depression in Late Life: Results of the NIH Consensus Development Conference. Edited by Schneider LS, Reynolds CF III, Lebowitz BD, et al. Washington, DC, American Psychiatric Press, 1994

Gilewski M, Farberow N, Gallagher D, et al: Interaction of depression and bereavement on mental health in the elderly. Psychol Aging 6:67–75, 1991

Grimby A: Bereavement among elderly people: grief reactions, post-bereavement hallucinations, and quality of life. Acta Psychiatr Scand 87:72–80, 1993

Grossberg GT, Zinny GH, Nakra BRS: Geriatric psychiatry consultations in a university hospital. Int Psychogeriatr 2:161–168, 1990

Harlow SD, Goldberg EL, Comstock GW: A longitudinal study of the prevalence of depressive symptomatology in elderly widowed and married women. Arch Gen Psychiatry 48:1065–1068, 1991

Horowitz MJ: Stress Response Syndromes. New York, Jason Aronson, 1976

Johnson RJ, Lund DA, Dimond M: Stress, self-esteem, and coping during bereavement among the elderly. Social Psychology Quarterly 49:273–279, 1986

Kalish RA: Older people and grief (special issue: Death and Bereavement). Generations 11:33–38, 1987

Kaplan C, Gallagher-Thompson D: The treatment of clinical depression in caregivers of spouses with dementia. Journal of Cognitive Psychotherapy 9:35–44, 1995

Kastenbaum RJ: Death, Society, and Human Experience, 2nd Edition. St. Louis, MO, CV Mosby, 1981

Lazarus RS, DeLongis A: Psychological stress and coping in aging. Am Psychol 38:245–254, 1983

Lieberman MA: Bereavement self-help groups: a review of conceptual and methodological issues, in Handbook of Bereavement. Edited by Stroebe MS, Stroebe W, Hansson R. Cambridge, UK, Cambridge University Press, 1993, pp 411–426

Lopata HZ: On widowhood: grief work and identity reconstruction. Journal of Geriatric Psychiatry 8:41–55, 1975

Lund DA (ed): Older Bereaved Spouses. New York, Hemisphere, 1989

Lund DA, Caserta M, Dimond M: Gender differences through two years of bereavement among the elderly. Gerontologist 26:314–320, 1986

Lund DA, Caserta M, Dimond M: Impact of spousal bereavement on the subjective well-being of older adults, in Older Bereaved Spouses. Edited by Lund DA. New York, Hemisphere, 1989, pp 3–15

Lund DA, Caserta M, Dimond M: The course of spousal bereavement in later life, in Handbook of Bereavement. Edited by Stroebe MS, Stroebe W, Hansson R. Cambridge, UK, Cambridge University Press, 1993, pp 240–254

Marmar C, Horowitz MJ, Weiss DS, et al: A controlled trial of brief psychotherapy and mutual-help group treatment of conjugal bereavement. Am J Psychiatry 145:203–212, 1988

Mawson D, Marks IM, Ramm L, et al: Guided mourning for morbid grief: a controlled study. Br J Psychiatry 138:185–193, 1981

McCrae RR: Age differences in the use of coping mechanisms. J Gerontol 37:454–460, 1982

McCrae RR, Costa PT: Psychological resilience among widowed men and women: a 10-year follow-up of a national sample, in Handbook of Bereavement. Edited by Stroebe MS, Stroebe W, Hansson R. Cambridge, UK, Cambridge University Press, 1993, pp 196–207

Middleton W, Raphael B, Martinek N, et al: Pathological grief reactions, in Handbook of Bereavement. Edited by Stroebe MS, Stroebe W, Hansson R. Cambridge, UK, Cambridge University Press, 1993, pp 44–61

Moss MS, Moss SZ, Rubinstein R, et al: Impact of elderly mother's death on middle-age daughters. Int J Aging Hum Dev 37:1–22, 1993

National Institutes of Health Consensus Conference: Diagnosis and treatment of depression in late life. JAMA 268:1018–1024, 1992

O'Neil M: Grief and bereavement in AIDS and aging. Generations 13:80–82, 1989

Osterweis M, Solomon F, Green M (eds): Bereavement: Reactions, Consequences, and Care. Washington, DC, National Academy Press, 1984

Parkes CM: Bereavement: Studies of Grief in Adult Life. New York, International Universities Press, 1972

Parkes CM, Weiss RS: Recovery from Bereavement. New York, Basic Books, 1983

Raphael B, Middleton W, Martinek N, et al: Counseling and therapy of the bereaved, in Handbook of Bereavement. Edited by Stroebe MS, Stroebe W, Hansson R. Cambridge, UK, Cambridge University Press, 1993, pp 427–453

Rees WD: The hallucinations of widowhood. BMJ 4:37–41, 1971

Reynolds CF III: Treatment of depression in special populations. J Clin Psychiatry 53 (9 suppl):45–53, 1992

Sable P: Attachment, loss of spouse, and grief in elderly adults. Omega: Journal of Death and Dying 23:129–142, 1991

Sanders CM: Risk factors in bereavement outcome, in Handbook of Bereavement. Edited by Stroebe MS, Stroebe W, Hansson R. Cambridge, UK, Cambridge University Press, 1993, pp 255–267

Shuchter S, Zisook S: The course of normal grief, in Handbook of Bereavement. Edited by Stroebe MS, Stroebe W, Hansson R. Cambridge, UK, Cambridge University Press, 1993, pp 23–43

Sireling L, Cohen D, Marks I: Guided mourning for morbid grief: a replication. Behavior Therapy 29:121–132, 1988

Stoddard J, Henry JP: Affectional bonding and the impact of bereavement. Advances 2:19–28, 1985

Stroebe MS, Stroebe W: The mortality of bereavement: a review, in Handbook of Bereavement. Edited by Stroebe MS, Stroebe W, Hansson R. Cambridge, UK, Cambridge University Press, 1993, pp 175–195

Stroebe MS, Stroebe W, Hansson R (eds): Handbook of Bereavement, Cambridge, UK, Cambridge University Press, 1993

Stylianos S, Vachon M: The role of social support in bereavement, in Handbook of Bereavement. Edited by Stroebe MS, Stroebe W, Hansson R. Cambridge, UK, Cambridge University Press, 1993, pp 397–410

Thompson LW, Gallagher-Thompson D, Futterman A, et al: The effects of late-life spousal bereavement over a 30-month interval. Psychol Aging 6:434–441, 1991

United States Bureau of the Census: Current Population Reports, Series P-23, 138: Demographic and Socioeconomic Aspects of Aging in the United States. Washington, DC, U.S. Government Printing Office, 1984

Vaillant GE: Adaptation to Life. Boston, MA, Little, Brown, 1977

Viney L: The construing widow: dislocation and adaptation in bereavement. Psychotherapy Patient 6:207–222, 1990

Worden JW: Grief Counseling and Grief Therapy, 2nd Edition. New York, Springer, 1991

Wortman C, Silver RC: Coping with irrevocable loss, in Cataclysms, Crises, and Catastrophes: Psychology in Action. Edited by VandenBos G, Bryant B. Washington, DC, American Psychological Association, 1987, pp 185–235

Wortman C, Silver RC: The myths of coping with loss. J Consult Clin Psychol 57:349–357, 1989

Zisook S, Shuchter SR: Time course of spousal bereavement. Gen Hosp Psychiatry 7:95–100, 1985

Zisook S, Shuchter SR: The first four years of widowhood. Psychiatric Annals 15:288–294, 1986

Zisook S, Shuchter SR, Sledge P, et al: Aging and bereavement. J Geriatr Psychiatry Neurol 6:137–143, 1993

CHAPTER 18

Sleep and Chronobiological Disturbances

Thomas C. Neylan, M.D.
Mary G. De May, M.D.
Charles F. Reynolds III, M.D.

Defining normal, age-related changes in sleep is as challenging as defining normal, age-related changes in memory and cognition. For example, memory difficulties are no longer considered to be an aspect of normal aging per se, and their appearance warrants evaluation and intervention. In the same way, nonrestorative sleep is not a normal part of aging, and its occurrence warrants careful diagnostic evaluation. Pursuing this analogy further, it is known that the speed of information processing decreases with age, but that the overall capacity to learn new information or to retrieve previously encoded information remains intact. Similarly, changes in sleep occur with age that affect the overall depth and length of the sleep period. However, in healthy older persons, the ability of sleep to restore functional daytime energy remains intact.

Many investigators have documented the dramatic rise in sleep-related complaints with age (for a review, see Reynolds et al. 1985b). Interestingly, studies in which investigators have attempted to control for comorbid medical and psychiatric disorders have shown that some aspects of insomnia, such as sleep latency, do not worsen with age (Gislason and Almqvist 1987). Thus, an approach to sleep disorders in the elderly must take into account the multiple factors that conspire against healthy sleep, including comorbid medical and neuropsychiatric disorders; psychosocial factors such as retirement, isolation, and bereavement; and normal age-related changes in sleep and circadian physiology.

A detailed understanding of sleep in elderly persons is essential for several public health reasons. For example, inability to sleep is often the precipi-

This project was supported in part by the following grants from the National Alliance for Research on Schizophrenia and Depression (NARSAD [TCN]) and the National Institute of Mental Health (NIMH): MH–00295 (CFR), MH–37869 (CFR), MH–30915 (CFR), and AG–06836 (CFR).

tating event that prompts family members to forgo caring for demented patients in the home (Pollack et al. 1990; Sanford 1975). Several longitudinal studies have documented the tight association between complaints of insomnia and depressed mood in community-dwelling subjects (Rodin et al. 1988; Vollrath et al. 1989). Further, studies from the Epidemiologic Catchment Area (ECA) survey have found that sleep complaints often predate the onset of a mood disturbance (Ford and Kamerow 1989). Hence, careful evaluation and early intervention for insomnia may prevent the subsequent occurrence of depression.

Sleep and Aging in Healthy Older Persons

Sleep in normal adult humans at all ages consists of recurring cycles of non–rapid eye movement (non-REM) and rapid eye movement (REM) sleep. Non-REM sleep is subdivided into stages 1, 2, 3, and 4, with stages 3 and 4 defined as slow-wave or delta sleep. In slow-wave sleep, the brain is the least metabolically active, the electroencephalograph (EEG) shows the slowest frequency of brain electrical activity, and the stimulus needed to arouse subjects from sleep is greatest (Carskadon and Dement 1994). REM sleep is an extraordinary sleep stage, with relatively increased brain electrical activity; increased cerebral blood flow above the awake state; fluctuations of eye movements, heart rate, and respiration; and a generalized muscle atonia in which the subject is paralyzed except for the diaphragm and the extraocular muscles. With healthy aging, this recurrent cycle remains intact.

The total time spent asleep decreases modestly between the third and ninth decades. The primary change consists of a reduction in EEG amplitude, a reduction and disappearance of visually scored slow-wave sleep, and an increased number of microarousals and awakenings. As a rule, older subjects tend to sleep less efficiently—that is, the percentage of time spent asleep while lying in bed decreases to a normal range of 70%–80% (Prinz et al. 1990). In addition, the elderly are more prone to awaken when there are changes in environmental noise or temperature (Zeppelin et al. 1984).

The most consistent change in sleep architecture is attributed to the reduction of EEG amplitude

of slow-wave sleep (for a review, see Bliwise 1993). Slow-wave sleep is defined by both frequency and amplitude parameters. With increasing age, a substantial reduction occurs in EEG amplitude, which accounts for the reduction or loss of visually scored slow-wave sleep (Webb and Dreblow 1982). Changes in other stages of sleep are less dramatic. The relative percentage of REM sleep changes little with age (Feinberg et al. 1967), although several studies have shown some reduction in REM percentage (Bliwise 1993). Interestingly, REM measures may have prognostic significance. There is a higher mortality rate in depressed, cognitively impaired elderly patients with reduced REM sleep (Hoch et al. 1989). The temporal distribution of REM sleep is flattened in healthy older persons, with a uniform percentage in both halves of the night (Hayashi and Endo 1982; Reynolds et al. 1985b). The elderly have more awakenings and thus have an increased percentage of stage 1 sleep.

Circadian Regulation of Sleep in Elderly Persons

Many investigators have suggested that the flattening in the sleep-wake rhythm in elderly persons is evidence of a fundamental change in circadian physiology. Specifically, the fact that elders have decreased nocturnal sleep, take more naps, and have more objective sleepiness as measured by the Multiple Sleep Latency Test (Carskadon et al. 1982) suggests that the segregation of sleep and wakefulness in the light-dark cycle breaks down with age. However, sleep-disordered breathing and nocturnal myoclonus were not measured in many of these studies. These disorders are extremely prevalent and may explain many of the findings in sleep architecture in the elderly (Bliwise 1993). For example, Reynolds and colleagues (1991a) demonstrated that healthy elderly subjects who have been screened for sleep apnea actually show less sleepiness as defined by the Multiple Sleep Latency Test (Reynolds et al. 1991a). Nevertheless, as a group, the healthy elderly tend to nap quite frequently. One study showed that greater than 80% of the elderly regularly nap (Tune 1968). It is possible that the elderly nap more frequently because they have more opportunities within their social matrix for daytime sleep (Buysse et al. 1992; Webb 1981a).

Multiple studies have shown that the elderly have a flattened circadian rhythm with respect to temperature and cortisol production. The flattening of the temperature rhythm is perhaps related to the increase in the temperature nadir in elderly subjects (Weitzman et al. 1982). In addition, there are data that suggest that temperature, REM sleep, and cortisol rhythms—all of which are thought to reflect the underlying circadian oscillator—are phase-advanced by approximately 90 minutes in elderly subjects compared with younger control subjects (Czeisler et al. 1980, 1986). This may explain, in part, the shortened REM latency and the increase in early-morning awakening that have been observed in elderly persons. Elderly individuals appear to be less tolerant of shifts in their sleep-wake schedules. For example, with age, healthy subjects become more intolerant of the effects of jet lag and shift work (Preston 1973). The response of elders to environmental cues that entrain circadian rhythms—that is, to *Zeitgebers*—may be affected by age. Thus, their reduced tolerance could be related to a decreased responsiveness or exposure to these time cues (Monk 1989).

Effect of Gender on Sleep in the Elderly

Several studies have shown that healthy elderly men have more awakenings and less slow-wave sleep than healthy aged-matched women (Reynolds et al. 1985b). Further, Reynolds and colleagues (1990b, 1991b), using computer-derived measurements, have found that men have onset of slow-wave sleep reduction sooner than women. These findings were somewhat unexpected, given the known increase in subjective insomnia complaints and use of sedative-hypnotic medications in elderly women (Mellinger et al. 1985).

Sleep Need Versus Sleep Ability

Whether older subjects have decreased ability or decreased need for sleep is controversial. This controversy likely will be unresolved as long as the essential function of sleep remains unknown. Hence, the concept of sleep need must be considered cautiously, given the ambiguity of what "need" is actually being served. There are intriguing data supporting both sides of the controversy. Studies

evaluating the effects of exercise on sleep have shown that healthy elderly persons exhibit less change in sleep after exercise than do younger subjects, implying a decreased ability for sleep (Montgomery et al. 1988). However, a stronger method for testing the homeostatic function of sleep is sleep deprivation. Multiple studies have shown that elders have an intact ability for recovery of slow-wave sleep after sleep deprivation (Webb 1981b). Interestingly, women have a more robust rebound of slow-wave sleep compared with male control subjects (Reynolds et al. 1986). Several studies suggest that older adults have a decreased sleep need compared with younger subjects, based on the older subjects' smaller neuropsychological performance decrement after sleep deprivation (Bonnet and Rosa 1987). However, elderly persons may have less of a decremental change because they perform less well at baseline on tasks of vigilance (Bliwise 1993).

Etiology of Sleep Disorders in Elderly Persons

Behavioral and psychosocial changes that occur in late life have a powerful modulating influence on sleep-wake function. For example, retirement eliminates the potent entraining influence of work life. The absence of a structured daytime schedule can facilitate the acquisition of behaviors such as napping, which can lead to increased complaints of nocturnal insomnia. There are intriguing data to suggest that social withdrawal and disenfranchisement can contribute to disruption in sleep-wake function. Hapte-Gabr and co-workers (1991) have found that social attachments are associated with a higher quality of sleep. Dew and colleagues (1994) showed that older subjects with superior sleep quality have more psychosocial support and stability at baseline and follow-up evaluation.

The higher prevalence of sleep-wake complaints in older adults may be related in large measure to the higher prevalence in this population of general medical disorders that adversely affect sleep. Such disorders include congestive heart failure, pulmonary disease, chronic arthritis, gastroesophageal reflux, and diabetes, among many others. Complicating this fact is that many treatments for these disorders adversely affect sleep—for example, diuretics, antihypertensive agents, theophylline,

L-dopa, and corticosteroids (Buysse 1991). Medical disorders and medications can lead to both objective and subjective complaints of insomnia and daytime sleepiness, as well as to the acquisition of new behaviors deleterious to sleep, such as napping or the use of caffeine and alcohol.

Sleep-Disordered Breathing

Sleep-disordered breathing is highly prevalent in the elderly. Approximately 24% of community-dwelling seniors and 42% of institutionalized elderly subjects have sleep-disordered breathing (Ancoli-Israel et al. 1991b). Obstructive sleep apnea appears to be the most prevalent respiratory disorder associated with sleep in this population. It involves a collapse of the oropharynx during respiration, resulting in hypoxia and sleep fragmentation. Obstructive sleep apnea can lead to symptoms of hypersomnolence, decreased alertness, diminished concentration and attention, systemic and pulmonary hypertension, and cor pulmonale. The number of obstructive events per hour of sleep has been found to be predictive of mortality in the elderly (Ancoli-Israel et al. 1989; Hoch et al. 1989). Older adults appear to be more susceptible to upper airway collapse because of anatomic factors such as the higher prevalence of obesity, as well as neurological factors that contribute to an increase in pharyngeal resistance (White et al. 1985). The treatment of obstructive apnea includes weight loss, avoidance of alcohol and other sedatives, sleep position training to avoid lying supine, oropharyngeal surgery, and nasal continuous positive airway pressure. Effective intervention can result in improved sleep and daytime alertness, and prevent the development of systemic and pulmonary hypertension.

Restless Legs/Nocturnal Myoclonus

Periodic leg movements are highly prevalent in healthy seniors, with incidence estimates ranging from 37.5% (Ancoli-Israel et al. 1991a) to 57% (Reynolds et al. 1985b). The clinical significance of an increase in periodic leg movements is not clear. Periodic leg movements can cause brief microarousals that decrease the depth and continuity of sleep. Leg movements that do not result in EEG arousal appear to have no clinical significance. Restless leg syndrome consists of disagreeable sensa-tions in the legs that provoke the patient to move about to obtain some relief. It can cause significant sleep-onset insomnia. Patients can also have significant sleep fragmentation secondary to the invariable presence of periodic limb movements. Restless leg syndrome is associated with iron deficiency anemia and a decline in central dopamine function. Both periodic leg movements and restless leg syndrome can be treated with L-dopa/carbidopa. Other therapies include benzodiazepines, synthetic opiates, iron supplements, and beta-blockers.

Bereavement

Spousal bereavement is associated with a high prevalence of depression and associated sleep disturbance. Reynolds and colleagues (1993a, 1993b) have hypothesized that the changes seen in sleep after a major life event, such as the death of a spouse, may be a marker of resilience or successful adaptation in elderly persons. For example, bereaved patients without major depression have been found to have a slight decrease in slow-wave sleep in the first non-REM period and an increase in phasic REM activity. However, they otherwise have a normal degree of sleep efficiency, total sleep time, and REM latency. In contrast, bereaved subjects with complicated depression have sleep disruption indistinguishable from that which occurs in patients with recurrent major depression (Pasternak et al. 1992; Reynolds et al. 1992, 1993a).

Late-Life Mood Disorders

A wealth of studies have documented the prevalence of sleep disruption in patients with major depression. Depressed patients have been found to have decreased slow-wave sleep, reduced REM latency, increased phasic REM activity in the first half of the night, and prominent sleep continuity disturbance (Kupfer and Reynolds 1992). The degree to which sleep in depressed patients differs from that in control subjects is a function of age. Knowles and MacLean (1990) performed a meta-analysis of published studies of sleep in the elderly that showed that the disparity between depressed patients and control subjects increases as a function of age. Some of the sleep parameters have prognostic significance. For example, reduced REM latency before treatment has been found to be a predictor of recurrence of depression (Giles et al. 1987). The ideal foundation of treatment of the sleep disturbance is optimal treatment of the underlying depressive disorder (see Chapter 13, "Mood Disorders").

Dementia

The study of sleep in patients with dementia is complicated by diagnosis and selection bias. Alzheimer's disease is believed to account for the majority of cases of irreversible dementia. However, it remains a diagnosis of exclusion, confirmable only at autopsy (Katzman 1976). In patients with probable Alzheimer's disease, sleep disturbance is common and often precipitates institutionalization, as families and caregivers become unable to manage nighttime arousal and behavior problems. Disturbed sleep-wake cycle, nighttime wandering, insomnia, and nighttime delirium ("sundowning") are quite common. One likely explanation involves degeneration of the brain stem region and associated pathways that are involved in the regulation of the sleep-wake cycle (Vitiello et al. 1992). Alzheimer's disease is known to affect hippocampal and cortical neurons. In patients with Alzheimer's disease, cortical presynaptic cholinergic neurons degenerate along with the reticular formation of the pons and medulla. It is believed that acetylcholine and the nucleus basalis of Meynert play an important role in sleep regulation and promotion. Thus, from a neuroanatomic and neurochemical perspective, it is not surprising that patients with cortical degeneration from Alzheimer's disease have sleep disturbance.

Specifically, one sees sleep-wake cycle disruption, which worsens with the severity of the dementia; frequent arousals and awakenings; more daytime naps; decreased slow-wave sleep; and decreased REM sleep (Prinz et al. 1982). Reynolds et al. (1985a) have described indeterminate non-REM sleep (fewer spindles and complexes). The disturbance in normal diurnal rhythm is usually partial and mild. Complete diurnal reversal is very rare, but changes in sleep-wake rhythm do correlate with the severity of the dementia.

The phenomenon of "sundowning" is exceedingly common in patients with dementia of any etiology. Sundowning is perhaps best conceptualized as transient nocturnal delirium. It is most commonly observed in evening and night hours with improvement during the day (sleep-wake cycle disturbance

is an essential feature) and is characterized by decreased ability to maintain attention, and by disorientation, disorganized thought and speech, restlessness, agitation, perceptual disturbances (hallucinations and illusions), anxiety, paranoia, and mood lability. It is not uncommon for patients with transient nocturnal delirium to become threatening and combative, symptoms that often necessitate pharmacological management.

The etiology of transient nocturnal delirium is not known. Simply awakening patients from sleep may precipitate such behavior (Evans 1987; Feinburg et al. 1967). Vitiello et al. (1992) cited a number of specific etiological hypotheses, including: 1) REM sleep behavior disorders; 2) partial complex seizures (common in advanced dementia); 3) sleep apnea and subsequent awakenings; 4) neuroleptic-induced akathisia; and 5) deterioration of the suprachiasmatic nucleus. The latter is intriguing in that some patients with Alzheimer's disease undergo deterioration of the suprachiasmatic nucleus (a putative biological clock), resulting in symptoms that reflect dysregulation of the circadian sleep-wake system. There is also some evidence that transient nocturnal delirium may be more frequent in winter compared with autumn (Bliwise 1993; Bliwise et al. 1989). The possible links between daylight exposure, seasonal variations in body temperature, and circadian and sleep-wake system warrant further exploration.

The evaluation and treatment of sundowning behavior is initially identical to that for any delirium: a thorough medical assessment for treatable causes, including those of infectious, toxic-metabolic, neoplastic, electrophysiologic, endocrinological, or pharmacological origin. Behavioral techniques—decreasing stimulation, reorientation and reassurance, low-level night lighting—can be helpful. Some researchers advocate scheduled middle-of-the-night activity for patients with intransigent nocturnal delirium. Bright-light exposure is also being evaluated for possible treatment of nocturnal delirium and sleep-wake cycle disturbance (Campbell et al. 1991). Low-dose, high-potency antipsychotic medications can often be helpful. Some patients may need more sedating antipsychotics, whereas others benefit from the judicious use of benzodiazepines and/or sedating antidepressant medications. Beta-blockers and mood stabilizers have been tried in more refractory cases, with variable results.

Cognitive Impairment of Depression and Dementia With Depression

A final problem common in the assessment of sleep in elderly patients involves concurrent symptoms of depression and cognitive impairment. Cognitive impairment is not uncommon in elderly depressed patients (so-called pseudodementia) and can present a diagnostic dilemma. A number of studies have addressed the sleep of depressed versus demented patients (Reynolds et al. 1987, 1990a). To summarize these findings, depressed patients have more marked sleep maintenance difficulty. They are observed to have shortened REM latency, longer first REM period, higher first REM period density of rapid eye movements, greater REM intensity, and higher REM sleep percentage. Buysse and co-workers (1988) used total versus REM sleep deprivation as probes to differentiate depressive syndromes from dementia in the elderly. Both groups showed rebound with increased sleep efficiency, but depressed patients had lower sleep efficiency after deprivation than did patients with dementia. REM latency was increased in both groups. In depressed patients, an increase in slow-wave sleep during recovery was related to clinical improvement (an antidepressant effect of sleep loss). REM sleep deprivation resulted in little REM rebound in depressed patients but a modest increase in REM in patients with dementia. A remaining question is whether characteristics of recovery sleep after sleep deprivation can differentiate these syndromes.

Parkinson's Disease

Sleep problems are common in patients with Parkinson's disease, affecting about 75% of patients; sleep problems worsen with progression of the disease (Aldrich 1994; Nausieda et al. 1984). Notably, patients with Parkinson's disease have difficulty initiating and maintaining sleep; they also experience nocturnal vocalizations, apneic episodes, spontaneous daytime napping, difficulty turning over in bed, and sometimes REM sleep behavior disorder (Factor et al. 1990; Hardie et al. 1986). The motor symptoms of Parkinson's disease do not completely remit during sleep. Tremor disappears with onset of stage 1 sleep, but may reappear during arousals and awakenings (Fish et al. 1991). For some patients, sleep may be beneficial, with an improvement in tremor noted for 1–2 hours after awakening.

When approaching the evaluation and treatment of sleep complaints in patients with Parkinson's disease, it is important to address the question of whether the sleep problems are related to the disease itself or to the pharmacological treatment under way. Dopaminergic medications such as L-dopa/carbidopa in low doses may promote sleep. High evening doses, however, increase sleep latency, disrupt sleep in the first half of the night, and promote sleep in the second half of the night (Ashkenasy and Yahr 1985). Dopaminergic medications may also cause vivid dreams, nightmares, and night terrors. Clonazepam and other short-acting benzodiazepines may be helpful in reducing sleep latency and in controlling periodic leg movements. Tricyclic antidepressants may be helpful as well, with additional benefit to Parkinson's disease symptoms derived from the anticholinergic side effects of these drugs.

Evaluation of Sleep-Wake Complaints in Elderly Patients

Elderly patients with chronic insomnia or daytime sleepiness should be thoroughly evaluated for medical and psychiatric disorders that can adversely affect sleep. A detailed history and physical examination and a comprehensive list of all medications is essential. An assessment of daytime activity and sleep-related behaviors can be obtained with the use of a 2-week sleep diary. Patients with excessive sleepiness should be referred for polysomnography for evaluation of possible sleep apnea or nocturnal myoclonus, given the high prevalence of these disorders in this population. Patients with insomnia that is not secondary to psychiatric or medical disorders or to medication or substance use are, by exclusion, given the diagnosis of primary insomnia.

Nonpharmacological Treatment of Insomnia and Sleep-Wake Schedule Disorders

Nonpharmacological treatment of insomnia is highly desirable and, ideally, should be the mainstay of therapy. Such treatment is time intensive for the clinician and involves short-term hardship for the patient, followed by long-term gains. It contrasts with pharmacotherapy, which is perhaps easier for the clinician, has short-term benefit for the patient, but can lead to long-term difficulties. An essential part of therapy involves educating the patient regarding what can be realistically expected from treatment. Often, patients who complain of light sleep but who otherwise have good daytime energy can be reassured by learning what is known about normal sleep patterns in late life. Further, patients may benefit from learning that intermittent sleep deprivation is not medically dangerous. Habits that promote healthy sleep, referred to as *sleep hygiene* (Hauri and Orr 1982), include adhering to a regular sleep-wake schedule, avoiding stimulants and alcohol, limiting daytime naps, and getting regular exercise. The effectiveness of these habits has been empirically demonstrated. For example, Vitiello et al. (1990) showed that a program of aerobic fitness training improves sleep quality.

Two strategies for promoting healthy sleep involve reducing the time spent awake in bed. Stimulus control behavior modification (Bootzin 1972) involves having the patient go to bed only when sleepy, limiting the use of the bed for sleep and intimacy, and having the patient get out of bed if sleep onset is delayed more than 15 minutes. Sleep restriction therapy (Spielman et al. 1987) reduces the awake time by a different method. Patients are asked to estimate their average total sleep time with the aid of a sleep diary. After that, they limit their time in bed to the estimated sleep time. Patients initially experience their usual difficulties with sleep onset and maintenance. However, over time, aided by rebound sleep from sleep deprivation, they begin to sleep more efficiently during the bed time. Both of these methods involve some initial hardship and frustration. Success with these methods requires that the clinician spend much time with the patient to set up reasonable expectations, particularly when initiating treatment (Glovinsky and Spielman 1991; Morin 1993). Controlled evaluations of stimulus control (Morin and Azrin 1988) and sleep restriction (Friedman et al. 1991) have demonstrated the effectiveness of these methods.

Phototherapy is potentially useful for treating sleep-wake schedule disorders as well as insomnia. Many institutionalized elderly patients have little exposure to natural sunlight, a factor that may contribute to a breakdown in the segregation between nocturnal sleep and daytime wakefulness (Ancoli-Israel and Kripke 1989). Timed exposure to bright light has been found to improve sleep maintenance in elderly subjects (Campbell and Dawson 1991).

Pharmacological Treatment of Insomnia

The pharmacological treatment of insomnia in elderly patients necessitates understanding of the principles of pharmacokinetics and pharmacodynamics. *Pharmacokinetics* refers to the effect of a patient on the metabolism of a drug. It involves processes of drug absorption, distribution, biotransformation, and elimination. *Pharmacodynamics*, succinctly, refers to the effect of a drug on the patient. For a review of these principles, see Chapter 20, "Pharmacological Treatment."

For insomnia in elderly patients that is unresponsive to nonpharmacological measures, several classes of medications are available. Individuals over the age of 65 consume up to 40% of all sedative-hypnotic medication (Miles and Dement 1980); 14% of elderly persons use sleeping medication on a daily basis (Baker 1985). Alcohol is the most common nonprescription medication used by patients for sleep. Although its use may decrease sleep latency, alcohol's distortion of sleep architecture and well-known deleterious long-term side effects render it a poor remedy.

Benzodiazepines are widely used in the treatment of insomnia and surpass barbiturates with regard to safety. In contrast to barbiturates, the benzodiazepines are not associated with any induction of hepatic enzymes, are safer in overdose, and are less likely to produce withdrawal seizures. Benzodiazepines with an intermediate half-life, especially those without active metabolites, include lorazepam, oxazepam, and temazepam. These drugs are generally safe and effective in the treatment of acute, time-limited insomnia. The half-life to elimination ($t_{1/2}$) is 8–15 hours in elderly persons, and there is usually little daytime sedation. Several years go, the lay media publicized the considerable controversy that arose regarding the short-acting benzodiazepine triazolam, citing reports of severe and untoward effects of this drug on memory (Cowley 1991). This medication has been banned in several countries. In the United States, the Food and

Drug Administration (FDA) reviewed the drug and recommended that it remain on the market with some labeling changes. A literature review by Rothschild (1992) does not reveal compelling evidence for any uniquely negative characteristics of triazolam relative to other benzodiazepines. The usual concerns regarding benzodiazepine effects on memory (see below) and the usual recommendations for dose reductions in the elderly are warranted.

The intermediate-$t_{1/2}$ benzodiazepines are felt to be superior to longer-$t_{1/2}$ benzodiazepines (such as diazepam and chlordiazepoxide), largely because the latter accumulate active metabolites, resulting in excessive sedation and cognitive or motor impairment. Risks of benzodiazepine treatment for insomnia in the elderly include rare disinhibition (probably dose related and linked to longer-$t_{1/2}$ benzodiazepines); memory problems (impairment in acquisition and recall of information, linked to route, dose, and pharmacokinetics—common to all agents in this class); oversedation, confusion, exacerbation of depressive symptoms and underlying cognitive impairment (particularly in patients with central nervous system [CNS] pathology); impairment of motor function and coordination and an increased risk of falls (related to dose; effects worse in mornings); and rebound insomnia after withdrawal (more pronounced with shorter-$t_{1/2}$ drugs).

Although the accumulation and prolonged effect of longer-acting benzodiazepines render these drugs less appropriate for use in elderly patients, some exceptions do occur. Clonazepam, with a $t_{1/2}$ of 38–100 hours in elderly individuals, is helpful in relieving nocturnal myoclonus, restless leg syndrome, and REM sleep motor disinhibition. When daytime agitation is a problem—for example, in agitated patients with dementia—or when next-day sedation may be desirable, longer half-life benzodiazepines may be indicated.

Cyclic antidepressants are relatively safe and effective for the pharmacological treatment of insomnia in older adults. In addition to being considered for use in the setting of a major depressive episode, these medications should be considered when a patient's insomnia appears likely to be chronic. Although amitriptyline is the most sedating of the tricyclic antidepressants, it is also the agent with the greatest anticholinergic effects and the one associated with a significant risk of orthostatic hypoten-

sion, falls, and other side effects. Secondary amine tricyclics, such as nortriptyline and desipramine, are safer in this regard. Nortriptyline is the best-studied tricyclic antidepressant in elderly populations, and in dosages required to treat insomnia it has been demonstrated to be safe and effective. Although doxepin has been used a good deal for insomnia, it, too, has considerable anticholinergic properties. Trazodone is a heterocyclic antidepressant with few anticholinergic but significant alpha$_1$-adrenergic properties. It usually causes few cardiac side effects. Trazodone is quite sedating and is associated with hypotension.

The benefits of antidepressants in the longer term treatment of insomnia in elderly patients include relative safety, efficacy, and lack of development of tolerance or dependence. These agents are unsafe in overdose and must be prescribed with caution for patients at risk for suicide and those with significant cardiac conduction disease or narrow-angle glaucoma.

Over-the-counter sleep medications (diphenhydramine and other antihistamines) are best avoided in the elderly. Although these medications reduce sleep latency, over time their use results in more frequent awakenings. They are universally associated with impairment in daytime functioning (performance and memory tasks), even at low doses. They are also frequently associated with delirium in elderly individuals, particularly when administered concomitantly with other CNS-active medications.

Zolpidem is a nonbenzodiazepine, imidazopyridine-class hypnotic agent that is effective in inducing and maintaining sleep. Zolpidem binds specifically to the type I (W1) benzodiazepine receptor, but has no myelorelaxant, anxiolytic, or anticonvulsant effects. The drug is rapidly absorbed and peaks in just over 2 hours. It is highly bound to plasma protein and does not accumulate. The $t_{1/2}$ is 2.9 hours in elderly patients, and there is no associated daytime sleepiness or memory effects (Kryger et al. 1991; Merlotti et al. 1989; Scharf et al. 1991). Although zolpidem requires further study in elderly patients with insomnia, it appears to be a promising new pharmacological treatment. The lack of myelorelaxant properties is an added benefit in those patients with sleep apnea, as there is no additional relaxation of the upper airway, in contrast to what occurs with benzodiazepine therapy.

Future Research Directions

The public health significance of sleep disorders in the elderly has been clearly demonstrated (Reynolds et al. 1995). More work is needed to clarify the pathophysiological significance of mild obstructive sleep apnea and periodic limb movements. In addition, much work is needed to demonstrate the effectiveness of current interventions. For example, there is a need for more randomized clinical trials of nonpharmacological therapies such as phototherapy, sleep restriction, and aerobic fitness. Similarly, much more information about the risks and benefits of chronic administration of hypnotic medication is needed. This might include comparisons between maintenance treatment with low-dose benzodiazepines versus nonbenzodiazepines such as trazodone. Finally, more work is needed to demonstrate the effectiveness of combined interventions.

References

Aldrich MS: Parkinsonism, in Principles and Practice of Sleep Medicine, 2nd Edition. Philadelphia, PA, WB Saunders, 1994, pp 783–789

Ancoli-Israel S, Kripke DF: Now I lay me down to sleep: the problem of sleep fragmentation in elderly and demented residents of nursing homes. Bulletin of Clinical Neurosciences 54:127–132, 1989

Ancoli-Israel S, Klauber MR, Kripke DF, et al: Sleep apnea in female nursing home patients: increased risk of mortality. Chest 96:1054–1058, 1989

Ancoli-Israel S, Kripke DF, Klauber MR, et al: Periodic limb movements in sleep in community dwelling elderly. Sleep 14:496–500, 1991a

Ancoli-Israel S, Kripke DF, Klauber MR, et al: Sleep disordered breathing in community-dwelling elderly. Sleep 14:486–495, 1991b

Ashkenasy JJM, Yahr MD: Reversal of sleep disturbance in Parkinson's disease by antiparkinsonian therapy: a preliminary study. Neurology 35:527–532, 1985

Baker T: Introduction to sleep and sleeping disorders. Med Clin North Am 69:1123–1152, 1985

Bliwise DL: Sleep in normal aging and dementia. Sleep 16:40–81, 1993

Bliwise DL, Lee K, Corroll JS, et al: A rating scale for assessing sundowning in nursing home patients. Sleep Res 18:111, 1989

Bonnet MH, Rosa RR: Sleep and performance in young adults and older normals and insomniacs during acute sleep loss and recovery. Biol Psychol 25:153–172, 1987

Bootzin RR: A stimulus control treatment for insomnia, in American Psychological Association Proceedings. Washington, DC, American Psychological Association, 1972, pp 395–396

Buysse DJ: Drugs affecting sleep, sleepiness and performance, in Sleep, Sleepiness and Performance. Edited by Monk TH. New York, Wiley, 1991, pp 249–306

Buysse DJ, Reynolds CF III, Kupfer DJ, et al: Electroencephalographic sleep in depressive pseudodementia. Arch Gen Psychiatry 45:568–575, 1988

Buysse DJ, Browman KE, Monk TH, et al: Napping and 24-hour sleep/wake patterns in healthy elderly and young adults. J Am Geriatr Soc 40:779–786, 1992

Campbell SS, Dawson D: Bright light treatment of sleep disturbance in older subjects. Sleep Res 20:448, 1991

Carskadon MA, Dement WC: Normal human sleep: an overview, in Principles and Practice of Sleep Medicine, 2nd Edition. Philadelphia, PA, WB Saunders, 1994, pp 16–25

Carskadon MA, Brown ED, Dement WC: Sleep fragmentation in the elderly: relationship to daytime sleep tendency. Neurobiol Aging 3:321–327, 1982

Cowley G: Sweet dreams or nightmare. Newsweek, August 19, 1991, pp 44–51

Czeisler CA, Weitzman ED, Moore-Ede MC, et al: Human sleep: its duration and organization depend on its circadian phase. Science 210:1264–1267, 1980

Czeisler CA, Rios CD, Sanchez R, et al: Phase advance and reduction in amplitude of the endogenous circadian oscillator correspond with systemic changes in sleep-wake habits and daytime functioning in the elderly. Sleep Res 15:268, 1986

Dew MA, Reynolds CF III, Monk TH, et al: Psychosocial correlates and sequelae of electroencephalographic sleep in healthy elders. J Gerontol 49:8–18, 1994

Evans LK: Sundown syndrome in institutionalized elderly. J Am Geriatr Soc 35:101–108, 1987

Factor SA, McAlarney T, Sanchez-Ramon JR, et al: Sleep disorder and sleep effect in Parkinson's disease. Mov Disord 4:280–285, 1990

Feinburg I, Koresko RL, Heller N: EEG sleep patterns as a function of normal and pathological aging in man. J Psychiatr Res 5:107–144, 1967

Fish DR, Sawyers D, Allen PJ, et al: The effect of sleep on the dyskinetic movements of Parkinson's disease and torsion dystonia. Arch Neurol 48:210–214, 1991

Ford DE, Kamerow DB: Epidemiologic study of sleep disturbances and psychiatric disorders: an opportunity for prevention? JAMA 262:1479–1484, 1989

Friedman L, Bliwise DL, Yesavage JA, et al: A preliminary study comparing sleep restriction and relaxation treatments for insomnia in older adults. J Gerontol 46:P1–P8, 1991

Giles DE, Jarrett RB, Roffwarg HP, et al: Reduced REM latency: a predictor of recurrence of depression. Neuropsychopharmacology 1:33–39, 1987

Gislason T, Almqvist M: Somatic diseases and sleep complaints. Acta Medica Scandinavica 221:475–481, 1987

Glovinsky PB, Spielman AJ: Sleep restriction therapy, in Case Studies in Insomnia. Edited by Hauri PJ. New York, Plenum, 1991, pp 49–63

Hapte-Gabr E, Wallace RB, Colsher PL, et al: Sleep patterns in rural elders: demographic, health and psycho-behavioral correlates. J Clin Epidemiol 44:5–13, 1991

Hardie RJ, Efthimiou J, Stern GM: Respiration and sleep in Parkinson's disease (letter). J Neurol Neurosurg Psychiatr 49:1326, 1986

Hauri P, Orr WC: The Sleep Disorders: A Current Concepts Monograph. Kalamazoo, MI, Upjohn, 1982

Hayashi Y, Endo S: All-night sleep polygraphic recording of healthy aged persons: REM and slow-wave sleep. Sleep 5:277–283, 1982

Hoch CC, Reynolds CF III, Houck PR, et al: Predicting mortality in mixed depression and dementia using EEG sleep variables. J Neuropsychiatry Clin Neurosci 1:366–371, 1989

Katzman R: The prevalence and malignancy of Alzheimer's disease: a major killer. Arch Neurol 33:217–218, 1976

Knowles JB, MacLean AW: Age-related changes in sleep in depressed and healthy subjects: a meta-analysis. Neuropsychopharmacology 3:251–259, 1990

Kryger MH, Steljes Z, Pouliot Z, et al: Subjective versus objective evaluation of hypnotic efficacy: experience with zolpidem. Sleep 14:399–406, 1991

Kupfer DJ, Reynolds CF III: Sleep and affective disorders, in Handbook of Affective Disorders, 2nd Edition. Edited by Paykel ES. London, Churchill Livingstone, 1992, pp 311–323

Mellinger GD, Balter MB, Uhlenhuth EH: Insomnia and its treatment: prevalence and correlates. Arch Gen Psychiatry 42:225–232, 1985

Merlotti L, Roehrs T, Koshorek G, et al: The dose effects of zolpidem on the sleep of healthy normals. J Clin Psychopharmacol 9:9–14, 1989

Miles LE, Dement WC: Sleep and aging. Sleep 3:119–120, 1980

Monk TH: Circadian rhythm. Clin Geriatr Med 5:331–346, 1989

Montgomery I, Trinder J, Paxton S, et al: Physical exercise and sleep: the effect of the age and sex of the subjects and type of exercise. Acta Physiol Scand Suppl 133:36–40, 1988

Morin CM: Insomnia: Psychological Assessment and Management. New York, Guilford, 1993, pp 83–155

Morin CM, Azrin NH: Behavioral and cognitive treatments of geriatric insomnia. J Consult Clin Psychol 5:748–753, 1988

Nausieda PA, Glantz R, Weber S, et al: Psychiatric complications of levodopa therapy of Parkinson's disease, in Advances in Neurology, Vol 40. Edited by Hassler RG, Christ JF. New York, Raven, 1984, pp 1271–1277

Pasternak RE, Reynolds CF III, Hoch CC, et al: Sleep in spousally bereaved elders with subsyndromal depressive symptoms. Psychiatry Res 43:43–53, 1992

Pollack CP, Perlick D, Linsner JP, et al: Sleep problems in the community elderly as predictors of death and nursing home placement. J Community Health 15:123–135, 1990

Preston FS: Further sleep problems in airline pilots on world-wide schedules. Aerospace Medicine 44:775–782, 1973

Prinz PN, Peskind ER, Vitaliano PP, et al: Changes in the sleep and waking EEGs on nondemented and demented elderly subjects. J Am Geriatr Soc 30:86–93, 1982

Prinz PN, Vitiello MV, Raskind MA, et al: Geriatrics: sleep disorders and aging. N Engl J Med 323:520–526, 1990

Reynolds CF III, Kupfer DJ, Taska LS, et al: EEG sleep in elderly depressed, demented and healthy subjects. Biol Psychiatry 20:431–442, 1985a

Reynolds CF III, Kupfer DJ, Taska LS, et al: Sleep of healthy seniors: a revisit. Sleep 8:20–29, 1985b

Reynolds CF III, Kupfer DJ, Hoch CC, et al: Sleep deprivation in healthy elderly men and women: effects on mood and on sleep during recovery. Sleep 9:492–501, 1986

Reynolds CF III, Kupfer DJ, Hoch CC, et al: Sleep deprivation as a probe in the elderly. Arch Gen Psychiatry 44:982–990, 1987

Reynolds CF III, Buysse DJ, Kupfer DJ, et al: Rapid eye movement sleep deprivation as a probe in elderly subjects. Arch Gen Psychiatry 47:1128–1136, 1990a

Reynolds CF III, Kupfer DJ, Thase ME, et al: Sleep, gender and depression: an analysis of gender effects on the electroencephalographic sleep of 302 depressed outpatients. Biol Psychiatry 28:673–684, 1990b

Reynolds CF III, Jennings JR, Hoch CC, et al: Daytime sleepiness in the healthy "old old": a comparison with young adults. J Am Geriatr Soc 39:957–962, 1991a

Reynolds CF III, Monk TH, Hoch CC, et al: Electroencephalographic sleep in the healthy "old old": a comparison with the "young old" in visually scored and automated measures. J Gerontol 46:M39–M46, 1991b

Reynolds CF III, Hoch CC, Buysse DJ, et al: EEG sleep in spousal bereavement and bereavement-related depression of late life. Biol Psychiatry 31:69–82, 1992

Reynolds CF III, Hoch CC, Buysse DJ, et al: Sleep after spousal bereavement: a study of recovery from stress. Biol Psychiatry 34:791–797, 1993a

Reynolds CF III, Hoch CC, Buysse DJ, et al: REM sleep in successful, usual, and pathological aging: the Pittsburgh experience 1980–1993. J Sleep Res 2:203–210, 1993b

Reynolds CF III, Buysse DJ, Kupfer DJ: Disordered sleep: developmental and biopsychosocial perspectives on the diagnosis and treatment of persistent insomnia, in Psychopharmacology: The Fourth Generation of Progress. Edited by Bloom FE, Kupfer DJ. New York, Raven, 1995, pp 1617–1629

Rodin J, McAvay G, Timko C: A longitudinal study of depressed mood and sleep disturbances in elderly adults. J Gerontol 43:45–53, 1988

Rothschild AJ: Disinhibition, amnestic reactions, and other adverse reactions secondary to triazolam: a review of the literature. J Clin Psychiatry 53 (12 suppl):69–79, 1992

Sanford JRA: Tolerance of debility in elderly dependents by supporters at home: significance for hospital practice. BMJ 3:471–473, 1975

Scharf MB, Mayleben DW, Kaffeman M, et al: Dose-response effects of zolpidem in normal geriatric subjects. J Clin Psychiatry 52 (2 suppl):77–83, 1991

Spielman AJ, Saskin P, Thorpy MJ: Treatment of chronic insomnia by restriction of time in bed. Sleep 10:45–56, 1987

Tune GS: Sleep and wakefulness in normal human adults. BMJ 2:269–271, 1968

Vitiello MV, Schwartz RS, Bradbury VL, et al: Improved subjective sleep quality following fitness training in healthy elderly males. Sleep Res 19:154, 1990

Vitiello MV, Bliwise D, Prinz P: Sleep in Alzheimer's disease and the sundown syndrome. Neurology 42:83–94, 1992

Vollrath M, Wicki W, Angst J: The Zurich study, VIII: Insomnia: association with depression, anxiety, somatic syndromes, and course of insomnia. European Archives of Psychiatry and Neurological Sciences 239:113–124, 1989

Webb WB: Patterns of sleep in healthy 50- to 60-year-old males and females. Research Communications in Psychology, Psychiatry, and Behavior 6:133–140, 1981a

Webb WB: Sleep stage responses of older and younger subjects after sleep deprivation. Electroencephalogr Clin Neurophysiol 52:368–371, 1981b

Webb WB, Dreblow LM: A modified method for scoring slow wave sleep of older subjects. Sleep 5:195–199, 1982

Weitzman ED, Moline ML, Czeizler CA, et al: Chronobiology of aging: temperature, sleep/wake rhythms, and entrainment. Neurobiol Aging 3:299–309, 1982

White DP, Lombard RM, Cadieux RJ, et al: Pharyngeal resistance in normal humans: influence of gender, age, and obesity. J Appl Physiol 58:365–371, 1985

Zeppelin H, McDonald CS, Zammit GK: Effects of age on auditory awakening thresholds. J Gerontol 39:294–300, 1984

CHAPTER 19

Alcohol and Drug Problems

Dan G. Blazer, M.D., Ph.D.

The problems of alcohol and drug abuse in late life are closely related. Of the two, alcohol abuse is the more publicized but not necessarily the more prevalent. Misuse of both alcohol and drugs derives from the context of Western society. Primary care physicians and geriatric psychiatrists cannot diagnose or treat these disorders without appreciating the milieu from which they emerge and the factors that reinforce the behaviors.

Use of alcohol has a long and complex history in human societies (Maddox and Blazer 1985). Among the ancients, alcohol was described as "the water of life" and given magical, symbolic significance in religious and social ceremonies that marked transitions over the life course from birth to death. In other words, alcohol is such a domesticated drug—the recreational beverage of choice—that it is difficult to discuss alcohol as a potentially addictive substance like those "other drugs," such as cocaine. Yet clinicians are ambivalent about alcohol, and with good reason. Alcohol is associated with a wide range of personal and social problems across the life span. For example, intoxication is involved in an estimated 50% of all traffic fatalities.

Drug abuse must also be considered within the context of its culture. Neither illegal nor prescription drugs are perceived as "recreational" by the vast majority of older adults. Admitted drug abuse is a rare phenomenon in the older adult. Nevertheless, 25% of drugs and drug sundries consumed in this country are consumed by those age 65 and older—2.5 times the proportion for the entire population. Older adults frequently suffer from one or more chronic illnesses. Most will take at least one prescription medication in any given year. Elders are comfortable taking medications, and many are skilled at detecting the optimal dose for certain types of subjective effects. They also recognize the nuances of side effects from one medication to the other. The veritable "pharmacy within the medicine cabinet" provides older persons with a wide selection of prescription and over-the-counter agents for treating a given malady. This fact, coupled with the decreased availability of primary medical care in some communities and the increased cost of such care, makes self-medication for physical and mental health problems a common occurrence. An inevitable outcome for older persons from an individualistic society with multiple barriers to appropriate medical and psychiatric care is the abuse of prescription and over-the-counter medications.

Both alcohol and drug problems confront clinicians who treat older adults. Occasionally, medication and alcohol misuse or abuse is the primary problem encountered. More often, however, this problem accompanies other disorders and complicates therapy. In this chapter, alcohol and drug problems will be reviewed separately. Although these disorders undoubtedly overlap, each has unique characteristics and deserves separate attention.

Alcohol Abuse and Dependence

Investigation of alcohol abuse and dependence among older adults has increased in recent years. The reason for this attention is not a dramatic or even a persistent increase in rates of alcohol problems in the elderly. As reviewed previously in this text (see Chapter 9), the current prevalence of alcohol abuse/dependence for persons 65 years of age and older ranges from 1.9% to 4.6% for men and from 0.1% to 0.7% for women (Myers et al. 1984). In other cultures, rates may be higher. For example, among men 70 years of age and older in Sweden, 10% abused alcohol or were heavy drinkers (Mellstrom 1981). Although no differences were found among racial/ethnic groups in the Epidemiologic Catchment Area (ECA) studies (Myers et al. 1984), some clinical studies have suggested that rates are higher in older African Americans than in whites (Blum and Rosner 1983). In the United States, even the lifetime prevalence of alcohol problems in older adults is lower than for younger persons in the population. This finding may partially be explained by cohort differences in drinking experiences and selective survival of more moderate drinkers. The risk factors for alcohol abuse in the elderly are similar to those for the general population—male gender, poor education, low income, and a history of other psychiatric disorders, especially depression. The comorbidity of alcohol problems and psychiatric illness in late life is 10%–15% (Finlaysen et al. 1988).

One explanation for the increased interest in alcohol problems among the elderly is that late life is perceived as a time of stressful events, such as retirement, widowhood, illness, and isolation. Alcohol use has traditionally been a culturally accepted strategy for stress reduction. With increased stress, older individuals may increase both their alcohol intake and their risk for alcohol-related problems. The decreased ability of the older adult to metabolize alcohol, coupled with concomitant medical problems, increases the risk of accidents, side effects, and overt toxicity. Alcohol abuse may first be noticed by family members as elders become less capable of living alone. Discovery that a parent has a long history of alcohol intake may offend the social sensibilities of middle-aged children and grandchildren, who have held their parents and grandparents in high esteem (Maddox and Blazer 1985). The potential for alcohol problems to emerge in individuals who have maintained a relatively constant intake of alcohol over the majority of their adult lives will increase as more older adults reach their 80s and 90s, for alcohol toxicity can increase with the decreased ability to metabolize alcohol in late-late life.

Despite the above scenario, the problem of alcohol abuse and dependence in late life, albeit serious, is not as severe as it is among young adults. Although the population at risk for late-life alcohol problems increases with each successive cohort ("the graying of the Western world"), the rate of increase has not been dramatic. In fact, most older persons living today were raised in a culture that included a strong tradition of temperance. In a national survey by Armor et al. (1977), 52% of elderly men and 68% of elderly women said they were abstainers. These percentages, however, will drop with those cohorts entering late life in the 21st century. The increased percentage of users does not necessarily suggest an increased percentage of those who abuse alcohol, although increased per capita consumption is usually associated with an increase in the magnitude of abuse (Faris 1974).

Longitudinal studies of risk factors for alcohol problems in the elderly are virtually nonexistent. Nevertheless, suggestive data from cross-sectional research may be informative in regard to potential etiological agents. For example, Glatt (1978) identifies three precipitating factors in late-onset alcoholism: a habitual drinking pattern before late life, personality factors, and environmental factors. Personality characteristics that predispose to late-life drinking problems include anxiety and worry about one's social environment, such as loss of a loved one and loneliness. Personality factors appear to be less related to late-onset alcoholism than they do to alcoholism onset at earlier stages of the life cycle. Instead, alcohol problems in the elderly may precipitate stressful events such as marital discord and social isolation (especially from family). In their survey of alcohol abuse among the elderly, Rathbone-McCuan et al. (1976) questioned 695 persons 55 years of age and older in Baltimore, Maryland. They found that older alcoholic individuals drank primarily to alleviate depression and to escape existing social problems. The older problem drinkers generally reported poorer health and had more physical problems than did the elderly normal drinkers. In addition, the older problem drinkers had more problems with finances and social isolation. Warheit and Auth (1984) found that, compared with a high-risk alcohol group of younger persons, those in a high-risk alcohol group who were 50 years of age and older were less likely to report difficulties in marital status and life satisfaction (although the trend was in a similar direction in the younger group).

Risk-factor studies of alcohol intake over time are relatively rare in the literature. Longitudinal studies for drinking patterns, however, are more common and provide insight into changing patterns of alcohol intake through the adult years. For example, more than 1,800 men ages 28–87 were studied for more than 10 years in the Veterans Administration's Normative Study of Aging (Glynn et al. 1984). In this panel there was almost no change in mean alcohol consumption during the follow-up period. In addition, rates of problems with drinking did not decline over time. These data do not support the findings from previous cross-sectional studies that aging modifies drinking behaviors. Men in their 40s and 50s in 1973 were especially persistent in their alcohol intake over time. In an earlier investigation, Gordon and Kannel (1983) found that participants in the Framingham Heart Study increased their alcohol consumption by more than 63% over a 20-year follow-up period (1952–1972). An increase in consumption from 1952 to 1972 is consistent with the stability in consumption reported in the Veterans Administration normative aging study if one recognizes that both cohorts were influenced by a national trend toward increased alcohol use. That is, the tendency to decrease alcohol consumption with age may have been counterbalanced by social forces encouraging greater consumption.

In a follow-up of nearly 1,300 adults treated for moderately severe to severe alcohol problems, Helzer and colleagues (1984) found few age differences that predicted outcome. There was some evidence that among the survivors, older alcoholic individuals are less likely to experience persistent, severe problems. At the same time, all-cause mortality was higher for older adults, and alcohol-related mortality was similar for both the young and the elderly. Among the predictors of continued alcoholism, social isolation was more strongly correlated in the older group. Organic brain syndrome was not associated with outcome for the younger sample, but its absence was associated with a good outcome for the older group. In summary, this sample of treated alcoholic patients followed for 6–10 years revealed a good outcome in a large proportion of the older subjects.

Pharmacological Properties of Alcohol

Ethyl alcohol is absorbed easily through the mucous membranes of the stomach, small intestines, and colon. Although peak blood levels are generally reached within 30–90 minutes after alcohol intake, complete absorption may take from 2 to 6 hours. Many factors alter the rate of absorption; some of these factors are age related. In general, alcohol absorption is as rapid in late life as it is at earlier stages of the life cycle. Most foods in the stomach retard absorption, especially milk and milk products. In contrast, because absorption from the small intestine is extremely rapid, patients who have undergone gastrectomy frequently complain that they quickly become intoxicated by small amounts of alcohol that would not have been a problem before the operation (Garver 1984; Muehlberger 1958; Ritchie 1981).

Once absorbed, ethanol is distributed throughout the body, but not evenly. Alcohol is not distributed to fatty tissues (Garver 1984). Older adults have less total body water per unit mass, less extracellular fluid, and higher body fat. The net result is that a standard ingested dose of ethanol will result in a higher blood level in an older adult than in a younger adult because of the lower effective fluid volume for distribution (Wiberg et al. 1971), due in part to an increased proportion of lipid tissue with aging.

More than 90% of the alcohol that enters the body is completely oxidized. This process takes place in the liver, primarily under the influence of the hepatic enzyme alcohol dehydrogenase. There is no evidence that the activity of this enzyme decreases as a function of aging in humans (Garver 1984). At all ages, the metabolism of alcohol is slow and constant. Therefore, a definite limit must be placed on the amount of alcohol that is consumed in a given period; otherwise, intoxication or more serious consequences may result secondary to an accumulation of alcohol. The small amount of alcohol not oxidized may be either excreted in the urine (or other body fluids) or diffused into the alveolar air and exhaled. In other words, the body must process virtually all the alcohol ingested.

The process of alcohol metabolism can lead to secondary problems for the older adult. Gastric secretions are mediated psychically by alcohol, for alcohol is a very strong stimulus if enjoyed by the individual. The presence of alcohol in the stomach in concentrations of about 10% results in gastric secretions rich in acid but poor in pepsin (in contrast to the reflex secretion, which is rich in both). At stronger concentrations (40% or over), alcohol is directly irritating to the mucosa and may cause congestive hyperemia and inflammation. As a result, plasma protein may be lost into the gastrointestinal lumen, and erosive gastritis may ensue (Chowdhury et al. 1977; Ritchie 1981). Alcohol may also facilitate constipation if ingested habitually in moderate amounts. The mechanism is probably secondary to inadequate food intake and insufficient bulk. Diarrhea, on the other hand, may result from the irritant action of alcohol.

The oxidation of alcohol in the liver leads to a change in the ratio of nicotinamide adenine dinucleotide (NAD) to a relative increase NAD's reduced form, NADH. This change, in turn, apparently enhances lipid synthesis by the liver. Alcohol may also indirectly promote the accumulation of fatty tissue in the liver. Acetylglycerophosphate increases in concentration with an accompanying stimulation of the esterification of fatty acids, which leads to a collection of fat in the liver (Kalant et al. 1980; Ritchie 1981). Accumulation of fat and an accompanying accumulation of protein may initially cause no difficulties, but eventually the process cannot be reversed, and the result is a progression to various stages of liver disease, especially cirrhosis. Alcoholic fatty liver and cirrhosis are diseases of middle and late life; these conditions are unlikely in persons who consume less than 80 g per day for 10–20 years.

Alcohol also exerts a diuretic effect on the kidneys. This effect appears to be above and beyond the large amounts of fluids that chronic alcohol abusers usually ingest with alcoholic beverages. This diuresis may be secondary to a decrease in the release of antidiuretic hormone from the posterior pituitary. The relative increase in urine formation can be a problem, especially for elderly men whose urine flow is compromised by prostatic difficulties (Garver 1984; Ritchie 1981).

Although alcohol is popularly thought to be a sexual stimulant, chronic ingestion of alcohol often results in decreased sexual interest, if not impotence. The mechanism by which this effect occurs is a decrease in the release of luteinizing hormone from the anterior pituitary. The older adult who already believes that his or her sexual functioning is compromised may enter a vicious cycle by drinking to avoid the anxiety of decreased sexual performance, yet enhancing the disability through alcohol intake.

The Physical Consequences of Alcoholism in Later Life

When evaluating alcohol intake over time, the clinician must attend to the interaction between alcohol use and chronic or periodic illness in the elderly. Although alcohol directly affects organ systems—alcohol increases cardiac rate and output secondary to its effect on cardiac muscle—the primary impact is cumulative. To illustrate this cumulative impact, consider the example of a person with chronic alcoholism who develops compromised hepatic functioning. This compromise in liver function may exacerbate osteomalacia secondary to decreased hepatic metabolism of vitamin D_3 to its more active 25-hydroxylated form.

Undernutrition that results from chronic alcohol intake, especially among those who use large amounts of alcohol over long periods (the "skid-row alcoholics"), commonly leads to cirrhosis. Cirrhosis is one of the eight leading causes of death among persons 65 years of age and older. Alcohol can damage the heart, resulting in alcohol-induced cardiomyopathies. In contrast, some investigators have reported an actual reduction in coronary artery disease in subjects who drink moderate quantities of alcohol over time (Yano et al. 1977). This does not mean, however, that older persons should be advised to drink alcohol to prevent coronary heart disease.

Chronic effects of alcohol intake on the gastrointestinal tract are well known to clinicians who work with older adults. In general, persons with chronic alcoholism have a lower gastric basal acid output, a maximal acid output, and an increased likelihood of developing chronic atrophic gastritis. The preexisting atrophic gastritis that is common in elderly alcoholic individuals may facilitate the formation of gastric mucosal lesions, which lead to upper gastrointestinal bleeding. Absorption of both folic acid and vitamin B_{12} declines with chronic alcohol use. Because these substances are essential to cognitive functioning, their loss through malabsorption or through decreased dietary intake among elderly alcoholic persons may lead to cognitive and psychological impairment as well as the resultant anemias. Peripheral neuropathy may occur in as many as 45% of chronic alcoholic patients due to deficiency of thiamine and other B-complex vitamins.

Nutritional requirements do not change dramatically with aging, although older persons may require more protein (Gersovitz et al. 1982). Chronic alcoholism is associated with a reduced intake of a number of nutrients, including protein. Protein malnutrition is manifested in individuals with alcoholism as muscle wasting, hypoproteinemia, and edema. Iron deficiency also occurs, but this is generally due to gastrointestinal blood loss rather than to decreased dietary intake or malabsorption. As noted above, older adults may be more subject to gastric lesions, which in turn may lead to chronic occult bleeding.

A concern equally as important as the medical consequences of late-life alcohol use is the interaction of aging, alcohol, and dementia. Many investigators report chronic alcoholism to be associated with a variety of neuropsychological and cognitive deficits. Although chronic alcoholism does not appear to disrupt cognitive and neuropsychological functioning diffusely, specific clusters of cognitive functions are affected in the older alcoholic individual. Most investigators agree that intelligence remains relatively unaffected, but deficits are known to occur in memory and information processing. These deficits are similar to the impairment seen in patients suffering from alcoholic amnestic dementia (Wernicke-Korsakoff's disease). Specifically, deficits most frequently found in alcoholic individuals are impaired performance in tasks involving visual-spatial analysis, tactual spatial analysis, nonverbal ab-

straction, and set flexibility. Although recovery of many of these functions may occur with abstinence from alcohol, recovery rarely leads to complete remission of symptoms.

Alcohol produces a range of impairment, from the subtle cognitive difficulties that can affect nonalcoholic heavy drinkers, to progressively greater impairment in older adults who drink heavily over short periods of time, to the "worst case scenario" of alcoholic amnestic dementia seen in those with long-term alcoholism. This chronic end-stage dementia is caused by thiamine deficiency as well as by the direct toxic effects of alcohol on brain tissue. Postmortem examination of the brains of persons with alcoholic amnestic dementia demonstrates widespread neuronal loss, especially in the frontal regions. Alcoholic patients also experience more rapid rates of cerebral atrophy and degeneration of the mammillary bodies. Clinically, the end stage of alcoholic dementia is characterized by relatively intact intellectual functioning associated with severe anterograde and retrograde amnesia. In contrast to patients with Alzheimer's disease, those with alcoholic dementia who abstain may exhibit stable or even improved short-term memory and motor performance over time.

To appreciate the scope of alcohol problems in the elderly, the risk of death from alcohol use should be explored. In the 8-year outcome study described by Helzer et al. (1984), 24% of the 234 alcoholic subjects who were age 60 or older at enrollment died before the study was completed, compared with 9% of the 1,048 subjects under the age of 60. The proportion of subjects reported to have died of alcohol-related causes was similar for younger and older alcoholic individuals. Although data from death certificates lead to an underestimation of the overall number of deaths due to alcohol, that bias is consistent across age groups.

Nashold and Naor (1981) observed that reports of alcohol as the cause of death in Wisconsin increased markedly between 1963 and 1977. In the older age group, the majority of alcohol-related deaths were due to an underlying cause involving alcohol—for example, cirrhosis. In another study, Edwards and colleagues (1983) followed for 10 years 99 married men diagnosed as having alcoholism. The increase in risk over the expected deaths in this group was 2.68; 5 patients died by suicide or circumstances suggesting suicide. Alcohol leads to an increased risk of mortality in middle life—thus limiting the number of alcoholic persons who survive to late life—but it is also associated with increasing mortality in late life. The causes of death among these individuals who drink chronically are varied and include suicide, accidents, cardiovascular and liver disease, and even cancer.

There are a number of parallels between the sleep characteristics observed in normal aging and those on the chronic alcoholic individual who is abstinent. For example, the sleep of chronic alcoholic patients who have withdrawn from alcohol is characterized by decreased slow-wave sleep, interruptions of sleep, and decreased or interrupted periods of rapid eye movement (REM) sleep (Adamson and Burdick 1973). Prolonged abstinence from alcohol in middle life, however, will lead to improved sleep over time. In other words, the central nervous system (CNS) abnormalities produced by alcohol apparently reverse. The older person who uses alcohol as a sedative experiences an additional sleep problem. The relatively rapid metabolism of alcohol, in contrast to most sedative-hypnotics, may produce a rebound awakening at a point 3–4 hours into sleep. Even though the older adult using alcohol may fall asleep without difficulty, his or her sleep is disrupted during the night.

Given the relatively large number of prescription and nonprescription drugs used by older adults, the interaction of alcohol with these drugs is of special importance to the elderly. The impairments produced by alcohol are augmented by drugs such as sedatives, anticonvulsants, antidepressants, major and minor tranquilizers, and analgesics (especially the opiates). Poor muscle coordination, impaired judgment, and slurred speech are common when these agents are used together. Other side effects are less frequent but can be equally serious. Older adults using oral hypoglycemic agents to treat adult-onset (type II) diabetes may experience unpleasant symptoms such as nausea and flushing, as do patients who combine disulfiram and alcohol use. Unpredictable fluctuations of plasma glucose concentrations are another potential adverse effect. The efficacy of some drugs, such as coumarin-type anticoagulants, is blocked by alcohol, because alcohol increases the metabolism of these drugs (Ritchie 1981). In contrast, plasma concentrations of alcohol are usually not changed by the use of other medications (Garver 1984).

Addiction, Tolerance, and Withdrawal

The most significant clinical problem faced by the clinician treating the older alcoholic individual is the potential for addiction and tolerance to the agent, with the concomitant problem of alcohol withdrawal. Since alcohol is the only readily available addictive agent in Western society, it is usually the drug of choice for individuals who wish to block unpleasant emotions with drugs.

Chronic use of high concentrations of alcohol will lead to addiction. Jaffe (1980) suggested that addiction can be defined operationally as "a behavioral pattern of drug use, characterized by overwhelming involvement with the use of a drug (compulsive use), the securing of its supply, and a high tendency to relapse after withdrawal" (p. 536). Older adults manifest their addiction when placed in a situation in which alcohol is not readily available. They may demonstrate increased anxiety and may pursue alcohol in order to decrease this anxiety. In addition, they experience sleep disturbance, nausea, and weakness, which are concomitants of a lowered blood-alcohol level. Addiction is unique as a problem for older adults for at least two reasons. First, patterns of drinking have continued for many years (often dating from early or middle life), and lifelong habits are often not associated with problems of recent onset. In addition, the relatively "quiet" use of alcohol over the years desensitizes both the older adult and the family to the problems with alcohol (Pascarelli 1974; Schuckit 1977).

Akin to addiction is the potential for tolerance with chronic use of alcohol. Not only can older adults become tolerant to alcohol, but they may also become cross-tolerant to drugs similar to alcohol. Despite the potential for relatively normal function among alcoholic individuals (even when ethanol blood levels are relatively high), the heavy use of alcohol associated with tolerance continues to create irreversible changes in the liver, the gastrointestinal tract, and the CNS (Bosmann 1984). Cross-tolerance, especially with benzodiazepines, is of major clinical concern. Given that older adults are more likely to take benzodiazepines than are younger persons, the potential for abuse of both agents—separately or in combination— increases dramatically (Mellinger et al. 1978).

Symptoms following alcohol withdrawal are not appreciably different across the life cycle. Nevertheless, the older adult may manifest these symptoms, especially the more severe ones, for a longer period after acute cessation of alcohol intake. Initial symptoms include tremors, anxiety, nausea, vomiting, and perspiration. If the withdrawal syndrome is allowed to continue without intervention with either a cross-tolerant drug (such as diazepam) or reinstitution of alcohol, the tremulous state will peak within 1–2 days after the onset of the withdrawal syndrome. This tremulous peak is accompanied by hallucinations and, in severe cases, withdrawal seizures. Confusion, agitation, and disorientation mark the individual's level of consciousness. In the older adult with compromised health, the severity of this withdrawal syndrome is naturally greater (Bosmann 1984; Mello and Mendelson 1977).

Diagnostic Workup

The diagnostic workup of the older adult in whom an alcohol problem is suspected hinges on a comprehensive history. Detailed information should first be obtained from the patient regarding specifics of the drinking behavior. This information must be supplemented by family members, preferably ones from two generations. Unfortunately, some alcoholic older adults have virtually no family or other social network (the "skid-row alcoholic"), and historical information is therefore limited.

Questions that should be asked include the following: Does the elder drink, and how often does he or she drink? Does the elder drink constantly? Is there a pattern of binge drinking? Elders who suffer from chronic problems with alcohol are usually regular drinkers. Tolerance for binges decreases with age. A lifetime history of alcohol use provides a background for present patterns of use.

The "CAGE" questions are commonly used for screening for alcohol problems:

[C]. " . . . felt the need to cut down on your drinking?"
[A]. " . . . ever felt annoyed by criticism of your drinking?"
[G]. " . . . had guilty feelings about drinking?"
[E]. " . . . ever take a morning 'eye-opener' ?"

The CAGE questions are not as useful in screening older persons as they are in helping to identify alcohol problems among the younger population. Because, given a persistent drinking pattern over time, older alcoholic individuals tend to have problems with emergent physical and psychological symptoms, personal guilt or concern about drinking is less common. In fact, the older adult may not recognize the connection between new symptoms and drinking habits that have continued for decades.

Additional data to identify drinking problems in the elderly should be derived from the following categories: personal health, family health problems, interpersonal difficulties, and work difficulties (Ewing 1985). Patients should be asked about gastrointestinal symptoms such as nausea, vomiting, diarrhea, abdominal pain, and unexplained gastrointestinal hemorrhages. Neurological problems should be reviewed, including episodes of amnesia, headaches, and peripheral neuropathy. Falls, lack of attention to personal health, bruises, cuts, sprains, cigarette burns, or skin diseases often result from excessive alcohol use.

A thorough review of psychiatric symptoms is essential, including a detailed evaluation of cognitive status, history of major depression, symptoms of generalized anxiety, and psychotic symptoms (delusions and hallucinations). Paranoid ideation regarding relatives or friends is not uncommon in the older person who is severely alcoholic. It is critical to document suicidal ideation, given the elevated risk for suicide in both elderly and alcoholic populations.

A genetic predisposition to alcohol problems is less likely to be a contributing etiological factor in the elderly alcoholic patient—especially if the onset of significant drinking problems occurs later in life. Moreover, a history of alcohol abuse in the family of the older adult is also prone to bias, because complete historical information from alcoholic elderly patients regarding parents and siblings is usually difficult or impossible to obtain. A documented family history of psychiatric disorder (especially major depression and schizophrenia) or alcohol abuse/dependence is important nonetheless, and the clinician should search medical records in addition to interviewing the elderly alcoholic patient.

An indicant of emerging alcohol problems among older persons is concomitant problems in interpersonal relations. Although such problems occur most often in the marriage, they can also occur between the older adult and children or, occasionally, friends. Family problems may be the result of the drinking behavior (such as arguments over an appropriate amount to drink) or may result from symptoms of the alcohol abuse (such as paranoid ideation or cognitive difficulties).

During the physical examination of the older adult with alcoholism, the clinician should screen for medical problems that may exacerbate alcohol problems—or that may be exacerbated by chronic alcohol use—as well as for evidence of alcohol abuse, such as signs of personal neglect of hygiene. The neurological examination should be performed in detail, with attention directed to the evaluation of peripheral neuropathy. Traditional signs of chronic alcohol abuse, such as flushing of the face, injected conjunctiva, tremors, and malnutrition, may merge with normal signs of aging or poor health status.

If evidence of cognitive abnormalities emerges during the mental status examination (and it often does), further cognitive workup is indicated. The clinician should make every effort to keep the alcoholic older adult abstinent for 2–3 weeks before a detailed cognitive evaluation. Psychological tests may be threatening to the older adult who fears that deficits will appear that have been previously undetected. Baseline cognitive scores, however, can be especially important in monitoring the longitudinal progress of the patient, as well as in providing additional force to the clinical admonition to abstain from further alcohol use. For example, Parker et al. (1982) found that alcohol use above usual consumption significantly increases problems with abstraction in formal testing.

Laboratory evaluation of the acutely alcoholic older adult should include thorough liver function evaluation—lactate dehydrogenase (LDH), serum glutamic-oxaloacetic transaminase (SGOT), serum glutamic-pyruvic transaminase (SGPT), and alkaline phosphatase. Given the potential for an electrolyte imbalance in this population, a screening chemistry is essential, with special attention to glucose. Low blood magnesium reflects a magnesium deficiency that may occur with alcohol use. Elevated serum and urine amylase suggests chronic pancreatitis. Alcoholic cardiomyopathy may be manifested on an electrocardiogram as frequent arrhythmias, especially atrial fibrillation.

Once the history, physical examination, and laboratory tests have been completed, the clinician

should assign a diagnosis. Schuckit et al. (1985) have reviewed the clinical implications of the diagnoses of alcohol abuse and dependence on the basis of DSM-III (American Psychiatric Association 1980). Ideally, a diagnostic system should provide etiological information, prognostic information, and information regarding response to treatment. Because etiological information is difficult to integrate into a diagnostic system—as is evidenced by the move away from etiology in DSM-III that was continued in DSM-III-R (American Psychiatric Association 1987)—more emphasis has been placed on prognosis. When Schuckit and co-workers reviewed the clinical significance of the DSM-III distinction between men who were diagnosed as suffering from either alcohol abuse or alcohol dependence, they found that the two groups were virtually identical. Subjects with alcohol dependence, however, took more drinks per drinking day and had more alcohol-related medical problems and past hospitalizations than those diagnosed as abusers. During the 1-year follow-up, those diagnosed as suffering from alcohol dependence were somewhat more likely to visit a public detoxification facility. Nevertheless, the authors did not support prognostic implications for the differentiation between alcohol abuse and alcohol dependence in alcoholic patients. These data should be considered within the context of the more dependent patterns of alcohol intake that emerge in late life.

Schuckit et al. (1985) also proposed that the criteria for alcohol dependence be changed to include more than just the accumulation of symptoms gathered retrospectively over the lifetime of the alcoholic person's drinking behavior. Specifically, they suggested that more objective criteria be established for tolerance and withdrawal. Schuckit and colleagues' definition of tolerance requires a history of being able to function despite relatively high alcohol concentration—for example, walking or talking coherently in the presence of high blood-alcohol levels. Their criteria for withdrawal are a hampered ability to work or to interact with peers, or the necessity of medical intervention. In summary, the clinician should adapt the symptom presentations of alcohol abuse/dependence in the elderly from DSM-III-R in order to make these criteria more relevant to clinical management. Documentation of these symptoms and signs, however, is critical regardless of the nomenclature used.

Treatment

The treatment of the older patient with alcohol abuse/dependence must include biological, psychological, and psychotherapeutic interventions within the patient's social milieu, especially the family. If the older adult suffers from acute intoxication that leads to a stuporous or comatose state, acute hospitalization must be instituted for withdrawal from alcohol and for institution of the therapeutic program (initially, pharmacological therapy). In milder cases of alcohol dependence, in which withdrawal is the first step, treatment may proceed in the outpatient setting. Outpatient withdrawal is possible only if the patient is highly motivated and is willing to allow open monitoring of the withdrawal program by the family, with frequent (often daily) contact with the clinician. Regardless, the initial step in the treatment of alcoholism is to stop alcohol intake. Attempts to work over longer periods of time with the alcoholic individual who continues to drink are doomed to failure.

In the treatment of the older patient who is severely alcoholic, restoration of fluid and electrolyte balance during the initial phase of withdrawal is essential. Complaints of thirst and dry mucous membranes may delude the clinician into accepting a diagnosis of dehydration when, in fact, drying results from alcohol expiration through the lungs. To avoid iatrogenic overhydration, the clinician should begin administration of 500–1,000 mL of a 5% normal saline solution while waiting for the results of the blood chemistry screen. Use of glucose solutions should be avoided; the older alcoholic patient may have subsisted on a diet high in carbohydrates, in addition to alcohol, which is metabolized almost entirely as a carbohydrate, and glucose solutions can lead to an iatrogenic increase in blood glucose to diabetic levels. Because of poor dietary nutritional intake, fluids should be supplemented with parenteral B vitamins. Individuals with chronic alcoholism, as noted above, may suffer from magnesium deficiency. Adding a deep intramuscular injection of magnesium at a dose of 0.10–0.15 mL/kg to the initial therapeutic regimen is an important adjunct to treatment (Blazer and Siegler 1984).

The next step in treatment is the institution of medications that are cross-tolerant with alcohol. Diazepam has been the drug of choice for managing patients in withdrawal because of its relatively extended half-life and cross-tolerance with alcohol. Initial doses depend on the patient's age, weight, and the amount of alcohol consumed over the week before admission. Even with these data, however, doses must be carefully titrated during the first 24–48 hours of withdrawal. The usual starting dosage is between 5 and 15 mg every 6–12 hours until the delirium, agitation, and/or hallucinations are sufficiently decreased. If therapy proceeds on an outpatient basis, careful monitoring is necessary to ensure that alcohol is not added to the regimen of the benzodiazepine. After the first day, the diazepam dose can usually be decreased at a rate of approximately 20% per day. Other medium- to long-acting benzodiazepines—such as chlorazepate—can be used as well.

When an overt delirium emerges with seizures and hallucinations, diazepam is the anticonvulsant of choice because of its rapid onset of effect. An increase in memory problems, the onset of dysarthria, and the development of ataxia in the elderly patient indicate that drug intoxication has developed secondary to excessive medication or as a result of the synergistic effects of the drug with alcohol. When such intoxication occurs, the drug should be discontinued for 24–36 hours and the patient should be carefully observed for a recurrence of the withdrawal symptoms; the drug can then be reinstituted. If persistent signs and symptoms of withdrawal are seen beyond 3 days after the last known drink, the clinician should suspect dependence on minor tranquilizers or hypnotics as well as alcohol.

Some withdrawal programs in communities encourage withdrawal within a social setting that is based on social support in the absence of drug use (a detoxification center). Although some rehabilitation centers in hospitals may overuse medication, the severe effects of withdrawal, such as delirium tremens, should dissuade the clinician from routinely using alternative withdrawal settings, especially for the older adult.

After detoxification, the long-term goals of treatment become paramount in the treatment process. First, the clinician should consider prophylaxis with disulfiram. If this drug is used, a contract must be established between the patient and the physician plus at least one family member. A family member (or possibly the emergency room of a local hospital) should have the responsibility for administering the daily dose of disulfiram to the elder. The patient, in turn, must agree to take the tablet when offered. Both the patient and family members must be warned of the potential effects if alcohol is ingested while the patient is taking disulfiram. Acetaldehyde increases in the blood when ethanol and disulfiram are present concurrently, and this leads to the "acetaldehyde syndrome"—a flushing of the face, intense throbbing in the head and neck (which may develop into a pulsating headache), difficulty breathing, nausea, vomiting, sweating, thirst, chest pains, hypertension, vertigo, blurred vision, and confusion. These symptoms are outlined on the package insert provided by the manufacturer. There is no evidence that disulfiram is contraindicated in late life. Nevertheless, if health status in the elder is compromised, the clinician must carefully weigh the benefits versus potential problems of prescribing disulfiram.

Therapeutic intervention with the family is essential. First, family members should be warned of the severe and potentially irreversible problems that alcohol can cause in the older adult, especially memory problems. Most families are more concerned with the immediate effects of intoxication. If the older family member drinks silently without overt signs of intoxication, this behavior may be tolerated. The threshold for concern in the family must therefore be lowered through the process of education. Patient, family, and clinician become a team as they seek to correct the problem.

Self-help groups are essential to the long-term support of the abstinent alcoholic person. The Alcoholics Anonymous (AA) program has proved over many years to be effective in encouraging abstinence for individuals throughout the life cycle. Support groups provide social support coupled with appropriate pressure from peers who have experienced similar problems. AA is complementary to the authority of the clinician and must not be considered a threat to medical authority. AA meetings may be especially beneficial to the older alcoholic individual who is discouraged and lonely secondary to isolation and feelings of uselessness. Involvement in the group setting, coupled with a sense of helping others and interaction with younger persons, may reintegrate the sober elder into society.

Many older persons resist the suggestion to join a self-help group, however. One reason is that elders continue to deny that they have a problem or believe themselves perfectly capable of correcting the prob-lem alone. The self-sufficient attitude of the current elderly cohort is one reason that such beliefs are so persistent in the elderly. More commonly, the older adult feels no "fit" with the environment of such self-help groups. The cohort of elderly alcoholic persons in the latter part of the 20th century have not experienced recovery groups and the self-help phenomena, unlike those who will reach old age in the early years of the 21st century. Given their frequent success, participation in self-help groups should be encouraged, but clinicians should not force the older adult to participate.

Support from family members and the clinician, as well as integration into more traditional social environments, may accomplish the same purpose as self-help and support groups (Butler and Lewis 1977). In mobilizing coping resources, the social environment (acute and chronic stressors, social network resources), the health care system (availability of health care services such as medical intervention, behavioral therapy, and educational programs), and coping strategies of the older patient can be woven into a unique matrix for a given elder. Such an integrated approach not only enables a more comprehensive evaluation of the diagnostic profile but also provides a framework from which successful treatment can be implemented. Intervention should target for change specific points within the system, but the strategy should also reflect the clinician's continuing recognition that the entire system is interdependent.

Drug Abuse

Drug abuse is usually associated with adolescents and young adults. Certainly the abuse of illicit drugs is uncommon in older adults. Nevertheless, the fact that drug abuse occurs among persons in later life must not be overlooked. The propensity of older adults to use prescription drugs inappropriately renders late life a period of high risk for the side effects of this misuse. Glantz (1981) suggested that the motivation for elderly persons to abuse drugs may be similar to the motivation for adolescents. Both must negotiate a period of uncertain and changing roles, as well as changes in self-concept. Older persons face step-downs on the economic ladder and disadvantages in the employment market. Friends and relatives may not be as available because of distance, or may be removed by death.

Although self-sufficiency continues to be a means of coping (adolescents and the elderly both strive for control), the ability of the impaired older adult to maintain self-reliance and independence is compromised. Drugs are easily available to both groups. The adolescent seeks illegal drugs on the street; the older adult obtains addictive drugs from local physicians. For example, Capel et al. (1972) discovered that the majority of drug-addicted persons who survive to late life continue their drug use via concealed habits, using substitute narcotics such as hydromorphone hydrochloride. Alcohol and barbiturates may be added to enhance the effects of this narcotic.

Even the progress from milder to more powerful drugs, frequently seen in the movement to addiction among adolescents, may have parallels among the elderly (Glantz 1981). Older persons begin taking mild analgesics and sedative-hypnotic agents but fail to obtain the relief they desire. Without realizing the danger of addiction, they progress to the use of narcotic analgesics for chronic pain problems and higher doses of tranquilizing and sedative-hypnotic agents. Once addiction and tolerance are established, older adults exhibit little initiative to reverse the problem. By obtaining medications from multiple physicians and borrowing medicines from family members, they feed their habit over time. Frequently, hospitalization uncovers the addiction, because withdrawal symptoms appear 3–4 days after admission.

Problems deriving from excessive and inappropriate prescription and over-the-counter drug use are well documented in the geriatric literature. Law and Chalmers (1976) estimated that 85% of older persons living in the community and 95% of those residing in long-term care facilities receive prescription drugs. In 1976, more than 12 prescriptions were written per person each year for those 65 years of age and older (Lamy and Vestal 1976). Undoubtedly, such estimates would be even higher today.

The Scope of the Problem

The frequency of excessive drug use in the elderly, especially the use of psychoactive drugs, is well-documented. From a household survey of more than 2,000 people, Mellinger et al. (1978) reported that among those persons over 60 years of age, 20% of women and 17% of men regularly used psychoactive drugs during the year preceding the survey, figures that were higher than those from any other age group. In the 60+ age group, 11% of the men and 25% of the women had used a minor tranquilizer and/or sedative at least once during the year preceding the survey—again, a rate higher than that for any other age group. These rates may be declining in community samples, since rates of antianxiety and sedative-hypnotic use have decreased in recent years (Hanlon et al. 1992). Heightened public awareness of problems secondary to benzodiazepines has probably contributed to this decline.

A report from the National Medical Care Expenditure Survey (Rossiter 1983) documented that persons 65 years of age and older were more likely to have used pain relievers (25.9%) prescribed by a physician during the past year. Except for cardiovascular medications, analgesic and psychotherapeutic agents were the drugs used the most by older adults. In a review of nursing home prescribing habits, Ray et al. (1980) found that in 173 Tennessee nursing homes, 43% of the patients had received antipsychotic medications during the year preceding the survey, and 9% were chronic recipients—that is, they received at least one dose for 365 days during the preceding year.

Christopher et al. (1978), reporting on 873 hospitalized persons in Dundee, Scotland, concluded that prescribing in this inpatient population was not excessive, with an average of three medications being received at any given time. Patients on the geriatric ward were receiving the highest number of drugs. However, certain drug groups, especially the sedative-hypnotics, were prescribed excessively, with few attempts made to reduce the dose with increasing age. The prevalence of hypnotic use ranged from more than 40% among the medical patients to more than 70% on the geriatric wards. In a survey involving 195 hospitalized persons over age 60, Salzman and van der Kolk (1980) found that one-third had received at least one psychotropic drug the day of the survey. Hypnotics were the most frequently prescribed drugs, with flurazepam being the drug of choice. The authors noted that each of the psychoactive drugs prescribed had potentially dangerous side effects, and dosing of these drugs did not reflect attention paid to the age of patients by the treating clinicians.

In the community, however, the evidence of significant abuse of illicit drugs in the elderly is remarkably absent. The best data available are those derived from the ECA studies. Myers et al. (1984) found no evidence of drug abuse in the 65+ age group at two of the three ECA sites surveyed, and a prevalence of just 0.2% at the third site. More than 3,000 persons age 65 and older were interviewed for this survey. Regarding the lifetime prevalence of drug abuse or dependence, fewer than 0.1% of the subjects at these three ECA sites reported any such history (Robins et al. 1984). These studies are subject to bias, given the subjects' difficulty in recalling information regarding drug abuse and/or their denial of such use. Nevertheless, denial and selective recall are probably no more a problem for the elderly than for persons at any other stage of life. What is more likely to contribute to the relatively low prevalence of current and lifetime drug abuse among the elderly is a cohort effect (older persons in the 1980s were never heavy users of drugs) and selective mortality (persons from the present generation of older adults who used illicit medications did not survive to late life). However, community surveys that rely on household data may underestimate drug abuse, especially by failure to include homeless and transient persons.

Behavioral and Social Correlates of Drug Abuse in Older Adults

Many psychosocial factors contribute to the potential toxicity and addictive potential of both prescription and illicit drugs among the elderly (Blazer 1983). Certain character traits of older adults contribute to increased drug use (Baldessarini 1977). The more passive older adult may use drugs prescribed by a number of physicians without question. Even "double prescribing," the prescription of the same drug by two or more physicians can go unchallenged by the dependent elder. Addiction accrues over time without being noticed by the patient, family, or physician. Only when such a patient is admitted to the hospital for an unrelated disorder do the symptoms of addiction become apparent. Once hospitalized, passive older adults often fail to report the medications they were taking before hospitalization, expecting the physician to "know" how to manage their problem. Those patients who appear most compliant could be the most prone to drug abuse in an outpatient medical or psychiatric practice.

In addition to character traits, the social setting surrounding the prescription of medications affects the patient's potential for abusing medications. Many psychosocial factors determine therapeutic drug abuse. Noncompliance, a most important factor in treating psychiatric disorders, usually does not contribute to drug abuse. Rather, older adults are more inclined not to take prescribed medications on schedule than to use prescribed drugs excessively. Blackwell (1973) estimated that up to 50% of patients do not take prescribed medications. The potential for addiction may be actualized, however, if the milieu for prescribing medications discourages communication between the older adult and the physician (Lamy 1980). In the distracting and hurried environment of the physician's office, proper use of a medication frequently is not communicated to older adults. Because older persons are hesitant to ask questions, they leave the office without understanding how a drug is to be used. To please the physician, they take the medication, but not at the dose required. The tendency for older persons to carry all of their medications in one container increases the potential for confusion regarding when a particular drug should be taken. Intoxication from excessive use of the benzodiazepines is not uncommon under these circumstances.

The practice of sharing and swapping medications among older adults is not infrequent as a precipitant of abuse or dependence. Friends, roommates, or spouses are treated by different physicians for similar problems. Through informal communication with one another regarding the effectiveness of individual drug therapies, the elder may mistakenly determine that a friend's physician has prescribed a better treatment than his or her own clinician. Because limited finances preclude obtaining a second opinion (or even an initial consultation), medications are informally shared. Through the additive effects of drugs, such as the sedative-hypnotics, evidence of addiction or abuse appears, often unexplained to the primary care physician. The diagnosis of the problem is further complicated because older adults are hesitant to reveal that they have obtained medications from another source.

Another contributor to problems of abuse is over-the-counter drug use. In Western societies, over-the-counter drugs are used even more often than prescription drugs. Chaiton et al. (1976) estimated that more than 50% of elders surveyed had used at least one over-the-counter drug during the 48 hours preceding the community survey. Most of these elders had not consulted a physician regarding the use of the drug or its potential interaction with prescription drugs. The most commonly used of the over-the-counter drugs are agents to improve sleep, to improve gastrointestinal symptoms such as constipation, and to relieve pain. The combination of nonprescription drugs with anticholinergic effects (such as diphenhydramine) with prescribed antidepressants and/or phenothiazines can lead to anticholinergic toxicity or even a full-blown central anticholinergic syndrome.

"Do-something" prescribing is an iatrogenic contributor to drug abuse in the elderly. If the older adult pays for a doctor's consultation, he or she expects a result—the result usually being a prescription. Physicians also gain some assurance that they have upheld their part of the patient-physician contract when they write a prescription. Drugs prescribed under these circumstances are often not prescribed to treat specific target symptoms. Benzodiazepines, sedative-hypnotic agents, tricyclic antidepressants, and even neuroleptics become the drugs of choice because of the mistaken view that the drugs promote the general well-being of the patient. Not only do such prescribing practices reinforce a pattern of medical care that discourages the physician from talking with the older adult, they also increase the likelihood of polypharmacy.

A variation on the theme of do-something prescribing that may contribute to drug addiction and/or abuse in the elderly is defensive prescribing. Those physicians who serve as medical directors of nursing homes or who have large consulting practices in long-term care facilities are frequently called by nursing staff and even family members about patients' disturbing and uncontrollable physical or behavioral symptoms. Agitation and sleep problems are among those most commonly encountered by a stressed nursing staff. Against his or her better judgment, a physician may prescribe medications, not so much to alleviate a specific symptom in an older adult as to reassure staff and family members. Defensive prescribing is not an indictment of the lack of care by a physician, nursing staff, or family. Rather, it is a symptom of a difficult situation—the management of an acutely agitated and cognitively impaired older adult in a facility with limited personnel. Nevertheless, such prescribing practices must be recognized as major contributors to addiction and abuse in older adults.

Diagnostic Workup

The diagnostic workup of the older adult in whom a diagnosis of drug abuse or dependence is suspected is similar to that described for the workup of suspected alcohol abuse and dependence. Many of the symptoms described earlier apply to prescription and nonprescription drug abuse as well. Although older adults may be seen after taking an overdose of a sedative, narcotic, or other agent, the most common presentations of drug misuse/abuse are symptoms of toxicity and/or withdrawal.

The benzodiazepines (both anxiolytic and sedative-hypnotics) are the most commonly prescribed drugs and are, therefore, the most likely to be abused. Symptoms characteristic of benzodiazepine toxicity include sedation, confusional states, "sundowning" (heightened agitation or frank delirium at night), ataxia, and even stupor or coma. The potential for a fatal overdose is low with these agents alone, but when benzodiazepines are combined with other agents, such as alcohol, this potential increases dramatically. Withdrawal symptoms, in contrast, may mimic the psychiatric disorder for which the drugs were originally prescribed. Anxiety and agitation, sleep problems, muscle cramps (especially in the legs), tremors, and perceptual distortions may emerge upon withdrawal. The most serious withdrawal symptom, however, is the onset of seizures.

Tricyclic antidepressants are frequently prescribed and may contribute to increased problems with memory, confusion, and sedation. Confusion and even fugue states are described in the morning after an excessive nighttime dose of tricyclic antidepressants; these symptoms are frequently accompanied by postural hypotension and excessive lethargy. In a patient with bipolar disorder, successful use of an antidepressant to reverse depressive symptoms may later trigger an elevation in mood and an increase in activity. Even a frank manic episode with delusions and hallucinations can be precipitated by these drugs.

Lithium carbonate, a most effective drug in the treatment of manic-depressive illness, can be especially problematic for older adults. Symptoms including dizziness, ataxia, drowsiness, and confusion may occur when serum levels are below 1.0 mEq/L. Older persons do not tolerate lithium therapy as well as persons in middle life, and therefore the drug must be prescribed with extreme caution. Self-abuse with lithium is uncommon, but the desire of the clinician to obtain therapeutic effect in a patient who suffers from rapid-cycling bipolar disorder or unipolar recurrent depression augments the potential for lithium toxicity.

When these or other symptoms emerge, a thorough history from the patient and family (similar to that described above for alcohol problems) is the next clinical step of importance. If the clinician questions the history provided by the patient, many laboratories provide a drug toxicity screen. Most of these laboratories can return results to the clinician within 6 hours. Specimens can be obtained from either urine or blood. Toxicity screens must be interpreted cautiously, for drugs are often cross-reactive to the probes used in the screen. Other ancillary laboratory procedures, such as electrophysiological tracing, cardiac monitoring, and radiologic examination (for problems deriving from drug use), can be obtained as well, but are usually not required.

Treatment of Drug Abuse/Dependence in Older Adults

Treatment approaches for drug abuse/dependence in the older adult are similar to those used for patients at other stages of the life cycle. Given that the older adult is frail, however, the clinician must be careful to err on the side of being conservative. Specifically, early hospitalization is indicated when evidence of abuse is present. For example, the older adult who chronically takes benzodiazepines and is found to be excessively lethargic should be hospitalized, despite the clinician's recognition of the cause of the problem and the family's insistence that the problem can be managed at home.

The immediate goal upon hospitalization is to remove the potential for acute toxicity from the medication. If drug ingestion is recent, gastric evacuation is indicated. In the elderly, however, special care must be taken to avoid aspiration. Activated charcoal (30 g) has been recommended along with the lavage to absorb barbiturates, alcohol, and propoxyphene (Ellinwood et al. 1985). Once the clinician is convinced that the potential for acute toxicity has been removed, the patient should be transferred to a ward where close monitoring is possible. Electrocardiographic monitoring is often indicated for the first 24–48 hours. Monitoring of respiration, however, is of most importance, especially if the patient shows evidence of slow, rapid, or shallow breathing. When improvement does not ensue, peritoneal dialysis or hemodialysis may be indicated.

Once the patient has survived the immediate problems of overdose, the next challenge presented to the clinician is to manage withdrawal symptoms. Depending on the half-life of the drug, withdrawal may last from 6 hours to 8–10 days (the half-life of flurazepam, for example, may exceed 200 hours in an older adult). Support with the medication or a substitute drug is indicated during this period. At the same time, the clinician must begin educating the patient and family regarding the cause of the hospitalization and the need to change the outpatient drug therapy significantly in order to prevent the recurrence of such a problem. With most elders, education and intervention during the course of an acute hospitalization for drug problems are effective. Older adults are often unaware of the potential problems of drug use and, when informed, are most happy to be free of the potential of future addiction or toxic reactions secondary to a medication.

In some cases, however, the older adult will continue to seek medications, especially analgesics and benzodiazepine-like compounds. In these cases, careful outpatient monitoring and work with the family provide the best means for successfully achieving a long-term abstinence from potentially abusable drugs. Because elders tend to use the same pharmacy despite having multiple physicians, contact with the pharmacist can be especially helpful in monitoring drug use.

References

Adamson J, Burdick JA: Sleep of dry alcoholics. Arch Gen Psychiatry 28:146–149, 1973

American Psychiatric Association: Diagnostic and Statistical Manual of Mental Disorders, 3rd Edition. Washington, DC, American Psychiatric Association, 1980

American Psychiatric Association: Diagnostic and Statistical Manual of Mental Disorders, 3rd Edition, Revised. Washington, DC, American Psychiatric Association, 1987

Armor D, Johnston D, Pollich S, et al: Trends in U.S. Adult Drinking Practices. Santa Monica, CA, Rand Corporation, 1977

Baldessarini RJ: Chemotherapy in Psychiatry. Cambridge, MA, Harvard University Press, 1977

Blackwell B: Drug therapy: patient compliance. N Engl J Med 289:249–252, 1973

Blazer D: Drug management in the elderly, in Experimental and Clinical Interventions in Aging. Edited by Walker RF, Cooper RL. New York, Marcel Dekker, 1983, pp 343–354

Blazer D, Siegler IC: A Family Approach to Health Care in the Elderly. Menlo Park, CA, Addison-Wesley, 1984

Blum C, Rosner F: Alcoholism in the elderly: an analysis of 50 patients. J Natl Med Assoc 75:489–495, 1983

Bosmann HB: Pharmacology of alcoholism in aging, in Alcoholism in the Elderly. Edited by Hartford JT, Samorajski T. New York, Raven, 1984, pp 161–174

Butler RN, Lewis MI: Aging and Mental Health: Positive Psychosocial Approaches, 2nd Edition. St. Louis, MO, CV Mosby, 1977

Capel WC, Goldsmith BM, Waddell KJ, et al: The aging narcotic addict: an increasing problem for the next decades. J Gerontol 27:102–106, 1972

Chaiton A, Spitzer WO, Roberts RS, et al: Patterns of medical drug use—a community focus. Can Med Assoc J 114:33–37, 1976

Chowdhury AR, Malmud LS, Dinoso VP: Gastrointestinal plasma protein loss during ethanol ingestion. Gastroenterology 72:37–40, 1977

Christopher LJ, Ballinger BR, Shepherd AMM, et al: Drug-prescribing patterns in the elderly: a cross-sectional study of in-patients. Age Ageing 7:74–82, 1978

Edwards G, Oppenheimer E, Duckitt A, et al: What happens to alcoholics? Lancet 2:269–271, 1983

Ellinwood EH, Woody G, Krishnan RR: Treatment for drug abuse (Chapter 90), in Psychiatry, Vol 2. Edited by Michels R, Cavenar JO. Philadelphia, PA, JB Lippincott, 1985, pp 1–12

Ewing JA: Substance abuse: alcohol, in Psychiatry, Vol 2. Edited by Michels R, Cavenar JO. Philadelphia, PA, JB Lippincott, 1985

Faris D: The prevention of alcoholism and economic alcoholism. Prev Med 3:36–48, 1974

Finlaysen RE, Hunt RD, Davis LJ, et al: Alcoholism in elderly persons: a study of the psychiatric and psychosocial features of 216 inpatients. Mayo Clin Proc 63:761–768, 1988

Garver DL: Age effects on alcohol metabolism, in Alcoholism in the Elderly. Edited by Hartford JT, Samorajski T. New York, Raven, 1984, pp 153–160

Gersovitz M, Motio K, Munro HN, et al: Human protein requirements: assessment of the adequacy of the current recommended dietary allowance for dietary protein in elderly men and women. Am J Clin Nutr 35:6–14, 1982

Glantz M: Predictions of elderly drug abuse. J Psychoactive Drugs 13:117–126, 1981

Glatt MM: Experiences with elderly alcoholics in England. Alcoholism 2:23–26, 1978

Glynn RJ, Bouchard GR, Locastro JS, et al: Changes in alcohol consumption behaviors among men in the normative aging study, in Nature and Extent of Alcohol Problems Among the Elderly (Research Monograph No 14). Edited by Maddox G, Robins LN, Rosenberg N. Rockville, MD, National Institute on Alcohol Abuse and Alcoholism, 1984, pp 101–116

Gordon T, Kannel WB: Drinking and its relation to smoking, blood pressure, blood lipids and uric acid: the Framingham study. Arch Intern Med 143:1366–1374, 1983

Hanlon JT, Fillenbaum GG, Burchett B, et al: Drug-use patterns among black and nonblack community-dwelling elderly. Annals of Pharmacology 26:679–685, 1992

Helzer JE, Carey KE, Miller RH: Predictors and correlates of recovery in older versus younger alcoholics, in Nature and Extent of Alcohol Problems Among the Elderly (Research Monograph No 14). Edited by Maddox G, Robins LN, Rosenberg N. Rockville, MD, National Institute on Alcohol Abuse and Alcoholism, 1984, pp 83–100

Jaffe JH: Drug addiction and drug abuse, in The Pharmacological Basis of Therapeutics, 6th Edition. Edited by Gilman AG, Goodman LS, Gilman A. New York, Macmillan, 1980, pp 535–584

Kalant H, Kahnna JM, Israel Y: The alcohols, in Principles of Medical Pharmacology, 3rd Edition. Edited by Seemen P, Sellars V, Roschlau WH. Toronto, Canada, University of Toronto Press, 1980, pp 245–253

Lamy PP: Prescribing for the Elderly. Littleton, MA, PSG Publishing, 1980

Lamy PP, Vestal RE: Drug prescribing for the elderly. Hosp Pract [Off Ed] 11:111–118, 1976

Law R, Chalmers C: Medicines and elderly people: a general practice survey. BMJ 1:565–568, 1976

Maddox GL, Blazer DG: Alcohol and aging. Center Reports on Advances in Research (Duke University Center for the Study of Aging and Human Development) 8:1–6, 1985

Mellinger GD, Balter MB, Manheimer DI, et al: Psychic distress, life crisis, and use of psychotherapeutic medications: national household survey data. Arch Gen Psychiatry 35:1045–1052, 1978

Mello NK, Mendelson JH: Clinical aspects of alcohol dependence, in Drug Addiction, I: Morphine, Sedative/Hypnotic and Alcohol Dependence. Edited by Martin WR. Berlin, Springer-Verlag, 1977, pp 613–666

Mellstrom D: Previous alcohol consumption and its consequences for aging, morbidity and mortality in men aged 70–75. Age Ageing 10:277–283, 1981

Muehlberger CW: The physiologic action of alcohol. JAMA 167:1840–1845, 1958

Myers JK, Weissman MM, Tischler GL, et al: Six-month prevalence of psychiatric disorders in three communities: 1980 to 1982. Arch Gen Psychiatry 41:959–967, 1984

Nashold RD, Naor EM: Alcohol-related deaths in Wisconsin: the impact of alcohol mortality. Am J Public Health 71:1237–1271, 1981

Parker ES, Parker DA, Brodie JA, et al: Cognitive patterns resembling premature aging in male social drinkers. Alcoholism 6:46–52, 1982

Pascarelli EF: Drug dependence: an age-old problem compounded by old age. Geriatrics 29:109–110, 1974

Rathbone-McCuan E, Lohn H, Levenson J, et al: Community Survey of Aged Alcoholics and Problem Drinkers. DHEW Grant #1R18 AAD 1734-01, Final Project Report to DHEW by Levindale Geriatric Research Center, June 1976

Ray WA, Federspiel CF, Schaffner W: A study of antipsychotic drug use in nursing homes: epidemiologic evidence suggesting misuse. Am J Public Health 70:485–491, 1980

Ritchie JN: The aliphatic alcoholics, in The Pharmacologic Basis of Therapeutics, 6th Edition. Edited by Gilman AG, Goodman LS, Gilman A. New York, Macmillan, 1981, pp 376–390

Robins LN, Helzer JE, Weissman MM, et al: Lifetime prevalence of specific psychiatric disorders in three sites. Arch Gen Psychiatry 41:949–958, 1984

Rossiter LF: Prescribed medicines: findings from the National Medical Care Expenditure Survey. Am J Public Health 73:1312–1315, 1983

Salzman C, van der Kolk B: Psychotropic drug prescriptions for elderly patients in a general hospital. J Am Geriatr Soc 28:18–22, 1980

Schuckit MA: Geriatric alcoholism and drug abuse. Gerontologist 17:168–174, 1977

Schuckit MA, Zisook S, Mortola J: Clinical implications of DSM-III diagnoses of alcohol abuse and alcohol dependence. Am J Psychiatry 142:1403–1408, 1985

Warheit GJ, Auth JB: The mental health and social correlates of alcohol use among differing life cycle groups, in Nature and Extent of Alcohol Problems Among the Elderly (Research Monograph No 14). Edited by Maddox G, Robins LN, Rosenberg N. Rockville, MD, National Institute on Alcohol Abuse and Alcoholism, 1984, pp 29–82

Wiberg GS, Samson JM, Maxwell WB, et al: Further studies on the acute toxicity of ethanol in young and old rats: relative importance of pulmonary excretion and total body water. Toxicol Appl Pharmacol 20:22–29, 1971

Yano K, Rhoads GG, Kajan A: Coffee, alcohol, and risk of coronary artery disease among Japanese men living in Hawaii. N Engl J Med 297:405–409, 1977

Treatment of Psychiatric Disorders in Late Life

CHAPTER 20

Pharmacological Treatment

Jonathan Davidson, M.D.

The number of aging individuals in the U.S. population continues to grow. In 1950, approximately 8% of the population was over age 65, a figure that is expected to grow to 12% of the population, or 32 million people, by the year 2000. There is a particular increase in the number of individuals over age 80, who are perhaps the most vulnerable group from the standpoint of health problems. Similar trends have occurred in other countries, such as Great Britain, where the number of people between the ages of 65 and 74 increased by one-third between 1950 and 1981, and the number of persons over 75 increased by 40%. Older people are more likely to experience bereavement, which also serves as a risk factor for illness. For example, Mor et al. (1986) found an increased use of antianxiety medication and alcohol and more physician visits after bereavement; bereaved spouses are twice as likely to be hospitalized. An idea of the kinds of illnesses that are commonly seen in older patients can be obtained from the Epidemiologic Catchment Area study (Weissman et al. 1984), which showed the following disorders to be most frequent in men over age 65: severe cognitive impairment, phobic anxiety, alcohol abuse, and dysthymic disorder. Older women most often presented with phobic anxiety, severe cognitive impairment, dysthymic disorder, and major depression without bereavement.

Treatment of psychiatric illness in the elderly is often difficult because of the greater likelihood of concomitant chronic physical illness, such as cardiovascular, cerebrovascular, and degenerative joint diseases, as well as malignant disease. More psychotropic prescriptions are given by primary care physicians than by any other group of health providers for patients over 55 years of age (Larson et al. 1991), and the importance of education remains clear for all medical specialties regarding geriatric psychopharmacology.

General Pharmacological and Physiological Considerations

In using pharmacotherapy, it is important to recognize that physiological changes in the elderly affect the pharmacokinetics and pharmacodynamics of drug activity. Patients often take multiple medications, which can lead to compliance problems, drug-drug interactions, and iatrogenic illness. In an elderly person, it is sometimes unnecessary to look further than the combination of drugs in order to explain the appearance of new symptoms. The physiological changes will often mean that a drug that might be well tolerated in a younger patient will produce a heightened effect at the same dose in an older person. It is usually preferable to initiate treatment at a dose no more than one-half the recommended adult dose, and then build up the dose slowly.

The four main processes involved in drug disposition are absorption, distribution, metabolism, and elimination. Drug absorption can be delayed in older people, as a result of any of the following factors: reduction of gastric and intestinal motility, impaired epithelial transport mechanism, or reduced intestinal blood flow. In addition, there is reduced blood flow to the liver relative to brain and coronary arteries in old age. These considerations may be of more theoretical than actual importance, because drug effects are often enhanced in older persons. Thus, any reduction of absorption can be more than offset by changes in other processes that affect drug disposition.

Many drugs are lipophilic, being taken up for storage in fatty tissue. The fraction of fat to total body weight increases with age from 25% to 45%. As a result, there is a relatively larger volume of distribution available for antidepressant, antipsychotic, and benzodiazepine drugs, all of which are lipophilic. Conversely, a hydrophilic drug like lithium will have a small volume of distribution. Another important change with respect to drug distribution relates to the declining amount of albumin, which is reduced by as much as 25% between the ages of 40 and 60. Many drugs are protein bound, and only a small fraction are transported in the active, or free, state. Even a limited reduction of the protein-bound fraction will increase the free fraction by a substantial amount, thereby effectively raising the amount of active drug.

Drug metabolism usually takes place in the liver; with reduced perfusion, the process of metabolism and inactivation will be delayed and/or reduced. Drugs that are inactivated by glucuronidation are less affected than drugs that are oxidized. Drugs having a higher potential for hepatotoxicity—for example, chlorpromazine and hydrazine monoamine oxidase inhibitors (MAOIs)—should be used more cautiously. As a general rule, it is preferable to choose the drug with the simplest metabolic profile. For example, haloperidol would be preferred over

thioridazine, desipramine over imipramine, and oxazepam over diazepam, all other things being equal. One of the newer selective serotonin reuptake inhibitors (SSRIs), fluoxetine, has a very long half-life and should therefore be used with more caution in elderly people.

Other concomitant medications can affect drug metabolism. Methylphenidate, propranolol, and neuroleptics may all increase the plasma level of tricyclic drugs by competing for the same metabolizing enzymes. Other drugs, such as phenytoin and barbiturates, can induce hepatic enzymes and thereby lower the plasma level of a tricyclic.

Elimination of drugs is related not only to liver function but also to renal function. Renal function and perfusion decline with age, and drugs like lithium, dextroamphetamine, fluvoxamine, and nortriptyline—for all of which renal excretion is a significant pathway—are likely to have a more prolonged effect in the elderly. Plasma levels of antidepressant drugs may be increased in the elderly because of impaired renal excretion (Richey 1975). Drug pharmacodynamics alter with age as a result of decreases in receptor number, neurotransmitter levels, and structural changes in the target organs. Monoamine oxidase, the catecholamine- and indolamine-metabolizing enzyme, increases after age 55, and this might partially account for the lowered concentration of norepinephrine and serotonin in old age.

Treatment of Patients in Psychotic States

Slater and Roth (1972) have described the development of first-onset schizophrenia-like psychosis in late life, sometimes referred to as late paraphrenia—a term that has not been sanctioned in DSM-IV (American Psychiatric Association 1994). Slater and Roth noted F. Post's (1962) belief that "paraphrenia" should be seen as a partial or incomplete form of schizophrenia, and observed that Post did not distinguish the two disorders on the basis of drug responsiveness. However, there appears to be some evidence from human lymphocyte antigen studies that paraphrenia differs genetically and biologically from schizophrenia (Naguib et al. 1987). It may account for 8%–9% of all first hospital admissions among women over 65 years of age. The disorder occurs characteristically in single women, being accompanied by paranoid delusions or hallucinations, but with little or no evidence of dementia. As many as one-third of patients have hearing impairment, and visual impairment is by no means rare; 5% have cerebral disease but lack organic features. The prognosis for survival is better than for the dementias, and the life expectancy is identical to that of the normal population (Kay 1959). In F. Post's study (1962), 27 out of 35 patients responded to adequate doses of phenothiazines for an extended period, but showed a high relapse rate when medication was stopped. If late paraphrenia is not properly treated by pharmacotherapy, the remission rate is as low as 7 out of 23, and the illness can pursue a chronic course. Many patients with late-onset paraphrenic illness have exhibited suspiciousness and a long-standing tendency to isolate themselves from others; therefore it is often important to mobilize all available support systems to ensure compliance with medication and to detect signs of relapse at the earliest opportunity.

Schizophrenia of early onset tends to change its presentation with age: rather than exhibiting the florid positive signs and symptoms of the disorder, the older patient will more often manifest withdrawal.

Mania can occur in the older individual, and it has been estimated that between 6% and 19% of consecutively admitted older patients with affective disorder carry a diagnosis of mania (F. Post 1984). The coexistence of perplexity in the symptom picture may lead to the mistaken impression of an organic state. Treatment of mania in an older person follows the same psychopharmacological principles that would apply to a younger patient, with due allowance being made for the need for dosage adjustment, the greater likelihood of side effects, reduced renal clearance in the case of lithium, and reduced rate of inactivation of neuroleptics and carbamazepine.

Organic psychoses are characteristically seen in elders. These can be produced by a number of pathological states, including electrolyte imbalance; alcohol withdrawal or hallucinosis; tumor; infection; and metabolic, endocrine, and iatrogenic causes (e.g., drugs such as anticholinergic compounds—including antihistamines, antidepressants, and antiparkinsonian drugs—and antiarrhythmics, steroids, bronchodilators, digitalis, diuretics, and analgesics). It is important to establish possible etiology before

embarking on a neuroleptic crusade. If there is some urgency to initiate neuroleptic treatment without knowledge of cause, the clinician should proceed with caution, remembering that it is better to use a drug with minimal anticholinergic properties. Dementia may lead to psychotic symptoms—such as paranoid delusions, hallucinations, or behavioral and psychomotor changes —that will respond to treatment with antipsychotic medication.

Antipsychotic Drugs

The same drugs that are used to treat psychosis in the younger adult are also used in the older patient, the primary drugs in this regard being the dopamine receptor–blocking neuroleptics. Other potentially useful—but less well-researched—drugs for treating psychosis in the elderly include lithium, benzodiazepines, and carbamazepine.

The major classes of neuroleptics are listed in Table 20–1. Aliphatic phenothiazines are of low potency and are nonspecific in their effect—that is, they have an impact on a number of other systems besides dopaminergic pathways. They have marked anticholinergic, anti-adrenergic, and sedative properties, and are more likely to produce organ toxicity than are other neuroleptics. The aliphatic drugs contain a three-ring nucleus and carbon atom side chain, similar to tricyclic antidepressants when viewed two-dimensionally but differing from the antidepressants when viewed in a three-dimensional or configurational way. Chlorpromazine and promazine belong to the aliphatic group. Piperidine phenothiazines also have low potency and resemble the aliphatic drugs in many ways. The piperidine phenothiazines include thioridazine and its metabolite, mesoridazine.

The dose range of each drug is given in Table 20–1. Although they are generally not the drugs of first choice, and despite having more side effects than other neuroleptics, the aliphatic and piperidine phenothiazines are in many cases the most effective drugs for older patients. The initial dose will be determined by a number of factors besides the patient's age; adequacy of hydration, degree of orthostasis, cardiac function, concomitant medications, and severity of psychotic symptoms are all important considerations. In almost all cases, the starting dose for older individuals will be lower than the starting dose for younger adults.

Table 20–1. Classes of neuroleptics and their dose ranges

Category	Drug name	Dose range (mg/day)[a]
Phenothiazines		
Aliphatic	Chlorpromazine	30–300
Piperidine	Thioridazine	30–300
Piperazine	Trifluoperazine	1–15
	Perphenazine	8–32
	Fluphenazine	1–10
Butyrophenones	Haloperidol	2–20
Thioxanthenes	Thiothixene	2–20
	Chlorprothixene	30–300
Dibenzoxapines	Loxapine	5–100
	Clozapine	25–500
Dihydroindolones	Molindone	5–100

[a]Although there is in reality a very wide dosage range, and dose selection should be determined on the basis of individual response, these ranges are sufficient for most older patients.

Other neuroleptic drug classes are of higher potency and do not have such a wide spectrum of activity—that is, they are less sedating and have weaker effects on the peripheral autonomic nervous system, but they are more likely to induce extrapyramidal reactions. However, tardive dyskinesia is equally likely to arise in association with any neuroleptic. These other classes of neuroleptics include 1) piperazine phenothiazines—trifluoperazine, fluphenazine, perphenazine, acetophenazine, and prochlorperazine (although the latter two are rarely used, and prochlorperazine has a poor antipsychotic effect); 2) thioxanthenes, such as thiothixene and chlorprothixene; 3) butyrophenones, including haloperidol; 4) dibenzoxapines, such as loxapine and clozapine; and 5) dihydroindolones, such as molindone. Clozapine has the advantages of being more clinically efficacious in treatment-resistant states and of producing fewer and less severe extrapyramidal side effects (EPS) and reducing the risk for tardive dyskinesia.

Side Effects of Antipsychotic Drugs

Anticholinergic effects of the aliphatic and piperidine phenothiazines include dry mouth, constipation, erectile impairment, urinary delay, tachycardia, impaired sweating, aggravation of narrow-angle glaucoma, impaired memory, and varying levels of delirium. If these are troublesome, the clinician has three options: lower the dose, change medication to one with fewer anticholinergic effects, or leave the dose and medication unchanged and add bethanechol, a drug with cholinergic effects.

Anti-adrenergic effects consist of orthostatic hypotension and ejaculatory impairment. The former can be managed by dose reduction or by changing the medication to a drug with higher potency. Very severe hypotension, which is more likely to happen after parenteral administration, can be treated by use of levarterenol or phenylephrine, but not with epinephrine (the unopposed beta-adrenergic effects of epinephrine will lower the blood pressure even further).

Extrapyramidal effects consist of dystonia, parkinsonian symptoms and signs (including tremor, rigidity, and rabbit syndrome), akathisia, akinesia, and tardive dyskinesia. Akinesia, parkinsonism, and acute dystonic reactions respond to the antiparkinsonian drugs described later in this chapter (see "Antiparkinsonian Medication"). Akinesia can present as drowsiness, lethargy, weakness, and fatigue and may be mistaken for psychosis or depression; the differential diagnosis is important, because treatment is different. Akathisia manifests as restlessness, muscle cramps, jitteriness, pacing, inner anxiety, or some combination of these. It is not always easy to recognize and should not be mistaken as being a manifestation of the illness. Although akathisia often responds to antiparkinsonian drugs, it may prove to be distressingly unresponsive and cause noncompliance with the antipsychotic drug regimen. Benzodiazepines and beta-blockers may be of help, however. In using anticholinergic compounds to treat these side effects, clinicians should always remember that such drugs can induce many other side effects, including psychotic symptoms and delirium.

Other neuroleptic side effects include an increased risk of seizures, agranulocytosis, cholestatic jaundice, photosensitivity, alterations of cardiac conduction, ocular damage, temperature disturbance, and the so-called neuroleptic malignant syndrome. Lowering of the seizure threshold is most severe with clozapine and chlorpromazine, but the overall risk of seizures due to neuroleptics in general is still low.

Agranulocytosis is a life-threatening, but fortunately rare, complication of neuroleptic drugs that is most likely to occur in the first few months of treatment; 75% of all cases have occurred in patients over 50 years of age (Holloway 1974). Clozapine can also produce agranulocytosis, and so use of this drug requires weekly blood count monitoring for the duration of treatment.

Cholestatic jaundice is also rare, occurring mostly with low-potency drugs. Although a 1% incidence figure has been given, it is generally held that this side effect has declined in frequency and that its appearance, rather than being intrinsic to the drug, may have been related to the manufacturing process.

Thioridazine is limited to an upper dosage of 800 mg/day; daily dosages exceeding this level are associated with an increased risk of retinal damage. Neuroleptic malignant syndrome, which carries a 20% mortality rate, is characterized by hyperthermia, hypertension, sweating, muscular rigidity, and alteration in level of awareness. Elevation of white cell count and creatinine phosphokinase levels are found. Dantrolene and bromocriptine are both effective in reversing this condition. Should it be necessary to reinstitute a neuroleptic, it is prudent to pick a low-potency drug, since neuroleptic malignant syndrome seems to be more likely to occur with a high-potency compound. Catatonia can develop as a result of neuroleptics and presents with rigidity, immobility, and waxy flexibility. This can lead to serious medical complications, and the reaction may be prolonged. Antiparkinsonian drug therapy is ineffective. Although most of these are rare reactions, they are among the more serious side effects.

Conduction changes are more likely to occur with the low-potency drugs, and there have been some reports of serious ventricular arrhythmias, including torsade de pointes, with thioridazine; high-potency drugs are safer in this regard.

Careful attention to side effects of neuroleptics is necessary. At this time there is evidence that these drugs are being widely used in rest home populations but with very little medical supervision (Avorn et al. 1989).

Forms of Administration

Although tablets or capsules will serve adequately in most cases, there are special circumstances in which it is preferable to administer antipsychotic drugs in liquid form or by injection. Liquid medication is advantageous when the patient's compliance is questioned or if swallowing pills or capsules presents a problem, and it can be given under supervision, thereby ensuring that the patient does in fact ingest the medication. All neuroleptics come either in concentrate or elixir form. Injectable preparations are formulated for all drugs except molindone and thioridazine. Depot-release, long-acting injectable haloperidol and fluphenazine are also available. Injectables are also useful in situations of noncompliance and when there is an urgent need to bring an acutely psychotic patient under control. Intramuscular administration is adequate in all except the most unusual situations, but intravenous haloperidol has been espoused for the very agitated intensive care unit patient. A suggested approach to managing an acutely psychotic, debilitated older patient, or one with organic brain syndrome, is to inject 0.5 mg of haloperidol two or three times a day, initially. A graduated insulin syringe will facilitate the use of such small doses (Granacher 1979). The dose can then be adjusted as necessary.

Once in vogue, the so-called rapid tranquilization approach is probably of no greater benefit than simply using conventional doses. In rapid tranquilization, the patient receives higher-than-usual intramuscular and/or oral doses of drug over a 24- to 48-hour period.

Intramuscular doses of a neuroleptic can be supplemented by parenteral use of a benzodiazepine, such as lorazepam, to control an acutely agitated, psychotic patient. Another indication for the use of intramuscular administration is when oral therapy has been ineffective. It is possible to tell this way if a patient's nonresponse to oral therapy is related to poor absorption through the gut or to a high first-pass effect. Generally, it may be assumed that a comparable intramuscular dose is one-half to one-third the oral dose. Before embarking on a full dose of a long-acting injectable neuroleptic, it is prudent to administer a test dose—2.5 mg (0.1 cc) of fluphenazine decanoate, or 5 mg of haloperidol decanoate. In older patients, the use of small doses of fluphenazine (2.5–5.0 mg) every 1–2 weeks is preferable to monthly injections. Some elderly patients with paranoid psychosis will respond to doses of depot fluphenazine as low as 5 mg, and they may need only a small number of injections.

Antidepressant Drug Therapy

Depression is common in older persons, who are more likely to experience bereavement, other personal loss, and decline in physical health. It has been estimated that the suicide rate at age 65 exceeds by fivefold the rate for younger age groups, and it continues to increase for men in their 70s. The majority of suicides among the elderly are related to problems associated with physical illness (Goodstein 1985). Deaths from reasons other than suicide are also increased among elderly persons with depression. Therefore, effective treatment of depression has a number of implications besides the short-term impact.

Before embarking on a course of drug therapy, the clinician should consider in the differential diagnosis a number of possible causes for a patient's depression; these may include endocrine, metabolic, cardiac, hematologic, infective, drug-induced, and other physical causes of the symptoms. In addition, other psychiatric states may induce symptoms of depression, including grief, dementia, and delirium. Atypical presentations of depression should also be recognized, such as alcohol abuse, violations of the law, and so forth.

In choosing an antidepressant medication, some general principles should be observed:

1. The clinician should inquire about previous treatments, paying close attention to degree of response, type and magnitude of side effects, and whether the medication was adequately tolerated. The word "allergy" is sometimes used without clear meaning, and the exact nature of the reaction should be identified, since it sometimes turns out that the reaction was not allergic in nature and was dose related.
2. If a family member has been treated with antidepressants, the response should be noted. This will give useful information as to which drug may help the patient.
3. It is important to identify what other medication a patient may be taking. This is not always an easy task, since an older individual may be on a variety of different drugs and may be unable to tell their names without help. It is advisable for patients to bring all the medicines they take to their appointment; enlisting the help of a family member in gathering the medications is helpful. The physician should specify the need to bring prescription as well as over-the-counter drugs, because patients and relatives may not think of nonprescription drugs as "medications." Questions should also be posed as to the use of alcohol and other chemical substances.
4. Older persons who are depressed may respond only partially or not respond at all to therapy with a single antidepressant, and there is greater likelihood that a combination of drugs will be needed to bring about the desired improvement. Therefore, the clinician must be familiar with the types of combinations that may be effective, how to apply them, and the problems that might arise with their use.

The principal drug groups are tricyclic and tetracyclic antidepressants, MAOIs, SSRIs, aminoketones, triazolopyrridines, lithium, stimulants, and, on rare occasions, azaspirones and triazolobenzodiazepines. All have their place, even though some are used only infrequently. Conventional doses and drug categories are listed in Table 20–2.

Tricyclic and Tetracyclic Antidepressants

The tricyclics can be subdivided into secondary and tertiary amines, according to the number of methyl groups on the side chain. Secondary amines are demethylated products of the parent tertiary drug. These are shown in Table 20–2, along with customary dose ranges. In older patients, the secondary amines are often better tolerated because of their lower side effect potential, although some patients complain that they do not sleep as well as they do when they take the tertiary drugs.

Only one tetracyclic drug is currently being marketed—maprotiline. It resembles more the secondary amine than the tertiary amine tricyclics in action. As described by Richelson (1982), the tetracyclic drugs have widely varied effects on different receptor systems, including antihistaminic, anticholinergic, anti-adrenergic, and antidopaminergic effects.

Amitriptyline, doxepin, trimipramine, and maprotiline all have marked antihistaminic effects, and as a result may produce sedation and weight gain. The extent to which marked weight gain occurs in older patients on these drugs needs further clarifi-

Table 20–2. Classes of antidepressants and stimulants and their dose ranges

Category	Drug name	Dose range (mg/day)[a]
Tricyclics	Amoxapine	50–300
	Desipramine	10–300
	Nortriptyline	10–150
	Protriptyline	10–40
	Amitriptyline	25–300
	Clomipramine	25–250
	Doxepin	10–300
	Imipramine	25–300
	Trimipramine	25–300
	Carbamazepine	Poorly defined
Tetracyclics	Maprotiline	25–150
Monoamine oxidase inhibitors	Phenelzine	15–90
	Tranylcypromine	10–60
	L-deprenyl	5–40
Selective serotonin reuptake inhibitors	Fluoxetine	5–60
	Paroxetine	10–40
	Sertraline	25–150
Triazolopyrridine	Trazodone	50–600
Aminoketone	Bupropion	75–450
Stimulants	Dextroamphetamine	2.5–30
	Methylphenidate	5–40
Azaspirone	Buspirone	20–60

[a]It is uncommon for high doses to be required, and they should be attained only very gradually, in keeping with patient tolerance.

cation, however, and it is my opinion that such a side effect is less common among the elderly.

The tertiary amine tricyclics imipramine, amitriptyline, and doxepin have marked anticholinergic properties, whereas the secondary amine drugs and maprotiline are relatively weak in this regard. Anticholinergic effects, which have been described previously, can pose major problems in older patients, most notably confusion, delirium, urinary retention, erectile impairment, constipation, paralytic ileus, and tachycardia. It is generally preferable to avoid a tertiary amine tricyclic as the first-line treatment in patients who are vulnerable to these complications.

Anti-adrenergic effects are thought to be related to the induction of orthostatic hypotension, although this is by no means the only factor. The degree of orthostasis present at baseline, the use of other concomitant hypotensive medication, and the dose of drug may all influence the degree of orthostasis. Nortriptyline is the least likely of the tricyclics to produce orthostatic drop. Roose et al. (1987) have shown 7% and 0% incidences of orthostatic hypotension, respectively, for imipramine and nortriptyline in patients with normal electrocardiograms, compared with frequencies of 32% and 5%, respectively, in patients with either conduction disease or cardiac failure. Orthostasis can be potentially serious in older patients because of the risk of falling and sustaining fractures or other injuries. Measures that can be taken to reduce the risk of orthostasis include ensuring adequacy of hydration; instructing the patient to change position slowly or to ingest caffeine; or using triiodothyronine or ephedrine. Administration of medication three or four times a day is preferred, on the grounds that blood pressure–altering effects of antidepressants are partly related to the peak drug plasma level attained. Administration of the full dose at bedtime may increase the chance of a patient getting out of bed during the night and falling. Although orthostatic hypotension is viewed as an unwanted effect of therapy, at least two studies have shown that in elderly patients with depression, the presence of a marked pretreatment orthostatic drop in systolic blood pressure predicts a high likelihood of recovery from tricyclic therapy.

Antidopaminergic effects of antidepressants are rarely a source for concern, with the exception of amoxapine, which has a dopamine receptor–blocking metabolite and can give rise to extrapyramidal symptoms.

There is a risk of seizures with tricyclic antidepressants. This risk ranges from 1 in 1,000 (0.1%) if there are no other predisposing factors to up to 3 in 100 (3%) under certain conditions (for example, the use of high-dose imipramine in patients with atypical depression). With maprotiline, the risk of seizures is about 0.2%–2%, and it is somewhat higher for clomipramine. In overdose, amoxapine, maprotiline, and desipramine are all more likely to cause seizures. There is some evidence that the seizure risk associated with antidepressants lessens with age (Davidson 1988).

Cardiac conduction changes will occur in some older patients, and it should be remembered that drugs in this class act as type 1 quinidine-like antiarrhythmics. Increased PR, QRS, and QT intervals appear on the electrocardiogram (ECG). In patients with normal cardiac function, imipramine and nortriptyline carry a 0.7% incidence of 2:1 atrioventricular block. When bundle-branch block is already present, as many as 18% of patients who are treated with imipramine may develop significant QRS prolongation or 2:1 atrioventricular block. Patients who are already on quinidine or procainamide will need to have their dose reassessed: sometimes it is possible to discontinue the antiarrhythmic medication and replace it with the antidepressant. The degree of drug-induced intraventricular conduction delay is related to plasma levels in the case of nortriptyline. As a procedural guide, it is recommended that all elderly patients have an ECG before starting on antidepressant drugs.

Skin rash, liver toxicity, hematologic changes, tinnitus, and myoclonus are all seen with the tricyclics. Rash is more commonly seen with maprotiline than with other drugs. Hematologic changes are a particular problem with carbamazepine, a drug reserved for more refractory states. Myoclonus is more common with drugs that have a serotonergic action, and it can be treated with quinine or with a benzodiazepine, by dose reduction, or by changing medication.

Measurement of plasma levels.   There is much interest in the use of plasma levels in patients who are undergoing antidepressant therapy. Therapeutic ranges have not been defined for most drugs, but measuring plasma levels is nonetheless useful; however, such measurements are not yet a routine part of patient management. The American Psychiatric Association's Task Force on the Use of Laboratory Tests in Psychiatry (1985) concluded that is worthwhile to obtain imipramine and nortriptyline levels in any patient who receives these drugs. The existence of a therapeutic window between 50 and 140 ng/mL for nortriptyline in patients with endogenous major depression is well documented. At levels below or above this window, clinical response is less satisfactory. If the dose is pushed too high, then deterioration may set in, and the appropriate course would be to lower the dose. A minimum combined imipramine and desipramine level of 180–200 ng/mL is associated with a high probability of success with imipramine therapy in patients with major depression. A minimum level of 120 ng/mL has been advanced in the case of desipramine. With respect to amitriptyline, the literature is contradictory, but in general it more convincingly argues against, rather than for, any consistent relationship between plasma level and therapeutic effect. There are few data for doxepin, trimipramine, protriptyline, amoxapine, and maprotiline.

There are a number of situations in which knowledge of the plasma level would be useful: 1) if there is nonresponse at a "reasonable" dose; 2) if unusually high doses are about to be or are being used; 3) if noncompliance is suspected; 4) when there is drug toxicity or overdose; 5) in the presence of side effects that may be related to plasma level, such as cardiac conduction defects with nortriptyline; 6) before introducing another drug that is known to affect plasma levels or metabolism of the tricyclic antidepressant; and 7) if change in clinical state occurs after switching to a generic brand of the same drug.

Procedurally, the optimum time for collecting samples to determine steady-state levels is 10–14 hours postdose when the drug is taken once a day, and just before the morning dose when the drug is taken in divided doses. The stopper of the collection tube should not contain trisbutoxyethyl, because this chemical elutes drug into the red cells and spuriously lowers plasma level. The dark-blue Becton-Dickinson stoppered tube and the Venoject Kimble-Terumo tubes are suitable.

Dose initiation of tricyclic and tetracyclic antidepressants.   Low starting doses are advisable— 25 mg of the tricyclics (except protriptyline) and maprotiline, or 5 mg of protriptyline. In some cases—for example, in patients above age 75, those who are in poor physical health, or those with a known history of sensitivity to the side effects of drugs—starting doses as low as 10 mg of a tricyclic drug are indicated. Frequent monitoring is required, as the dose is slowly raised every 2–3 days. Lying and standing pulse rate and blood pressure, sensorium, and urinary and bowel function should all be checked. Dose increases should continue until there is evidence of improvement or until side effects occur. It may take several weeks for full response to occur, and the physician should not succumb to impatience. The patient and his or her family should be instructed that this delay is to be expected, and at the same time told that side effects may precede improvement. Despite advertised claims, there is no solid evidence that any particular tricyclic acts more rapidly than any other. Some sign of response by 2 weeks is thought to predict good ultimate outcome, and if there is absolutely no improvement after 3 weeks, then little is to be gained by persisting any longer. In a study of depressed patients in general (that is, not specifically in the elderly), improvement of the following symptoms at the end of 1 week distinguished responders from nonresponders: depressed mood, anxiety, hostility, and depressed appearance (Bowden 1984). Initial signs of improvement are often more apparent to staff and family members than they are to the patient. Such observations, when made by others, can be shared with the patient, who may still be doubting whether improvement can occur.

Some symptoms are viewed as having predictive value for successful outcome with tricyclic therapy. These include the "endogenous" symptoms, such as greater initial severity of psychomotor retardation, anhedonia, weight loss, and early-morning wakening. However, it should be noted that in its pure form, endogenous depression is uncommon, and the prominence it has received in textbooks echoes a bygone era in psychiatry when the concept of depression was more narrow. Marked hypochondriasis, delusions, and "hysterical" symptoms are thought to predict a poor response. However, a tricyclic in combination with a neuroleptic is more likely to be successful in patients with psychotic depression (Spiker et al. 1985). Poststroke depression is responsive to tricyclic antidepressants such as nortriptyline.

Duration of therapy. Duration of drug therapy is longer in older patients, because depression generally runs a more protracted course in this population. In patients between the ages of 31 and 50, the natural length of depression varies from 9 to 18 months, whereas after age 50, its cycle lasts for an average of 3–5 years (Ayd 1983). Premature discontinuation of therapy or overenthusiastic dose reduction may cause depressive relapse. The desired length of therapy and the relapse rates upon discontinuation have not been well studied in the elderly, but a minimum of 6 months is recommended (Flint 1992).

Combination therapy with tricyclic antidepressants. Tricyclic drugs may need to be combined with other drugs in order to overcome nonresponse or partial response. The addition of lithium at full doses can translate partial response into full response, especially in patients with melancholic presentations (Price et al. 1986). It may be necessary to persist with lithium for 3–4 weeks until improvement sets in. There are few guidelines in the literature (Austin et al. 1991), perhaps because it is not easy to study a large number of such patients; however, there is some evidence that lithium add-on therapy is more likely to be effective in older patients with depression. An advantage of this treatment approach is its relative safety.

Triiodothyronine, 25 µg daily, can be added; this approach is as effective as adding lithium to the tricyclic drugs (Joffe et al. 1993). However, there is little information to help the clinician in the selection of appropriate patients. An SSRI may be added to potentiate the effects of a partially effective tricyclic antidepressant drug. Care should be taken, however, lest there be untoward potentiation of tricyclic antidepressant side effects, the occurrence of which is probably related to the marked rise in plasma levels that can result when fluoxetine is added.

Monoamine Oxidase Inhibitors

The efficacy of phenelzine compared with that of nortriptyline and placebo has been demonstrated in older depressed patients (Georgatas et al. 1986). MAOIs such as phenelzine and tranylcypromine are a valuable down-the-line treatment for the older person. However, offsetting the undoubted benefit of MAOI therapy in previously nonresponsive depressed patients is the knowledge that these drugs are potentially more dangerous and have a lower safety margin than all other antidepressant drugs.

The MAOIs can be grouped into the hydrazine and nonhydrazine types. Phenelzine belongs to the first category, and tranylcypromine and deprenyl belong to the second. Hydrazines are purportedly more hepatotoxic than the nonhydrazine MAOIs, but the risks appear to be exceedingly low. There is no overall difference in efficacy between the two groups, but individual patients sometimes respond better to one drug than to another; sometimes the side effects of one drug are tolerated less well than those of another.

The MAOIs inhibit monoamine oxidase, an enzyme that is an important regulator of biogenic amine activity. These agents are irreversible inhibitors—that is, they permanently inactivate the available enzyme supply. Once an MAOI is stopped, the body must synthesize new enzyme before MAOI effects will wear off. This may take 10–14 days, although by the end of 1 week the supply of monoamine oxidase may be back to 50% of the baseline level as a result of new synthesis. These considerations are important from the safety perspective, since dietary and medication restrictions must remain in force for this time period even though the patient is no longer taking the MAOI. Deprenyl is an MAO-B–selective inhibitor at low doses, and it is therefore considered to be somewhat safer. However, at these doses, deprenyl is a less effective antidepressant. At higher doses, it works more effectively, but then does not offer any safety advantages.

The anticholinergic effects that often bedevil tricyclic therapy are of less concern with MAOIs, except at high doses. Therefore, MAOI therapy is sometimes indicated when a tricyclic drug has failed due to anticholinergic side effects. Impaired sexual arousal, constipation, and urinary delay do occur with higher doses of MAOIs, however. Anticholinergic effects are much more pronounced when an MAOI is used in conjunction with tricyclics, antihistamines, and antiparkinsonian drugs.

Blood pressure changes are problematic with MAOIs: both lying systolic and orthostatic blood pressure may drop, manifesting as dizziness, weakness, or inability to stand up. Sometimes these blood pressure changes may be asymptomatic, and for that reason it is important to check blood pressure at each visit. I have found that isocarboxazid-induced hypotension is dose related, although this is not the case for orthostatic drop. These changes do not occur immediately and may not become apparent until after 3 weeks of therapy. A sodium chloride supplement, 2–3 g/day, can be helpful in counteracting hypotension, although this treatment is contraindicated if there is evidence of heart or kidney disease or if the patient must restrict sodium intake. Other measures that can be taken are those described above for tricyclic drugs, although great caution should be used with regard to concomitant use of ephedrine, because this combination can lead to a hypertensive reaction. As with the tricyclics, pre-treatment systolic orthostasis is related to outcome, at least for isocarboxazid.

Increased blood pressure from pressor agents, such as tyramine, phenylephrine, phenylpropanolamine, pseudoephedrine, and amphetamine, can lead to a hypertensive crisis in patients undergoing MAOI therapy. The incidence may be as high as 8% (Rabkin et al. 1984), although in my experience it is far lower. The fatality rate is estimated at 1 in 100,000 patients who experience hypertensive crisis as a result of a pressor agent–tranylcypromine interaction. A hypertensive reaction due to any MAOI–pressor agent interaction may be treated with intravenous administration of 5 mg of the alpha-blocker phentolamine, 300 mg iv of diazoxide, or sodium nitroprusside infusion. The practice of having patients carry around 50 mg of chlorpromazine "just in case" is not advisable because of the possibility of marked hypotension if the self-made diagnosis is incorrect. The risk of hypertensive crisis cannot be eliminated altogether, but it can be substantially lowered through proper counseling, patient selection, and family involvement. A more reasonable recommendation is to give patients nifedipine (10 mg) with instructions to chew and absorb sublingually in the event of a possible hypertension reaction.

Impaired sleep, weight gain, myoclonus, memory impairment, headache, restlessness, and anorexia may all occur as side effects with MAOI therapy. Tranylcypromine is more likely than the hydrazine drugs to cause weight loss, anorexia, agitation, headache, and insomnia. Dietary and drug instructions and contraindicated medications for patients on MAOIs are described by Davidson et al. (1984); issues of compliance and patient education are described by Walker et al. (1984). Before any elective operative procedure, MAOIs should be discontinued for at least 2 weeks. In an emergency, however, a patient can undergo surgery, with due precaution being taken by the anesthesiologist. Further suggestions as to patient management are given elsewhere (Churchill-Davidson 1965).

Extrapyramidal symptoms from MAOIs are rare, but these drugs do potentiate the extrapyramidal effects of neuroleptics. Monitoring of platelet monoamine oxidase activity is not routinely indicated, and there is little evidence for a relationship between enzyme inhibition and clinical response to an MAOI, other than for phenelzine in younger patients with atypical depression. In the case of tranyl-cypromine, it appears that full monoamine oxidase inhibition occurs at doses below those needed for an antidepressant effect.

Dose is a critical determinant of outcome with MAOI therapy, in that an increase of 15 mg of phenelzine, 5 mg of isocarboxazid, or 10 mg of tranyl-cypromine may be pivotal. In patients who are unable to tolerate the side effects but who relapse when the dose is lowered by one tablet, a half-tablet decrease can be sufficient. Isocarboxazid has an advantage in this case, since it is the only scored MAOI tablet; coated tablets are more difficult to break. Recommended doses are given in Table 20–2, and the importance of reaching the maximum tolerated dose is stressed. It is recommended that the initial dose be low—10 mg of isocarboxazid or tranyl-cypromine, 5 mg of deprenyl, or 15 mg of phenelzine. The dose can then be increased every few days, one tablet at a time, up to four or five tablets a day. If side effects become a problem, the dose can be lowered, but if there is neither response nor side effect, then further dose increases can be undertaken. Duration of therapy is similar to that of the tricyclics. The response to phenelzine is sustained during maintenance therapy with the elderly; however, because many patients only receive an MAOI because they have a chronic depression that has been resistant to treatment with other drugs, they may need a longer period of maintenance therapy.

Features that should cause a clinician to consider the use of an MAOI in an elderly patient include phobic anxiety, nonpsychotic agitation, somatic anxiety, anergia, reserpine-induced depression, or a previous history of panic attacks or chronic anxiety. A number of older patients with depression have been noted to develop psychotic symptoms, such as paranoid delusions, or to stop eating and become mute or withdrawn within 2 weeks of beginning treatment, usually at high doses of the drug (50–60 mg of isocarboxazid, 75–90 mg of phenelzine). In such cases, the patient has had a history of previous psychotic depression or may have presented with psychomotor retardation. The degree to which each of these features contributes to overall variance in outcome may be relatively small, and in general an MAOI should be thought of as potentially helpful in practically any form of major depression. Some hold the opinion that tranylcypromine is the most effective MAOI in older patients with depression.

Selective Serotonin Reuptake Inhibitors

Since 1988, the use of antidepressant drugs has undergone a fundamental change in that many practitioners now adopt an SSRI as first- or second-line treatment for depression. Fluoxetine first became available on the market in 1988, followed some years later by sertraline and paroxetine. These drugs are free of many of the cardiovascular and autonomic side effects associated with MAOIs and tricyclic antidepressants and represent an important advance in therapy. However, fluoxetine and its active metabolite, norfluoxetine, have exceptionally long half-lives. As a result, some side effects that do occur may persist for a long time in elderly patients. There is also a problem with medication interactions, in that fluoxetine significantly potentiates the effects of tricyclic antidepressants and some benzodiazepines. Fluoxetine-induced weight loss in the elderly can also be a vexing problem (Brymer and Winegrad 1992). Other interactions may occur between fluoxetine and valproic acid, phenelzine, buspirone, and neuroleptics. Experience with sertraline and paroxetine is more limited at this time.

Aminoketones

At the same time as fluoxetine appeared on the market, a nonserotonergic alternative, bupropion, also became available. This catecholaminergic drug is well tolerated in the elderly and has a favorable cardiovascular profile in that it causes minimal hypotension or conduction change. The risk of seizures, present at high doses of 450 mg and above, may be lower in older patients (Davidson 1988), and the drug is well suited as an antidepressant in the elderly. Its principal drawback is the need for thrice-daily administration at the upper dosage range of 400–450 mg/day.

Other Antidepressant Therapy

Trazodone has a definite role in the treatment of older depressed patients. Its freedom from anticholinergic effects gives it a major advantage over tricyclic and tetracyclic drugs. Side effects include sedation, hypotension, and dizziness; priapism is a rare but serious risk. A low starting dosage of 50 mg/day is recommended, with progressive increases up to a maximum of 600 mg/day, which would correspond roughly to a tricyclic dosage of 225 mg/day.

With trazodone, the hypnotic dosage is often below the antidepressant dosage; this is an important point, because there may be a tendency to rest content with a suboptimal antidepressant dose once the patient starts to sleep better.

The antianxiety agent alprazolam has been documented to have antidepressant effects equivalent to those of tricyclics, and greater than those of placebo. However, it may be that the drug is less effective in patients with melancholia or in cases of marked vegetative change. A potential advantage of alprazolam is its lack of autonomic and cardiovascular properties. The chief drawbacks are sedation, interference with memory, and possible withdrawal effects. Although the recommended dosage range is 0.5–4 mg/day, the upper range has not been fully explored, and there are anecdotal reports indicating that substantially higher dosages may be needed. The long-term effects of alprazolam need to be better understood. Withdrawal of the drug must always be approached with caution, and the patient and family should be warned about the possibility of withdrawal seizure upon abrupt discontinuation. In one study (Weissman et al. 1992), alprazolam was found to be as effective as imipramine (and placebo) in elderly patients with depression, but was associated with fewer side effects; relapse was also greater on discontinuation of therapy.

Buspirone, an azaspirone anxiolytic drug, can also have antidepressant effects at higher dosages—for example, 40–60 mg/day. It is generally free of the problem side effects that characterize tricyclics and MAOIs but may cause agitation, nausea, headache, or lightheadedness. Buspirone can serve as a useful alternative, or adjuvant, in patients with depression who prove difficult to treat.

The tricyclic anticonvulsant carbamazepine possesses some mood-elevating effects and can be used in treatment-refractory depression (R. M. Post et al. 1986). Use of the drug should be preceded by a complete blood count (CBC) and differential, liver function tests, electrolyte levels, and an ECG to rule out arrhythmia or a conduction disorder. The starting dosage of 200 mg twice daily may be gradually raised by 200-mg increments up to as high as 1,200 mg/day. Blood level monitoring is recommended, more for safety than for efficacy reasons, with the range being 8–12 µg/mL. Regular blood counts should be performed, and the drug should be discontinued if red cells fall below 4,000,000/mm^3,

if hematocrit falls below 32%, if leukocytes fall below 4,000/mm^3, if platelets are less than 100,000/mm^3, or if reticulocytes are below 0.3%. The patient and family members should also be told to report immediately if the patient develops fever, sore throat, mouth ulcers, bleeding, or any infection; in such cases, further hematologic assessment should be undertaken and the drug stopped until the cause has been established.

Stimulants

Almost consigned to the scrap heap of psychopharmacology, stimulants can have a useful role in treating depression in older patients that is not sufficiently realized. The main reservations relating to these drugs have traditionally centered around risks of abuse, dependency, and assumed inefficacy. In medically ill patients with depression, in patients in withdrawn postoperative states, and in those with poststroke depression, stimulant drug therapy is often beneficial. A stimulant drug is also indicated when tricyclic antidepressants, SSRIs, or other drugs produce unacceptable side effects. Response to drugs in this class is characteristically rapid, with improvement being noted within 48 hours. In fact, if there is no response to a sufficient dose within 3 days, the drug trial can be considered as having failed.

There is an impression that methylphenidate is preferable in adjustment disorder whereas dextroamphetamine is more effective in major depression, but these contentions require more rigorous testing. Double-blind studies do not, in general, conclusively show efficacy for stimulant drugs, but this question still remains little studied. Recommended starting doses are 5 mg of dextroamphetamine and 10 mg of methylphenidate. Dextroamphetamine has a longer half-life than methylphenidate and can be given once in the morning, whereas methylphenidate is best given on a twice-daily basis. The total daily dosages range from 2.5 to 30 mg for dextroamphetamine and from 5 to 40 mg for methylphenidate. In one survey (Woods et al. 1986), the mean maximal daily dosages were 12 mg and 13.5 mg for dextroamphetamine and methylphenidate, respectively. Mood, motivation, psychomotor state, sleep, and appetite all improved, and the overall improvement often permitted improvement in the underlying medical disorder once the patient's depression had lifted.

It is best to administer the last dose of methylphenidate in the afternoon, since insomnia can be a side effect, but in general the psychostimulants are remarkably free of unwanted effects in older patients. At high doses there is a risk of agitation. Many clinicians agree that therapy can be discontinued shortly after the patient has become asymptomatic.

Psychostimulant therapy may also be indicated for potentiating the effect of a tricyclic drug or to counteract the hypotensive effects of antidepressants. This can lead to potentially dangerous hypertension in conjunction with an MAOI, but it is nonetheless noted that such therapy may have a place in carefully selected patients who are refractory to treatment (Feighner et al. 1985).

Mood-Stabilizing Therapy

Lithium

Lithium is indicated to treat patients with acute mania, hypomania, and some schizoaffective states; it is also indicated for regulation and prophylaxis in recurrent unipolar and bipolar disorders. Lithium is excreted through the kidney; therefore in older patients, whose renal clearance of lithium will be reduced, the half-life will be longer, averaging 36 hours.

Before starting a patient on lithium, a pretreatment workup should be performed, including CBC and differential, urinalysis, thyroxine and triiodothyronine uptake, free thyroxine index, thyroid-stimulating hormone assay, electrolytes, creatinine, and ECG. If renal function is thought to be impaired, a 24-hour creatinine clearance test may be performed.

It is recommended that lithium be started at a low dose and slowly increased as tolerated. In an acutely manic elderly patient, 300 mg is usually well tolerated, and this can be increased up to 900 mg in most cases. Because of the 36-hour half-life, it can take as long as 180 hours before the steady state has been reached, and it will take this long before a blood level measurement is meaningful. In older and/or medically compromised patients, a small initial dose of 75 mg or 150 mg can be used. In manic patients, the desired blood lithium level is in the range of 1.0–1.4 mmol/L. In patients with acute mania, the onset of lithium's effects will take several days, and so concomitant neuroleptic therapy is

usually needed. In patients with hypomania, lithium alone is sufficient. If lithium is being administered for prophylaxis to a patient who is not acutely symptomatic, then plasma levels of 0.4–0.7 mmol/L may be adequate. Monthly or bimonthly lithium levels are suggested for older patients. To properly interpret a lithium level, the blood sample should be drawn 12 hours after the last dose.

Debate exists as to whether lithium is best given in a single daily dose or in divided doses. There is some evidence that once a-day dosing is associated with less polyuria and less structural damage to the kidney.

Benign side effects may appear early in lithium therapy, such as fine tremor, nausea, headache, tiredness, and polyuria. Other side effects include memory impairment, weight gain, thyroid enlargement, hypothyroidism, diabetes insipidus, psoriasis, skin infection, and sinus arrhythmia.

At blood levels in excess of 1.5 mmol/L, lithium's toxic effects are likely to supervene. These consist of coarse tremor, slurred speech, ataxia, nystagmus, hyperreflexia, weakness, drowsiness, muscle fasciculations, and vomiting. If unchecked, toxicity can progress to impaired consciousness, clonus, seizures, EEG slowing, electrolyte imbalance, coma, and death. Prompt recognition and management of a toxic reaction is therefore most important. In such a situation, lithium should be stopped and the patient monitored on a daily basis with ECG and lithium and electrolyte measurements. Fluid intake should be increased to 5–6 liters per day. Twice-daily administration of urea, 20 g iv, or 50–100 g/day iv of mannitol, will increase the clearance of lithium through diuresis. Intravenous aminophylline, administered slowly, increases tubular blood flow and decreases tubular reabsorption of lithium. Sodium lactate increases lithium excretion. Hemodialysis may be indicated in cases of refractory lithium toxicity.

Lithium interacts with a number of drugs, resulting in either a decrease or an increase of lithium blood levels. Drugs that can raise the plasma lithium level and/or reduce renal excretion include thiazide diuretics, spironolactone, triamterene, nonsteroidal antiinflammatory drugs (except aspirin), and possibly tetracycline. Any of these drugs can therefore lead to a state of lithium toxicity. Theophylline drugs have been reported to lower lithium levels.

Other drugs that do not directly alter the disposition of lithium can still lead to lithium toxicity. A lithium-neuroleptic interaction may lead to confusion, EPS, and cerebellar signs; this is rare, however, and should not deter the clinician from using such combinations. Increased neurotoxicity can result from lithium and phenytoin, and from lithium and carbamazepine. High-dose combinations of an MAOI and lithium can produce a serotonin syndrome, with muscular overactivity and temperature increase.

It is sometimes necessary to combine lithium and a diuretic in elderly patients. If the patient is already on lithium, then it is best to check the level and lower the dose by half. Lithium levels and electrolytes should then be monitored at least twice weekly at first, and the dose adjusted according to side effects and blood indices. Potassium supplementation is generally advisable with thiazides. Loop diuretics such as furosemide and ethacrynic acid cause less retention of lithium than do the thiazides.

Patient and family education is an important part of lithium management. Reliability and possession of the requisite information are required to obtain the maximum benefit and avoid potentially serious side effects. One consideration is that manic patients are not always willing to accept the need for lithium, and a good doctor-patient relationship will go some way toward forestalling this problem. Family support, good dietary habits, supervision of other medications, and adequate care of coexisting physical pathology are also major considerations. In a geriatric patient on lithium, any gastrointestinal upset, change in salt intake, or change in dietary plan should signal the need to consult with a physician or temporarily curtail medication.

Carbamazepine

The tricyclic drug carbamazepine has been demonstrated to have antimanic effects, as well as providing interepisode prophylaxis. Some patients with bipolar disorder respond to carbamazepine alone, whereas others fare better when it is combined with another mood stabilizer. Rapidly cycling bipolar patients may respond better to carbamazepine than to lithium, and patients with angry, paranoid mania may respond better than those with euphoric mania. The role of carbamazepine in treating depression is less well established.

When combined with neuroleptics and antidepressants, carbamazepine may lower the levels of drugs in these groups, an effect that also can occur with oral contraceptives, steroids, theophylline, and warfarin. Some drugs—including propoxyphene, diltiazem, verapamil, and erythromycin—cause an increase in carbamazepine levels. A starting dosage of 100 mg/day may be increased carefully every 2–3 days to produce a drug level of 6–8 ng/mL, provided there are no problematic side effects. The induction of carbamazepine's own drug-metabolizing enzymes may require a later dosage increase at about 6 weeks.

There is no general agreement as to the schedule for obtaining blood counts in patients on carbamazepine. Agranulocytosis occurs in 1 in 125,000 patients on the drug. A baseline CBC and differential should be obtained, with subsequent monitoring at intervals of 4–8 weeks. Of more importance is the need to quickly respond if the patient develops fever, sore throat, or bruising, which may indicate bone marrow suppression. Hepatotoxicity is rare, rashes occur in about 5% of cases, and other side effects include diplopia, sedation, headache, nausea, ataxia, and impaired memory.

Valproate

Valproic acid (which dissociates to valproate after ingestion) is an acyclic anticonvulsant, with additional uses including control of acute mania and prevention of recurrences. Its antimanic properties are evident within 2 weeks of initiating treatment, and it may be beneficial in lithium-resistant rapid cyclers. Valproic acid has generally been used in combination with other mood stabilizers and antidepressants, and its role as monotherapy is unclear.

Of the three available forms of valproic acid, the enteric-coated divalproex sodium is the most widely used because it causes less gastrointestinal distress.

Dosage ranges from 125 to 2,500 mg/day, and plasma levels should be within the range of 50–100 ng/mL, although this recommendation rests upon extrapolation from the therapeutic range for the drug's anticonvulsant activity.

Sedation, alopecia, weight change, gastrointestinal distress, tremor, and ataxia sometimes occur. Hepatotoxicity is very rare, but liver function tests should be obtained every 1–2 months. Minor elevations of liver test results are of little consequence, although elevation of bilirubin may be more significant (Schatzberg and Cole 1991). Liver function tests, CBC and differential, and blood valproate levels should be rechecked at intervals (e.g., every 2–4 months).

Valproate can be combined with other mood stabilizers, although the combination with clonazepam can potentially lead to status petit mal. Fluoxetine and erythromycin both may potentiate valproate's effects.

Valproate may also be useful in treating elderly patients with organic brain syndrome who develop an agitated psychosis (Mazure et al. 1992).

Other Mood-Stabilizing Drugs

Phenytoin has been promoted in the past as having mood-stabilizing effects, but there are no convincing data to support its use in patients with bipolar disorder. Some supportive data, however, favor use of the calcium channel blocker verapamil in younger patients with mania, in whom it was shown to be as effective as lithium in one study (Garza-Trevino et al. 1992). Other calcium channel blockers, such as nifedipine, may also be useful.

Pharmacological Treatment of Anxiety

Antianxiety and Hypnotic Medications

The benzodiazepines have almost entirely supplanted barbiturates and propanediols for treating anxiety, although today there are still some older patients who have been well stabilized on a barbiturate for many decades and in whom there is little to be gained by tampering; indeed such patients may rightly resist any attempt at altering their medication regimen. Other drug groups have a place in treating older individuals with anxiety disorder, including the antidepressants, antihistamines, neuroleptics, and beta-blockers. The new azaspirone drug buspirone may also be especially useful in treating the older patient.

Benzodiazepines

It is always important to rule out other causes of anxiety, which can be the presenting symptom of numerous physical and psychiatric disorders. Precipitating factors should be looked for, identified, and dealt with as appropriate. The first-line choice of drug therapy in primary anxiety is a benzodiazepine. Although all benzodiazepines are equally effective, there are important differences in metabolism and side-effect profiles. It is also possible that the triazolobenzodiazepines (e.g., alprazolam) differ from other benzodiazepines with respect to cross-tolerance, which would have practical importance in managing withdrawal reactions.

Triazolam is a short-acting drug, with a half-life of up to 4 hours. Short- to intermediate-acting drugs include alprazolam, lorazepam, oxazepam, and temazepam. Long-acting drugs include flurazepam, diazepam, chlordiazepoxide, clorazepate, and prazepam. Oxazepam and lorazepam, which are metabolized by conjugation, do not yield active metabolites and are less likely to produce cumulative side effects. Although short-acting benzodiazepines provide an advantage over long-acting drugs in this regard, they have some disadvantages, such as the potential for withdrawal effects and rebound insomnia, and the need to administer the drug in divided doses instead of as a single daily dose.

Side effects of benzodiazepines consist of sedation, drowsiness, lethargy, memory and cognitive impairment, ataxia, paradoxical hostility, aggravation of sleep apnea, nightmares, hallucinations, dysarthria, diplopia, nystagmus, weakness, and depression. Anxiety may be intensified if the drugs interfere with respiration. Benzodiazepine effects will be potentiated by alcohol, other sedatives, anticonvulsants, MAOIs, sedating tricyclics, sedating neuroleptics, and antihypertensives.

Clinical indications for benzodiazepines include insomnia (see below), generalized anxiety disorder, posttraumatic stress disorder, panic disorder, acute states of anxiety or agitation, and alcohol withdrawal. Benzodiazepines are sometimes useful as an adjunct to antidepressant therapy in anxious or agitated depressed patients or in depressed patients who require treatment with a secondary amine tricyclic but who are not sleeping adequately. Insomnia induced by an MAOI may also respond to a benzodiazepine. In controlling panic attacks, alprazolam and clonazepam may be particularly beneficial.

Starting dosages in the elderly will be one-half to one-third those used in younger individuals. Illustrative starting dosages are 2–5 mg/day of diazepam, 10 mg/day of oxazepam, 0.25–0.5 mg/day of alprazolam, and 2 mg/day of lorazepam. The doses can be raised every few days until the desired effect is obtained or side effects appear. It is recommended that attempts be made to reduce the dose or discontinue medication after a few weeks and to present the treatment as either a short-term measure or, if the patient has a chronic anxiety state, as an intermittent treatment to be used in conjunction with other approaches. It is questionable whether daily long-term benzodiazepine therapy is either effective or indicated, except in rare cases, and there is a real risk in the elderly of producing cumulative toxicity. There is a chance of withdrawal symptoms, psychosis, or other major decompensation in a significant number of patients who have taken long-term benzodiazepines at standard doses (Tyrer et al. 1983). A daily dose reduction at the rate of 10% per day is recommended for drug withdrawal.

Other Anxiolytics

Buspirone is an anxiolytic drug that differs in many respects from the benzodiazepines. It is nonsedating, does not interact with alcohol, and has no abuse liability; it may take somewhat longer to relieve symptoms, at least as far as patient perception is concerned. The starting dosage is 5 mg twice a day, to be increased as needed up to 60 mg/day. Some patients who have become used to and responded well to benzodiazepines do not feel that buspirone is as helpful.

Because the full implications of long-term benzodiazepine use are unknown, consideration should be given to the advantages of low doses of tricyclic antidepressants, such as doxepin, trimipramine, or nortriptyline, which frequently provide adequate anxiety relief.

Beta-blockers can be useful for managing somatic anxiety, although side effects to be concerned about in older patients include dizziness, hypotension, depression, aggravation of respiratory distress, diabetes, bradycardia, and heart failure. However, some individuals who receive beta-blockers for other reasons still complain of anxiety; thus, the role of beta-blockers as anxiolytic agents appears to be limited in this age group.

Patients with organic brain disease who exhibit nonpsychotic anxiety or agitation may respond better to a neuroleptic than to a benzodiazepine. High-potency, nonsedating drugs such as haloperidol (starting at 0.5 mg) and thiothixene (starting at 1 mg) are well tolerated and are unlikely to produce troublesome extrapyramidal effects. Low-potency drugs are more likely to affect autonomic function.

An alternative approach is available with the antihistamines, which may be indicated in patients with chronic obstructive pulmonary disease. Daily doses of 10–25 mg of hydroxyzine or diphenhydramine can be used. Side effects include those associated with all anticholinergics, as described in earlier sections of this chapter.

Pharmacological Management of Insomnia

When deciding whether to use a hypnotic drug, and how long to use it for, the clinician should consider the following points: 1) Has the cause been adequately identified? If polysomnography is available, has it been used? 2) Is the patient taking other medication that might interact with a hypnotic? Could medication be the cause of insomnia? 3) Is a sleep apnea syndrome present? 4) What side effects may the hypnotic produce, and what is the drug's metabolic profile? What is known of the patient's physical state that might have an impact on drug effects? 5) The following are relative contraindications to benzodiazepine therapy in older patients: previous substance abuse; lack of adequate support systems; heavy snoring; impaired renal, liver, and pulmonary function; and suicide potential (Reynolds et al. 1985).

For short-term management, a benzodiazepine is indicated, and an agent from this class may also be useful in patients with chronic insomnia that is clearly part of a generalized anxiety disorder. Maintenance doses of benzodiazepines in older persons should be kept at lower levels than in younger people. The medication should be taken 30–60 minutes before bedtime, and instructions can be given to omit doses at least 1–2 nights per week. It is important to provide information as to possible daytime complications, such as hangover, sedation, forgetfulness, and so forth.

The nonbenzodiazepine drug zolpidem, an imidazopyridine, is a short-acting hypnotic without muscle relaxant and anticonvulsant effects. It is an effective hypnotic at a dose of 5 mg/day. Studies of zolpidem in the elderly reveal a delay in elimination and low overall incidence of sedation and ataxia. Other side effects include nausea, diarrhea, dizziness, headache, and perceptual distortions.

Other approaches to sleep hygiene should be used, such as instructing the patient not to use the bed for activities antithetical to sleep, such as paying the bills, preparing the grocery list, and so forth. Other nonpharmacological approaches have been outlined by Reynolds and colleagues (1985).

Antiparkinsonian Medication

Opinion is divided about whether medication should be given routinely to prevent neuroleptic-induced EPS. With low-potency neuroleptics, the frequency of EPS is not appreciably different as a result of prophylaxis (Stramek et al. 1986), but with high-potency drugs such as haloperidol, the frequency of EPS is reduced threefold by routine prophylaxis (Stramek et al. 1986; Winslow et al. 1986). Whether a patient develops EPS will be determined by age, physical and central nervous system condition, and selection and dosage of drug, to name only a few factors. In general, about 20%–40% of all neuroleptic-treated patients will experience EPS.

Most antiparkinsonian agents have anticholinergic side effects, although amantadine is an exception in this regard. Anticholinergic, antihistamine, beta-blocker, and benzodiazepine drugs are all effective in treating EPS.

For example, the following drugs are classified as anticholinergic: benztropine (1–4 mg/day), biperiden (2–6 mg/day), ethopropazine (50–600 mg/ day), procyclidine (5–15 mg/day), and trihexyphenidyl (2–15 mg/day). Two antihistamine drugs are diphenhydramine (25–150 mg/day) and orphenadrine (50–200 mg/day). Any one of these drugs is likely to be effective in most cases of EPS.

Second-line antiparkinsonian agents are propranolol (10–40 mg/day) and diazepam (2–10 mg/ day) for akathisia that has not responded to other drugs. Akathisia can sometimes be difficult to recognize. Amantadine (100–300 mg/day) is a nonanticholinergic drug that has dopaminergic effects and is a useful, if expensive, alternative treatment.

Injectable forms of benztropine, diphenhydramine, and orphenadrine are available for severe EPS. Also, in acute dystonia, intramuscular lorazepam or intravenous diazepam can be used.

Pharmacotherapy for Dementia: Brain Stimulants and Vasodilators

Loss of brain-tissue functioning results in organic brain syndrome, characterized by a decrease in intellectual ability, memory loss, disorientation, and impaired judgment. In contrast to acute organic brain syndrome, which is reversible when the precipitating cause is removed, chronic organic brain syndrome is insidious, and its treatment is empirical and less successful.

Poor nutrition contributes to impaired cognition in the elderly. The plasma lipids play a major role in the development of organic brain syndrome secondary to atherosclerosis, so that serum cholesterol should not exceed 220 mg/dL and the triglyceride level should remain below 150 mg/dL (Frederickson 1974). A low-cholesterol diet containing no more than 30% of daily calories as fat is beneficial. Saturated animal fats should be eliminated as far as possible, and steady exercise, cessation of smoking, and control of blood pressure are all important (Walker and Brodie 1980). A majority of elderly hospitalized patients were found in one study (Whanger and Wang 1974) to have inadequate diets, low folate, and low vitamin B_{12}. Daily vitamin supplements have been recommended for all patients over the age of 65 (Verwoerdt 1976).

Vasodilators may have some limited effect in patients with early to mild dementia of vascular origin, but have no impact in those with more severe forms of the disorder. Cyclandelate (800–1,200 mg/day) and papaverine (150 mg/day) are smooth-muscle vasodilators, which can cause flushing, hypotension, and headaches. Nicotinic acid (0.5–3 g/day) dilates cutaneous blood vessels. Nylidrin (9–48 mg/day) and isoxsuprine (30–60 mg/day) are beta-agonists, which increase blood flow. Although they are indicated as being possibly effective for symptoms associated with cerebrovascular insufficiency, there is no conclusive evidence that these drugs are useful in patients with Alzheimer's disease.

Ergoloid mesylates, marketed as the combination drug Hydergine, appear to be somewhat more effective than other vasodilators. Hydergine is a mixture of four ergot alkaloids and was originally marketed as an alpha-adrenergic antagonist vasodilator, but the combination possesses other attributes, including agonist activity at serotonin and dopamine receptor sites. When given for 12 weeks at doses of up to 7.5 mg/day, ergoloid mesylates have been found to reduce confusion, recent memory impairment, depression, and emotional lability (Dysken 1987). Even further improvement in comparison with placebo was noted over a total of 6 months; in that period, no patient on ergoloid mesylates deteriorated, whereas many patients on placebo did do so. The drug is currently being tested further in patients with Alzheimer's disease. Although the recommended dosage range is 1 mg three times a day, this may not be adequate for all patients; in some, higher doses of 9 mg may be needed. Side effects are rarely troublesome. Sublingual irritation can occur with the sublingual preparation, and nausea and gastrointestinal disturbances can also result at times. The medication comes in tablet, liquid capsule, liquid, and sublingual tablet forms.

Other treatments have been used in patients with dementia, all of which must still be considered as experimental and of unproved efficacy. These include physostigmine, choline, lecithin, and tetrahydroaminoacridine (THA). Each of these therapies is discussed in Chapter 12 in the section on cognitive-enhancing drugs in patients with Alzheimer's disease. Still other therapies, including opiate antagonists and hyperbaric oxygen, have been tried but not proved successful.

Gerovital H_3 is an interesting compound that is no longer available, but did show some promise for improving memory, attention span, and concentration (for more detail, see the section on Gerovital H_3 in Chapter 1). The use of piracetam, a cyclic gamma-aminobutyric acid (GABA) derivative, has resulted in some overall general improvement in patients diagnosed as having organic brain syndromes.

Special Considerations

It is important for the physician to understand those factors that determine *compliance* and *drug-taking behavior,* as outlined by Salzman (1982).

Poor vision can make it difficult to read the label and can lead a patient to mistake one pill for another that may visually resemble the first one. Arthritic changes can make it hard to open a safety-capped bottle, to cut a pill in half, or to measure out liquid. Nevertheless, compliance is probably higher in older patients, but it can be adversely affected by the appearance of side effects and also by the fact that many patients are on multiple medications, because compliance is inversely related to the number of medications a person takes. The most commonly used drugs in the older age groups are digoxin, hydrochlorothiazide, hydrochlorothiazide-triamterene, propranolol, diazepam, aspirin, and multiple vitamins (Stewart 1986).

The following example of an outpatient's medication profile, taken from my own clinical practice, illustrates the issues and problems surrounding the question of compliance and the fact that a substantial amount of time needs to be given to medication management at each visit. A 66-year-old man was receiving the following medications: aspirin, 325 mg, 1–2 qid prn; Cerumenex, 1 drop in the ear prn; potassium chloride 10%, 1 teaspoon in the morning; nitroglycerin, 0.4 mg, 1 tablet sublingually prn; diltiazem, 30 mg, 1 tablet qid; tetracycline, 250 mg, 1 capsule q12h; sulfamethoxazole, 500 mg, 2 tablets bid; Xylocaine 5%, administered prn; oxybutynin, 5 mg, 1 tablet tid, prn; L-tryptophan, 500 mg, 3 tablets qhs; phenelzine, 15 mg, 2 tablets bid; trifluoperazine, 2 mg, 2 tablets bid; and chlordiazepoxide, 10 mg, 1 tablet qid, prn. The patient was married, but his wife was unable to play an important role in helping him to keep his medication organized—she was being treated with medication for depression and had health problems of her own, which meant that the patient had to care for her over a protracted period of time. A significant other can definitely assist with medication compliance, but at times such help can give rise to difficulty relinquishing control to another person in the matter of taking medication. A look at this list also illustrates the problems faced by a patient in having to judge whether and when to take some as-needed medications, having to take medicines according to many different schedules, and having to maintain constant awareness as to the dietary and medication precautions that are necessary with the use of an MAOI. The use of a written list and instructions were of great help in managing this case. It has been observed that verbal instructions alone are associated with lower compliance as compared with written guidelines (Wandless and Davie 1977).

The issue of *medication cost* is inadequately appreciated by many physicians, and it is not always easy for either the patient or the doctor to obtain comparative prices. This topic was studied by Weiner et al. (1983), and the reader is referred to this paper for a more complete discussion, but some of the principles can be summarized here:

I Generic products are less expensive than the original brand.

I New drugs cost more than medications that have been marketed for some time.

I Newer drugs that are the sole representatives of their chemical class are usually sold at premium prices, because the manufacturers attempt to recoup high development costs.

I Preparations containing larger doses cost less per milligram than those containing lower doses.

I Prescriptions containing orders for large quantities of medication can often be filled in the pharmacy at a less expensive rate than can prescriptions written for a smaller amount.

Some drugs, such as chlorpromazine and lithium, are remarkably inexpensive, whereas L-tryptophan, the indications for which are less clear, is highly priced. A downside to the use of generic drugs is that, on occasion, they are not bioequivalent for a particular patient who had previously been well stabilized on the brand-name product.

In prescribing for the elderly, it is necessary to begin with *low doses*, as was described for each of the main drug groups in this chapter, and to increase the dose slowly, paying close attention to the symptom picture, to the patient's physiological state, and to the emergence of side effects. Under careful control, many older patients can, in fact, ultimately take full therapeutic drug doses. In patients over age 70, however, dose requirements may be less than those in younger patients. An example of this is the finding that therapeutic levels of nortriptyline can be achieved with dosages of only 30 mg/day in older patients (Dawling et al. 1981). It may often be necessary to adjust the dose of other medications or even to discontinue them as part of psychotropic management.

Coordination with other physicians is sometimes important and should not be overlooked. *Frequent review* is needed, and it is appropriate to periodically reaffirm with patients and/or their relatives that they understand any special conditions and restrictions about their medicine. Although one strives to give medication for the shortest time possible, it must be recognized that older patients very often require long-term medication.

Just as it is essential to medicate when the need exists, so is it important not to medicate unnecessarily. It has been shown, for example, that dementia-related behavior problems can be treated effectively by educational procedures with a resultant 72% decline in antipsychotic drug use and a 36% decline in the use of restraints (Ray et al. 1993).

To obtain the best results from pharmacotherapy in older patients, more than usual care and skill are generally needed; when these are applied, even the most difficult challenges can yield rewarding results.

References

American Psychiatric Association: Diagnostic and Statistical Manual of Mental Disorders, 4th Edition. Washington, DC, American Psychiatric Association, 1994

Austin MVP, Souza FGM, Goodwin GM: Lithium augmentation in antidepressant-resistant patients: a quantitative analysis. Br J Psychiatry 159:510–514, 1991

Avorn J, Dreyer P, Connelly K, et al: Use of psychoactive medication and the quality of care in rest homes: findings and policy implications of a statewide study. N Engl J Med 320:227–232, 1989

Ayd F: Continuation and maintenance antidepressant drug therapy, in Affective Disorders Reassessed 1983. Edited by Ayd FJ, Taylor I, Taylor B. Baltimore, MD, Ayd Medical Communications, 1983, pp 73–99

Bowden CL: Early signs of response to antidepressants. International Drug Therapy Newsletter 10:5–6, 1984

Brymer C, Winegrad CM: Fluoxetine in elderly patients: is there cause for concern? J Am Geriatr Soc 40:902–905, 1992

Churchill-Davidson HC: Anesthesia and monoamine oxidase inhibitors. BMJ 1:520, 1965

Davidson JRT: Seizures and bupropion: a review. J Clin Psychiatry 50:256–261, 1988

Davidson JRT, Zung WWK, Walker JI: Practical aspects of MAO inhibitor therapy. J Clin Psychiatry 45 (7, Sec 2):78–80, 1984

Dawling S, Crome P, Braithwaite RA, et al: Nortriptyline therapy in elderly patients: dosage prediction from plasma concentrations at 24 hours after a single 50-mg dose. Br J Psychiatry 139:413–416, 1981

Dysken M: A review of recent clinical trials in the treatment of Alzheimer's dementia. Psychiatric Annals 17:179–196, 1987

Feighner JP, Herbstein J, Damlooji N: Combined MAOI, TCA and direct stimulant therapy of treatment-resistant depression. J Clin Psychiatry 46:206–209, 1985

Flint A: The optimum duration of antidepressant treatment in the elderly. International Journal of Geriatric Psychiatry 7:617–619, 1992

Frederickson D: Atherosclerosis and other forms of arteriosclerosis, in Principles of Internal Medicine, 7th Edition. Edited by Wintrope MW, Thorn GW, Adams RD, et al. New York, McGraw Hill, 1974, pp 1225–1235

Garza-Travino E, Overall JE, Hollister LE: Verapamil versus lithium in acute mania. Am J Psychiatry 149:121–122, 1992

Georgatas A, McCue RE, Hapworth W, et al: Comparative efficacy and safety of MAOIs versus TCAs in treating depression in the elderly. Biol Psychiatry 21:1155–1166, 1986

Goodstein RK: Common clinical problems in the elderly. Psychiatric Annals 15:299–312, 1985

Granacher RP: Titrating intramuscular dosages for elderly patients (letter). Am J Psychiatry 136:997, 1979

Holloway D: Drug problems in the geriatric patient. Drug Intelligence and Clinical Pharmacy 8:632–642, 1974

Joffe RT, Singer W, Levitt A, et al: A placebo-controlled comparison of lithium and triiodothyronine augmentation of tricyclic antidepressants in unipolar refractory depression. Arch Gen Psychiatry 50:387–393, 1993

Kay DWK: Observations on the natural history and genetics of old age psychoses: Stockholm material 1931–1937. Proceedings of the Royal Society of Medicine 52:791, 1959

Larson DB, Lyons JS, Hollmann AA, et al: Psychotropics prescribed to the US elderly in the early and mid 1980s: prescribing patterns of primary care practitioners, psychiatrists, and other physicians. International Journal of Geriatric Psychiatry 6:63–70, 1991

Mazure CM: Valproate treatment of older psychotic patients with organic mental syndromes and behavioral dyscontrol. J Am Geriatr Soc 40:914–916, 1992

Mor V, McHonrey C, Sherwood S: Secondary morbidity among the recently bereaved. Am J Psychiatry 143:158–163, 1986

Naguib M, McGriffin P, Levy R, et al: Genetic markers in late paraphrenia—study of HLA antigens. Br J Psychiatry 150:124–127, 1987

Post F: The impact of modern drug treatment on old age schizophrenia. Gerontologia Clinica (Basel) 4:137–141, 1962

Post F: Affective disorders in old age, in Handbook of Affective Disorders. Edited by Paykel ES. New York, Guilford, 1984, pp 393–402

Post RM, Uhde TW, Roy-Burne P, et al: Antidepressant effects of carbamazepine. Am J Psychiatry 143:29–34, 1986

Price LH, Charney DS, Heninger GR: Variability of response to lithium augmentation in refractory depressions. Am J Psychiatry 143:1387–1392, 1986

Rabkin J, Quitkin FM, Harrison W, et al: Adverse reactions to monoamine oxidase inhibitors, I: a comparative study. J Clin Psychopharmacol 4:279–288, 1984

Ray WA, Taylor JA, Meador KG, et al: Reducing antipsychotic drug use in nursing homes: a controlled trial of provider education. Arch Intern Med 153:713–721, 1993

Reynolds CF III, Kupfer DJ, Hoch CC, et al: Sleeping pills for the elderly: are they ever justified? J Clin Psychiatry 46 (2, Sec 2):9–12, 1985

Richelson E: Pharmacology of antidepressants in use in the United States. J Clin Psychiatry 43 (11, Sec 2):4–1, 1982

Richey DP: Effects of human aging on drug absorption and metabolism, in The Physiology and Pathology of Human Aging. Edited by Goldman R, Rockstein M, Sussman ML. New York, Academic Press, 1975, pp 59–94

Roose SP, Glassman AH, Giardina EGV, et al: Tricyclic antidepressants in depressed patients with cardiac conduction disease. Arch Gen Psychiatry 44:273–280, 1987

Salzman C: Basic principles of psychiatric drug prescription for the elderly. Hosp Community Psychiatry 33:133–136, 1982

Schatzberg AF, Cole JO: Manual of Clinical Psychopharmacology. Washington, DC, American Psychiatric Press, 1991

Slater E, Roth M (eds): Aging and the mental disorders of the aged, in Clinical Psychiatry. London, Balliere, Tindall & Cassell, 1972, pp 580–586

Spiker DG, Weiss JC, Dealy RS, et al: The pharmacological treatment of delusional depression. Am J Psychiatry 142:430–436, 1985

Stewart RB: Applied pharmacology in the elderly: an overview of the Dunedin program, in Dimensions of Aging. Edited by Bergener M, Ermini M, Staehlin HB. New York, Academic Press, 1986, pp 221–226

Stramek JJ, Simpson GM, Morrison RL, et al: Anticholinergic agents for prophylaxis of neuroleptic-induced dystonic reactions: a prospective study. J Clin Psychiatry 47:305–309, 1986

Task Force on the Use of Laboratory Tests in Psychiatry: Tricyclic antidepressants–blood level measurements and clinical outcome: an APA Task Force Report. Am J Psychiatry 142:163–169, 1985

Tyrer PJ, Owen R, Dowling S: Gradual withdrawal of diazepam after long-term therapy. Lancet 1:1402–1406, 1983

Verwoerdt A: Clinical Geropsychiatry. Baltimore, MD, Williams & Wilkins, 1976

Walker JI, Brodie HKH: Neuropharmacology of aging, in Handbook of Geriatric Psychiatry. Edited by Busse EW, Blazer DG. New York, Van Nostrand Reinhold, 1980, pp 102–124

Walker JI, Davidson JRT, Zung WWK: Patient compliance with MAO inhibitor therapy. J Clin Psychiatry 45 (8, Sec 2):78–80, 1984

Wandless I, Davie JW: Can drug compliance in the elderly be improved? BMJ 1:359–361, 1977

Weiner RD, Coffey CE, Campbell CP, et al: The price of psychotropic drugs: a neglected factor. Hosp Community Psychiatry 34:531–535, 1983

Weissman MM, Tischler GL, Holzer CE, et al: Six-month prevalence of psychiatric disorders in three communities. Arch Gen Psychiatry 41:959–971, 1984

Weissman MM, Prusoff B, Sholomskas A, et al: A double-blind clinical trial of alprazolam, imipramine, or placebo in the depressed elderly. J Clin Psychopharmacol 12:175–182, 1992

Whanger AD, Wang HS: Vitamin B_{12} deficiency in normal aged and psychiatric patients, in Normal Aging, Vol 2. Edited by Palmore E. Durham, NC, Duke University Press, 1974, pp 63–72

Winslow RS, Stillner V, Coors DJ, et al: Prevention of acute dystonic reactions in patients beginning high-potency neuroleptics. Am J Psychiatry 143:706–710, 1986

Woods SW, Tesar GE, Murray GB, et al: Psychostimulant treatment of depressive disorders secondary to medical illness. J Clin Psychiatry 47:12–15, 1986

CHAPTER 21

Diet, Nutrition, and Exercise

Robert J. Sullivan Jr., M.D.

Simply by achieving old age, an individual can be assured that the diet he or she has consumed has been sufficiently nutritious to support life. This is no mean feat in a period when the longevity of human survival has reached limits previously unknown in history. As age increases, lifelong eating habits need periodic reevaluation. Deterioration in taste buds and olfactory sensation makes some foods less palatable. Changes in living habits can alter dietary requirements. The onset of illness creates special diet demands. Both the elderly person and those responsible for the care of elderly individuals must be aware of potential problems with nutrition and diet in order to respond appropriately to challenges of late life.

Exercise habits, like dietary patterns, are easily taken for granted. Few individuals comprehend how vigor declines with each hour of indolence. But decline it does until it adversely affects one's ability to respond to the demands of daily life. The gradual reduction in physical activity that often accompanies late life is also associated with a diminution in appetite. Because a balanced nutrient intake depends on eating a variety of foods, subtle nutrient deficits may follow a faltering intake. This chapter explores how diet, nutrition, and exercise contribute to vigor in late life.

Nutrition

The science of nutrition involves the study of food intake to promote growth and to replace worn or injured tissues. Elderly individuals are vulnerable to nutrition problems as a result of health problems that are unique to their age. In this section, established standards of nutrition are explained, and results of assessments made using those standards are presented.

Documenting Nutritional Status

Clinicians who care for older adults are usually called upon to assess nutritional status in situations in which a *diet history* reveals inadequate intake. In addition to the history, several tools are available to quantitate a deficit. Standard *height/weight tables*, which serve well for nutritional assessment in young and middle-aged individuals, are less reliable in the elderly because of a loss of height due to vertebral compression fractures, kyphosis, and spinal disc collapse. Accordingly, geriatricians instead turn to documenting reserves of protein and fat and to assessing immune function.

Assessment of *body protein stores* involves two components. Somatic protein stores are measured by recording the midarm circumference to assess muscle mass, although this takes some skill and experience to accomplish with accuracy (Grant et al. 1981). Visceral protein stores are determined by measuring serum levels of various marker substances; of these, serum hemoglobin and albumin are the most widely accepted.

Assessment of body *fat stores* permits determination of energy reserves. Water immersion studies (Jackson et al. 1985) are accurate, but difficult and time-consuming to accomplish. Newer techniques using bioelectric impedance, tritium dilution, and dual-photon absorptiometry (Sergi et al. 1993) are technically interesting for research studies, but they involve complex equipment and are costly. Skin-fold measurement by caliper is easily done in the office or at the bedside and remains the standard for daily clinical work (Clark et al. 1993).

Skin tests to ascertain lymphocyte T-cell activity are useful to assess *immune system function.* Intradermal injection of fungal antigens such as Candida or Trichophytin, to which virtually every healthy person is reactive, are commonly utilized. Fresh antigens for injection must be available, and the test takes 48 hours to interpret (Grant et al. 1981). A total lymphocyte count below 1,500/mL is useful as evidence of an inadequate diet and can be quickly determined from routine blood counts.

For the majority of people, a diet history, coupled with documentation of weight, triceps skinfold thickness, midarm circumference, hemoglobin level, albumin level, and a total lymphocyte count will permit adequate evaluation of nutritional status. When applied to healthy elderly persons, these parameters are found to be in close agreement with national norms for all age groups (Burns et al. 1986), suggesting that when abnormalities occur, they do present a true indication of malnutrition and are not simply changes related to aging.

Caloric Intake Profile Over a Lifetime

A fascinating series of studies of rats done more than five decades ago suggested that diet modification can prolong life (McCay et al. 1939). Spartan fare helped these rats to live longer. Total calorie limitation was more important than fat or protein limitation alone, and there could be no deficit of essential nutrients. The ideal program began with limitation in youth and extended throughout the life of the laboratory animal. The precise reason for improved longevity is not yet clear. From recent analysis of longitudinal study data in humans, it is apparent that low weight in the elderly is not necessarily beneficial, but that obesity is a significant problem as well (Andres 1980). Thus, there is active interest in determining the ideal weight for humans throughout life (Andres 1985).

Variation of Nutritional Needs With Age and Health

Based on current data, it appears that for most persons, growing old is not associated with a need for special diet supplements. Caloric needs vary with individual activity level and should be adjusted accordingly. Regular weight checks are the best means of monitoring caloric intake. A stable weight customarily signifies continuing good health.

When illness strikes, nutritional demands can change dramatically. Most individuals compensate spontaneously or have sufficient reserves to tide themselves over acute situations. Should a chronic illness develop, as often happens with elderly persons, specific attention will be needed to ensure adequate nutrition. Heart failure, lung failure, renal failure, chronic infection, and depression all result in weight loss, sometimes of substantial proportions. Studies in cancer patients have implicated humoral substances as being partially responsible for the anorexia that accompanies, and often precedes, overt clinical manifestations of neoplasia (Odell 1978). Dementia is accompanied by weight loss, but the etiology of this process remains unknown. The underlying mechanisms for appetite modulation need further elucidation in order that we might exert a greater influence on this vital function.

Nutrition is often compromised in the course of acute illness. Malnourishment has been found in hospitalized patients at rates varying from 17% to 44% for medical patients and from 30% to 65% for surgical patients (Bienna et al. 1982). Impaired wound healing (Irvin 1978) and reduced immunocompetence (Mullen 1980) have been attributed to malnutrition. Because of the ubiquity of nutrition problems among hospitalized patients, it is essential to record weight on admission and every 3 days thereafter. Laboratory tests to be followed include albumin levels and lymphocyte counts. Nutrition deprivation reaches critical proportions when a patient has been without substantial intake for a period of 10 days or suffers a weight loss exceeding 10% of baseline weight.

Diet

Building on the preceding discussion of nutrition, diet recommendations can be made for daily food consumption to achieve specific health goals. Diet manipulation falls within the tradition of primary, secondary, and tertiary preventive medicine. A well-proportioned diet can prevent the occurrence of malnutrition, obesity, or cachexia (primary prevention). In disease states such as iron deficit, a diet supplement can cure an illness already present (secondary prevention). In diseases such as heart failure, dietary modification can control the course of an illness not otherwise curable by diet alone (tertiary prevention). The following discussion explores diet alternatives in sickness and in health.

Achieving an Adequate Diet

People live to old age in many societies throughout the world despite dietary habits that vary widely. Studies of disease patterns show that dietary preferences affect the kinds of illness experienced by members of a population. Information gleaned from these "natural experiments" has led to specific diet recommendations to capture the beneficial aspects of a particular cuisine. Each new generation has access to dietary alternatives that its predecessors could not have imagined. Frozen foods, irradiated foods, hybrid vegetables, and fast foods were not available in the recent past. Population mobility has expanded the mingling of cultures, with the result that foods from many corners of the earth are widely known and appreciated. These trends yield expanded opportunities to achieve a healthful diet.

Barriers to an adequate diet.   Throughout their lives, people seek to satisfy their basic needs of shelter, food, and security. At times, they encounter unforeseen difficulties in securing these necessities. In terms of diet, there are both major and minor events that pose potentially threatening problems.

Often cited as exerting an important influence on the diets of elderly persons are *social barriers.* In-

adequate financial reserves, poor housing, and limitations in benefit programs make pursuit of a balanced diet difficult (Massachusetts Department of Public Health 1976). Safety of access and distance to food markets are problems for residents of major cities. Those living in rural areas experience similar isolation when the ability to drive is lost or family members depart. The death of a spouse or housemate who prepared meals may be a devastating blow. Without the means for getting food to the table, no one can consume a balanced diet.

Even when adequate food is available, *sensory changes* can interfere with adequate dietary intake. People who eat alone often fail to prepare sophisticated or varied fare, with a resultant decline in consumption volume and variety. Dental problems reduce the types of food that can be masticated (Wayler et al. 1984). Vision limitations due to cataracts or glaucoma make food preparation and consumption problematic. Fear of a public display of food-soiled clothes or a messy table can lead vision-impaired individuals to withdraw from congregate meals and associated social interactions. With increasing age, subtle shifts in gustatory senses occur. Disease or medication use can have a similar impact. Particularly distressing are the effects of dysosmia or dysgeusia (altered smell and taste), whereby common aromas or flavors are perceived as distinctly unpleasant (Schiffman 1983). Substantial changes in food preference are an inevitable consequence.

Medications can enhance the need for specific dietary supplements (Watkin 1983). Trimethoprim and dilantin are associated with increased need for vitamins D and K and folic acid. The use of barbiturates, cholestyramine, and aspirin calls for extra folic acid, iron, and vitamin C in the diet. Alcohol, neomycin, cholestyramine, and cholchicine influence fat-soluble vitamin absorption. The list goes on and on. Because treatments are usually brief, and nutrients are abundant in a normal diet, deficits are rarely encountered.

Because it is chronic and progressive, altered *anatomic function* with age may alter dietary requirements in ways that are not easily overcome with a normal diet. Atrophic gastritis, often clinically undetected, affects the absorption of several nutritional factors, with both reductions and elevations documented (Krasinske et al. 1986). Altered intestinal transit time with aging is a factor of importance. Fortunately, in the absence of surgical removal or alteration of intestinal integrity, elderly persons usually absorb sufficient nutrients to remain healthy if their diet contains a reasonable blend of needed components.

Diet as Preventive Therapy (Primary Prevention)

In some circumstances, diet modification is capable of disease alleviation, if not outright cure. With the passage of time, more health problems can be expected to join the list, of which a few examples follow.

Dehydration. The elderly lose sensitivity to dehydration (Phillips et al. 1984), especially if they become demented (Seymour et al. 1980) or are being treated with diuretics. Therapy requires maintenance of sufficient water intake so that the body can perform normal adjustments to maintain renal integrity and electrolyte balance. A fluid intake of 2,000 mL/day is recommended as a minimum. Juice, coffee, tea, milk, and other liquids constituting the daily diet are combined in calculating total consumption.

Atherosclerosis. The value of a normal serum cholesterol level in reducing cardiovascular disease risk is well established (Kuske and Feldman 1987). Diet modification can play a major role in reducing body cholesterol levels, yielding involution in atherosclerotic lesions (Kannel 1986). Stroke, myocardial infarction, claudication, renal failure, visual decline, and other degenerative processes are favorably influenced in the bargain. Alcohol will raise the high-density lipoprotein ratio favorably if consumed in modest amounts of 2 ounces or less daily (Friedman and Lieber 1983).

Although cholesterol control has known value for younger individuals, there is uncertainty about emphasis on this modality for the elderly. It is possible that vigorous dietary modifications will lead to diminished palatability and a reduction in intake or an unbalanced program of nutrition in elderly individuals. It is reasonable to permit cholesterol elevations to rise over published norms for those in their eighth and ninth decades.

Diverticulosis. In the past, fiber was thought to irritate colons with diverticulae. However, intraluminal recording devices subsequently revealed that enhanced dietary fiber intake actually reduced pressure and therefore could contribute to a reduction in diverticulae formation. Epidemiological studies of populations known to consume high-fiber diets support this conclusion. For this reason, and for reasons mentioned elsewhere in this chapter, dietary fiber now is emphasized as a daily dietary constituent.

Cancer. Some diet components are known carcinogens. Nitrosamines, produced by fats dripping on hot coals and redeposited with smoke on barbecued or charred meat, are considered examples. Salt-preserved foods are also suspect (Sugimura and Sato 1983). Stomach cancer is on the decline in the United States, where smoked or salted foods are infrequently consumed in comparison with foods preserved by other methods.

Fiber in the diet may protect against cancer by several mechanisms. It speeds transit of fecal material through the body while it binds noxious elements (including deoxycholic acid and lithocholic acid), thus reducing gut contact time (Hill et al. 1971). The relatively low incidence of colon cancer in developing countries is explained in part by the high fiber content of primitive diets (Armstrong and Doll 1975). High fiber consumption can cause problems for some people, however. Some minerals and drugs are bound by dietary fiber, thus reducing their absorption. Enhanced gas production resulting from bacterial action on gut fiber may be physically uncomfortable and socially inhibiting. On the whole, though, the advantages of increasing dietary fiber outweigh the problems.

Despite scientific evidence suggesting correlations between dietary constituents and cancer, there is no unanimity of opinion about specific dietary modifications for cancer risk reduction (Committee on Diet, Nutrition and Cancer 1982). Factors such as smoking or environmental pollutants and carcinogens may wield a much greater influence than does diet (Pariza 1984).

Diet as Therapeutic Intervention (Secondary Prevention)

In disease states that involve discrete nutrient deficits, it is sometimes possible to cure the condition by supplementing intake of the needed item.

Iron deficiency. Iron is found in red meat and certain vegetables. Most older persons easily maintain sufficient iron reserves through consumption of their normal diet. Acute blood loss such as that resulting from trauma, or chronic blood loss such as occurs with occult gastrointestinal bleeding, are common reasons for an iron deficit. Whenever iron-store depletion is found, it is essential to seek a reason for blood loss. Once a diagnosis is made and effective treatment has returned the body to stability, an iron deficit can be treated by dietary supplements. The usual course of therapy returns iron stores to normal within 3–6 months.

Lactase deficiency. Many adults gradually lose the ability to digest lactose, the milk sugar, as a result of the steady decline in intestinal lactase levels with each passing year. Lactase deficiency creates uncomfortable symptoms of gas production, diarrhea, and cramping within an hour or two of eating dairy products. The degree of lactase decline is variable, and some people must avoid all foods containing lactose.

Alleviation of symptoms is achieved with total elimination of milk products for a period of 3 days. A reintroduction of foods will then delineate the level at which symptoms reappear. Acidophilus milk and yogurt contain bacteria that digest the lactose molecule, thus bypassing the need for endogenous lactase. Some cheeses are also low in lactose. Many persons find specific dairy products that can be consumed without discomfort.

Diet and Disease Control (Tertiary Prevention)

In certain disease states, nutritional changes can have a positive influence in controlling the impact or progression of a pathological process.

Osteoporosis. The cause of osteoporosis is unclear. It is related to a complex interaction of vitamin D, calcium, and estrogen within the body, coupled with weight-bearing activity. Kyphosis, hip fractures, and collapse of spinal vertebrae are among the common sequelae of this disease, which is estimated to result in over 70,000 fractures yearly. Very few people want to look old and bent, and so the search for a control of osteoporosis is driven by both cosmetic and medical considerations.

Dietary calcium deficiency among older persons is commonly found when community surveys of eating habits are undertaken. Since bones deficient in calcium are weak, logic suggests that calcium supplements could reduce the impact of osteoporosis. Regrettably, however, there may be adverse consequences of calcium supplementation. Intestinal discomfort is common, with symptoms of bloating or stomach pain. Constipation may develop, sometimes of major proportions. Absorption of excessive calcium can lead to renal stone formation. These side effects perhaps are acceptable if bone integrity is maintained in the bargain.

The administration of fluoride has been found to influence calcium balance favorably by creating an increase in bone density. High-dose fluoride supplementation causes irritation to the stomach lining. Regrettably, new bone formed in response to supplemental fluoride intake is somewhat brittle and may fail to improve weight-bearing ability or resistance to fracture as much as originally hoped (Bernstein and Cohen 1967).

Glucose regulation. Diabetics need multiple interventions to successfully control their disease, and one of the most important interventions involves diet. Achieving an ideal weight through a reduction of total calorie intake is important in cases due to insulin resistance in which obesity is a contributing factor. Maintenance of blood sugar levels as close to normal as possible is essential to avoid microvascular deterioration. Attention to dietary balance and timing is the foundation of all therapeutic efforts for sugar regulation and thus a reduction in disease complications.

Vascular volume modification. In patients with heart failure and some forms of hypertension, an attempt is made to modify intravascular volume by limiting dietary sodium intake. Edema may be reduced and blood pressure normalized by this relatively simple intervention. Unfortunately, sodium is found in many foods and so intake is difficult to avoid. Many persons find foods devoid of sodium to be lacking in flavor and therefore unappetizing. When intake cannot be lowered or proves ineffective, diuretic therapy may be necessary to alter sodium balance.

In patients with renal failure who develop edema, sodium restriction may be detrimental if it creates a reduction in vascular volume that leads to a loss of renal perfusion pressure. Such an illness requires skilled care with precise diet adjustment to optimize function.

Systemic illness. In the preceding examples, discrete dietary components are supplemented or altered to manage specific deficits. Many illness conditions call for broad dietary interventions to stem a tide of adverse effects set in motion by the underlying pathological process. Systemic infections create metabolic demands at a time when the patient may not wish to eat. Patients who have had a stroke may be unable to eat because of paralysis, confusion, or unconsciousness. Comprehensive diet augmentation is necessary to offset the demands of illness in these settings. Fortunately, food supplements are available that feature a balanced array of nutrients suitable for consumption as a beverage, for infusion through a feeding tube, or for infusion directly into a vein if required. Hospitals and long-term care facilities employ nutritionists who are skilled at recognizing and treating deficits associated with dietary limitations imposed by ill health and at recommending solutions.

Specific Dietary Recommendations

Drawing on the preceding discussions, a number of dietary suggestions can be made for healthy individuals. Adjustments can then be made to meet the special requirements imposed by disease states.

Calories and water. The total fluid intake should be over 2,000 mL/day. Calories from all sources should be about 30 kcal/kg, with attention to weight change as an indication of success in management.

Protein. The daily protein intake should be approximately 12.5% of total calories. High levels of protein consumption have been shown to lower body calcium by increasing renal exertion (Marsh et al. 1980), and may contribute to a gradual decline in renal function as well (Brenner et al. 1982).

Fat. Consumption of fats should be modest to keep weight within accepted limits and should emphasize the polyunsaturated forms when possible. A diet with about 10% of calories as monounsaturated

fat, 10% as polyunsaturated fat, and 10% saturated fat—and with less than 300 mg/day of cholesterol—is ideal.

Carbohydrates. Carbohydrates consisting of refined sugars and complex carbohydrates, starches, and fiber complete the daily diet. The major role of sugar is to provide energy, whereas the more complex carbohydrate molecules provide dietary fiber.

Fiber. Dietary fiber includes cellules and fibrils of vegetable origin, including cellulose, hemicelluloses, and pectins. Gums and mucilage from plant secretory cells represent another portion of the fiber spectrum. Although they are not absorbed as nutrients, these carbohydrate molecules exert numerous beneficial effects, as previously mentioned. Figs, prunes, raisins, fresh fruits, and vegetables are particularly rich sources of fiber and are recommended for daily consumption. Vegetarians, who necessarily consume substantial fiber daily, have excellent lipid profiles (Fisher et al. 1986).

Minerals. Recommendations regarding the mineral content of the diet usually start with *sodium*. About 2 g daily is adequate for health, a level that can be found easily in the ordinary diet without the addition of salt. In bygone days, salt supplementation of food was rare, except among the wealthy. Nowadays, with salt shakers found on the table wherever food is served, salt is overused. Fortunately, in the absence of disease, the body is capable of discarding excess sodium in the urine, where it does no harm.

Iron is found in abundance in a balanced diet and is readily absorbed. In the absence of iron-loss disease, no supplemental sources are required.

Calcium intake for older men and women should be in the neighborhood of 1,500 mg/day, primarily from natural foods. For most adults, this means consuming some dairy products daily. Calcium carbonate tablets are an alternative supplemental source for people who are unable to consume dairy products. Calcium citrate is used if achlorhydria is present. Fluoride supplements are not recommended due to toxicity and the absence of proven value (Riggs et al. 1980).

The *zinc* content of a regular diet meets bodily requirements with ease. Zinc supplementation has been touted as a means to encourage wound healing and to stimulate immune cell function (Sandstead et al. 1982), and is often considered for individuals suffering from chronic decubitus ulcers. If the dietary intake is balanced and adequate for maintenance of a normal weight, especially when patients are using commercial liquid dietary supplements, zinc needs should be easily achieved without additional supplementation.

Iodine is needed for normal thyroid function. Commonly found in soil, iodine is consumed in adequate quantities with vegetables and fruits. Where the soil is iodine depleted, supplementation is necessary. Since iodized salt is widely available, iodine depletion is now virtually nonexistent throughout the United States.

Trace elements, including magnesium, copper, chromium, silicone, manganese, cobalt, and selenium, are readily available in a mixed diet, and supplements are not currently recommended. The role of these minerals in hypertension and heart disease is receiving close attention, which may lead to dietary recommendations in the future (Kannel 1986).

Vitamins. Most vitamins that are necessary for the maintenance of metabolism are readily found in the food of a balanced diet. Although vitamin supplements are often recommended to alleviate fatigue or malaise, there is little likelihood that a significant improvement will be appreciated at intake beyond the minimum daily requirements. This has not stopped the widespread promotion of vitamin supplements by salespersons who represent various retail outlets for such products.

After vitamin C, *vitamin A* is the second most popular vitamin purchased as a specific supplement. The closely related compound *beta-carotene* is currently under active investigation. It may reduce cancer incidence throughout the body by favorably influencing host defenses or by trapping free radicals that would otherwise induce cell damage (Krinsky and Deneke 1982). Sufficient quantities of vitamin A are present in yellow vegetables to meet our nutritional needs. Although excessive carotene consumption does not result in toxic effects, vitamin A itself can cause adverse effects when taken in large quantities.

Individual components of the *vitamin B group* are often sold in drug and nutrition stores in combination or individual formulations. *Vitamin B$_{12}$* and

folic acid are among the best known of this collection. A balanced diet has more than adequate resources to meet dietary minimums of all these substances. Alcoholic individuals may require folic acid supplements, particularly when their habit prevents adequate dietary intake. Persons deficient in vitamin B$_{12}$ will need intramuscular injections or concentrated oral supplements, as their absorption is often impaired.

Vitamin C has been in the headlines for years since Dr. Linus Pauling promoted its value as a cold remedy. Regrettably, overuse of this vitamin has toxic effects. It has the potential to create renal oxalate stones, diarrhea, and vitamin B$_{12}$ absorption difficulties if used in excess (Chalmers 1975). Recent advances in understanding the role of antioxidants in the aging process may alter our appreciation of the role of this vitamin. Vitamin C may be protective due to its influence on immune mechanisms, inhibition of nitrosamine formation in the stomach, and antioxidative effects (Willett and MacMahon 1984). Reliance on a balanced diet alone is sufficient for maintenance of needed tissue levels.

Vitamin D is synthesized in the body wherever sunlight is available. As little as 15 minutes of sun exposure twice weekly is enough to meet bodily demands. Where no sunlight is available, oral supplementation with 400 units of vitamin D daily is sufficient. Amounts in excess of that level may lead to renal stone formation (Weisman et al. 1984).

Vitamin E is known to serve as an intracellular antioxidant and may prove to be protective against cancer (Bieri et al. 1983; Willett and MacMahon 1984). Vitamin E is found in adequate amounts in a regular diet, and supplements have no proven value.

Summary

A balanced diet can be selected that meets nutritional needs quite well, even late in life. Acute nutritive deficiencies are uncommon in the United States, although the incidence and impact of lifelong marginal deficiencies remain to be delineated. Cultural differences have provided insights regarding components of diets that yield the greatest benefit for disease prevention and therapy. Adoption of those specific components as part of one's daily intake can be expected to pay long-term dividends in terms of overall health.

Exercise

Along with diet, exercise receives insufficient attention in terms of its potential contribution to a healthy and full life. Exercise is a subcategory of physical activity that is planned, structured, repetitive, and purposive (Caspersen et al. 1985). If regularly done, it contributes to the development of physical fitness—defined as the ability to carry out daily tasks with vigor and alertness, without undue fatigue, and with ample energy to enjoy leisure-time pursuits and meet unforeseen emergencies (President's Council on Physical Fitness and Sports 1971). In the following discussion we explore the value of, and the problems associated with, an exercise program.

Correlation of Age and Inactivity

There is a remarkable similarity between growing old and being inactive (Bortz 1982). When forced to be immobile, the body of a youth will quickly lose vigor and begin to look old. Balance becomes unsteady, and strength declines in any adult who withdraws from an active lifestyle. This apparent correlation between aging and inactivity is remarkable. The value of such an observation lies in the opportunity to recover lost function (Posner et al. 1986). Although one can never reclaim lost years of age, lost physical conditioning due to inactivity that mimics aging can be reversed, with remarkable benefits (Larson and Bruce 1987).

Etiology of Inactivity

When the opportunity arises to participate in exercise programs, older persons are less likely than their more youthful counterparts to step forward (Ades et al. 1987). Several possible reasons for this reluctance can be postulated, as outlined below.

Lack of knowledge regarding exercise value or methods. In the past, the conception of exercise as an enjoyable activity was eclipsed by one equating it with painful exertion or competitive endeavors. Changes in the understanding of physical conditioning have altered that image considerably. It is now appropriate for persons of all ages and both genders to exercise. Sport and competition may be engaged in if desired, but numerous noncompeti-

tive options are also available. This new perception of exercise has not been embraced by many elderly people.

Fear of injury. Among the concerns voiced by older persons when contemplating an exercise program are fears of muscle injury or of falling and possibly sustaining a bone fracture. Many worry about triggering a heart attack if they exert themselves. The key to avoiding such risks is to engage only in fitness activities that are within the limits imposed by disease, disuse, or inherited conditions. Virtually everyone can undertake a properly tailored program with the confidence that no harm will be done. Preexercise evaluation by a physician will delineate the limits that an individual should observe. Within those limits, regular exercise will maintain physical capacity, yielding significantly improved resources for participation in the activities of daily life.

Lack of time. A lack of time to participate in exercise activities is frequently cited as a critical factor by youthful persons eligible for fitness programs (Godin et al. 1985). Before retirement, work demands may indeed impose substantial limits on time availability. After retirement, even with involvement in numerous activities, most individuals have sufficient flexibility that they can establish their own priorities and place exercise among the items they consider essential, should they choose to do so.

Lack of access to resources. One problem encountered by all individuals who are interested in a physical conditioning program is access to suitable resources. The cost of membership at an exercise facility, the distance from home to the facility, the presence of exercise periods specifically dedicated to older members at the facility, and companionship while exercising are important considerations that affect participation.

There are many alternatives to a facility-centered exercise program. Often, one can make use of resources close at hand to accomplish similar physical development. Rapid walking is an extremely effective, inexpensive, and enjoyable exercise that can be done in the immediate home environment. When coupled with stretching and upper body exercises, such a program can be used to achieve and maintain a remarkable level of fitness.

Lack of interest in exercise. There is a large group of individuals who simply lack the motivation to be active (Dishman et al. 1985). Physical inactivity among the elderly is not unique to modern Western society and may represent a cross-cultural phenomenon (Beall et al. 1985). Because exercise programs are voluntary, people who join them are self-selected as perceiving significant value in the undertaking, and studies utilizing such groups are subject to bias.

To minimize participant dropout and maximize attendance, emphasis on companionship among the participants and close attention to graded advancements of effort is helpful. Inclusion of an education component, with attention to the special needs of smokers or obese patients, is also beneficial (Moritznik et al. 1985).

Types of Activity

Exercise program components have evolved over a number of years and continue to change as research indicates special value for particular aspects. Flexibility, strength, and endurance are the three elements around which any program is built. Although an individual exercise may target only one of these elements, there is considerable overlap in the end result. Thus, a weight-lifting program designed to build strength also produces enhanced endurance and flexibility.

Limbering and flexibility. First among the activities that any individual should do at the start of an exercise session are limbering and warm-up exercises, followed by gentle stretching and flexing. The goal is to prepare ligaments and muscles for the strengthening and endurance activities to follow. Injuries are much less likely to occur if a proper warm-up is undertaken.

Limbering and warm-up exercises can be done in any open space. Chair exercises are available for those incapable of standing because of balance problems or weakness. Floor mats are useful, as many of the activities require lying on one's side or back. When available, a pool with water at chest height is a great asset for flexibility training. The maintenance of flexibility has daily value for activities such as donning clothes, trimming toenails, and attending to personal hygiene.

Strength. Physical conditioning programs traditionally emphasize development of specific muscle groups for a particular sport or event. The same concept applies to conditioning programs for life. An individual must have sufficient strength to carry out daily activities. Muscle cells developed in youth persist throughout life, representing banked reserves waiting to be used. Building muscle strength is accomplished by contraposing muscle contraction against resistance. Weight lifting is the traditional method used for this purpose. Machines have been devised that permit every muscle fiber in the body to be selectively laden with precisely the ideal pull to extract maximum development. Resistance devices using hydraulic pistons are available in which the load can be adjusted by twisting a dial. Hydraulic apparatus can resist motion in two directions, thereby speeding reciprocal muscle development in one exercise effort.

Homegrown alternatives to professional weight equipment are legion. Sacks filled with sand, strips of rubber tubing, and water-filled bags lifted by ropes on pulleys fastened to doors are but a few of the ingenious ways to provide resistance for muscle development. Vigorous walking or regular stair-climbing are remarkably effective, inexpensive, and available methods to encourage musculoskeletal development.

Endurance. The third part of a fitness program involves enhancement of the cardiovascular system to improve endurance. *Aerobic conditioning* is the term used to describe training that requires an individual to stay within limits that permit inhaled oxygen to fully supply the needs of the body during exercise. The body responds by increasing its efficiency of oxygen transport and use from the lungs to each individual cell component. Improved oxygen use permits extended periods of muscle activity without fatigue. This aspect of physical conditioning is documented by measuring oxygen consumption during maximum exercise exertion (VO_2 max).

Endurance and strength aspects of conditioning are distinct. One has only to compare a wrestler and a long-distance runner to see the archetypes of these two concepts. Most elderly individuals will benefit more from a track-style development program than from a wrestler approach: a person can always get help to move the sofa, but no one can help him or her walk briskly down the sidewalk in time to catch the next bus.

Activity Initiation

Getting involved in exercise after years of inconsistent exertion calls for careful planning. Injuries to the musculoskeletal or cardiovascular system should be avoided while precariously balanced medical conditions are managed effectively. Physical limitations must be identified, specific exercises selected, monitoring parameters chosen, and exertion ranges established. Regular reassessment is then needed to upgrade the program in response to participant progress.

Injury risk assessment.   Medical investigation should focus on identifying occult problems such as diabetes, thyroid conditions, anemia, or electrolyte imbalance. The circulatory system, orthopedic conditions, and any physical deformities must receive particular attention because of the limits they may impose on exertion. Lung disease and asthma may restrict needed ventilation, whereas neurological disease can alter balance, coordination, or muscle use. Dementia of a severity that precludes the understanding of exercise limits must disqualify an exercise applicant unless a sponsor will always be on hand to provide guidance. Medication review must document items that will alter performance indicators. Beta-blocker medications, for example, will lower pulse rates; this must be taken into account in establishing a proper training range for the pulse. Medication review occasionally uncovers the presence of a disease not previously documented that might affect an exercise prescription, and such a review provides an index of disease severity.

Fitness assessment.   Initial evaluation should include a flexibility assessment to evaluate the applicant's ability to participate in established workout routines and to identify any need for special attention. Muscle strength can be measured accurately by means of devices developed for disability determination. Although such baseline data will provide a satisfying measure of progress for the participant, they are rarely obtained in community exercise programs outside of the medical care system. More commonly, strength is assessed in terms of adequacy to accomplish daily tasks. If specific activities cannot be performed, such as rising from a chair, then strengthening of the involved muscle groups is undertaken.

Endurance assessment involves simultaneous performance by two interrelated body functions. First, the individual must have musculoskeletal strength and flexibility to do physical work. Second, the cardiovascular system must be able to respond to the oxygen transport challenge imposed by that work. Bicycle ergometry and treadmill testing are two standard means of assessing endurance, which is valuable for establishing the limits of a safe exercise program. Endurance is measured in terms of metabolic equivalents (METS), where sitting is given a value of 1 and top exertion, 24. Older persons commonly enter a program with a performance level of 6–8 METS.

Program organization.   The value of group versus solo exercise programs is the subject of some debate (Miller et al. 1984). Exercising by oneself yields the maximum versatility in terms of scheduling and privacy with generally good results (DeBusk et al. 1985). Group exercise programs are widely available at fitness centers, community agencies such as the YMCA/YWCA, and city recreation departments. The majority cater to persons with no known physical impediments. Some programs are tailored exclusively to special needs of those recovering from an illness such as myocardial infarction. All supervised programs incorporate many weeks of gradually increasing exertion with careful observation for untoward events. During this time, the participant is taught principles of safe and effective exercise that can be applied throughout the remainder of the participant's life.

Many people skip preevaluation and plunge into a self-designed exercise program without hesitation. Of course, the majority do very well with this approach, especially when they are prudent in listening to signals that their bodies convey about exercise limits. An ideal program includes a 5-minute limbering and warm-up period, followed by a 30-minute exercise period during which the heart rate is kept in a target training range previously determined as ideal. This is followed by a gradual cooldown period for an additional 10 minutes. Each part of this sequence is important for safe and effective exercise.

One aspect of exercise that is often misunderstood is the tremendous value that accrues at submaximal exertion levels (Badenhop et al. 1983). One need not punish the body to vastly improve physical performance (Sidney and Shephard 1978). A person should be comfortable at all times and easily able to converse while exercising. Most important of all, the person should enjoy the process.

Benefits of Exercise

The benefits of exercise are thought to reach beyond the simple enhancement of muscle performance. Self-image and emotional stability, although reported to improve by some investigators (Taylor et al. 1985), may not change much (Blumenthal et al. 1982). Whereas weight control is facilitated by an increase in caloric consumption related to exercise, obesity is ultimately determined by food intake (Blair et al. 1985). Nutrition can be enhanced by physical exertion, provided that an increased caloric intake is associated with greater variety in the diet. Weight-bearing activity improves bone calcium metabolism and strength. Control of hypertension and diabetes may be favorably affected as well (Siscovick et al. 1985). Oxygen use is improved, and the circulatory system receives substantial benefit (Cunningham et al. 1987; deVries 1970). Serum lipid reduction, collateral development in the peripheral and coronary circulation, and increased cardiac muscle reserve are noted to occur (Bortz 1980).

Virtually all who partake of regular exercise programs report an improved ability to manage their activities of daily living. They are less dependent on motorized resources such as elevators or automobiles and can participate in more activities without fatigue. Moreover, they are delighted to find that former vigor can be successfully recalled.

Hazards of Exercise

The majority of older persons experience few problems as they undertake exercise as part of a fitness program. The benefits are assumed to outweigh the risks, provided that appropriate limits are set and cautious advances are undertaken (Koplan et al. 1985).

Of greatest concern is the possibility of sudden death induced by exercise. If a careful physical evaluation has been made in advance and the patient cooperates by observing established limits, there is little likelihood that the exercise will constitute a significant risk (VanCamp and Peterson 1986). In the long run, there will be a risk reduction resulting from the program (Siscovick et al. 1985).

The risk of musculoskeletal injuries can be kept to a minimum by attending to proper warm-up routines, using good equipment during the workout, and avoiding overexertion. Osteoarthritis flares are a constant concern that may limit or terminate the experiment. For many, exercise will strengthen supporting muscles and yield improved joint use. Pool exercises with motion against water resistance are remarkably effective and safe for arthritic patients. When arthritis flares do occur, rest and antiinflammatory medication are the only recourse. Restarting exercise later with altered routines may protect fragile joints.

Osteoporosis presents significant risks for the elderly patient. Falls of any nature can lead to fractures, particularly of the hip and wrist. Vertebral collapse can be terribly painful. When fractures occur, total cessation of exercise is required until healing is complete. In most cases, reinstitution of exercise is then appropriate. There is some comfort in knowing that weight-bearing activity will strengthen bone. Some particularly fragile persons must limit exercise to a pool, where falls are impossible and stress is greatly reduced.

Thermal condition during exercise requires attention, because older persons often fail to appreciate extremes of heat or cold. Avoiding outside exercise in freezing weather is essential. Warm clothing is needed whenever the temperature is below 60 °F. Temperatures above 80 °F are likewise troublesome, especially if the humidity is high. Brisk walking in shopping malls has become popular because of year-round stable temperatures, an interesting environment, solid footing, and the availability of help if problems occur.

Fatigue may be a complaint of the exercise program participant. This usually represents an overly vigorous approach to physical exertion. However, close watch must be kept for congestive heart failure or other medical conditions that have become unbalanced and are manifesting as systemic complaints. Prior screening of exercise candidates should exclude those whose medical status is too precarious to undertake an active fitness program. The risks are minimized by maintaining the target intensity of 60%–70% of maximal heart rate (Larson and Bruce 1987). Within this range, comfortable, safe, and effective programs can be created to keep most of us feeling far younger than our chronological years of age would suggest.

Conclusions

Intensive efforts are under way to find the optimum nutrition elements throughout life that will reduce the likelihood of developing disease. At this time, there are a number of trends worth following, of which limitation of fat intake and regular consumption of fiber seem of greatest value. Provided that we are able to eat a balanced diet, our nutrition status should maintain itself with no need for supplementation. Supplements, if used at all, should include only calcium. With disease states, special attention to nutrition is essential for recovery or control. Numerous helpful diet modifications can be prescribed that may control illness with little or no need for medications.

Physical exertion, when enjoyed as part of an ongoing fitness program, can make older persons feel and act younger than their chronological years. Care is necessary when initiating any activity change, but experience has shown that reserves from early life can be recalled to active service without undue hardship. The improvement in activities of daily living and the potential for expanding one's resources for dealing with stress or illness make exercise an attractive element in a program of health promotion or maintenance.

References

Ades PA, Hanson JS, Gunther PGS, et al: Exercise conditioning in the elderly coronary patient. J Am Geriatr Soc 35:121–124, 1987

Andres R: Influence of obesity on longevity in the aged. Advances in Pathobiology 7:238–246, 1980

Andres R: Impact of age on weight goals. Ann Intern Med 103:1030–1033, 1985

Armstrong B, Doll R: Environmental factors and cancer incidence and mortality in different countries with special reference to dietary practices. Int J Cancer 15:617–631, 1975

Badenhop DT, Cleary PA, Schaal SF, et al: Physiological adjustments to higher- or lower-intensity exercise in elders. Med Sci Sports Exerc 15:496–502, 1983

Beall CM, Goldstein MC, Feldman ES: Social structure and intracohort variation in physical fitness among elderly males in a traditional third world society. J Am Geriatr Soc 33:406–412, 1985

Bernstein DS, Cohen P: Use of sodium fluoride in the treatment of osteoporosis. J Clin Endocrinol Metab 27:197–210, 1967

Bienna R, Ratcliff S, Barbour GL, et al: Malnutrition in the hospitalized geriatric patient. J Am Geriatr Soc 30:433–437, 1982

Bieri JG, Coras L, Hubbard VS: Medical uses of vitamin E. N Engl J Med 308:1063–1071, 1983

Blair SN, Jacobs DR, Powell KE: Relationships between exercise or physical activity and other health behaviors. Public Health Rep 100:172–180, 1985

Blumenthal JA, Schocken DD, Needles TL, et al: Psychological and physiological effects of physical conditioning on the elderly. J Psychosom Res 26:505–510, 1982

Bortz WM: Effect of exercise on aging—effect of aging on exercise. J Am Geriatr Soc 28:49–51, 1980

Bortz WM: Disuse and aging. JAMA 248:1203–1208, 1982

Brenner BM, Meyer TW, Hostetter TH: Dietary protein intake and the progressive nature of kidney disease: the role of hemodynamically mediated glomerular injury in the pathogenesis of progressive glomerular sclerosis in aging, renal ablation and intrinsic renal disease. N Engl J Med 307:652–659, 1982

Burns R, Nichols L, Calkins E, et al: Nutritional assessment of community-living well elderly. J Am Geriatr Soc 34:781–786, 1986

Caspersen CJ, Powell KE, Christenson GM: Physical activity, exercise, and physical fitness: definitions and distinctions for health-related research. Public Health Rep 100:126–131, 1985

Chalmers TC: Effects of ascorbic acid on the common cold: an evaluation of the evidence. Am J Med 58:532–536, 1975

Clark RR, Kuta JM, Sullivan JC: Prediction of percent body fat in adult males using dual energy x-ray absorptiometry, skinfolds, and hydrostatic weighing. Med Sci Sports Exerc 25:528–535, 1993

Committee on Diet, Nutrition and Cancer: Diet nutrition and cancer. Washington, DC, National Academy Press, 1982

Cunningham DA, Rechnitzer PA, Howard JH, et al: Exercise training of men at retirement: a clinical trial. J Gerontol 42:17–23, 1987

DeBusk RF, Haskell WL, Miller NH, et al: Medically directed at-home rehabilitation soon after clinically uncomplicated acute myocardial infarction: a new model for patient care. Am J Cardiol 55:251–257, 1985 deVries HA: Physiological effects of an exercise training regimen upon men aged 52 to 88. J Gerontol 25:325–336, 1970

Dishman RK, Sallis JF, Orenstein DR: The determinants of physical activity and exercise. Public Health Rep 100:158–171, 1985

Fisher M, Levine PH, Weiner B, et al: The effect of vegetarian diets on plasma lipid and platelet levels. Arch Intern Med 146:1193–1197, 1986

Friedman HS, Lieber CS: Alcohol and the heart, in Nutrition and Heart Disease (Contemporary Issues in Clinical Nutrition, Vol 6). Edited by Feldman EB. New York, Churchill Livingstone, 1983, pp 145–164

Godin G, Shephard RJ, Colantonio A: The cognitive profile of those who intend to exercise but do not. Public Health Rep 100:521–526, 1985

Grant JP, Custer PB, Thurlow J: Current techniques of nutritional assessment. Surg Clin North Am 61:437–463, 1981

Hill MJ, Crowther JS, Drasar BS, et al: Bacteria and aetiology of cancer of large bowel. Lancet 1:95–100, 1971

Irvin TT: Effects of malnutrition and hyperalimentation on wound healing. Surg Gynecol Obstet 146:33–36, 1978

Jackson AS, Pollock ML: Practical assessment of body composition. Phys Sportsmed 13:76–90, 1985

Kannel WB: Nutritional contributors to cardiovascular disease in the elderly. J Am Geriatr Soc 34:27–36, 1986

Koplan JP, Siscovick DS, Goldbaum GM: The risks of exercise: a public health view of injuries and hazards. Public Health Rep 100:189–195, 1985

Krasinske SD, Russell RM, Samloff IM, et al: Fundic atrophic gastritis in an elderly population: effect on hemoglobin and several serum nutritional indicators. J Am Geriatr Soc 34:800–806, 1986

Krinsky NI, Deneke SM: The interaction of oxygen and oxy-radicals with carotenoids. Journal of the National Cancer Institute 69:205–210, 1982

Kuske TT, Feldman EB: Hyperlipoproteinemia, atherosclerosis risk, and dietary management. Arch Intern Med 147:357–360, 1987

Larson EB, Bruce RA: Health benefits of exercise in an aging society. Arch Intern Med 147:353–356, 1987

Marsh AG, Sanchez RB, Mickelsen O: Cortical bone density of adult lacto-ovo-vegetarian and omnivorous women. J Am Diet Assoc 76:148–151, 1980

Massachusetts Department of Public Health: Determining the needs of the elderly and chronically disabled. N Engl J Med 294:110–111, 1976

McCay L, Maynard L, Sperling G, et al: Retarded growth, life span, ultimate body size and age changes in the albino rat after feeding diets restricted in calories. J Nutr 18:1–13, 1939

Miller NH, Haskell WL, Berra K, et al: Home versus group exercise training for increasing functional capacity after myocardial infarction. Circulation 70:645–649, 1984

Moritznik J, Speedling E, Stein R, et al: Cardiovascular fitness program: factors associated with participation and adherence. Public Health Rep 100:13–18, 1985

Mullen JL: Reduction of operative morbidity and mortality by combined preoperative and postoperative nutritional support. Ann Surg 192:604–610, 1980

Odell WD, Wolfson AR: Humoral syndromes associated with cancer. Annu Rev Med 29:379–406, 1978

Pariza MW: A perspective on diet, nutrition and cancer. JAMA 251:1455–1458, 1984

Phillips PA, Rolls BJ, Ledingham JGG, et al: Reduced thirst after water deprivation in healthy elderly men. N Engl J Med 311:753–759, 1984

Posner JD, Gorman KM, Klein HS, et al: Exercise capacity in the elderly. Am J Cardiol 57:52c–58c, 1986

President's Council on Physical Fitness and Sports: Physical Fitness Research Digest, Series 1, No 1. Washington, DC, U.S. Government Printing Office, 1971

Riggs BL, Hodgson SF, Hoffman DL, et al: Treatment of primary osteoporosis with fluoride and calcium: clinical tolerance and fracture occurrence. JAMA 243:446–449, 1980

Sandstead HH, Henriksen LK, Greger JL, et al: Zinc nutriture in the elderly in relation to taste acuity, immune response and wound healing. Am J Clin Nutr 36:1046–1059, 1982

Schiffman S: Taste and smell in disease. N Engl J Med 308:1275–1279, 1337–1343, 1983

Sergi G, Perini P, Bussolotto M, et al: Body composition study in the elderly: comparison between tritium dilution method and dual photon absorptiometry. J Gerontol 48:M244–M248, 1993

Seymour DG, Henschke PJ, Cape RDT, et al: Acute confusional states and dementia in the elderly: the role of dehydration/volume depletion, physical illness and age. Age Ageing 9:137–146, 1980

Sidney KH, Shephard RJ: Frequency and intensity of exercise training for elderly subjects. Med Sci Sports Exerc 10:125–131, 1978

Siscovick DS, LaPorte RE, Newman JM: The disease-specific benefits and risks of physical activity. Public Health Rep 100:180–188, 1985

Sugimura T, Sato S: Mutagens-carcinogens in foods. Cancer Res 43 (suppl):2415S–2421S, 1983

Taylor CB, Sallis JF, Needle R: The relation of physical activity and exercise to mental health. Public Health Rep 100:195–202, 1985

VanCamp SP, Peterson RA: Cardiovascular complications of outpatient cardiac rehabilitation programs. JAMA 256:1160–1163, 1986

Watkin DM: Handbook of Nutrition, Health and Aging. Park Ridge, NJ, Noyes Publications, 1983

Wayler AH, Muench ME, Kapur KK, et al: Masticatory performance and food acceptability in persons with removable partial dentures, full dentures and intact natural dentition. J Gerontol 39:284–289, 1984

Weisman Y, Schen RJ, Eisenberg Z, et al: Single oral high-dose vitamin D_3 prophylaxis in the elderly. J Am Geriatr Soc 34:515–518, 1984

Willett WC, MacMahon B: Diet and cancer—an overview. N Engl J Med 310:633–638, 697–703, 1984

CHAPTER 22

Psychotherapy

Keith G. Meador, M.D., M.P.H.
Claudia D. Davis, R.N., M.S.N.

▌ Psychotherapy in Later Life

The current decade is one in which rapid advances in the scientific knowledge underlying psychiatric treatment are occurring. In this, "the decade of the brain," increasing evidence is emerging detailing the biophysiological aspects of a variety of psychiatric disorders, and new psychopharmacologic treatments continue to exert increasing influence on treatment perspectives. Mental health disciplines are being confronted with important challenges in combining the developing biological perspectives with psychological and social perspectives into an integrated biopsychosocial model for understanding and treating mental illness.

Fogel et al. (1990) emphasized the "risks to the mind" as major concerns for the elderly and their families. They identified seven major risks to the elderly mind: 1) dementia, 2) depression, 3) schizophrenia and other chronic mental illnesses, 4) behavioral and emotional consequences of nondementing brain disease, 5) prescription drug and alcohol abuse, 6) maladaptive emotional responses to predictable crises of late life, and 7) prescription drug psycho-

toxicity. While delineating these concerns, these risk factors also highlight an underlying problem: although public awareness of the mental disorders of late life has grown substantially, medical practice, medical education, and health care financing are still a long way from fully incorporating a sophisticated understanding of mental and behavioral issues into the health care of the elderly (Fogel et al. 1990).

An American Psychiatric Association (APA) Task Force on Models of Practice in Geriatric Psychiatry (1993) has underscored the need for attention to models of psychiatric care for the elderly, observing that mental health needs in the elderly and their families are often overlooked, trivialized, or ignored by primary care providers and others.

Reconsideration of psychotherapy and psychosocial interventions has begun to raise questions about old assumptions that psychotherapy was not a usual and necessary part of the treatment of the elderly patient. Recent attempts to formulate guidelines for the treatment of depression have given an important emphasis to psychotherapeutic interventions. The National Institutes of Health (NIH) Consensus Development Panel on Depression in Late

Life (1992) concluded that psychosocial interventions were a crucial part of the treatment of depression in the elderly. Cognitive-behavior therapy, interpersonal therapy, and short-term dynamic therapy constitute the recommended psychotherapeutic modalities for treatment of depressed elderly persons. In addition, marital and family interventions, as well as community-based psychosocial intervention systems, should be considered.

The APA's "Practice Guideline for Major Depressive Disorder in Adults" (APA Work Group on Major Depressive Disorder 1993) stresses that therapists actually often use a combination or synthesis of various approaches and strategies. The importance of individually tailoring psychotherapy to each patient's particular condition and coping capacities is vital. The indications for psychotherapy in elderly persons are essentially the same as for younger patient populations.

Treatment of the elderly has been influenced not only by burgeoning scientific knowledge of psychiatric disorders and treatment and the emergence of new models of intervention, but also by the demands of a rapidly changing health care delivery system. From the deinstitutionalization movement in the 1960s and 1970s, through the major Medicare change with the diagnosis-related group (DRG) system in the 1980s, to the current national attempt to redesign the health care delivery system, almost every aspect of health care delivery is being reassessed, with emphasis on outcomes and the cost-effectiveness of care. These evolving changes will shape psychiatric interventions in ways that will demand a greater ability to demonstrate results of treatment and more creativity in types of services, settings, and providers offered.

All of these trends influence psychotherapy as one of the treatment modalities for the elderly. In this chapter we review historical biases against undertaking psychotherapeutic work with the elderly, discuss limitations in our understanding of human development in the elderly, and describe challenges inherent in psychotherapy with the elderly. We also examine and discuss a variety of psychotherapeutic modalities: individual psychotherapies, including dynamic (insight-oriented, supportive, and brief dynamic), cognitive-behavior, existential, and life review modalities; group, marital, and family therapies; and the combination of pharmacotherapy and psychotherapy.

Historical Perspectives Against Psychotherapy

The elderly have traditionally been labeled as poor candidates for psychotherapy. This idea stems from the writing of Freud, who believed that those over 40 years of age were not good candidates for psychoanalysis. Freud did not believe that elderly adults possessed the elasticity of mind necessary for psychotherapy. He also questioned what he saw as the unmanageable length of time required to deal with all of the historical data in the elderly, and he was skeptical of the economic and long-term value of treatment in late life (Freud 1924/1966). It is interesting to note, however, that Freud himself continued his own analysis until the time of his death, at 83. Abraham (1949) was less pessimistic, arguing that the age at onset of the neurosis was more crucial than the age of the patient. In her journal, *The Measure of My Days,* Florida Scott-Maxwell (1968), herself an analytical psychologist, vividly recounted the intense emotional life she experienced while in her 80s.

Chaisson-Stewart (1985) summarized other potential problems with the idea of age-related rigidity in conducting psychotherapy with elderly persons. These included beliefs that elders have decreased capacity for abstraction and new learning; perceptions that defenses, style, and personality characteristics are fixed and immutable in older adults; and recognition of limitations in internal and external resources and choices that may be available to elderly persons. However, these possible difficulties were not seen as insurmountable obstacles but instead as challenges requiring development and selection of therapeutic modalities tailored to the unique needs of individuals and groups of elderly patients.

Human Development in Elders

One underlying problem that influences psychotherapeutic work with elderly persons has been the limitations in theory and research related to human development in this population. Although significant work has been done in recent years, there is still controversy and a lack of consensus about normative psychological and emotional development during this period of life. Differing yet complementary perspectives have been used to examine the developmental tasks and challenges of later life.

A number of intrapsychic issues are inevitably confronted in old age. Elders need to find restitution and compensation for the stresses and losses associated with aging. From an intrapsychic perspective, there is continued struggle to maintain self-esteem at a time when one has diminishing ego resources, and when there are increasing narcissistic threats and losses. Mental status changes, sexual changes, retirement, and changing economic resources all threaten the elderly. Disappointment with one's achievements and/or those of one's adult children may present itself as a narcissistic injury for some. Failing health and illness in older adults as well as those around them may heighten a sense of vulnerability.

Jung viewed the second half of life in a far different way than did earlier psychoanalytic perspectives. Jung was more focused on the second half of life, the "afternoon" and "evening," as a time of opportunities. He contrasted the first half of life, in which the focus was outward in work, family, and involvement with society, with the shift inward as one grows older, with the goal becoming that of mature individuation (Jung 1939).

Erickson and colleagues (1986) have applied a developmental approach to understanding the psychological issues in later life. Erickson explains personality development as involving the resolution of eight developmental stages from infancy to old age. The eighth stage, occurring in old age, is characterized by resolution of the conflict between ego integrity and despair. If elderly individuals have built a secure sense of ego and knowledge of their legacy through their children or work, they attain ego integrity, whereas failure to resolve this conflict results in both disappointment with one's self and despair (Kimmel 1974; Woods and Witte 1981).

Atchley (1982) suggested that elderly persons can defend against loss of self-esteem by means of a variety of strategies. These include focusing on past successes, rejecting input that does not fit their existing self-concept, and refusing to apply myths to themselves. Choosing to interact with those who can provide self-esteem–building, supportive contact facilitates maintenance of positive self-esteem.

Social science approaches to understanding the developmental challenges of elderly persons have taken three divergent views. *Disengagement theory* has stressed the gradual withdrawal from social roles, which is argued to be mutually beneficial to the individual and society as the individual ages. *Activity theory*, in contrast, suggests the importance of replacing social roles and relationships with new roles and relationships as transition occurs across the life span. *Continuity theory* proposes, instead, that the individual maintains whatever pattern of social involvement has characterized earlier life periods. Clearly, from the perspectives of these divergent theories, therapeutic efforts would be quite dissimilar.

Several authors have stressed the positive opportunities within more existential perspectives of aging. Tournier (1972) combined insights from psychotherapy and theology. He suggested that old age can be a new beginning filled with purpose and hope, and emphasized the role of activity and leisure, new interests, and spiritual involvement as strategies for growth. Tournier proposed that individuals must learn to grow old, and that in order for this to be successfully accomplished, the aging process must be planned and prepared for throughout life. Thibault (1993) emphasizes that old age can be a unique time for spiritual inner work, and that empowerment can occur through this process. Freidan (1993) challenges the "age mystique" and advocates a radical paradigm shift in the way aging is perceived. She suggests that old age be viewed not in terms of deterioration, decline, and loss, but instead as a unique stage of life with its own patterns for relationships, career, sex, family, and involvement. The potential for growth within individuals and their society is stressed.

It is important to note that, for most of recorded history, life after age 40 was a reality for only a few. However, with changing life span demographics, this period of life is in flux. Many current elders are pioneers in creating new models for aging, as will be the "baby boomers" as they move into this age. Emerging and evolving views of the opportunities/tasks of old age will exert an impact on the kinds of therapies that are designed for the future.

Challenges Inherent in Psychotherapy With Older Adults

Most authors agree that there are challenges inherent in psychotherapy late in life. These challenges or barriers to therapy can be divided into four categories: caregiver-/patient-related issues, family-related issues, physician-related barriers, and societal/systems barriers (Lazarus and Sadavoy 1988).

Caregiver/patient challenges include the belief that unhappiness, depression, and anxiety are expected concomitants of old age. Psychiatric symptoms are often attributed to physical health issues and are considered immutable to treatment; consequently, psychiatric care may not be sought. Also, elderly persons, particularly those in the current 65-year-old and over cohort, may shun psychiatric intervention because of the stigma that was attached to psychiatric care during most of their lives. Many psychiatric problems, particularly depression, manifest as hopelessness, apathy, cognitive impairment, and anergy, which may limit treatment seeking or be interpreted as representing a general lack of motivation.

In addition to these issues, changes in vision or hearing may create special problems for therapy, as do language problems such as aphasias. Limited endurance and strength, particularly in very old persons who have coexisting medical problems, may limit emotional and physical energy available for therapeutic work. Also, lack of awareness of resources for psychological treatment may result in failure to seek treatment. There are also pragmatic problems related to sites of service, transportation, and reimbursement constraints that affect treatment seeking.

Family-related challenges to psychotherapy include mistaken beliefs that psychiatric symptoms are a normal part of aging, with resultant minimization of symptoms. Also, when the elderly individual does not initiate treatment, families may be hesitant and ambivalent about encouraging therapy. This ambivalence may reflect a variety of issues related to patient-child roles, caregiving, and the need to maintain an idealized view of one's parents. Ambivalence, conflict, and old resentments rooted in long-standing family dynamics may limit care seeking, as can negative family views toward psychiatric intervention.

Therapist-related challenges include the presence of negative, stereotypical attitudes toward elderly persons, particularly in our youth-oriented society. The aged in our society have been a stigmatized group during recent decades. Goffman (1963) pointed out that a part of the social process that occurs in the response of others to a stigmatized individual is the construction of a stigma theory through which stereotypes are created and undesirable traits are

imputed to the stigmatized individual. For the elderly individual experiencing psychological distress or an actual psychiatric illness, there is the double effect of the stigmas of aging and mental illness, both of which are prevalent in our culture. It may be difficult for the therapist to remain uninfluenced by these culturally contingent stereotypes. Therapists may also feel frustration and therapeutic nihilism because of the chronic illnesses of and imminent death anticipated in many older patients. Such responses may be particularly problematic for the younger therapist who has difficulty understanding the experiential reality of these phenomena, or for the older therapist who may feel threatened because of overidentification.

Countertransference issues are also commonly mentioned as therapist-related challenges. Unresolved conflicts with parents or grandparents may be reactivated. Also, the therapist's unresolved issues around his or her own personal aging may be triggered and result in countertransference difficulties.

Historically, psychiatrists have been resistant to working therapeutically with elders. However, the increasing development of postresidency fellowships, along with innovative programs in hospital, community, and nursing home settings, indicates that trends are changing in this area. The proliferation of literature in the field and the attention given to geriatric mental health issues by a variety of task forces likewise reflect hopeful changes. Other mental health disciplines such as nursing and social work continue to contribute substantially to this process.

Health care delivery system and societal issues have also created challenges to providing psychotherapeutic intervention. Medicare and other third-party reimbursement for outpatient psychotherapy is inadequate. Also, in many areas there are only limited services specifically designed for older adults. The health care delivery system for psychotherapy services is modeled on traditional office visits or mental health center visits, but services may need to be delivered in more diverse and accessible sites. Societal and system biases have also resulted in differential treatment for "mental" versus "physical" illnesses. However, alternative health care plans that have recently been discussed have begun to emphasize parity for the treatment of mental disorders, although the lack of inclusion of psychotherapeutic interventions within parity plans continues to be a point of discouragement and contention.

Individual Psychotherapies for Elders

Psychodynamic Therapy

Psychodynamic psychotherapy tends to be insight oriented or supportive in its orientation, although some combination of the two is usually a pragmatic necessity in the clinical setting. The balance on this continuum is particularly weighted toward the supportive end of the spectrum in working with elderly individuals, due to the physical frailty, limitations (as described in the earlier section on challenges to psychotherapy), and concomitant need for pharmacotherapy that are frequently encountered in this population. When approaching the elderly patient with a psychodynamic therapeutic model, the clinician's consideration of the degree of emphasis to place on insight versus supportive work is a crucial part of the initial assessment. The patient's history of and current capacity for object relatedness, along with his or her psychological mindedness and depth of motivation for change, are valuable indicators in this decision (Myers 1991). If one assumes an optimal assessment of these parameters and minimal characterological deficits, the elderly patient's aptitude for insight-oriented psychotherapy should be viewed positively within the acknowledged limitations for many older persons (such as limited resources and physical constraints).

Muslin (1992) noted the potential for resistance specific to the aging person, such as the "resistance to aging" syndrome, to be encountered within a dynamic self psychology framework. Although resistance is inevitable in a dynamic psychotherapeutic process, Yesavage and Karusa (1982) emphasized that older persons frequently show a decreased resistance to change and increased motivation for therapy due to their anticipation of a shorter life span in the context of their life experiences.

Although transference and countertransference issues are an important part of any psychotherapy, they are particularly central to the dynamic psychotherapeutic process. Transference is multigenerational in the elderly person, with "reverse transference," as delineated by Grunes (1987), being specific to therapy with older persons. Grunes described this phenomenon as the therapist's being viewed as the child of the patient, with corresponding expectations and powers projected onto the therapist. The countertransference in psychotherapy with the elderly is distinguished by the therapist's typically being younger than the patient. Idealization, unconscious hostility due to anger with one's parents, and avoidance of conflictual material due to deferential respect for the patient are examples of possible consequences of countertransference specific to the older patient–younger therapist context. Although cognizance of these dynamics on the part of the therapist is vital, Meerloo (1955) allowed for less emphasis on interpreting the transference in psychotherapy with the elderly. The constructive potential for the therapist to serve in the transferential role may be greater than the therapeutic benefit derived from interpretation of the transference. This perspective advocated by Meerloo leads to the consideration of supportive psychotherapy as a complement to insight-oriented therapy within the dynamic framework.

Supportive psychotherapy as a legitimate, systematic therapeutic approach has gained increasing credibility in the last decade. Werman's (1984) description of a model for the practice of supportive psychotherapy emphasized the assessment of ego functioning and the restraint required by the therapist in supportive psychotherapy, with the necessity of more discernment when taking a more active therapeutic posture. Supportive psychotherapy frequently provides reassurance for the elderly patient, attempting to decrease anxiety and enhance the patient's feeling of being understood. Psychoeducational components may be included at times as the therapist attempts to enhance the elderly patient's ego strength so as to foster adaptation and gain of symptomatic relief. Somatic preoccupations of the elderly will frequently necessitate a more active, supportive role by the therapist in order to establish a therapeutic alliance and identify the cause of the somatic complaint. Although the goal is ultimately to reduce the frequency of sessions, some form of sustained therapeutic relationship is not uncommon in a supportive psychotherapeutic framework. The contemporary significance of supportive psychotherapy within the practice of psychotherapy (Rockland 1993) will only be enhanced by health care policy changes, because of its emphasis on adaptation and focused symptom relief.

Time-limited psychotherapeutic modalities have emerged in the last 20 years. Brief dynamic therapy attempts to resolve core conflicts based on a dynamic understanding of personality and historical relationships in the context of situational variables, with the goals being symptomatic relief and enhanced self-esteem. Achievement of insight or structural characterological change should not be expected. A brief, time-limited psychodynamic approach would be applicable in elderly patients when there are clearly delineated, circumscribed problems that can be expected to resolve in a limited period of time, such as an unresolved grief reaction or an adjustment disorder.

A number of advantages have been ascribed to brief dynamic therapy, including that it 1) recognizes the finitude of the older person's life, 2) conveys a message that acknowledges current stressors and recognizes past mastery, with the goal of a short-term intervention, 3) reduces fear of dependency on the therapist, and 4) reduces the financial burden of therapy (Lazarus et al. 1987).

Brief dynamic psychotherapy models use the therapist's understanding of the patient and the transference to clarify and interpret the patient's emotional responses to current life issues in a more timely fashion. Changes that occur in brief psychodynamic therapy are in the area of symptom improvement and problem resolution rather than in character structure and personality.

One study of the process and outcome of brief psychodynamic psychotherapy (Lazarus et al. 1987) revealed interesting data about how patients use the psychotherapy. Findings were consistent with earlier research indicating that symptomatic and focal problem improvement occurred in the relative absence of increased insight or self-understanding. Patients were noted to use the therapeutic relationship to reestablish a sense of self or to bring together diverse, disparate aspects of self into a more positive configuration. The therapist was used for validation of normalcy and competency and to assist in restoration of a positive sense of self. Previously suppressed or newly emerged aspects of self were incorporated into a more cohesive positive sense of self. It is interesting to note a distinctive finding in this study. Compared with men, women were found to show improvement earlier and to a greater extent, and to maintain improvement longer. They also differed from men in their relationship with the therapist, use of defense, and manner of conflict resolution.

Silberschatz and Curtis (1991) presented a time-limited psychodynamic therapy for older adults and challenged historical assumptions about elders' rigidity and inability to accomplish therapeutic work. These authors suggested that a patient can profit from such a therapeutic model if the therapist adequately evaluates the patient's treatment goals and develops interventions in accordance with these goals. They argued that what is often perceived as being rigidity and defensiveness are actually what Weiss (1986) called *tests of the therapist*. For example, one patient's request for medication, although seemingly justified, actually represented a test by that patient of whether palliative measures would be assumed to be the only alternative. *Survivor guilt* is also a dynamic to be explored in elderly persons as they observe the decline of friends and relatives.

Brief dynamic psychotherapy is based on dynamic concepts of conflict and transference, but its time-limited, focused approach is particularly useful with the elderly population when this framework is desired. The literature reflects an overall efficacy for brief dynamic therapy of 35%, which is slightly less than for other therapies (APA Task Force on Models of Practice in Geriatric Psychiatry 1993); however, studies to date have been limited and contain methodological problems. Additional research is needed to explore the techniques used and outcome of brief therapy models.

Cognitive-Behavior Therapy

Gallagher and Thompson (1982) established cognitive-behavior therapy as a primary psychotherapy for elderly persons through their modifications of Beck's seminal work in this area. Cognitive-behavior therapy is a time-limited, focused psychotherapy developed primarily for use with patients with depressive illness. The negative cognitive triad of Beck's model (Beck et al. 1979) includes a negative view of self, the world, and the future, with negative thought patterns manifested in a variety of cognitive distortions. These cognitive distortions present as exaggerations, overreactions, and automatic assumptions despite evidence to the contrary. The process of cognitive therapy has five primary components. It includes 1) learning to identify negative thought patterns, 2) making the connection between negative thoughts and depressive feelings, 3) examining automatic thought patterns and their validity, 4) learning to identify and change distorted thought patterns that sustain negative feelings, and

5) incorporating the above-described process into developing a less distorted and more adaptive view of one's self, the world, and one's future.

Gallagher and Thompson (1982) suggested the need for elderly persons to be socialized to the treatment process because of the distrust of psychotherapy frequently encountered in this population. This socialization process can be an opportunity for rendering supportive care and encouragement regarding the patient's capacity to improve. When working with older persons with possible perceptual deficits and cognitive limitations, the therapist should utilize multiple modes of learning. Examples specific to the older person's age should be used, and the therapist should consider the increased time requirements for processing and implementation.

Thompson and colleagues (1987) found that 75% of patients studied over a 10-year period had shown clear improvement or full remission by the end of their outpatient course of therapy, which usually included approximately 15–20 hour-long sessions. The greatest improvement was found in patients for whom a clear precipitant for a reactive depression was linked to a specific event or situation. For patients with more chronic problems, which are not uncommon in the elderly, 30–40 sessions proved to be more efficacious. Although cognitive-behavior therapy alone is most useful in elders without melancholic symptoms, the combination of cognitive-behavior therapy and desipramine proved to be more efficacious than desipramine alone in elderly outpatients in this study by Thompson et al.

Despite the fact that the more cognitive components of the cognitive-behavior model become less useful with advanced cognitive impairment in the elderly, behavioral methods continue to be effective (Teri and Gallagher-Thompson 1991). Lewinsohn et al. (1985) proposed a behavioral model of depression on which Gallagher and Thompson (1981) based a behavioral treatment plan for use with elders. This model included the following components:

1. Tracking of behavior (pleasant and unpleasant events) and mood
2. Establishing the relationship between behavior and mood
3. Targeting aspects of the client's life that are realistic to change
4. Learning of social skills to foster capacity to experience pleasant events and avoid unpleasant

ones. Skills that are central include a) progressive relaxation techniques for stress management; b) assertiveness training; c) cognitive skills, primarily learning to avoid or to decrease the frequency of negative or self-destructive thoughts; d) social/communication skills; and e) time management. The client and therapist select those skills that are most pertinent to the specific clinical situation.
5. Initiating a concrete plan for change and measuring progress through tracking of behavior and mood
6. Assuming more self-initiated changes
7. Generalizing and transferring skills learned to a broader array of situations

Teri and Gallagher-Thompson (1991) modified this model for use with outpatients with Alzheimer's disease, incorporating the primary caregiver into the treatment process. Behavioral therapy has been useful in managing behavioral disorders in cognitively impaired nursing home residents and in allowing for reductions in their antipsychotic medications (Ray et al. 1993). Modifications for the nursing home include parallel processes for variable levels of cognitive functioning. For the cognitively impaired resident, changing the psychosocial environment and improving care provider experiences correspond to skills acquisition and generalization for the cognitively intact elderly. As the numbers of oldest-old elderly continue to increase, the further development of behavioral therapies for use in outpatient and residential care settings will become more important.

Interpersonal Psychotherapy

In addition to short-term dynamic therapy and cognitive therapies, interpersonal psychotherapy has been found to be moderately successful in treating older adults (NIH Consensus Development Panel on Depression in Late Life 1992). Interpersonal psychotherapy has a long history, extending back to the work of Harry Stack Sullivan, who theoretically diverged from the classical view and its emphasis on intrapsychic processes. Sullivan recognized the important role of social relationships and redefined a view of psychotherapy that focused on social relationships throughout the various developmental phases. Sullivan's therapeutic model stressed corrective interpersonal experiences. Contemporary interpersonal therapy for depression is described as seeking "to recognize and explore depressive precipitants that involve interpersonal losses, role disputes and transactions, social isolation, or deficits in social skills" (APA Work Group on Major Depressive Disorder 1993, p. 5). The therapeutic task is for the therapist and patient to define the nature of the interpersonal problem and develop a plan to resolve it. From the perspective of interpersonal therapy, interpersonal difficulties may be causal, concomitant, or exacerbating/maintaining factors for depression or other illnesses.

Sholomakas et al. (1983) described a series of cases in which older persons were treated with interpersonal therapy; they concluded that this modality was useful for treating depressed older adults. These authors based their short-term interpersonal treatment on the premise that, regardless of other factors, depression occurs in a psychosocial and interpersonal context and that understanding and intervening in this context can be important in recovery and prevention of relapse. The therapy has two goals: 1) relieving depressive symptoms, and 2) helping the patient develop more effective strategies for dealing with the interpersonal issues associated with the onset of depression.

The therapist role is that of patient advocate, with the therapist being nonjudgmental while communicating warmth and unconditional positive regard. The therapist also takes an active stance in helping the patient focus on current interpersonal problem areas and guiding the patient in resolution of the problem areas.

Sholomakas and colleagues (1983) identified four problem areas that are common in the elderly and that identify relevant treatment goals:

1. *Grief.* Grief is a central feature for the elderly, as multiple losses are experienced and result in failure to negotiate the normal mourning process. Goals focus on facilitation of mourning and helping the patient to establish relationships to substitute for the loss.
2. *Interpersonal role disputes.* These situations are characterized by the elderly individual and at least one other person being involved in discrepant, nonreciprocal expectations for roles. Goals in this context are to help the patient identify the dispute, make choices about a plan of action, and

modify maladaptive communication patterns or unrealistic expectations.
3. *Role transitions.* Role transition problems are associated with a life change that is perceived as a loss. Retirement or a change in function or status due to illness are examples of role transition. Goals include helping the patient to perceive the transition in a more positive manner and restoring self-esteem by developing a sense of mastery about the demands of the new role.
4. *Interpersonal deficits.* Interpersonal deficits occur when a patient has developed inadequate or unsustaining interpersonal relationships. The deficit can result from social isolation, decreased quantity of relationships, or deficiencies in social skills. The goal of treatment is to reduce the patient's social isolation. The relationship with the therapist is pivotal, as past relationships are reviewed and new relationships are developed.

The primary characteristics of interpersonal therapy are identified as time-limited, not long-term; focused, not open-ended; emphasizing current, not past, relationships; interpersonal, not intrapsychic; and interpersonal, not cognitive/behavioral; personality is recognized but not focused on (Klerman et al. 1984). Klerman and colleagues identified four elements of assessment in the interpersonal therapy model. First, an inventory of current and past relationships is made. Second, the quality and patterning of interactions over time in interpersonal relationships is reviewed, looking for issues such as relationship to authority, dominance versus submission, dependency versus autonomy, intimacy, trust, and confiding. Third, cognitions are reviewed as they relate to the individual and others, their roles, and relationship history; this also includes norms, expectations, and meanings associated with roles. Fourth, the associated emotions that the individual experiences are reviewed.

Klerman et al. (1984) identified the same four key issues as did Sholomakas and colleagues: grief, interpersonal role disputes, role transitions, and role deficits. For role transition, for example, four tasks are identified: 1) facilitate evaluation of the role that has been lost, 2) encourage expression of emotions, 3) develop social skills suitable for the new role, and 4) establish new interpersonal relations, attachments, and social supports. The basic structure of interpersonal therapy, with its focus on grief, interpersonal role disputes, role transitions, and role deficits, addresses interpersonal events common among elderly individuals, making this model particularly appropriate for use with elderly patients.

Life Review/Reminiscence Therapy

Systematic life review therapy was first described by Butler (1963) as an extension of a natural developmental process in late life. Butler and Lewis (1977) defined the life review as "a universal mental process brought about by the realization of approaching disillusion and death that marks the lives of all older persons in some manner as their myths of invulnerability or immortality give way and death begins to be viewed as an imminent personal reality" (p. 165). Viney (1993) described a "personal construct therapy with the elderly" that builds on the life review tradition. The four primary assumptions of her personal construct model of psychological functioning in the elderly are as follows: 1) Persons consistently try to make sense of what is happening and what is anticipated in the future; 2) Both the internal, subjective experience and the external, objective perspective are considered to be important; 3) Psychological development progresses as experiences are serially interpreted and reinterpreted; and 4) The primary characteristic of psychological development is the integration of these reinterpretations. Viney's model offers a theoretical construct for the therapeutic benefit derived from life review and reminiscence. Life review therapy will be discussed further in the group psychotherapy section of this chapter.

Existential Psychotherapy

Existential psychotherapy arose from dissatisfaction with classical analytic and behavioral approaches to therapy. According to May and Yalom (1989), it started with an awareness that people are living in an age of transition, with almost everyone experiencing significant anxiety. Existential psychotherapy is not a specific technical approach with specific rules for therapy. Instead, it is a method of exploration that focuses on the nature of the human being and the nature of the individual's experience of anxiety, despair, grief, loneliness, and isolation. The existential therapist attempts to see the individual actuality without the distortion of projecting theories about the patient.

Existential psychotherapy emphasizes anxiety as a core problem confronted in therapy. For the existential therapist, anxiety has a broader definition than for other psychotherapeutic frameworks. According to May and Yalom (1989), "Anxiety arises from our personal need to survive, to preserve our being, and to assert out being" (p. 364). The existentialist sees two types of anxiety—normal anxiety and neurotic anxiety. The existentialist deals with the "I-Am" or basic experience of being, with guilt, and with "being-in-the-world" (p. 364). The existentialist also emphasizes an awareness that time is an important aspect of most human experiences.

Existential psychotherapy makes a unique assumption about the basis of inner human conflicts. It does not relate these conflicts to drives or early childhood experience, but rather to the conflict between the individual and the "givens" of human existence. Yalom (1985) identified four ultimate concerns that have importance for psychotherapy: death, freedom, isolation, and meaninglessness. He explored death as a primary source of anxiety and as a boundary situation and discussed the roles of life satisfaction and death desensitization. In exploring freedom, the issue of responsibility and its limits are considered. Isolation involves consideration of one's basic existential aloneness and looking at isolation and relationships.

McDougall (1992) called this model "the most useful theoretical basis for counseling the geriatric client because the existential approach emphasizes the present instead of the past, quality rather than quantity, subjective rather than objective awareness" (p. 3). He commented further that

> [e]xistential models of psychotherapy typically espouse the actualization of potential in order to obtain a sense of completeness and personal dignity. The aim of therapy is to assist older adults to understand their unconscious conflict, to diminish secondary anxiety by ordering maladaptive modes of dealing with themselves or others, and to develop adaptive ways of coping with primary anxiety. These mechanisms occur as they embark on a course of self-investigation by exploring four ultimate concerns—namely death, freedom, isolation, and meaninglessness. Undoubtedly, many elderly who seek out mental health professionals do so because they are facing such an existential crisis. (p. 3)

Alternative Modalities

Group Therapy

Group therapy has been used with elderly individuals in varied settings, including hospitals, residential facilities, nursing homes, and outpatient environments. Lazarus and Sadavoy (1988) identified the following as purposes of group therapy with the elderly: socialization; enhancing attitudinal changes; personal development; learning and education; behavior change using behavior modification, reality orientation, and reality therapy; emotional catharsis and life review; and problem solving.

Yalom (1985) has identified factors that are linked to therapeutic effectiveness or change in group therapy. These include instillation of hope, universality, imparting of information, altruism, corrective recapitulation of the primary family group, development of socializing techniques, imitative behavior, interpersonal learning, group cohesiveness, catharsis, and existential factors. Of these factors, Moberg and Lazarus (1990) focused on the ones that are especially applicable to the elderly. Providing basic information on a variety of subjects, including medication, social services, and recreational activities, is important. The opportunity for personal feedback is important because of the tendency of older persons to emphasize faults and minimize strengths. Resocialization and remotivation are useful to combat loneliness and isolation and to reinforce the ability to develop significant relationships. Enhancement of self-esteem occurs in the context of the realization that problems of aging are not unique to oneself. Emotional catharsis is helpful in allowing the isolated elderly individual to express feelings of self-pity, guilt, and failure. Finally, Moberg and Lazarus stated that the opportunity to express existential concerns—including dealing with losses and anxiety about death, and the wish to find meaning in life—is of particular value. Universality and instillation of hope are particularly curative factors in inpatient settings, where patients often feel isolated and hopeless in the midst of severe mental illnesses (C. D. Davis and E. Williams, "The Support Group in an Inpatient Geropsychiatric Setting" [unpublished manuscript], 1994).

Lazarus and Sadavoy (1988) have identified a variety of goals that groups, particularly in institutions, may strive to meet: halting regression; resocialization; reengagement; problem solving; and

information exchange. These goals will vary according to the composition, purpose, and setting of the group and will complement and overlap with the goals of other therapies.

A variety of group approaches are used with elderly persons, including group psychotherapy, activity groups (music, dance and movement, art, dramatics, and writing groups), oral-history groups (reminiscence and life review groups), reality orientation and remotivation/resocialization groups, and validation groups. Issue-focused groups such as widows' groups, retirement groups, and support groups for family caregivers are also used. These groups have different purposes and goals. They involve different leadership styles and even different disciplines functioning in the leadership roles. Burnside and Schmidt (1994) provide a comprehensive review of the variety of group approaches used with elderly populations.

Psychodynamic, interpersonal, supportive, cognitive-behavioral, and expressive models are all used in group psychotherapy with the elderly. Ingersoll and Silverman (1978) described an insight-oriented, time-limited group they referred to as the "There and Then Group." The group focused on helping individuals bridge the past and present and emphasized life review and reminiscing. Patients also kept a journal and completed a family genogram. The therapy was divided into eight sessions with the following foci: 1) orientation, 2) commencement of life review, 3) early-life experience, 4) introduction of the genogram, 5) loss and grief, 6) family patterns, 7) polarities (balance between painful and pleasurable memories), and 8) closure. Participants in this group showed overall improvement in self-esteem, anxiety, and somatic complaint measures. It is notable that the participants showed limited interest in journal writing but significant interest in the genograms.

Cognitive-behavior group therapy continues to grow in significance. Yost and Corbishley (1985) suggested that cognitive-behavior therapy is particularly appropriate for treatment of depressed elders because it deals with potentially depressive aspects of life unique to old age. It directly attacks negative beliefs that produce and maintain depression. The therapy requires the participant to act in ways that ultimately extinguish depressive attitudes. There are many potentially depressive life situations that confront elderly persons, including loss of health and mobility, friends and family, role satisfaction, and autonomy. In addition, limited economic resources may affect diet and environment. Often the changes/losses come suddenly and accumulate more rapidly in old age, allowing little time for adjustment. Many older persons also have beliefs that make them vulnerable psychologically. Most notably, they may share the negative societal stereotype of old age.

Brief dynamic group therapy models have been used in both inpatient and outpatient settings. Deutsch and Kramer (1977) implemented a program of five brief therapy groups meeting for 12 consecutive weeks. The purpose of these groups was to emphasize the aging process as a normal part of the life cycle, to generate positive attitudes, and to help members become involved in meaningful activities and substitutive new behaviors to increase self-worth. The groups focused on physical, economic, and social losses, with further examination of the resultant grief and depression. Outcomes reported included increases in coping skills, involvement in volunteer and part-time work, renewed family contact, and development of new friendships among the group members.

The expressive psychotherapy groups are dynamic in orientation, being neither didactic nor heavily structured. Group boundaries are rigorously maintained, with members added systematically and therapists utilizing transference interpretations. The expressive model is useful in assessing elderly individuals. As noted by Berland and Poggi (1979), "What is true is that our experience demonstrates the elderly's wish and ability to confront the great issue of their life stage and to do so with energy, great insight, and benefit to themselves" (p. 706). These authors also reported that members were able to deal with themes of death and loss effectively.

A variety of group approaches have emerged that involve creative expression, including activity groups, music groups, dance groups, movement groups, art groups, and dramatic groups. Groups may be largely physical, as in the dance and movement groups, or may involve more subtle expression, as in art groups. These groups attempt to restore the elders' self-confidence in their ability to perform, produce, and learn (Yost and Corbishley 1985). They provide the opportunity to reexperience old interests or to learn new ones, and to broaden the elder's world. There is also significant opportunity for social interaction in such groups, which are often less formal and structured than other groups. The elder is able to realize that new interests can still be acquired and new relationships formed. Group leaders may come from a variety of disciplines, including activity therapy, art therapy, music/dance therapy, and nursing or social work, along with psychiatry or psychology.

Another approach that is used in group work with the elderly is groups based on the use of memories. Reminiscence, life review, and guided autobiographical groups can all be modalities used in group therapy. Reminiscence-based activities have been used in a wide variety of settings, including residential homes, hospitals, and day care environments. Reminiscence was at one time seen as a negative behavior, but it is now seen as a means of preserving mental functioning and self-identifying in old age (Coleman 1988). Burnside and Haight (1994) pointed out that a reminiscence group should be planned with attention to detail, and each member must receive attention from the leader. An important goal in the group is to build new relationships based on present positive experience. Through the sharing of reminiscences, members affirm both their own lives and those of others in the group. Burnside and Haight developed detailed protocols for group reminiscence and for use in one-to-one reminiscence. Reminiscence therapy has the advantage of being usable with both moderately cognitively impaired and cognitively intact individuals.

Life review therapy is a specific type of therapy that is related to but different from reminiscence. The concept of life review was introduced by Butler (1963), who perceived life review as a task to be accomplished in the final stage of life. Life review is described as a process of reviewing, organizing, and evaluating one's life with the purpose of increasing integrity by seeing one's own unique life story (Woods et al. 1992). Life review can be used as an individual or group intervention. Woods and colleagues (1992) have developed four tools to assist in life review: 1) an intensive questionnaire covering 14 aspects of one's life; 2) a condensed guideline questionnaire, with key questions as a checklist covering 14 subsections of life history; 3) a general life-course trajectory checklist; and 4) a historical setting graph. Peachey (1992) has developed a short life-review question list with questions covering three areas: 1) ego differentiation versus work-role preoccupation, 2) body transcendence versus body preoccupation, and 3) ego transcendence versus ego preoccupation. Life review, like reminiscence models, can be used with partially demented as well as cognitively intact individuals.

Birren and Deutchman (1994) have developed a technique called *guided autobiography groups,* which draws from both reminiscence and life review concepts. Members are asked to write and share autobiographical material. Nine autobiographical areas are explored: major branching points in life; family history; career; role of money in life; health and body image; loves and dislikes; sexual identity; roles and experiences with death and ideas about dying; and aspirations, life goals, and the meaning of life. Guided autobiography may be particularly helpful to elders living in a society in which social change makes it difficult for individuals to integrate their lives as part of a natural progressive process.

Other therapeutic group approaches have focused on the here and now. *Reality orientation (RO) groups* are groups developed to rehabilitate confused geropsychiatric clients. RO groups have been used in hospitals, nursing homes, and day care programs. In addition, RO strategies can be used by individual caregivers. RO groups usually meet daily. A variety of props are used, including a calendar, clock, name tags, and an RO board—a large, movable board that can be used to post date, time, place, weather, next holiday, or other information helpful for reorienting group members. A variety of activities may be used, including current events, cooking, discussion groups, and reminiscence. RO programs can increase social interaction and involvement in activities. Burnside and Haight (1994) point out that RO works best in the context of a cheerful, cue-filled environment in which activities are performed that stimulate the senses.

Feil (1992) has developed a therapeutic approach called *validation therapy* for use with patients with late-onset dementia. This model is now used in more than 6,000 facilities in the United States and abroad. The goals of validation therapy are to stimulate verbal and nonverbal communication and to help restore feelings of dignity and well-being. Validation therapy includes 1) a way of categorizing behavior of disoriented elders into four discrete stages, 2) a method of communication (verbal and nonverbal) with persons in each stage, and 3) a theory of late-onset disorientation in previously healthy elders. Validation therapy accepts the losses in the oldest old of social control, cognitive thinking, sensory acuity, reflective self-awareness, speech, and mobility. Emphasis is placed on attending to verbal and nonverbal cues to find patterns in behavior. Techniques used include touch; close eye contact; a low, caring tone of voice; linking nonverbal behavior to unmet needs; mirroring nonverbal behavior; and matching rhythms and repeated movements with one's own. The four stages of behavior are malorientation, time confusion, repetitive motion, and the vegetative state. (Feil uses the term *malorientation* to refer to elderly persons in the early stage of dementia who have no previous history of mental illness, who are oriented to time and place, but who have occasional memory loss and mild disinhibition. The maloriented person experiences reactivation of unresolved conflicts during the period of memory decline and deals with these issues by blaming, accusing, and complaining.) Characteristics of individuals in each stage and helper responses are identifiable (Feil 1989, 1992). Validation therapy is an approach that provides an alternative to RO for the confused old-old, with whom RO may no longer be appropriate.

An additional approach to group work with elderly persons is the use of issue- or problem-focused support or self-help groups. *Retirement adjustment groups* assist individuals in the transition from life dominated by a work identity to other forms of self-identity and self-esteem. Crouch (1990) described a widowhood group that was based on Bowen's family systems theory and that used the concepts of triangling, differentiation of self, multigenerational transmission process, emotional cutoff, and sibling position to assist in understanding the individual widow's experience. Other widows' groups have been developed that focus on an educational model, assisting individuals in understanding the grief process. The National Association of Retired Teachers and the American Association of Retired Persons have developed support groups for widowed persons that employ a self-help approach (Burnside and Schmidt 1994). Groups have also been used extensively to assist individuals who are caregivers for Alzheimer's patients. These groups use an educational model, a mutual support model, or a combination of the education and mutual support emphases. Support groups can provide significant assistance in helping individuals deal with caregiver burden, which can have an impact on both physical and psychological health.

Family and Marital Therapy

Although limited work has been done in the area of family and marital therapy, the intergenerational issues manifested in late life as well as the changes in marital relationships necessitate consideration. Direct intervention with the children or spouse of an elderly patient is frequently an important part of the treatment process. This may primarily involve psychoeducational work around an illness process, or it may be dynamically oriented family or marital therapy working with long-standing issues and themes, with conflictual patterns being exacerbated by stressors of the present context. The deterioration that occurs in patients with progressive cognitive impairment frequently requires a role reversal in family interpersonal patterns. The family member who assumes a new role will benefit from supportive psychotherapy that deals with the new role and his or her feelings regarding the decline of the identified elderly patient. A multidisciplinary approach is useful in dealing with such situations, allowing for different care providers to meet the needs of the varied members of the family system. Capacity to meet the individual needs represented is frequently vital to providing adequate care for the systemic unit and the identified elderly patient. Knight (1986) emphasized the need for a conscious awareness on the part of the therapist regarding the competing interests represented by the different family members, and the potential for the therapist to perhaps unconsciously become imbalanced regarding these interests (or at least to be perceived in this way). Gallagher-Thompson et al. (1991) advocated cognitive-behavior therapy and time-limited psychodynamic therapy with families of elderly patients for assistance with their own affective responses to the illness of the identified elderly patient. This psychotherapeutic intervention ultimately benefits the elderly patient as well as the family member(s).

Pharmacotherapy With Psychotherapy

The particulars of psychopharmacotherapy in the elderly are comprehensively discussed in other chapters, but we emphasize here that the interface of pharmacotherapy and psychotherapy is particularly important in the total treatment of elderly individuals. Old assumptions regarding medications—particularly antidepressant medications—interfering with the psychotherapeutic process are increasingly acknowledged to be invalid.

When making clinical choices about treatment options, there are some clear guidelines for selecting a psychotherapy/pharmacotherapy combination. Combined treatment is indicated for patients whose depression is more severe and is associated with melancholia, or those who have only partial responses to either treatment alone. Those persons with a more chronic history or poor interepisode recovery should also receive combined therapy (Depression Guideline Panel 1993). If significant psychosocial or interpersonal problems remain after primary symptom remission with pharmacotherapy, psychotherapy should be added as an adjunctive therapy. For patients who are being treated solely with psychotherapy, the addition of medication should be considered if there is poor response to psychotherapy after 6 weeks or only partial response after 12 weeks (Depression Guideline Panel 1993). Patients with sleep and/or concentration difficulties may be less likely to make optimal use of psychotherapeutic efforts than are those who have attained some stabilization of such symptoms.

Concurrently, it is important that pharmacotherapy with psychotropic medications be initiated with elderly persons in a context that reflects recognition of supportive psychotherapeutic and psychoeducational needs. Compliance and general appropriate use of medications is more likely if a therapeutic alliance has been established and a supportive psychotherapeutic approach is being used. Frequently, older persons take multiple medications and will view as supportive a therapist's interest in interactions of their medications as well as concerns regarding side effects and their perceptions regarding their medications. If the psychotherapist is a nonphysician, basic interest and concern regarding medication use will still usually be appreciated, along with encouragement to consult the appropriate physician if indicated. In some instances in which side effects or possibly toxic effects are acute and the patient is reticent to contact the physician, the psychotherapist should obtain consent to make this contact to facilitate optimal pharmacological management.

Unconscious avoidance, neglect, or abuse of medications by an elderly patient is a potential dynamic in the relationship between a younger physician and an older patient. Hesitancy to explore this possibility and to intervene may be secondary to countertransference issues discussed earlier in this chapter. It is also important to consider the patient who responds well to medication and supportive therapy in the hospital setting but rapidly deteriorates after discharge, with recurrent admissions. In these instances, it may be useful to explore family and environmental factors that may require intervention beyond the scope of previously used medication and supportive therapy.

Practical Considerations in Therapy With the Elderly

Therapy with the elderly patient requires therapist sensitivity to some of the unique needs of older adults. The setting for the therapeutic contact should reflect attention to the special needs of many elderly persons. Offices should provide seating with adequate seat height, firmness, and arm rests to assist the elder who has mobility problems in getting in and out of the chair. Lighting should reflect the elder's need for two to three times the usual lighting for adequate visual acuity. The therapist should consider visual and/or hearing deficits in positioning the therapist's and patient's chairs. Closer proximity and face-to-face presentation may facilitate adequate hearing, and maximal use of nonverbal cues (such as facial expressions and gestures) should be made to enhance understanding. When the patient's hearing is impaired, the therapist may need to speak slowly and loudly or may at times have to use written modalities. Written materials for patients should be available in larger size type to accommodate those with decreased visual acuity. Ideally, offices should be handicapped accessible to allow for the wheelchair-bound client.

It is particularly important with the elderly, who are subject to many actual or potential ego threats, to convey respect, approval, and affirmation. The therapist, who is often decades younger than the patient, should address the patient as "Mr.," "Mrs.," or by another, appropriate honorific (such as an aca-demic or military title by which the patient is customarily addressed) unless the patient specifically requests to be addressed by his or her first name. The patient should generally be interviewed first and alone, even when it is clear that extensive family interviewing will be necessary to obtain adequate data. The therapist must also be sensitive to patient fears related to seeing a psychiatrist and try to make the patient's initial experience nonthreatening and helpful. Finally, although family contact may be a necessity, the patient's confidentiality must be respected.

Lazarus and Sadavoy (1988) emphasized that in working with the elderly, the therapist may assume different roles in the course of therapeutic work, including those of primary care physician, psychopharmacologist, individual or family therapist, and member of the health care team. With the elderly patient, who often has multiple medical problems and complex medication and treatment regimens, ongoing communication and coordination of treatment with other health care professionals involved in the patient's care is imperative.

To maximize therapeutic outcome, it is important that the treatment plan be individualized and explained in language the patient and family can understand. It is crucial that treatment goals be realistic, taking into account patient limitations to avoid setting the patient up for failure. However, therapeutic goals should not be limited by the therapist's preconceptions about the potential for change in the elderly patient.

Common Themes and Issues in Therapeutic Work With Elders

A number of authors have addressed common issues and themes encountered in therapeutic work with older adults (Butler et al. 1991; Colarusso and Nemiroff 1991; Knight 1986; Lazarus 1989; Steuer 1982). Although the number of issues or themes identified is lengthy, common areas of concern can be identified. The literature addressing the problems confronting elderly persons consistently identifies *loss in multiple spheres of life* as a central issue. These losses include health, physical and cognitive abilities, work roles, relationships, possessions, financial security, social position, and even the impending loss of life itself. For the purpose of this discussion, issues will be divided into three areas: intrapersonal issues, interpersonal/social issues, and issues related to one's own personal death. It is important to note that the issues in each area are conceived of as presenting not only challenges but also opportunities.

All elderly persons at some point confront the reality of growing old. Whereas growing up in our society has many positive connotations, growing old is viewed culturally in a far more negative, stigmatized way (Steuer 1982). Basic developmental issues include dealing with the maintenance of bodily integrity and reacting to physical infirmity and permanent impairment (Colarusso and Nemiroff 1991). Searching for signs of health may be an issue for the elder who is grappling with the realities of physical aging (Butler et al. 1991).

The maintenance of self-esteem and ego integrity become increasingly important as abilities and roles change. With retirement comes the need to define a new non–work-related identity. Even for the older woman who has not worked outside the home, home and social roles will change with the emancipation of children and change in the spouse's work role. The basic need to maintain empowerment versus helplessness and capacity for enjoyment versus lack of enjoyment of life become crucial (Knight 1986). From a more positive perspective, this period can be experienced as a time for new starts and second chances (Butler et al. 1991).

Interpersonal/social factors also present significant issues for the elderly. Role loss may occur through retirement, death of spouse or friends, or a general change in regular activities. In addition to role loss, role conflict may occur with children and with spouse as individual needs, capacities, and roles change. One specifically problematic role change is the role reversal that may occur when adult children assume responsibilities for elderly parents. Underlying all of these issues is the broader need to maintain companionship and connectedness as opposed to moving toward isolation and loneliness. Of importance in maintaining companionship amidst changing relationships is the ability to form new ties and to see oneself as continuing to possess the capacity for forming relationships.

In addition to intrapersonal and social issues, the elderly person must also deal with an awareness of the increasing proximity to his or her own death. At this stage of life, previous strategies of denial of death may fail. Patients may present with many issues that reflect "death in disguise" (Butler et al. 1991). The older person often experiences a need for life review and reflection, with a keen awareness of time, while at the same time tending to focus on the present and the past but not the future. This process may be one of searching for the meaning and purpose of one's life while dealing with issues such as guilt and atonement related to one's perceived failures. The individual may struggle with the process of dying and permitting death at some point (Butler et al. 1991). Beyond death itself, the need for support for the surviving spouse and children may be a concern for an older adult.

The intrapersonal, social, and death-related issues confronting elderly individuals are all important components of the experiential context that the elderly patient brings to any therapeutic contact. It is important to recognize the specific issues confronting any individual or family in a therapeutic context and to recognize that there may be great diversity in patient experiences. It is critical that the therapist not become overwhelmed and demoralized with the multiple issues confronting many elderly patients so that he or she remains able to actively assist in identifying opportunities and positive coping strategies.

Conclusions

Psychotherapy with older persons continues to develop with regard to techniques used and practice settings. This diversity is driven by the needs of an ever-growing elderly population whose personal psychiatric needs, as well as the psychological needs of their families, are being gradually, increasingly acknowledged. Meeting these needs optimally will require practitioners from multiple disciplines with varying expertise to coordinate their efforts, communicate better, and deliver a seamless continuum of care, with some form of psychotherapeutic intervention being part of the treatment process for many of the elders. Psychotherapy always occurs in a biopsychosocial context, and decisions regarding modality of therapy are dependent on the other variables within this context. The potential for elders to make good use of psychotherapy and to gain significant benefit from this process, albeit with adjustments made according to their stage in life, is being increasingly acknowledged. Systematic outcome research, carried out by investigators from multiple disciplines in a variety of care settings, will serve both the practitioner of psychotherapy and the elderly patient in continuing to maximize the appropriate and necessary use of psychotherapy in later life.

References

Abraham K: The applicability of psychoanalytic treatment to patients at an advanced age, in Selected Papers of Psychoanalysis. London, Hogarth Press, 1949, pp 312–317

American Psychiatric Association Task Force on Models of Practice in Geriatric Psychiatry: Selected Models of Practice in Geriatric Psychiatry. Washington, DC, American Psychiatric Association, 1993

American Psychiatric Association Work Group on Major Depressive Disorder: Practice guidelines for major depressive disorder in adults. Am J Psychiatry 150 (suppl):1–21, 1993

Atchley RC: The aging self. Psychotherapy: Theory, Research and Practice 9:388–396, 1982

Beck A, Rush J, Shaw B, et al: Cognitive Therapy of Depression. New York, Guilford, 1979

Berland DI, Poggi R: Expressive group psychotherapy with the aging. Int J Group Psychother 29:87–108, 1979

Birren JE, Deutchman DE: Guided autobiography groups, in Working with Older Adults: Group Process and Techniques. Edited by Burnside I, Schmidt MG. Boston, MA, Jones & Bartlett, 1994, pp 179–191

Burnside I, Haight B: Reminiscence and life review: therapeutic interventions for older persons. Nurse Pract 19:55–61, 1994

Burnside I, Schmidt MG (eds): Working With Older Adults: Group Process and Techniques. Boston, MA, Jones & Bartlett, 1994

Butler RN: The life review: an interpretation of reminiscence in the aged. Psychiatry 26:65–76, 1963

Butler RN, Lewis MI: Aging and Mental Health: Positive Psychosocial Approaches, 2nd Edition. St. Louis, MO, CV Mosby, 1977

Butler RN, Lewis MI, Sunderland T: Aging and Mental Health: Positive Psychosocial and Biomedical Approaches, 4th Edition. New York, Merrill, 1991

Chaisson-Stewart GM: Psychotherapy, in Depression in the Elderly: An Interdisciplinary Approach. New York, Wiley, 1985, pp 263–284

Colarusso CA, Nemiroff RA: Impact of the adult developmental issues on treatment of older patients, in New Techniques in the Psychotherapy of Older Patients. Edited by Myers WA. Washington, DC, American Psychiatric Press, 1991, pp 245–264

Coleman P: Issues in the therapeutic use of reminiscence with elderly people, in Mental Health Problems in Old Age: A Reader. Edited by Gearing B, Johnson M, Heller T. Chichester, UK, Wiley, 1988, pp 177–184

Crouch LR: Putting widowhood in perspective: a group approach utilizing family systems principles, in Caring for the Elderly in Diverse Settings. Edited by Eliopoulos C. Philadelphia, PA, JB Lippincott, 1990, pp 318–328

Depression Guideline Panel: Depression in Primary Care, Vol 2: Treatment of Major Depression (Clinical Practice Guideline No 5; AHCPR Publ No 93-0551). Rockville, MD, U.S. Department of Health and Human Services, Public Health Service Agency for Health Care Policy and Research, April 1993

Deutsch CB, Kramer N: Outpatient group psychotherapy for the elderly: an alternative to institutionalization. Hosp Community Psychiatry 28:440–441, 1977

Erickson EH, Erickson JM, Kivnick HQ: Vital Involvement in Old Age. New York, WW Norton, 1986

Feil N: V/F Validation: The Feil Method. Cleveland, OH, Edward Feil Productions, 1989

Feil N: Validation therapy with late-onset dementia populations, in Care Giving in Dementia. Edited by Jones GMM, Miesen BML. London, Tavistock/Routledge, 1992, pp 199–218

Fogel BS, Gottlieb GL, Furino A: Minds at risk, in Mental Health Policy for Older Americans: Protecting Minds at Risk. Edited by Fogel BS, Furino A, Gottlieb GL. Washington, DC, American Psychiatric Press, 1990, pp 1–22

Freidan B: Fountain of Age. New York, Simon & Schuster, 1993

Freud S: On psychotherapy (1924), in The Standard Edition of the Complete Psychological Works of Sigmund Freud, Vol 1. Translated and edited by Strachey G. London, Hogarth, 1966, pp 249–263

Gallagher DE, Thompson LW: Depression in the Elderly: A Behavioral Treatment Manual. Los Angeles, CA, University of Southern California Press, 1981

Gallagher DE, Thompson LW: Treatment of major depressive disorder in older adult outpatients with brief psychotherapies. Psychotherapy 19: 482–490, 1982

Gallagher-Thompson DE, Lovett S, Rose J: Psychotherapeutic interventions in stress of family caregivers, in New Techniques in the Psychotherapy of Older Patients. Edited by Myers WA. Washington, DC, American Psychiatric Press, 1991, pp 61–78

Goffman E: Stigma: Notes on the Management of Spoiled Identity. New York, Simon & Schuster, 1963, 1974

Grunes J: The aged in psychotherapy: psychodynamic contributions to the treatment process, in Treating the Elderly with Psychotherapy. Edited by Sadavoy J, Leszcz M. Madison, WI, International Universities Press, 1987, pp 31–44

Ingersoll B, Silverman A: Comparative group psychotherapy for the aged. Gerontologist 18:201–206, 1978

Jung C: The Integration of the Personality. New York, Farrar & Reinhart, 1939

Kimmell D: Adulthood and Aging: An Interdisciplinary Developmental View. New York, Wiley, 1974

Klerman GL, Weissman MM, Rounsaville BJ, et al: Interpersonal Psychotherapy of Depression. New York, Basic Books, 1984

Knight B: Psychotherapy with Older Adults. Beverly Hills, CA, Sage, 1986

Lazarus LW: Psychotherapy with geriatric patients in the ambulatory care setting, in Geriatric Psychiatry. Edited by Busse EW, Blazer DG. Washington, DC, American Psychiatric Press, 1989, pp 567–591

Lazarus LW, Sadavoy J: Psychotherapy with the elderly, in Essentials of Geriatric Psychiatry: A Guide for Health Professionals. Edited by Lazarus LW. New York, Springer, 1988, pp 147–172

Lazarus LW, Groves L, Gutmann D, et al: Brief psychotherapy with the elderly: a study of process and outcome, in Treating the Elderly with Psychotherapy. Edited by Sadavoy J, Leszcz M. Madison, WI, International Universities Press, 1987, pp 233–264

Lewinsohn PM, Hoberman H, Teri L, et al: An integrative theory of depression, in Theoretical Issues in Behavior Therapy. Edited by Reiss S, Bodzin PR. Orlando, FL, Academic Press, 1985, pp 331–359

May R, Yalom I: Existential psychotherapy, in Current Psychotherapies, 4th Edition. Edited by Corsini RJ, Wedding D. Itasca, IL, FE Peacock, 1989, pp 363–401

McDougall CJ: What role philosophy in psychotherapy? Perspect Psychiatr Care 28:3, 1992

Meerloo JAM: Psychotherapy with elderly people. Geriatrics 10:583–587, 1955

Moberg PJ, Lazarus LW: Psychotherapy of depression in the elderly. Psychiatric Annals 20:92–96, 1990

Muslin HL: The Psychotherapy of the Elderly Self. New York, Brunner/Mazel, 1992

Myers WA: Psychoanalytic psychotherapy and psychoanalysis with older patients, in Newer Techniques in the Psychotherapy of Older Patients. Edited by Myers WA. Washington, DC, American Psychiatric Press, 1991, pp 265–279

National Institutes of Health (NIH) Consensus Development Panel on Depression in Late Life: Diagnosis and treatment of depression in late life. JAMA 268:1018–1024, 1992

Peachey NH: Helping the elderly person resolve integrity versus despair. Perspect Psychiatr Care 28:29–30, 1992

Ray W, Taylor J, Meador K, et al: Reducing antipsychotic drug use in nursing homes: a controlled trial of provider education. Arch Intern Med 153:713–721, 1993

Rockland LH: A review of supportive psychotherapy, 1986–1992. Hosp Community Psychiatry 44:1053–1060, 1993

Scott-Maxwell F: The Measure of My Days. New York, Penguin Books, 1968

Sholomskas AJ, Chevron ES, Prusoff BA, et al: Short-term interpersonal therapy (ITP) with the depressed elderly: case reports and discussion. Am J Psychother 37:552–566, 1983

Silberschatz G, Curtis JT: Time-limited psychotherapy with older adults, in Newer Techniques in the Psychotherapy of Older Patients. Edited by Myers WA. Washington, DC, American Psychiatric Press, 1991, pp 95–100

Steuer J: Psychotherapy for depressed elders, in Treatment of Late Life Depression. Edited by Blazer DG. St. Louis, MO, CV Mosby, 1982, pp 195–220

Teri L, Gallagher-Thompson D: Cognitive-behavioral interventions for treatment of depression in Alzheimer's patient. Gerontologist 31:413–416, 1991

Thibault JM: A Deepening Love Affair: The Gift of God in Later Life. Nashville, TN, Upper Room Books, 1993

Thompson LW, Gallagher D, Steinmetz-Breckenridge J: Comparative effectiveness of psychotherapies for depressed elders. J Consult Clin Psychol 55:385–390, 1987

Tournier P: Learn to Grow Old. Louisville, KY, Westminister/John Knox Press, 1972

Viney LL: Life Stories: Personal Construct Therapy with the Elderly. Chichester, UK, Wiley, 1993

Weiss J: Part 1: Theory and Clinical Observation in the Psychoanalytic Process: Theory, Clinical Observation, and Empirical Research. Edited by Weiss J, Sampson H, Mount Zion Psychotherapy Research Group. New York, Guilford, 1986, pp 3–138

Werman DS: The practice of supportive psychotherapy. New York, Brunner/Mazel, 1984

Woods B, Portnoy S, Head D: Reminiscence and life review with persons with dementia: which way forward?, in Care Giving and Dementia. Jones GMM, Miesen BML. London, Tavistock/Routledge, 1992, pp 137–161

Woods N, Witte K: Life satisfaction, fear of death, and ego identity in elderly adults. Bulletin of Psychonomic Society 18(U):165–168, 1981

Yalom ID: The Theory and Practice of Group Psychotherapy. New York, Basic Books, 1985

Yesavage JA, Karusa TB: Psychotherapy with the elderly. Am J Psychother 36:41–55, 1982

Yost EB, Corbishley MA: Group Therapy in Depression and the Elderly: An Interdisciplinary Approach. Edited by Chaisson-Stewart GM. New York, Wiley, 1985, pp 288–315

CHAPTER 23

Clinical Psychiatry in the Nursing Home

Joel E. Streim, M.D.
Ira R. Katz, M.D., Ph.D.

Nursing homes provide long-term care for elderly patients with chronic illness and disability as well as rehabilitation and convalescent care for those recovering from acute illness. As documented in recent reviews (Rovner and Katz 1993; Streim et al. 1996), clinical studies have consistently provided evidence that the diagnosis, management, and treatment of mental disorders is an important component of nursing home care. At present, the delivery of mental health services is being shaped by a number of factors, including growing scientific knowledge, federal legislation and evolving regulations, and changes in the medical marketplace. In this chapter we review current information on the psychiatric problems that are common in the nursing home, discuss current trends affecting clinical care, and present a conceptual model for the organization of mental health services.

Nursing Home Populations

According to the 1985 National Nursing Home Survey (National Center for Health Statistics 1987),

approximately 5% of Americans 65 years of age or older—1.5 million people—resided in more than 20,000 long-term care facilities; 88% of all nursing home residents were 65 years of age or older. The proportion of individuals living in nursing homes increased with age and included 1% of those between 65 and 74 years of age, 3% of those between 75 and 84 years of age, and 22% of those 85 years of age and older. Persons living in these institutions tend to be very disabled: 91% of residents required assistance in bathing; 78% needed help with dressing; 63% needed assistance in both toileting and transferring; and 40% required help with eating. A total of 55% of nursing home residents were incontinent. Only 8% of these residents were independent in all activities of daily living (ADL). The mean length of stay in a nursing home was 2.5 years; 67% of the residents had lived in a home for at least 1 year. Projections have been made that 25% of Americans will spend part of their lives in nursing homes (Campion et al. 1983) and that the number of nursing home residents will more than triple by the year 2020 (McCarthy 1989).

Clinical Features of Psychiatric Disorders

Recent studies have uniformly reported high prevalence rates for psychiatric disorders among nursing home residents. Rovner and colleagues (1990a) reported a prevalence of 80.2% among persons newly admitted to a proprietary chain of nursing homes. Parmelee and associates (1989) found DSM-III-R (American Psychiatric Association 1987) psychiatric disorders in 91% of the residents of a large urban geriatric center. Other investigators, on the basis of psychiatric interviews of subjects in randomly selected samples, found prevalence rates of DSM-III (American Psychiatric Association 1980) or DSM-III-R disorders as high as 94% (Chandler and Chandler 1988; Rovner et al. 1986; Tariot et al. 1993). Although some studies have reported lower rates, those investigations used less rigorous methods for sampling or diagnosis (Burns et al. 1988; Custer et al. 1984; German et al. 1986; National Center for Health Statistics 1987; Teeter et al. 1976).

Dementia

In all studies, the most common psychiatric disorder has been dementia, with prevalence rates of 50%–75% (Chandler and Chandler 1988; Katz et al. 1989a; Parmelee et al. 1989; Rovner et al. 1986, 1990a; Tariot et al. 1993; Teeter et al. 1976). An Epidemiologic Catchment Area (ECA) study showed a lower prevalence of cognitive impairment, but the more severely impaired patients who could not complete testing procedures were excluded from the sample (German et al. 1986). Alzheimer's disease (DSM-III-R primary degenerative dementia) accounts for approximately 50%–60% of cases of dementia, and multi-infarct dementia for about 25%–30% (Barnes and Raskind 1980; Rovner et al. 1986, 1990a). Other causes of dementia are reported with lower prevalence and greater variability between sites.

Delirium is common in nursing homes and occurs primarily in patients made more vulnerable by a dementing illness. Available studies have indicated that approximately 6%–7% of residents were delirious at the time of evaluation (Barnes and Raskind 1980; Rovner et al. 1986, 1990a). However, this figure probably underestimates the number of patients who have reversible toxic or metabolic components to their cognitive impairment. In one study, investigators found that nearly 25% of impaired residents had potentially reversible conditions (Sabin et al. 1982), and in another, that 6%–12% of residential care patients with dementia actually improved in cognitive performance over the course of 1 year (Katz et al. 1991). In the nursing home, as in other settings, the most common reversible cause of cognitive impairment may be cognitive toxicity from drugs used to treat medical or psychiatric disorders.

The clinical features of dementing disorders include treatable components, such as hallucinations, delusions, and depressions, that can contribute to disability. Psychotic symptoms have been reported in approximately 25%–50% of residents with a primary dementing illness (Berrios and Brook 1985; Chandler and Chandler 1988; Rovner et al. 1986, 1990a; Teeter et al. 1976). Clinically significant depression is seen in approximately 25% of demented patients; one-third of such patients exhibit symptoms of a secondary major depression (Parmelee et al. 1989; Rovner et al. 1986, 1990a).

Behavioral disturbances may be present in as many as two-thirds to three-fourths of residents, and multiple behavior problems in half (Chandler and Chandler 1988; Cohen-Mansfield 1986; National Center for Health Statistics 1979; Rovner et al. 1986, 1990a; Tariot et al. 1993; Zimmer et al. 1984). Disturbances of behavior, in addition to impaired ability to perform ADL, have been identified as the most common reasons that patients with dementia are admitted to nursing homes (Steele et al. 1990), and disruptive behaviors frequently complicate care after admission (Cohen-Mansfield et al. 1989; Teeter 1976; Zimmer et al. 1984). The majority of psychiatric consultations in long-term care settings are for the evaluation and treatment of behavioral disturbances such as pacing/wandering, verbal abusiveness, disruptive shouting, physical aggression, and resistance to necessary care. As demonstrated by Loebel and co-workers (1991), there are frequent, but not invariable, associations between the nature of the behavioral problems that lead to psychiatric consultation and the underlying diagnosis. Behavioral disturbances most frequently occur in patients with dementia, often in those whose illness includes psychotic symptoms (Rovner et al. 1990b). Agitation and hyperactivity can also be caused by agitated depression, delirium, sensory deprivation or overload, occult physical illness, pain, constipation, urinary retention, and adverse drug effects including akathisia due to neuroleptics (Cohen-Mansfield and Billig 1986).

Cohen-Mansfield and co-workers (1989) made major contributions to the characterization, description, and measurement of agitation and related behavioral disturbances as these occur among patients with dementia. They identified three distinct types of agitated behaviors: verbally agitated behavior, physically nonaggressive behavior, and aggressive behavior. The verbally agitated behaviors most frequently observed were constant requests for attention, negativism, repetitive sentences and questions, screaming, and complaining. The physically nonaggressive behaviors most often seen were pacing, inappropriate robing/disrobing, trying to get to a different place, handling things inappropriately, general restlessness, and inappropriate mannerisms.

In addition to agitation, symptoms such as apathy, inactivity, and withdrawal occur among nursing home residents. Although these symptoms are less disturbing to staff and less frequently lead to psychiatric consultation, they can be disabling and may be associated with decreases in socialization and self-care. As reviewed by Marin (1990, 1991), apathy can be a symptom of depression, a component of dementia, or, possibly, a separate syndrome. Kaplitz (1975) suggested that the apathy associated with dementia may be treatable, and that it may respond to methylphenidate.

Depression

Depressive disorders represent the second most common psychiatric diagnosis in nursing home residents. The epidemiology and clinical features of these disorders were recently reviewed by Ames (1991) and by Katz and Parmelee (1993). Most studies in U.S. nursing homes show depression prevalence rates of 15%–50%, depending on the population studied and the instruments used, whether major depression or depressive symptoms are being reported, and whether primary depression and depression occurring secondary to dementia are considered together or separately (Baker and Miller 1991; Chandler and Chandler 1988; Hyer and Blazer 1982; Katz et al. 1989a; Lesher 1986; Parmelee et al. 1989; Rovner et al. 1986, 1990a, 1991; Tariot et al. 1993; Teeter et al. 1976). Studies from other countries have shown similar rates (Ames 1990; Ames et al.

1988; Harrison et al. 1990; Horiguchi and Inami 1991; Mann et al. 1984; Snowdon 1986; Snowdon and Donnelly 1986; Spagnoli et al. 1986; Trichard et al. 1982). Thus, the high rates of depression cannot be attributed solely to problems in this country's approach to long-term care for the elderly. Approximately 20%–25% of those residents who are cognitively intact meet DSM-III or DSM-III-R criteria for major depression; this figure is an order of magnitude greater than rates in the community-dwelling elderly (Blazer and Williams 1980; Kramer et al. 1985). The prevalence of other, less severe, forms of depression is even higher. In one study, Parmelee and associates (1992a) reported that the 1-year incidence of major depression was 9.4% and that patients with preexisting minor depression were at increased risk; the incidence of minor depression among those who were euthymic at baseline was 7.4%. Other, smaller scale studies have shown comparable rates (Foster et al. 1991; Katz et al. 1989a).

Depressions among nursing home residents tend to be persistent. Although there may be moderate decreases in self-rated depression in the initial 2 weeks after nursing home admission (Engle and Graney 1993), Ames et al. (1988) found that only 17% of patients with diagnosable depressive disorders had recovered after an average 3.6 years of follow-up. Evidence for morbidity associated with depression comes from studies showing an increase in pain complaints among residents with depression (Parmelee et al. 1991) and an association between depression and biochemical markers of subnutrition (Katz et al. 1993). In addition to its association with morbidity, depression has been found to be associated with an increase in mortality, with effect sizes ranging from 1.6 to 3 (Ashby et al. 1991; Katz et al. 1989a; Parmelee et al. 1992b; Rovner et al. 1991). There is, however, controversy about the mechanism involved. Whereas Rovner and colleagues (1991) reported that the increased mortality remained apparent after controlling for the patients' medical diagnoses and level of disability, Parmelee and associates (1992a) found that the effect could be attributed to the interrelationships among depression, disability, and physical illness. Resolution of this issue will require further study.

It has been demonstrated that major depression in long-term care patients is a treatable disorder. Katz and co-workers (1989b, 1990) conducted a double-blind, placebo-controlled study of the treatment of major depression in a study population (average age 84) from a large nursing home and congregate apartment facility. Subjects received either placebo or nortriptyline with dosages adjusted to achieve plasma levels within the therapeutic range. Among study completers ($n = 23$), 58% of patients taking active medication, but only 9% of those taking placebo, were rated "much" or "very much" improved; 83% of those given the drug, but only 22% of those given placebo, exhibited improvement of any degree. Thus, even a small-scale study demonstrated a significant drug-placebo difference.

This study by Katz and co-workers is valuable primarily because the patients' response to treatment serves as a probe of the nature of the psychopathology that occurs in long-term care patients. The literature on depression as it presents in patients with significant medical illness is marked by recurring questions about the extent to which diagnostic criteria developed in younger and healthier adults remain valid among patients with significant psychiatric-medical comorbidity. A priori, it may have appeared reasonable to hypothesize that the somatic and vegetative symptoms that characterize major depression in other populations were likely to lose their diagnostic value among long-term care residents; and that long-term care patients who have symptoms consistent with a diagnosis of major depressive disorder may, in fact, be experiencing a combination of medical symptoms and an existential reaction to disability, disease, and residential care placement. The results of the Katz et al. trial, however, demonstrated that DSM-III-R approaches to diagnosis remain valid as predictors of treatment response and suggest that the symptoms of major depression in frail elderly patients characterize a disease similar to that which occurs among younger adult psychiatric patients.

Although the available research literature demonstrates that major depression remains a specific psychiatric disorder among elderly patients who require residential care, the findings illustrate that such cases are highly complex and that essentially all patients have concurrent medical illnesses and disabilities that complicate diagnosis and treatment planning. Moreover, clinical experience indicates that the frequent occurrence of intercurrent illnesses over time complicates the long-term management of these patients and can make it difficult to deliver continuation or maintenance treatment. Thus, the concomitant occurrence of depression and medical illness among elderly persons in residential care settings presents a series of complex problems, the solutions to which require substantial clinical expertise. In addition to the high level of complexity that characterizes major depression among nursing home residents, there is evidence for heterogeneity in these patients that may reflect the existence of clinically relevant subtypes of depression. The treatment study of Katz and colleagues (1989b, 1990) demonstrated that measures of self-care deficits and serum levels of albumin were highly intercorrelated, and that both predicted a failure to respond to nortriptyline treatment. Thus, although the primary conclusion from this study must be that major depression remains a specific, treatable disorder, even in long-term care patients with significant medical comorbidity, there is also evidence for a treatment-relevant subtype of depression, characterized by high levels of disability and low levels of serum albumin, that appears to emerge specifically in this setting. This latter condition may be related to "failure to thrive," as discussed by Braun and colleagues (1988) and by Katz et al. (1993).

Problems Related to the Lack of Mental Health Services in Nursing Homes

Although psychiatric disorders are extraordinarily common among nursing home residents, psychiatric services are often not adequate. It has been estimated that as many as two-thirds of nursing home residents with psychiatric disorders are misdiagnosed (German et al. 1986; Sabin et al. 1982) and that as little as 5% of the needs of nursing home residents for mental health services are currently being met (Burns and Taube 1990). A major mismatch has existed between the needs of the residents and the types of care provided by nursing homes. Facilities designed primarily for the treatment of "uncomplicated" medical or surgical cases have in fact been serving patients with dementing disorders and with medical disorders complicated by depressions. Historically, this mismatch led not only to neglect but also to inappropriate treatment in which psychiatric problems were often mismanaged by use of physical or chemical restraints.

Use of Physical Restraints

Discussion of the use of mechanical restraints for the control of behavior makes the most dramatic case for increased mental health services in the nursing home. The 1977 survey of American nursing home residents showed that 25% of 1.3 million people were restrained by geriatric chairs, cuffs, belts, or similar devices, primarily in an attempt to control behavioral symptoms (National Center for Health Statistics 1979). Other surveys have demonstrated prevalence rates as high as 85%. In addition to agitation and behavior problems, patient factors predicting the use of restraints include age, cognitive impairment, risk of injuries to self or others (for example, from falls or combative behavior), physical frailty, presence of monitoring or treatment devices, and the need to promote body alignment. Institutional and system factors associated with restraint use include pressure to avoid litigation, staff attitudes, insufficient staffing, and the availability of restraint devices. Potential adverse effects include an increased risk of falls and other injuries, functional decline, skin breakdown, physiological effects of immobilization stress, disorganized behavior, and demoralization. Although mechanical restraints have frequently been used to control disruptive behavior, very little research has been devoted to evaluating the benefits versus the risks of the use of restraints or systematic investigations of alternatives. Werner et al. (1989) have suggested that use of mechanical restraints does not, in fact, decrease behavioral disturbances, and cross-national studies have indicated that it is possible to manage nursing home residents without such measures (Cape 1983; Evans and Strumpf 1989; Innes and Turman 1983).

Misuse of Psychotropic Drugs

There has also been widespread concern regarding the overuse of psychotropic drugs in nursing home residents. Historically, there is evidence that approximately 50% of residents have orders for these agents, with 20%–40% taking neuroleptics, 10%–40% taking anxiolytics or hypnotics, and 5%–10% taking antidepressants (Avorn et al. 1989; Beers et al. 1988; Buck 1988; Burns et al. 1988; Cohen-Mansfield 1986; Custer et al. 1984; DeLeo 1989; Ray et al. 1980; Teeter et al. 1976; Zimmer et al. 1984). Psychotropic drugs have frequently been prescribed without adequate consideration of the residents' psychiatric or medical status. In one study, Zimmer and co-workers (1984) reported that only 15% of residents being given psychotropic drugs had received a psychiatric consultation. Others have reported that 21% of patients with no psychiatric diagnosis were receiving psychotropic medication (Burns et al. 1988), that physician—as opposed to patient—characteristics predicted drug dosages (Ray et al. 1980), and that psychotropic drugs were often prescribed in the absence of any charted reference to the patients' mental status (Avorn et al. 1989).

The greatest concerns about inappropriate overuse of medications are related to neuroleptics administered to control behavioral symptoms. Although evidence exists for the efficacy of neuroleptics in managing agitation and related symptoms in nursing home residents with dementia, the effects of these agents are often not dramatic, and placebo responses may be common (Barnes et al. 1982; Schneider et al. 1990). Other medications or behavioral or environmental treatments may be equally effective. Moreover, it is important to note that whereas all of the evidence for the efficacy of antipsychotic medications comes from short-term studies, these medications are frequently prescribed for long-term treatment. One classic double-blind study of neuroleptic withdrawal showed that only 16% of patients who had been receiving medications on a chronic basis exhibited significant deterioration when the drugs were withdrawn (Barton and Hurst 1966). A more recent, small-scale withdrawal study in patients who had been receiving neuroleptics for several months showed that 22% experienced increased agitation upon withdrawal, 22% were unchanged, and 55% actually showed improvement (Risse et al. 1987).

Although the overprescription of antipsychotic medications in patients with dementia has been a major issue, the misuse of psychotropic drugs in the nursing home is not limited to excesses. The Institute of Medicine (1986) report, "Improving the Quality of Care in Nursing Homes," which did much to stimulate nursing home reform, highlighted problems both in the overuse of antipsychotic drugs and in the underuse of antidepressants for treatment of affective disorders. Similarly, in reviewing epidemiological studies on the use of psychotropics in nursing homes, Murphy (1989) noted that antidepressants were the one class of drugs that appeared to be underused, and that as a result, much of the major depression present in patients in nursing homes went untreated.

Federal Regulations and Psychiatric Care in the Nursing Home

The misuse of physical and chemical restraints was among the concerns emphasized by advocacy groups in urging the federal government to institute a process of nursing home reform. In addition, the U.S. General Accounting Office was concerned that states may have been admitting patients with chronic and severe psychiatric problems to Medicaid-certified nursing homes, not because patients needed this type of care but because admission would shift a substantial portion of the costs of their care from the state to the federal government. Apparently in response to both sets of concerns, Congress enacted Nursing Home Reform Amendments as part of the Omnibus Budget Reconciliation Act (OBRA) of 1987, Public Law 100-203. This legislation provided for government regulation of the operation of nursing facilities and of the care that they provide (Elon and Pawlson 1992). The legislation enacted by Congress mandated that the Health Care Financing Administration (HCFA) issue regulations (HCFA 1991) designed to operationalize the laws that, in turn, required that HCFA develop guidelines to assist federal and state surveyors in interpreting the regulations (HCFA 1992a). Mental health screening, assessment, care planning, and treatment are addressed under sections of the regulations that pertain to resident assessment, resident rights and facility practices, and quality of care.

The regulations include provisions for Preadmission Screening and Annual Resident Review (PASARR) that require assessment of each resident before admission to any nursing facility that receives federal funds (HCFA 1992b). When an initial first-stage screening reveals that a serious mental disorder (other than dementia) may be present, a second-stage evaluation requiring a psychiatric evaluation is mandated to ascertain whether the patient has a mental disorder, to make a specific psychiatric diagnosis, and to determine whether there is a need for acute psychiatric care that precludes adequate or appropriate treatment in a nursing home. Thus, preadmission screening is intended to prevent inappropriate admission of patients with severe psychiatric disorders to nursing homes and to help ensure that patients with disabilities due in large part to treatable psychiatric disorders (such as depression) are not placed in long-term care facilities before they receive the benefits of adequate psychiatric treatment. For eligible patients who are admitted to a nursing home, annual reassessment is required to determine whether nursing home care remains appropriate.

Regulations requiring comprehensive assessment for all residents (HCFA 1991) have led to guidelines for the administration of the Minimum Data Set (MDS) (Morris et al. 1990) or an equivalent instrument on a regular basis by members of an interdisciplinary health care team, usually with a nurse—and ultimately with the nursing home administrator—responsible for its completion (HCFA 1992c). Areas of assessment relevant to mental illness and behavior include mood, cognition, communication, functional status, medications, and other treatments. Responses on the MDS suggesting that there may be a need to reevaluate a patient's clinical status and treatment plan serve as triggers for Resident Assessment Protocols (RAPs) that define medical conditions, psychiatric disorders, adverse treatment effects, functional impairments, and disabilities that are common among nursing home residents; note differential diagnoses and potential causal and aggravating factors; outline procedures for evaluation; and list key elements of management or treatment (HCFA 1992c). The MDS and RAPs together are designed as a two-stage assessment system, with a screening survey followed by a focused clinical evaluation. RAP problem areas related to mental disorders and behavior include delirium, cognitive loss/dementia, psychosocial well-being, mood state, behavior problems, psychotropic drug use, and physical restraints. The individual RAPs are designed to help nursing home staff recognize common signs and symptom clusters that are indicators of clinically significant problems; to conduct indepth evaluations following standardized algorithms; and to determine whether it is necessary to alter the treatment plan. The regulations hold facilities responsible for ensuring that RAPs are followed appropriately. Although physicians have no mandated role in this process, physician involvement is clearly necessary for proper diagnosis and treatment of conditions covered by the RAPs (Elon and

Pawlson 1992). Psychiatrists may be involved in this process, either if they are delegated by the facility to coordinate RAPs relevant to mental disorders and behavior problems or if they are consulted regarding patients for whom the RAPs indicate a need for reevaluation.

Regulations related to resident rights and facility practices restrict the use of physical restraints and antipsychotic drugs when they are "administered for purposes of discipline or convenience and not required to treat the resident's medical symptoms" (HCFA 1991, p. 48,875 [tag F204]). Regulations related to quality of care further require that residents do not receive "unnecessary drugs" and specify that antipsychotic drugs may not be given "unless these are necessary to treat a specific condition as diagnosed and documented in the clinical record" (p. 48,910 [tag F307]). An unnecessary drug is defined as any drug used 1) in excessive dose (including duplicate therapy), 2) for excessive duration, 3) without adequate monitoring, 4) without adequate indications for its use, 5) in the presence of adverse consequences that indicate that it should be reduced or discontinued; or 6) for any combination of the reasons above (HCFA 1991). The guidelines based on these regulations further limit the use of antipsychotic drugs, antianxiety agents, sedative-hypnotics, and related drugs (HCFA 1992a). For each of these classes, the guidelines specify a list of acceptable indications, maximum limits for daily doses, requirements for monitoring treatment and adverse effects, and time frames for attempting dose reductions and discontinuation. To minimize concerns about federal interference with medical practice, the current guidelines include qualifying statements that recognize cases in which strict adherence to prescribing limits is "clinically contraindicated." Although the emphasis remains clearly on limiting the use of psychotropic drugs, the guidelines acknowledge that appropriate medical treatment can entail psychotropic drug regimens that depart from these limits. The guidelines instruct surveyors to allow nursing facilities the opportunity to present a rationale for the use of drugs prescribed contrary to the guidelines and to explain why such use is in the best interest of the resident before finding that the facility is not in compliance with regulations. Thus, the physician's options for treating nursing home residents need not be restricted by the regulations as long as clinical reasoning demonstrating that the

benefits of treatment (in terms of symptom relief, improved health status, or improved functioning) outweigh the risks is clearly documented in the clinical record. Although the facility, not the physician, is accountable for compliance with the regulations, the physician's clinical reasoning and judgment still play a critical role in the process of ensuring quality care.

In addition to addressing the use of psychotropic drugs, the interpretive guidelines also outline conditions for the use of physical restraints. According to the guidelines, restraints may not be used unless there is documentation that 1) efforts were made to identify and correct preventable or treatable factors that cause or contribute to the problem; 2) prior attempts to use less restrictive measures failed; and 3) use of restraints enables the resident to achieve or maintain the highest practicable level of function. Physical or occupational therapists must be consulted if restraints are deemed necessary to enhance body positioning or improve mobility.

Under the provisions designed to ensure quality of care, federal regulations define a need for geriatric mental health services in nursing homes, requiring that "the facility must ensure that a resident who displays mental or psychosocial adjustment difficulties receives appropriate services to correct the assessed problem" (HCFA 1991, p. 48,896 [tag F272]). Despite the attempt to promote case finding through screening and assessment, and provisions for mental health services under quality-of-care requirements, OBRA legislation and regulations thus far have not addressed deficiencies in access to mental health services for nursing home residents (Conn et al. 1992) or problems related to inadequate funding for such services (Borson et al. 1987; Kane 1991).

Other Trends Affecting the Nursing Home Environment

Evidence is beginning to accumulate that the federal initiative in nursing home reform is influencing the processes of long-term care and that significant reductions in the use of antipsychotic drugs and physical restraints can be accomplished without adverse effects. At the same time, the nursing home environment is being affected by a number of other factors, including the development of special care units for the treatment of patients with Alzheimer's disease and the growing impact of changes in the medical marketplace.

Special Care Units

Special care units (SCUs) have evolved in an attempt to address the specific needs of nursing home residents with dementia. By 1991, 10% of all U.S. nursing homes had established an SCU. The Office of Technology Assessment (OTA 1992) commented on this development, stating that existing special care units vary in virtually every respect, including their patient-care philosophies and goals, physical design features, staff-to-resident ratios, activity programs, use of psychotropic medications and physical restraints, admission and discharge practices, and charges. On the basis of both this variability and the limited research on the outcomes of care in these units, the OTA report found little evidence for the effectiveness of SCUs and suggested that it is not yet known exactly what constitutes effective nursing home care for individuals with dementia. Research designed to define the elements of treatment in SCUs and to determine their effectiveness is currently under way to improve the quality of care for nursing home residents and to inform public policy (Berg et al. 1991).

Changes in the Medical Marketplace

The institution in 1983 of the Medicare Prospective Payment System (PPS) established reimbursement for acute-care hospitals on the basis of diagnosis-related groups (DRGs) rather than lengths of stay, and led to significant "trickle-down" effects on nursing homes. It began a process in which hospitals have become ever more concerned with limiting the duration and costs of each hospital admission and in which they increasingly discharge patients to nursing homes as relatively short-term "step-down" facilities that provide subacute medical treatment, convalescent care, and rehabilitation services. Since the initiation of Medicare's PPS, it was estimated that such patients constitute approximately one-third of nursing home admissions. More recently, the trend toward decreasing lengths of stay in hospitals and the transfer of subacute patients to nursing homes has been reinforced as a result of additional cost-containment efforts on the part of insurers and health maintenance organizations

(HMOs). Depending on the extent to which these trends affect the policies of specific institutions, the clinical characteristics of patients who are admitted to nursing homes and their needs for mental health care will change. In general, short-stay residents—those patients who are discharged to the community or who die after relatively brief stays in nursing homes—differ from long-term care patients in that they are younger, more likely to be admitted directly from an acute-care hospital, less likely to have irreversible cognitive impairment or incontinence, and more likely to have a primary diagnosis of hip fracture, stroke, or cancer. The objectives of mental health care for short-stay patients are less related to managing behavior problems associated with dementia and more related to helping patients cope with disease and disability; to searching for reversible causes of cognitive impairment; and to treating disorders such as depression and anxiety that can be impediments to recovery. In short, the objectives of mental health care for these patients are similar to the goals of classical consultation-liaison psychiatry in the general hospital. If pressures related to decreasing lengths of stay "squeeze" the opportunities for psychiatric interventions out of the acute-care hospital, they may shift these interventions into nursing homes. The services required may be more intensive than those usually available to long-term care residents, but the enhanced mental health services will increase opportunities for tradeoffs in which an investment in psychiatric care can lead to more independent functioning and more rapid discharge to the community. It is hoped that the benefits of mental health care, in terms of both cost offsets and improved quality of life, will provide a strong incentive for insurers, public and private, to establish reimbursement policies that facilitate such treatment.

Mental Health Care in Nursing Homes: A Model for Service Delivery

The high prevalence of psychiatric disorders in nursing homes argues for the importance of establishing procedures and policies that incorporate mental health into the basic services provided. In addition, the complex nature of the psychiatric disorders exhibited by nursing home residents, the need to evaluate medical as well as social and environmental factors as causes of mental health problems, the potential benefits of specific treatments, and the need for careful monitoring to prevent serious adverse effects of medications all argue for the importance of specific professional components of care. Thus, clinical needs demand that mental health services in nursing homes have two distinct but interacting systems: one that is intrinsic to the facility and contextual, and another that is professional and concerned primarily with the delivery of specific treatments. It has been suggested that mental health training should be provided to facility staff to help them develop skills in assessment and clinical management to compensate for problems that occur when specific professional services are lacking. However, it is important to recognize that the intrinsic and professional systems cannot readily replace each other, and that adequate care requires both. Although the need for such staff training is very real, the goal should be to develop staff expertise to complement rather than replace the activities of mental health professionals. This two-system model has obvious implications with respect to the financing of mental health services in nursing homes: it demonstrates the need for funding for mental health care both as a necessary part of the per diem costs for nursing home care and as a reimbursable professional service.

Although the intrinsic and professional systems for mental health services are distinct, they must interact. Geriatric psychiatrists and psychologists can play important intrinsic roles as administrative and staff consultants, in-service educators, moderators of case conferences, participants in interdisciplinary team meetings, and contributors in other activities familiar to the consultation-liaison psychiatrist. Conversely, the facility staff must be effective in recognizing problems, facilitating referral, supporting treatment, and monitoring outcome to allow the professional system to function optimally.

Intrinsic System

The intrinsic system for mental health care in nursing homes can be conceptualized as including a number of components ranging from design of the environment, through formulation of institutional policies and procedures, to optimization of the manner in which staff and residents interact. The impor-

tance of the intrinsic system is recognized in nursing home regulations that require training of nursing aides; in the nursing staff assessments required to complete the MDS and RAPs; and in OBRA requirements that nursing homes provide assessments, treatment planning, and services to attain or maintain the highest practicable level of mental and physical well-being for each resident. Because psychiatric disorders are common in nursing homes, nurses and aides should be knowledgeable about the nature of the cognitive and functional deficits associated with dementia and the manifestations of delirium and depression. Staff members should understand how to modify their approach to working with residents when cognitive impairment or communication deficits interfere with care. They should also know how to apply basic principles of behavioral psychology to identify causes of agitation and related behavioral symptoms in patients with dementia and how to plan environmental and behavioral interventions. A number of approaches to providing such staff training have been developed. Evaluation studies have demonstrated that improved mental health care through staff training is an attainable goal, and have identified barriers that must be overcome before such an objective can be accomplished (Smyer et al. 1992). As mental health care is incorporated into the basic fabric of the nursing home, it must include provisions for patients with variable degrees of cognitive impairment and depression in both the design of activities and the formulation of policies regarding decision-making capacity.

The concept that a key component of mental health services is intrinsic to the nursing home is perhaps best developed in the design of SCUs for patients with dementing illnesses; nonetheless, the need for these services applies to all patients, not just those with dementia. Moreover, the potential benefits of such services are not limited to their effects on established disorders; there is, in addition, the potential for prevention. For example, evidence indicates that contextual interventions designed to encourage a sense of empowerment in residents can have positive effects on both mental and physical health. Knowledge of the benefits of encouraging autonomy is derived from the classic studies of Langer and Rodin (1976), who evaluated a controlled intervention designed to increase nursing home residents' sense of control over day-to-day events. Residents were randomized either to a treatment group in which staff gave the message that they were expected to be responsible for making decisions for themselves, or to a control condition in which the message conveyed was that staff were responsible for residents' care. Both immediately after the intervention and at 18 months' follow-up, the treatment groups exhibited benefits in mood, alertness, and active participation. The effects of control-enhancing interventions have been confirmed in a number of other studies (for example, Banziger and Roush 1983; Thomasma et al. 1990) and have been discussed in terms of "learned helplessness" models (Avorn and Langer 1982). In another classic study, Schulz (1976) examined the effects of interventions designed to make the interpersonal environment of nursing home residents either more controllable or more predictable. Residents were randomized to a control condition or to groups that received visits from college student volunteers. The visits were provided under a number of conditions: at random, or when their frequency and duration could, within limits, be either controlled or predicted by the resident. At the conclusion of the study, benefits were apparent when residents could either predict or control the visits; the random-visit and no-visit groups exhibited poorer outcome. The benefits of interventions designed to enhance the predictability of the environment were confirmed in subsequent research that randomized new residents to a number of different orientation programs (Krantz and Schulz 1980). In summary, these studies demonstrate that the social environment within which care is provided can have a significant impact on nursing home residents; its design should be viewed as a component of mental health care.

Professional System

The intrinsic system for mental health services as described above is necessary, but it is not sufficient to meet the needs of nursing home residents. In addition, the services of mental health professionals are important to evaluate the interactions between medical and mental health problems, to establish psychiatric diagnoses, and to both plan and administer specific treatments for mental disorders. This component of the professional system must encompass medically oriented psychiatric care, including psychopharmacological treatment. A recent Position Statement by the major provider groups in this field (American Association for Geriatric Psychiatry et al. 1992) acknowledged a history of misuse of psychotropic drugs in nursing homes but emphasized the principle that psychopharmacological treatment of diagnosed mental disorders is an important part of the medical and mental health care of nursing home residents. Several reviews (Devanand et al. 1988; Sunderland and Silver 1988) and a meta-analysis of placebo-controlled studies (Schneider et al. 1990) have documented the modest but real efficacy of neuroleptics for treating agitation and related behavioral symptoms in patients with dementia. A review of more limited research (Schneider and Sobin 1992) suggests that other agents also show promise. Although only a limited number of randomized, placebo-controlled clinical trials of psychopharmacological treatments have been conducted in nursing homes and related settings, the available data (Table 23–1) suggest that these treatments are effective in patients in nursing homes as well as in other settings. Two trials of antidepressant medications have been conducted in nursing home residents (Table 23–1). The researchers in one study (Dehlin et al. 1985) investigated the effectiveness of the serotonin uptake inhibitor alaproclate in patients with dementia who were not selected for the presence of affective symptoms; the largely negative results in this investigation were thus not informative regarding the efficacy of drug treatment for depression. However, as discussed above, other research has demonstrated the effectiveness of nortriptyline treatment for major depression in nursing home residents. Although further research on the psychopharmacological treatment of patients in nursing homes is obviously needed, it is clear that such treatment constitutes an important part of psychiatric care in nursing facilities. The complexity of psychopharmacological treatment in frail nursing home residents with medical comorbidity requires that the skills of psychiatrists knowledgeable in geriatrics be an integral part of the professional system.

The professional system should include care with a psychosocial as well as a biomedical focus. For example, psychiatrists or psychologists with specific expertise in behavioral treatment may be successful both in evaluating the antecedents and causes of agitation and related symptoms in patients with dementia and in developing environmental and behavioral interventions, even when efforts by the facility's nursing staff have proven ineffective. In addition,

Table 23–1. Placebo-controlled outcome studies of psychoactive medications in nursing home residents

Study	Medication (mg/day)	Sample	Outcome measures	Results/comments
Beber 1965	Oxazepam (10–80) vs. placebo	$N = 100$ mean age = 79 years; nonpsychotic with chronic brain syndrome ($n = 28$), mixed anxiety/depression ($n = 26$), anxiety ($n = 43$), or depression (n = 3)	Anxiety and tension Depression, lethargy, and autonomic reactions Irritability, insomnia, agitation, phobic reactions	Improvement in all parameters was significantly greater in oxazepam-treated group than in placebo-treated group 44 subjects received concomitant treatment with other drugs, including neuroleptics, antidepressants, hypnotics, antiparkinsonian agents, and analgesics
Barnes et al. 1982	Thioridazine (mean = 62.5) vs. loxapine (mean = 10.5) vs. placebo	$N = 53$ mean age = 83 years; dementia and ≥ 3 behavioral symptoms	BPRS SCAG NOSIE CGI	Total scores and global ratings showed modest efficacy with thioridazine and loxapine, not statistically better than placebo Prominent placebo effect Significant improvement in anxiety, excitement, emotional lability, and uncooperativeness in active treatment groups, but no significant differences in overall efficacy between thioridazine and loxapine Significant improvement on BPRS and SCAG only in subjects with high-severity baseline scores
Stotsky 1984	Thioridazine (10–200) vs. diazepam (20–40) vs. placebo	$N = 237$ nursing home patients mean age ≈ 80 years; all nonpsychotic with cognitive impairment, emotional lability, and ADL dysfunction; and agitation, anxiety, depressed mood or sleep disturbance (also studied 273 patients on geriatric wards of state hospitals)	Modified HAM-A Modified NOSIE Global evaluations	Thioridazine was well tolerated with few side effects Thioridazine-treated group improved significantly more than placebo group on all HAM-A items and global evaluations Thioridazine-treated group improved significantly more than diazepam group on NOSIE and global ratings Insomnia responded better to diazepam, but there was more overall improvement on HAM-A rating with thioridazine

(continued)

Table 23–1. Placebo-controlled outcome studies of psychoactive medications in nursing home residents *(continued)*

Study	Medication (mg/day)	Sample	Outcome measures	Results/comments
Dehlin et al. 1985	Alaproclate (400) (serotonin uptake inhibitor) vs. placebo	*N* = 40 mean age = 82 years; primary degenerative, multi-infarct, or mixed dementia; not selected on the basis of affective or behavioral symptoms	Intellectual function Motor function (ADL) Emotional function (including depressive symptoms) Clinical global evaluation	No difference in efficacy between alaproclate and placebo Severity of dementia ranged from mild to severe Behavioral problems not described
Katz et al. 1990	Nortriptyline (mean = 65.25) vs. placebo	*N* = 30 residents of nursing home or congregate housing mean age = 84 years; major depression (HAM-D scores ≥18)	HAM-D GDS CGI	Significant improvement in patients treated with nortriptyline compared with placebo on HAM-D and CGI, but not on GDS Location (in nursing home vs. congregate housing) not significantly related to response Trend toward decreased nortriptyline response in the nursing home related to higher levels of disability and lower serum albumin in nursing home patients

Note. ADL = activities of daily living; BPRS = Brief Psychiatric Rating Scale (Overall and Gorham 1962); CGI = Clinical Global Impressions (Guy 1976); GDS = Global Deterioration Scale (Reisberg et al. 1988); HAM-A = Hamilton Anxiety Scale (Hamilton 1959); HAM-D = Hamilton Rating Scale for Depression (Hamilton 1960); NOSIE = Nurses' Observation Scale for Inpatient Evaluation (Honigfeld et al. 1966); SCAG = Sandoz Clinical Assessment—Geriatric (Shader et al. 1974).

Table 23–2. Randomized, controlled studies of the outcomes of psychotherapy interventions in elderly nursing home residents

Study	Type of intervention	Sample	Outcome measures	Results/comments
Moran and Gatz 1987	Task-oriented group vs. insight-oriented group vs. waiting-list control group	$N = 59$ mean age = 76.3 years; conversant, mobile	Self-reported psychosocial competence (a) sense of control (b) trust (c) active coping (d) striving for social approval Life satisfaction	Task group improved on all measures except trust Task group had significant increase in life satisfaction compared with insight and control groups Insight group improved on sense of control and trust
Baines et al. 1987	Reality orientation crossover with reminiscence therapy vs. no-therapy control group	$N = 15$ mean age = 81.5 years; moderate–severely cognitively impaired	Cognitive function Life satisfaction Communication Behavior Staff knowledge of residents	Group that received reality orientation first, followed by reminiscence therapy, showed sustained improvement in communication and behavior, and non-sustained improvement in cognitive function (information/orientation) Intervention was associated with improved staff knowledge of residents
Goldwasser et al. 1987	Reminiscence group therapy vs. supportive group therapy vs. no-treatment control group	$N = 27$ demented (MMSE range = 1–22, mean = 10.4)	Depression Cognitive function Behavioral/ADL function	Reminiscence group showed nonsustained improvement in self-reported depression on BDI Neither intervention showed significant effects on cognitive or behavioral function
Orten et al. 1989	Reminiscence group vs. control group	$N = 56$ mean age = 82.6 years; moderately confused	Social behavior ADL function Agitation Somatic complaining Attitude	Significant improvement for 1 of 3 experimental groups; no improvement when all groups analyzed together Investigators suggest that therapist skills are an important variable
Rattenburg and Stones 1989	Reminiscence group vs. current topics discussion group vs. no group	$N = 24$ mean ages of groups = 83–87 years; judged by nursing home staff not to be cognitively impaired	Psychological well-being (happiness-depression scale) Activity level Functional level Mood	Both intervention groups improved on happiness-depression scale No improvement on other measures, including mood scale Positive correlation between happiness scores and ↑ verbal activity level between 1st and 4th weeks

(continued)

Table 23–2. Randomized, controlled studies of the outcomes of psychotherapy interventions in elderly nursing home residents *(continued)*

Study	Type of intervention	Sample	Outcome measures	Results/comments
Youssef 1990	Group reminiscence counseling for young-old vs. group reminiscence counseling for old-old vs. control group	*N* = 60 all women; young-old = 65–75 years old-old ≥ 75 years	Depression	Young-old group had significant improvement in depression scores on BDI Old-old group showed improvement only on social withdrawal and somatic preoccupation items, but not on total BDI scores Control condition was not described
Ames 1990	Psychogeriatric team recommendations vs. routine clinical care	*N* = 93 mean age = 82.3 years	Depression ADL performance	No difference between intervention and control groups Only 27 of 81 recommended interventions were actually implemented (e.g., medication changes, referral for mental health services) Role of psychogeriatric services in management of the homes and medical care of the residents was not clearly defined
Zerhusen et al. 1991	Group cognitive therapy vs. music group (control) vs. routine care (control)	*N* = 60 mean age = 77 years	Depression Performance ratings of group leaders	Cognitive therapy group had improvement in self-rated depression scores on BDI; no significant improvement in control subjects Group gains did not vary with group leader ratings
Williams-Barnard and Lindell 1992	Group therapy with high nurse prizing vs. group therapy with low nurse prizing vs. control group (met for 3 meetings vs. 16 meetings for experimental groups)	*N* = 73 age ≥ 65 years	Self-concept	Self-concept improved in 68.4% of residents in high-prizing group, 29.4% of residents in low-prizing groups, and 10.8% of residents in control group Self-concept declined in 40% of low-prizing group and 5.3% of high-prizing group
Bensink et al. 1992	Progressive relaxation (PR) group vs. activity group (control)	*N* = 28 age ≥ 65 years; mean age = 77 years; MMSE ≥ 20	Locus of control Self-esteem	Only PR group showed increase in perceived internal locus of control Both PR and activity groups showed increase in self-esteem with greater effect in PR group

Reference	Intervention	Sample	Outcome measures	Results
Abraham et al. 1992	Cognitive-behavior (CB) group therapy vs. focused visual imagery (FVI) group therapy vs. educational discussion (ED) control groups	N = 76 mean age = 84 years; depressed and mildly-moderately cognitively impaired	Cognitive function Depression Hopelessness Life satisfaction	No effects of group therapy on geriatric depression, hopelessness, or life satisfaction Both CB and FVI groups showed improved cognitive function on modified MMSE, with greater gains in FVI participants No significant cognitive change in ED control groups
McMurdo and Rennie 1993	Exercise sessions vs. reminiscence groups	N = 49 mean age = 81 years	Physical function ADL performance Depression Life satisfaction Cognitive function	Physical function improved in exercise group, declined in reminiscence group Self-reported depression (BDI scores) declined in both groups, with exercise group showing significantly greater improvement than reminiscence group

Note. ADL = activities of daily living; BDI = Beck Depression Inventory (Beck et al. 1961); MMSE = Mini-Mental State Exam (Folstein et al. 1975).

psychotherapy may be of value for residents whose cognitive abilities allow them to participate. Although there is growing evidence for its efficacy with older patients in other settings, only been a limited amount of research has been done on psychotherapy in the nursing home, and knowledge of its benefits remains rudimentary. A search of the *MEDLINE* and *PsycLit* databases for the terms *psychotherapy* and *nursing homes* for the period from 1987 until the present identified a number of controlled studies of psychosocial interventions (Table 23–2). With the exception of the study by Abraham and colleagues (1992), however, most of the studies selected patients on the basis of age, cognitive status, or degree of disability rather than on the basis of specific psychiatric symptoms. Most of the reports described nursing research designed to test the benefits of programs administered by the intrinsic care staff. Although in this context the results are encouraging, this literature review also demonstrated a critical gap in current knowledge: virtually no research has evaluated the outcomes of specific psychotherapies—modalities demonstrated to be efficacious in the treatment of older adults in other settings—for use with nursing home residents who have well-characterized psychiatric disorders. Although reports and demonstration projects by experienced clinicians have documented the value of psychotherapy in the treatment of depressed nursing home residents (Leszcz et al. 1985; Sadavoy 1991), further research is needed to determine how existing treatments should be modified and how they can be administered to optimize their effectiveness in the nursing home. In spite of the need for more research, psychotherapy for the more cognitively intact nursing home residents with depression should be considered as an important part of the professional mental health services made available to nursing home residents.

References

Abraham IL, Neundorfer MM, Currie LJ: Effects of group interventions on cognition and depression in nursing home residents. Nurs Res 41:196–202, 1992

American Association for Geriatric Psychiatry, American Geriatrics Society, American Psychiatric Association: Position Statement: Psychotherapeutic medications in the nursing home. J Am Geriatr Soc 40:946–949, 1992

American Psychiatric Association: Diagnostic and Statistical Manual of Mental Disorders, 3rd Edition. Washington, DC, American Psychiatric Association, 1980

American Psychiatric Association: Diagnostic and Statistical Manual of Mental Disorders, 3rd Edition, Revised. Washington, DC, American Psychiatric Association, 1987

Ames D: Depression among elderly residents of local-authority residential homes: its nature and the efficacy of intervention. Br J Psychiatry 156:667–675, 1990

Ames D: Epidemiological studies of depression among the elderly in residential and nursing homes. International Journal of Geriatric Psychiatry 6:347–354, 1991

Ames D, Ashby D, Mann AH, et al: Psychiatric illness in elderly residents of part III homes in one London borough: prognosis and review. Age Ageing 17:249–256, 1988

Ashby D, Ames D, West CR, et al: Psychiatric morbidity as prediction of mortality for residents of local authority homes for the elderly. International Journal of Geriatric Psychiatry 6:567–575, 1991

Avorn J, Langer E: Induced disability in nursing home patients: a controlled trial. J Am Geriatr Soc 30:397–400, 1982

Avorn J, Dreyer P, Connelly K, et al: Use of psychoactive medication and the quality of care in rest homes: findings and policy implications of a statewide study. N Engl J Med 320:227–232, 1989

Baines S, Saxby P, Ehlert K: Reality orientation and reminiscence therapy. Br J Psychiatry 151:222–231, 1987

Baker FM, Miller CL: Screening a skilled nursing home population for depression. J Geriatr Psychiatry Neurol 4:218–221, 1991

Banziger G, Roush S: Nursing homes for the birds: a control-relevant intervention with bird feeders. Gerontologist 23:527–531, 1983

Barnes RD, Raskind MA: DSM-III criteria and the clinical diagnosis of dementia: a nursing home study. J Gerontol 36:20–27, 1980

Barnes R, Veith R, Okimoto J, et al: Efficacy of antipsychotic medications in behaviorally disturbed dementia patients. Am J Psychiatry 139:1170–1174, 1982

Barton R, Hurst L: Unnecessary use of tranquilizers in elderly patients. Br J Psychiatry 112:989–990, 1966

Beber CR: Management of behavior in the institutionalized aged. Diseases of the Nervous System 26:591–596, 1965

Beck AT, Ward CH, Mendelson M, et al: An inventory for measuring depression. Arch Gen Psychiatry 4:561–571, 1961

Beers M, Avon J, Soumerai SB, et al: Psychoactive medication use in intermediate-care facility residents. JAMA 260:3016–3020, 1988

Bensink GW, Godbey KL, Marshall MJ, et al: Institutionalized elderly: relaxation, locus of control, self-esteem. Journal of Gerontological Nursing 18:30–36, 1992

Berg L, Buckwalter KC, Chafetz PK, et al: Special care units for persons with dementia. J Am Geriatr Soc 39:1229–1236, 1991

Berrios GE, Brook P: Delusions and psychopathology of the elderly with dementia. Acta Psychiatr Scand 75:296–301, 1985

Blazer DG, Williams CD: Epidemiology of dysphoria and depression in an elderly population. Am J Psychiatry 137:439–444, 1980

Borson S, Liptzin B, Nininger J, et al: Psychiatry and the nursing home. Am J Psychiatry 144:1412–1418, 1987

Braun JV, Wykle MH, Cowling WR: Failure to thrive in older persons: a concept derived. Gerontologist 28:809–812, 1988

Buck JA: Psychotropic drug practice in nursing homes. J Am Geriatr Soc 36:409–418, 1988

Burns BJ, Taube CA: Mental health services in general medical care and in nursing homes, in Mental Health Policy for Older Americans: Protecting Minds at Risk. Edited by Fogel BS, Furino A, Gottlieb GL. Washington, DC, American Psychiatric Press, 1990, pp 63–84

Burns BJ, Larson DB, Goldstrom ID, et al: Mental disorder among nursing home patients: preliminary findings from the National Nursing Home Survey Pretest. International Journal of Geriatric Psychiatry 3:27–35, 1988

Campion EW, Ban A, May M: Why acute-care hospitals must undertake long-term care. N Engl J Med 308:71–75, 1983

Cape RD: Freedom from restraint. Gerontologist 23:217, 1983

Chandler JD, Chandler JE: The prevalence of neuropsychiatric disorders in a nursing home population. J Geriatr Psychiatry Neurol 1:71–76, 1988

Cohen-Mansfield J: Agitated behaviors in the elderly: preliminary results in the cognitively deteriorated. J Am Geriatr Soc 34:722–727, 1986

Cohen-Mansfield J, Billig N: Agitated behaviors in the elderly: a conceptual review. J Am Geriatr Soc 34:711–721, 1986

Cohen-Mansfield J, Marx MS, Rosenthal AS: A description of agitation in a nursing home. J Gerontol 44:M77–M84, 1989

Conn DK, Lee V, Steingart A, et al: Psychiatric services: a survey of nursing homes and homes for the aged in Ontario. Can J Psychiatry 37:525–530, 1992

Custer RL, Davis JE, Gee SC: Psychiatric drug usage in VA nursing home care units. Psychiatric Annals 14:285–292, 1984

Dehlin O, Hedenrud B, Jansson P, et al: A double-blind comparison of alaproclate and placebo in the treatment of patients with senile dementia. Acta Psychiatr Scand 71:190–196, 1985

DeLeo D, Stella AG, Spagnoli A: Prescription of psychotropic drugs in geriatric institutions. International Journal of Geriatric Psychiatry 4:11–16, 1989

Devanand DP, Sackheim HA, Mayeux R: Psychosis, behavioral disturbance and the use of neuroleptics in dementia. Compr Psychiatry 29:387–401, 1988

Elon R, Pawlson LG: The impact of OBRA on medical practice within nursing facilities. J Am Geriatr Soc 40:958–963, 1992

Engle VF, Graney MJ: Stability and improvement of health after nursing home admission. J Gerontol [Soc Sci] 48:S17–S23, 1993

Evans LK, Strumpf NE: Tying down the elderly: a review of the literature on physical restraint. J Am Geriatr Soc 37:65–74, 1989

Folstein MF, Folstein SE, McHugh PR: Mini-Mental State: a practical method for grading the cognitive state of patients for the clinician. J Psychiatr Res 12:189–198, 1975

Foster JR, Cataldo JK, Boksay IJE: Incidence of depression in a medical long-term care facility: findings from a restricted sample of new admissions. International Journal of Geriatric Psychiatry 6:13–20, 1991

German PS, Shapiro S, Kramer M: Nursing home study of eastern Baltimore epidemiologic catchment area, in Mental Illness in Nursing Homes: Agenda for Research. Edited by Harper MS, Lebowitz BD. Rockville, MD, National Institute of Mental Health, 1986, pp 21–40

Goldwasser AN, Auerbach SM, Harkins SW: Cognitive, affective, and behavioral effects of reminiscence group therapy of demented elderly. Int J Aging Hum Dev 25:209–222, 1987

Guy W (ed): ECDEU Assessment Manual for Psychopharmacology, Revised (DHEW Publ No ADM 76-388). Rockville, MD, U.S. Department of Health, Education and Welfare, 1976

Hamilton M: The assessment of anxiety states by rating. Br J Med Psychol 32:50–55, 1959

Hamilton M: A rating scale for depression. J Neurol Neurosurg Psychiatry 23:56–62, 1960

Harrison R, Savla N, Kafetz K: Dementia, depression, and physical disability in a London borough: a survey of elderly people in and out of residential care and implications for future developments. Age Ageing 19:97–103, 1990

Health Care Financing Administration: Medicare and Medicaid: Requirements for Long Term Care Facilities, Final Regulations. Federal Register 56(187):48865–48921, September 26, 1991

Health Care Financing Administration: State Operations Manual: Provider Certification (Transmittal No 250). Washington, DC, U.S. Government Printing Office, April 1992a

Health Care Financing Administration: Medicare and Medicaid Programs: Preadmission Screening and Annual Resident Review. Federal Register 57(230):56450–56504, November 30, 1992b

Health Care Financing Administration: Medicare and Medicaid: Resident Assessment in Long Term Care Facilities. Federal Register 57(249):61614–61733, December 28, 1992c

Honigfeld G, Roderic D, Klett JC: NOSIE-30: a treatment-sensitive ward behavior scale. Psychol Rep 19:180–182, 1966

Horiguchi J, Inami Y: A survey of the living conditions and psychological states of elderly people admitted to nursing homes in Japan. Acta Psychiatr Scand 83:338–341, 1991

Hyer L, Blazer DG: Depressive symptoms: impact and problems in long term care facilities. International Journal of Behavioral Gerontology 1:33–44, 1982

Innes EM, Turman WG: Evolution of patient falls. Q Rev Biol 9:30–35, 1983

Institute of Medicine, Committee on Nursing Home Regulation: Improving the Quality of Care in Nursing Homes. Washington, DC, National Academy Press, 1986

Kane RL, Garrard J, Buchanan JL, et al: Improving primary care in nursing homes. J Am Geriatr Soc 39:359–367, 1991

Kaplitz SE: Withdrawn, apathetic geriatric patients responsive to methylphenidate. J Am Geriatr Soc 23:271–276, 1975

Katz IR, Parmelee PA: Depression in the residential care elderly, in Diagnosis and Treatment of Depression in Late Life: Results of the NIH Consensus Development Conference. Edited by Schneider LS, Reynolds CF, Lebowitz BD, et al. Washington, DC, American Psychiatric Press, 1993, pp 437–461

Katz IR, Lesher E, Kleban M, et al: Clinical features of depression in the nursing home. Int Psychogeriatr 1:5–15, 1989a

Katz IR, Simpson GM, Jethanandani V, et al: Steady state pharmacokinetics of nortriptyline. Neuropsychopharmacology 2:229–236, 1989b

Katz IR, Simpson GM, Curlik SM, et al: Pharmacological treatment of major depression for elderly patients in residential care settings. J Clin Psychiatry 51 (suppl):41–48, 1990

Katz IR, Parmelee PA, Brubaker K: Toxic and metabolic encephalopathies in long term care patients. Int Psychogeriatr 3:337–347, 1991

Katz IR, Beaston-Wimmer P, Parmelee PA, et al: Failure to thrive in the elderly: exploration of the concept and delineation of psychiatric components. J Geriatr Psychiatry Neurol 6:161–169, 1993

Kramer M, German PS, Anthony JC, et al: Patterns of mental disorders among the elderly residents of Eastern Baltimore. J Am Geriatr Soc 33:236–245, 1985

Krantz DS, Schulz PR: Personal control and health: some applications to crises of middle and old age. Advances in Environmental Psychology 2:23–57, 1980

Langer E, Rodin J: The effects of choice and enhanced personal responsibility for the aged: a field experiment in an institutional setting. J Pers Soc Psychol 34:191–198, 1976

Lesher E: Validation of the Geriatric Depression Scale among nursing home residents. Clinics in Gerontology 4:21–28, 1986

Leszcz M, Sadavoy J, Feigenbaum E, et al: A men's group psychotherapy of elderly men. Int J Group Psychother 33:177–196, 1985

Loebel JP, Borson S, Hyde T, et al: Relationships between requests for psychiatric consultations and psychiatric diagnoses in long term care facilities. Am J Psychiatry 148:898–903, 1991

Mann AH, Graham N, Ashby D: Psychiatric illness in residential homes for the elderly: a survey in one London borough. Age Ageing 13:257–265, 1984

Marin RS: Differential diagnosis and classification of apathy. Am J Psychiatry 147:22–30, 1990

Marin RS: Apathy: a neuropsychiatric syndrome. J Neuropsychiatry Clin Neurosci 3:243–254, 1991

McCarthy P: Why one nursing home and not another? Senior Patient May/June:97–102, 1989

McMurdo MET, Rennie L: A controlled trial of excercise by residents of old people's homes. Age Ageing 22:11–15, 1993

Moran JA, Gatz M: Group therapies for nursing home adults: an evaluation of two treatment approaches. Gerontologist 27:588–591, 1987

Morris JN, Hawes C, Fries BE, et al: Designing the national resident assessment instrument for nursing homes. Gerontologist 30:293–307, 1990

Murphy E: The use of psychotropic drugs in long-term care (editorial). International Journal of Geriatric Psychiatry 4:1–2, 1989

National Center for Health Statistics: The National Nursing Home Survey (DHEW Publ No PHS 79-1794). Washington, DC, U.S. Government Printing Office, 1979

National Center for Health Statistics: Use of nursing homes by the elderly: preliminary data from the 1985 National Nursing Home Survey (DHHS Publ No PHS 87-1250). Hyattsville, MD, NCHS, 1987

Office of Technology Assessment: Special Care Units for People With Alzheimer's and Other Dementias: Consumer Education, Research, Regulatory, and Reimbursement Issues (OTA-H-543). Washington, DC, U.S. Government Printing Office, August 1992

Orten JD, Allen M, Cook J: Reminiscence groups with confused nursing center residents: an experimental study. Soc Work Health Care 14:73–86, 1989

Overall JE, Gorham DR: The Brief Psychiatric Rating Scale. Psychol Rep 10:799–812, 1962

Parmelee PA, Katz IR, Lawton MP: Depression among institutionalized aged: assessment and prevalence estimation. J Gerontol 44:M22–M29, 1989

Parmelee PA, Katz IR, Lawton MP: The relation of pain to depression among institutionalized aged. J Gerontol [Psychol Sci] 46:P15–P21, 1991

Parmelee PA, Katz IR, Lawton MP: Depression and mortality among institutionalized aged. J Gerontol [Psychol Sci] 47:P3–P10, 1992a

Parmelee PA, Katz IR, Lawton MP: Incidence of depression in long term care settings. J Gerontol [Med Sci] 47:M189–M196, 1992b

Rattenburg C, Stones MJ: A controlled evaluation of reminiscence and current topics discussion groups in a nursing home context. Gerontologist 29:768–771, 1989

Ray WA, Federspiel CF, Schaffner W: A study of antipsychotic drug use in nursing homes: epidemiologic evidence suggesting misuse. Am J Public Health 70:485–491, 1980

Reisberg B, Ferris SH, deLeon MJ, et al: Global deterioration scale. Psychopharmacol Bull 24:661–663, 1988

Risse SC, Cubberley L, Lampe TH, et al: Acute effects of neuroleptic withdrawal in elderly dementia patients. Journal of Geriatric Drug Therapy 2:65–77, 1987

Rovner BW, Kafonek S, Filipp L, et al: Prevalence of mental illness in a community nursing home. Am J Psychiatry 143:1446–1449, 1986

Rovner BW, German PS, Broadhead J, et al: The prevalence and management of dementia and other psychiatric disorders in nursing homes. Int Psychogeriatr 2:13–24, 1990a

Rovner BW, Lucas-Blaustein J, Folstein MF, et al: Stability over one year in patients admitted to a nursing home dementia unit. International Journal of Geriatric Psychiatry 5:77–82, 1990b

Rovner BW, German PS, Brant LJ, et al: Depression and mortality in nursing homes. JAMA 265:993–996, 1991

Rovner BW, Katz IR: Psychiatric disorders in the nursing home: a selective review of studies related to clinical care. International Journal of Geriatric Psychiatry 8:75–87, 1993

Sabin TD, Vitug AJ, Mark VH: Are nursing home diagnosis and treatment inadequate? JAMA 248: 321–322, 1982

Sadavoy J: Psychotherapy for the institutionalized elderly, in Practical Psychiatry in the Nursing Home: A Handbook for Staff. Edited by Conn DK, Herrman N, Kaye A, et al. Toronto, Canada, Hogrefe & Huber, 1991, pp 217–236

Schneider LS, Sobin PB: Non-neuroleptic treatment of behavioral symptoms and agitation in Alzheimer's disease and other dementia. Psychopharmacol Bull 28:71–79, 1992

Schneider LS, Pollack VE, Lyness SA: A meta-analysis of controlled trials of neuroleptic treatment in dementia. J Am Geriatr Soc 38:553–563, 1990

Schulz PR: Effect of control and predictability on the psychological well-being of the institutionalized aged. J Pers Soc Psychol 33:563–573, 1976

Shader RI, Harmatz JS, Salzman C: A new scale for clinical assessment in geriatric populations: Sandoz Clinical Assessment—Geriatric (SCAG). J Am Geriatr Soc 22:107–113, 1974

Smyer M, Brannon D, Cohn M: Improving nursing home care through training and job redesign. Gerontologist 32:327–333, 1992

Snowdon J: Dementia, depression, and life satisfaction in nursing homes. International Journal of Geriatric Psychiatry 1:85–91, 1986

Snowdon J, Donnelly N: A study of depression in nursing homes. J Psychiatr Res 20:327–333, 1986

Spagnoli A, Forester G, MacDonald A, et al: Dementia and depression in Italian geriatric institutions. International Journal of Geriatric Psychiatry 1:15–23, 1986

Steele C, Rovner BW, Chase GA, Folstein MF: Psychiatric symptoms and nursing home placement in Alzheimer's disease. Am J Psychiatry 147:1049–1051, 1990

Stotsky B: Multicenter study comparing thioridazine with diazepam and placebo in elderly, nonpsychotic patients with emotional behavioral disorders. Clin Ther 6:546–559, 1984

Streim JE, Rovner BW, Katz IR: Psychiatric aspects of nursing home care, in Comprehensive Review of Geriatric Psychiatry—2, 2nd Edition. Edited by Sadavoy J, Lazarus LW, Jarvik LF, et al. Washington, DC, American Psychiatric Press, 1996, pp 907–936

Sunderland T, Silver MA: Neuroleptics in the treatment of dementia. International Journal of Geriatric Psychiatry 3:79–88, 1988

Tariot PN, Podgorske CA, Blazina L, et al: Mental disorders in the nursing home: another perspective. Am J Psychiatry 150:1063–1069, 1993

Teeter RB, Garetz FK, Miller WR, et al: Psychiatric disturbances of aged patients in skilled nursing homes. Am J Psychiatry 133:1430–1434, 1976

Thomasma M, Yeaworth R, McCabe B: Moving day: relocation and anxiety in institutionalized elderly. Journal of Gerontological Nursing 16:18–24, 1990

Trichard L, Zabow A, Gillis LS: Elderly persons in old age homes: a medical, psychiatric and social investigation. S Afr Med J 61:624–627, 1982

Werner P, Cohen-Masfield J, Braun J, et al: Physical restraint and agitation in nursing home residents. J Am Geriatr Soc 37:1122–1126, 1989

Williams-Barnard CL, Lindell AR: Therapeutic use of "prizing" and its effect on self-concept of elderly clients in nursing homes and group homes. Issues in Mental Health Nursing 13:1–17, 1992

Youssef FA: The impact of group reminiscence counseling on a depressed elderly population. Nurse Pract 15:32–38, 1990

Zerhusen JD, Boyle K, Wilson W: Out of the darkness: group cognitive therapy for depressed elderly. J Psychol Nurs 29:16–21, 1991

Zimmer JG, Watson N, Treat A: Behavioral problems among patients in skilled nursing facilities. Am J Public Health 74:1118–1121, 1984

CHAPTER 24

The Continuum of Care:
Movement Toward the Community

George L. Maddox, Ph.D.
Karen Steinhauser, M.A.
Elise Bolda, M.S.P.H., Ph.D.

In recent decades, public discussion of care for older persons has continually concentrated on what has come to be called "the alternatives issue." The attention of congressional committees initially focused on alternatives to institutionalization, particularly nursing home care, because older persons consume public health and related welfare resources at a higher rate than do adults in general, and nursing home care is an expensive component of total cost. Older persons, therefore, provide a very visible illustration of the general problem of securing quality care at bearable cost. What has clearly concerned the U.S. Congress about care of older people is the very high cost of services that appear to be poorly distributed, and inappropriate care of debatable quality (U.S. Senate Special Committee on Aging 1977). However, public discussion of efficient and effective alternative forms of care for older people, while generating a great deal of rhetoric over the past two decades, has produced surprisingly little definitive evidence that would inform choices among a bewildering array of competing options.

In revising this chapter, we have deliberately retained older references in order to illustrate an important point about how public policy on home and community-based care has continued to muddle through in recent decades. Americans are ambivalent about whether—if noninstitutional care is really a priority—we should allocate resources differently in order to provide care effectively in the long term. One important source of our ambivalence is the value we place on individual responsibility for health and welfare and our preference for minimizing the intervention of government in ensuring care. Another source of ambivalence is that our preference for high-technology medicine in hospital settings leads us to question the effectiveness of nonhospital alternatives. We continue to put our money where our preferences are—in hospital medicine (Maddox 1992). Research on home and community care over the past two decades has been plagued both by single-minded pursuit of the wrong question and by methodologically flawed evidence. The wrong question policy analysts have insisted on attempting to answer is, "Are home- and community-based long-term care cheaper?" That question is not effectively addressed without determining what constitutes a fair comparison among alternatives. A fair comparison requires the specification of assessed need for definable services, over what periods, in defined service settings. The more nearly the condition of fair comparisons are met, the more likely the conclusion that home and community care are not inevitably cheaper. But such care is often no more costly in the short run, and may eventually be less costly in the long run (Davies 1992). In the meantime, and equally important, home and community settings are clearly the preferred sites for care in the long term by older adults and their families. Further, as functional assessment techniques become more reliable, a substantial minority of disabled adults now cared for in institutional settings will be effectively cared for at home and in the community.

The need for fundamental reform of health care in the United States, particularly long-term care, has become increasingly obvious (Eisdorfer et al. 1989). The initial statement of the President's Health Security Plan (White House Domestic Policy Council 1993) proposed greater emphasis on home and community care. Although this proposal does not review the evidence that would justify the confidence that such care leads to cost savings, this is certainly the inference invited. Such a conclusion, however, may be warranted, and is certainly consistent with recent reforms of long-term care provision in Europe, particularly in the United Kingdom and Nordic countries. In these countries, current policies are emphasizing decentralized, case-managed social care for dependent older adults in home and community settings involving innovative uses of private-sector providers (Davies 1992).

Alternatives to Institutionalization

At the beginning of the 1970s, discussion began to focus on alternatives to institutionalization. A consensus emerged among both professionals and the lay public that too many older people were being inappropriately and unnecessarily institutionalized in mental hospitals and nursing homes. This consensus unquestionably had some basis in fact; however, because no definitive consensual procedures existed for determining appropriate levels and locales for care, estimates of the number of older people who were inappropriately institutionalized or receiving too much care varied from as little as 6% to as much as 40% or more. The confidence that too many people were receiving care, and perhaps too much care, in the wrong care settings, was matched by confident assertions that care in the community and, if possible, at home, provided obviously preferable alternatives at obviously lower costs. The obviousness of these conclusions has repeatedly been confronted by a troublesome fact: the efficiency and effectiveness of alternatives to the current organization of services continue to be asserted rather than systematically demonstrated. Some relevant evidence has accumulated, however; options have been more clearly defined, and systematic evaluation is increasingly possible. Yet in the 1990s, some of the current issues have the familiar look of old questions that have not been definitively resolved. The search for the optimal solution in organizing and financing long-term care has not been rewarded. An important observation about the organization and financing of health care in democratic, market-oriented societies is suggested by this outcome. The dominant values in the civic culture of a society—or at least those of the individuals who are empowered to make decisions for that society—determine the political feasibility of arrangements proposed by the planners of health and welfare services. The technical feasibility of a plan to organize health and welfare services for older adults is not the only or even the prime consideration. Assessment of political feasibility is a major consideration. In our view, the relevant dimensions of the civic culture include strong preferences for individual responsibility for personal welfare, for decentralization in decision making, for location of care services in the private sector, and for the provision of health care services primarily by physicians. In such a political environment, comprehensive planning for care services and consensus about who needs what services at whose expense are unlikely in the absence of effective political leadership dedicated to reform of long-term care (Maddox 1971, 1992; Rodwin 1984).

Structuring the Issues

The development of scientific knowledge, the transfer of that knowledge to professionals through training, and the translation of the knowledge into professional practice take place in the context of organizations intended to implement socially legitimate objectives. Therefore, an understanding of the delivery of care to a population benefits from a sociological understanding of how organizations intended to provide care define the roles and rules that structure the interactions of the professional helpers and those they help, and of how societies and communities allocate resources among such organizations.

More than three decades ago, Charles Perrow (1965) wrote a very insightful sociological analysis of key factors that influence the behavior of organizations whose product is personal care. His analysis provides a conceptual structure for thinking about some basic issues in the organization of helping resources. Perrow concentrated on three interactive societal factors: 1) the cultural system of a society embodying values and beliefs that influence the setting of legitimate organization goals, 2) the available technology that determines the means for goal attainment, and 3) the social structure of organizations in which specific techniques are embedded in ways that facilitate or inhibit goal attainment. Perrow's illustration of these three factors focused on care in mental hospitals. His basic argument, however, is broadly applicable to an understanding of how care is organized in response to impairment generally.

Culture is a shared, socially transmitted construction of reality. The concept refers broadly to the goals members of a society value and pursue; to the rules and roles that structure social life; and to the technologies and the material and symbolic products of group life. Through processes of socialization and social control, most shared cultural expectations are transmitted from generation to generation. Consequently, conformity to social expectations is the common experience of everyday life. Most members of most social groups want to become and be what they are expected to become and be. Dissents, conflict, and nonconformity do occur and are considered normal in democratically organized societies. When they take place, cultural belief systems provide plausible explanations and suggest corrective measures to ensure an acceptable level of social integration and cohesion.

Illness is a case in point. Illness has social as well as personal significance in all societies. This is so because illness typically impairs the performance of social roles. There are, therefore, social as well as personal reasons for limiting the impact of illness. Illness typically elicits temporary exemption from usual role obligations and helpful social response, but generally with the expectation that the sick individual wants to limit the debilitating effects of illness as much as possible. Modern societies attach considerable importance to controlling the effects of illness. In American society, for example, one of our largest industries, to which we in the 1990s have devoted more than 12% of our annual gross national product (GNP), is health care. Scientific medicine and its related technologies, human capital, and organization are integral parts of our culture. This is so much the case that some observers have referred to our belief in the "Great Equation"—that is, that medical care equals health (Wildavsky 1977). Others have described the dominance of physicians in the provision and control of health care as "the medicalization of care" (Fox 1977).

There is no question that in the last half-century, advances in medical technology have raised public expectations regarding the conquest of disease. Average life expectancy has increased dramatically worldwide (Maddox 1977, 1994). Sick people, for the most part, expect to receive care and be cured. Unfortunately, very high expectations encounter substantial obstacles. Health resources, particularly those for primary health care, are not equally distributed geographically and hence are not equally accessible. Moreover, as Wildavsky contended, the Great Equation is probably wrong; medical care does not equal health (Ingelfinger 1978; Saward and Sorensen 1978). The medical system doctors, other health professionals, hospitals, and drugs may account for and deal with only a small proportion of the factors affecting health. A much larger proportion appears to be determined by factors over which the medical system has little or no control—factors such as lifestyle (smoking, eating, drinking, worrying, inactivity), social conditions (income, inheritance), and social environment (air, water, noise, safety). This is why Wildavsky and others (Enthoven 1980; Hollingsworth et al. 1990; Ingelfinger 1978; Institute of Medicine 1991; Maddox 1971, 1994; Rodwin 1984; Saward and Sorensen 1978) continue to feel that a medical system cannot ensure health at *any* cost, much less at a politically bearable cost. Even in a society accustomed to high inflation, the total cost of health care has continued to escalate more rapidly than the cost of other goods and services (Culliton 1978; Hahn and Lefkowitz 1992; Walsh 1978). The result is a widespread sense of concern that reflects, according to public-opinion polls, a crisis less in confidence in the value of medical care than in the belief that appropriate care will not be received at a bearable cost without significant health care reform (Aaron 1991; Blendon and Taylor 1989; Lewis et al. 1976). Or, in terms of the three interacting factors stressed by Perrow, cultural beliefs and expectations about health care are mismatched with both the available technology and the organization of care for achieving shared goals ensuring health care. The medical technology available for diagnosis and treatment is impressive, although it is directed primarily toward diagnosis and acute illness. The organization for health care delivery concentrates on medical care dependent on high technology and controlled by highly specialized personnel centralized in or near hospitals. Financing of health care is directed primarily to medical care and to care that must be certified by, if not provided by, medical practitioners. There is a growing body of opinion that Wildavsky's extreme conclusion regarding the important but modest contribution that medicine can make in ensuring health is more right than wrong (Hollingsworth et al. 1990; Ingelfinger 1978; Saward and Sorensen 1978). Hence, increasing amounts of resources poured into health services as they are currently organized are likely to produce decreasing marginal returns on investments and less satisfaction with outcomes (Aaron 1991). In regard to health services, doing better in many ways but feeling worse (Knowles 1977) has been a likely outcome (Aaron 1991). Problems related to the health care of older persons are specific and instructive illustrations of why there is a continuing sense of crisis regarding our capacity to achieve adequate health care at a bearable cost and a continuing interest in "alternatives to institutionalization" (Harrington et al. 1985; Hawes et al. 1988; Kane and Kane 1978, 1985; Maddox 1977, 1992; Meltzer et al. 1981; Vogel and Palmer 1983).

Health Care for Older Persons

The cultural beliefs and values regarding the care of older persons in the United States are most accu-

rately described as complex, ambiguous, and contradictory. All citizens, including older ones, have a right to the best available care. What is best tends to be associated with high technology—that is, sophisticated equipment operated by specialized personnel, centralized in hospitals and medical centers. In recent decades, the short-stay hospital has come to be associated with curative therapies, which tends to evoke a positive image. This positive image has been tempered somewhat by concerns about the high cost of care. Long-stay institutions, on the other hand, evoke a very negative image, as indicated by public attitudes toward mental hospitals and nursing homes. Such institutions have been the focus of social concern and have provided the illustrations of unnecessary and inappropriate custodial, as distinct from curative, service. Nursing homes, as they have developed extensively in this country since the advent of Medicare and Medicaid programs, are clearly extensions of a medical model of care. Access to and continuation in nursing homes is contingent on both medical certification and, for many older adults, eligibility for Medicaid. In addition, critics of the very extensive development of nursing homes (more than 16,500 homes, 1.5 million beds, and a $38 billion annual cost in 1986) usually comment that the care provided does not emphasize enough the social components of care. Nursing homes suffer from the perception of being second-rate, understaffed, and underfunded hospitals (Kane and Kane 1978, 1985).

Deinstitutionalization of the mentally ill, including many older persons, has been the intention of public policy as well as the cultural preference in this country for more than two decades (Lamb 1981; Maddox 1972, 1975). Both public policy and cultural preference regarding deinstitutionalization reflect evidence as well as emotion. Media coverage of dramatic events involving older persons in long-term care institutions—events such as deaths resulting from fires, incidents involving abuse and inadequate care, and evidence of fiscal mismanagement—provide fuel for strong emotional responses. But there is also evidence of what appears to be unnecessary institutionalization, dependency-producing overcare, and questionable effectiveness of high-cost services (Kane and Kane 1978; Maddox 1972). A large number of persons, including many older persons, have been removed from mental institutions. Hospital censuses and lengths of stay have been reduced. Between 1955 and 1980, for example, the censuses of state hospitals declined nearly 75% (Goldman et al. 1983). There is little definitive evidence, however, with regard to the selection procedure used to determine who would be placed in the community, the fate of older individuals who have been so placed, or the impact of this placement on neighborhoods and communities. The best evidence indicated a decade ago that many of the "deinstitutionalized" are reinstitutionalized in less publicly visible long-term care facilities in the community (Kane and Kane 1978). Current evidence does not change that conclusion. Some observers have suggested that the reimbursement structure of Medicaid is an important factor in a process that is better described as a transfer between institutions than as deinstitutionalization (Gronfein 1985). Occasionally those who rally behind the philosophy of deinstitutionalization make extravagant claims about the proportion of older individuals who are inappropriately institutionalized, with estimates running as high as 40%. In fact, we do not have definitive evidence on this point. There is some evidence indicating that the great majority of individuals in, for example, nursing homes are significantly impaired, that 13%–14% might be cared for appropriately in a situation providing less intensive care, and that perhaps another 10% who probably benefit from institutionalization overall receive more care than their functional impairments require (Laurie 1978; Maddox 1977). This question has emerged again with some urgency as analysts have attempted to cost out the long-term care service reforms proposed in President Clinton's Health Security Plan. How many dependent older adults who are currently institutionalized might be appropriately treated at home or in the community? At present, no one has a definitive answer, although the social and medical processes used to allocate functionally impaired persons to various forms of care are sufficiently crude to virtually ensure debatable care placement for a substantial minority of older adults requiring care.

In the absence of a definitive technology in long-stay institutions that affords reasonable assurance of achieving the restoration of functioning, the inference is invited not only that such institutions are primarily custodial, focusing on maintenance rather than rehabilitation, but also that the organization of life within them unnecessarily increases the depen-

dence of residents. Unlike hospitals and medical centers, where high cost at least is associated with the hope for restoration of function, high cost in long-stay institutions has come to be associated with the expectation of increased dependence in a custodial environment. The organization of long-term care in the United States continues to be dominated by and to suffer from the consequences of what has been called "a medical model" of care, a model symbolized by a specialized physician in a hospital supported by technicians and technology. Although the continuing dominance of a medical model of long-term care might be interpreted as additional evidence of medicine's control of health care, this dominance actually reflects continuing hope that current medical technology and organization of care can effect cures for the chronically ill elderly in the face of discouraging evidence to the contrary. The persistent search for alternatives to institutionalization and preference for deinstitutionalization of health care for older persons are therefore hampered by the lack of demonstrably effective, efficient, and adequately distributed organizations for care in communities whose performance is superior to the overall performance of medical institutions (see, for example, Lamb 1981; Rowland and Lyons 1991).

Nevertheless, both professional and public opinion increasingly reflect a belief in the desirability and feasibility of providing more long-term care in the community rather than in institutional settings. This opinion is buttressed with increasing experience of satisfactory care outside institutions that is—at least, in fair comparisons—no more expensive than institutional care and possibly less expensive in the long term (Davies 1992; Hurtado et al. 1971; Maddox 1977; U.S. Department of Health and Human Services 1986). Consequently, the United States has entered an era in which experimentation with alternative organization and financing of care will continue to increase. The actual transformation of the care system to emphasize community-based rather than hospital-based care has moved slowly and will probably continue to move slowly, at least in the foreseeable future (Kavesh 1986; Koren 1986; Leader 1986). This is the case, in part, because reliable and valid procedures for determining the proper level and locale for care and for measuring outcome are inadequately developed and are neither routinely available nor consistently applied when available (Hawes et al. 1988; Maddox 1972; Maddox and Dellinger 1978; Maddox and Karasik 1975; Meltzer et al. 1981; Weissert et al. 1988). The implications of a substantial reorientation of care to emphasize community-based services for professional training and personnel development are also not yet well understood. It is not at all clear that public preference for high-technology medicine will be significantly reduced by the addition of opportunities for care in the community, or that the total cost of care will be reduced by additional forms of care unless the alternative forms are a substitute for existing forms. Some evidence indicates that an increasing number of highly technical medical procedures are being introduced into community care (Koren 1986) and hospice care, which in its initial stages of development was strongly antitechnology but is under pressure—after inclusion of the hospice as a service under Medicare—to become more like mainstream institutional care (Paradis and Cummings 1986). Although some hospices have incorporated more technical care procedures, largely related to pain control, hospice care still does not use technology whose sole purpose is extension of the length of life. The Patient Self-Determination Act of 1990 requires hospitals, nursing homes, and home health care agencies to inquire whether patients have advance directives and to document their existence. This process has been hailed by some as increasing the self-determination of patients by guaranteeing their right to forgo medical treatment or the use of advanced technologies. It is unlikely that significant changes in care practices will be forthcoming, because preliminary reports indicate that only a small percentage of patients have such plans at the time of admission to a health care facility (see High 1993). And, finally, although we have learned that more and better formal care does not diminish the commitment of kin and friends to care for older adults for whom they are responsible, we understand too little about the impact on kin and friendship networks of placing more responsibility for care in the community (George and Gwyther 1986; Laurie 1978; Maddox 1975). But these constraints notwithstanding, extensive development of community-based care for older persons will continue to be an issue in health care policy in the foreseeable future. Some observers believe that alternative forms of long-term care will be the dominant issue in the organization and financing of health care (see, for example, Maddox 1992; Vogel and Palmer 1983).

The Case for Community-Based Care

The case for increasing the probability that the locale for care will be outside institutions and that the care offered will stress social and psychological as well as medical components is outlined briefly here and developed in the sections that follow. In brief, it is argued first that community and home care for impaired older persons are commonsense responses to common problems of dependency in late life. Historically, these forms of care preceded institutionalization and continue today to provide most of the services required. Community and home care are old ideas that are currently being rediscovered or reaffirmed (Davies 1992; Maddox 1975, 1977; Rowland and Lyons 1991). Public attitudes and public policy regarding appropriate sources of and locations for care have typically reflected high regard for professional expertise and limited confidence in the competence and responsibilities of families to deal with impaired members. The transfer of presumed responsibility for impaired members of families from families to professional family surrogates has been pronounced (Fox 1977). Nevertheless, a substantial majority of the care provided to impaired older persons is supplied not by public agencies but by a network of kin and friends (Branch and Jette 1983; Health Policy Analysis Program 1978; Laurie 1978; Maddox 1975; U.S. General Accounting Office 1988). Community and home care are hardly novel ideas or unusual experiences.

Second, a wide array of community and home services (for example, home health and home help in the public and private sector) already exist (Comptroller General of the United States 1977a, 1977b; Health Policy Analysis Program 1978; Medicus Systems Corporation 1977; Rowland and Lyons 1991; Vogel and Palmer 1983; Weiler and Rathbone-McCuan 1978). The feasibility of establishing a wide variety of community-based services is not at issue. However, services for community and home care, like health and social services, generally are fragmented, uncoordinated, and not routinely accessible to or used by a majority of impaired adults (National Center for Health Statistics 1986).

Third, discussions of the economics of community and home services continue to be inconclusive. Intuitively, offering services outside institutions where high technology is concentrated ought to achieve economies. This has not been demonstrated to be the case, particularly when the quality and quantity of professionally prescribed services are also considered (Mor and Kidder 1985; U.S. Department of Health and Human Services 1986). In any case, the crucial economic issue in assessing alternative types of care services is the total cost of all services to the care system of acceptable levels and quality of care, not the cost of a discrete subset of services. The reduction of total service system cost attributable to community and home services has not been demonstrated (Hawes et al. 1988; Hurtado et al. 1971; Kemper et al. 1987; Maddox 1977; Ruchlin et al. 1989; Sager 1977; U.S. Department of Health and Human Services 1986; Weissert et al. 1988).

Fourth, concentration of public discussion on the cost-effectiveness of community and home services probably is an interesting diversion from a more basic issue. The basic issue is the fragmented, unsystematic organization of care and of the public financing of care. Only comprehensive, integrated care delivery systems at local levels offer any prospect for achieving cost-effectiveness for community and home care. And the most significant contribution of community and home care to the achievement of economy, according to some analysts, may be the removal of patients from exposure to high-technology, high-cost health care centers (Aaron 1991; Ball 1978; Enthoven 1978) and the requirement that care organizations deliver specified services for fees set prospectively (Enthoven 1980; Harrington et al. 1985).

Fifth, achieving an appropriately comprehensive, integrated system of care delivery at the local level will probably take the form of current proposals for a type of care system illustrated by health maintenance organizations (HMOs) (Garfield 1970; Lewis et al. 1976; see also White House Domestic Policy Council 1993). This type of care system as a prototype may continue to emphasize predominantly the medical as distinct from social and psychological aspects of care for older persons. Yet the emerging tradition of the HMO may offer a significant opportunity for melding the strengths of medical and social/psychological components of care in a manner that is publicly and politically appealing, as well as viable, as illustrated by a current demonstration in a social HMO (or SHMO), which features as standard services home- and community-based care (Greenberg et al. 1988). Evaluations of SHMOs may provide useful information about the cost-effectiveness of melding social and medical models of prepaid care for older adults. The HMO offers an opportunity for local variations in the specific organization of a care system, while providing for both prepayment and a relatively comprehensive, integrated, and controllable system of care. Personnel development and training, financing, and procedures for assignment to alternative types of care within any care system are critical problems, the solutions to which will determine how adequate, effective, and efficient that system of care will be. Recent evidence has suggested that the use of HMOs and SHMOs for geriatric care is not, however, risk free or automatically effective (Greenberg et al. 1988; Iglehart 1987).

Rediscovering Community and Home Care

Scientific medicine in the United States and optimism about the beneficial effects of exposure to physicians and hospitals date only from the second decade of this century (Ingelfinger 1978). Care of impaired individuals in general and of elderly individuals in particular tended to be a family, a neighborhood, or a community responsibility. Until World War II, federal spending for health care was largely confined to investment in traditional public health activities such as immunization. In the postwar era, a change in public attitudes and policy occurred, resulting in federal programs of increasing variety and scale. Before 1965, the federal investment in health care for the aged and poor was $4.4 billion. By 1977, that investment was $49.6 billion, of which Medicare and Medicaid accounted for $35.7 billion and the Department of Defense and the Veterans Administration for another $6 billion (Walsh 1978). By 1985, long-term care alone cost $45 million annually, with slightly more than half this amount coming from public funds. The financing of long-term care by Medicare and Medicaid was a prime factor in promoting the development of a nursing home industry, which, by the mid-1980s, included some 16,500 nursing homes with 1.5 million beds, at a cost of more than $38 billion annually in 1986 (National Center for Health Statistics 1988; Rabin and Stockton 1987). Long-term care beds are typically occupied by very elderly impaired persons—75% of them are over the age of 75, most having multiple impairments and more than half having significant mental impairment. In the 1970s, persons 65 years of age and older accounted for an average of 79 million hospital days annually, and on average, each of these persons visited a physician almost seven times annually; the total health cost for older persons was about three times higher than that for adults generally (Shanas and Maddox 1977; U.S. Department of Health, Education and Welfare 1977a). In the 1980s, older adults continued to use various health services at a rate higher than that of other adults. Personal annual per capita dollar expenditures for hospital care, physicians' visits, and drugs tend to average about three times higher for adults over 65 years old compared with younger adults (U.S. Senate Special Committee on Aging 1985). A relatively stable estimate of 5% of persons 65 years of age and older tend to be institutionalized at any given time in the United States in recent decades, and the estimated probability of a period of long-term institutionalization in late life is about 25% (Palmore 1976).

These widely quoted statistics are impressive and invite the incorrect inference that medical and institutional care have supplanted traditional community and home care. This is far from being the case. Epidemiological surveys provide evidence that although an estimated 80% of older adults have at least one chronic condition, about 60% of older persons are not significantly impaired in five important dimensions of functioning: social support networks, economic security, physical health, mental health, and the capacity for performing basic physical and management activities of daily living (Comptroller General of the United States 1977a; Maddox and Dellinger 1978; National Center for Health Statistics 1983). More than 9 out of 10 older adults will live most of their later years in the community. And for the approximately 12%–15% of older persons in the community who are seriously impaired, approximately 80% of the services they receive are provided by kin and friends, not by a public agency (Comptroller General of the United States 1977b; Health Policy Analysis Program 1978).

The fact that currently an estimated 20% of health and social services provided to seriously impaired older individuals have a public source of financing surely constitutes a change and a historical trend worth noting. Federal funding of total national health expenditures increased from 13% in 1965 (the year Medicare was enacted) to 23% 2 years later and to 29% of total expenditures by 1983 (Rabin and Stockton 1987). The federal share of national health expenditures remained relatively stable from 1983 to 1990, when the federal percentage of total national health expenditures was 29.2%. This change challenges both a cultural and a political preference for asserting the primacy of familial responsibility for older persons and activates anxieties about the weakening of family ties and related social obligations. Social theorists have accentuated this concern with discussions of what may be called the "consequences of modernization" thesis, which contends that the inevitable price of industrialization, urbanization, and rapid social change is the weakening of familial and community ties. The dependent old, in turn, would obviously be vulnerable to isolation, social irrelevance, and neglect. There is evidence that family structure and function have changed in recent decades. The divorce rate is high, single-parent families are now common, alternative family lifestyles are more visible, and families have access to and use an increasing array of experts to help in resolving personal and familial problems. Yet the fact remains that most older people are not isolated from kin and friends; impressive majorities of adult children indicate a continuing willingness to care for an older adult family member (Kane and Kane 1978; Maddox 1972; Maddox and Lawton 1993; Maddox and Wiley 1977; U.S. Department of Health and Human Services 1986). In sum, community and home care of dependent, impaired older individuals have been and continue to be the rule, not the exception. Therefore, current discussions of community and home care appropriately stress a long-established pattern that may be in need of rediscovery and revitalization but that is certainly not a daring new adventure.

Proliferation of Community Services

Community and home services, both public and voluntary, have been widely available and widely used in Western European countries for many years. In European settings, particularly those with comprehensive care systems, public debate focuses not on whether community and home services are feasible and desirable, but rather on how to increase their availability to and appropriations for underserved and unserved populations. On the basis of such experience, a considerable body of documentation and expertise exists regarding the organization, training, staffing, and performance of noninstitutional services for older persons. In general, such services have high social visibility, are integrated into comprehensive care systems, and are reasonably well financed. Experience in Europe suggests that one community or home care worker to help with household maintenance and personal care is required for every 100 older persons, a rate that is currently approximated in the Nordic countries. The United Kingdom has achieved a rate of one worker per 750 older persons. In the United States the current rate is about one worker per 5,000 older persons (Davies 1992; Maddox 1977, 1992).

Contemporary health care in the United States is characterized by a high degree of specialization of information, personnel, therapeutic procedures, and locales for delivering services (Eisdorfer et al. 1989; Vogel and Palmer 1983). This specialization includes community and home care (Kavesh 1986; Koren 1986; Leader 1986). The permutations and combinations of specialized people, activities, and locales have no known limits and therefore generate acute problems of fragmentation, require organizational coordination, and tend to have gaps in coverage (Harrington et al. 1985). Early in this century, health care was considerably less specialized in terms of knowledge, personnel, techniques, and locale of service. Hence, one encountered general practitioners and general nurses offering services primarily in homes and incidentally in hospitals. If one disaggregates the process of general medical care into specialized components, the logical possibilities are numerous medical specialists, physician extenders, hospital nurses, public health nurses, practical nurses, home health aides, home helpers, and so on. Similarly, if one observes a family caring for an impaired older member, this holistic process can be disaggregated into a large number of basic components, each of which can be the basis for a specialized activity for one or another category of professional or quasi-professional persons.

Let us assume a society concludes 1) that a number of impaired older persons need supportive health and welfare services, 2) that these services can be and should be offered outside institutions (that is, in the community or at home), and 3) that there should be some public support for these services when individuals do not have the informal social support ordinarily provided by kin and friends. What one would expect to develop is what one currently observes—a specialized service system that reflects the disaggregation of the holistic process into components and the development of specialized programs to deal with these components. Specialized systems of community and home care are emerging for each element of service ordinarily provided by kin and friend networks—for example, adult family homes, day care, day health, personal care, continuing supervision, congregate care, meals/nutrition, household maintenance, home health, social interaction/recreation, physical therapy, education, housing, transportation, information and referral, special income maintenance, and protective services (Health Policy Analysis Program 1978; Weiler and Rathbone-McCuan 1978). The process of disaggregation of care services could logically go on and on. The availability and use of such services has been relatively limited currently: less than 1% of Medicare expenditures in the 1970s and less than 3% currently have been, for example, directed to community and home care (Leader 1986; U.S. Department of Health, Education and Welfare 1977b). Nevertheless, many components of a noninstitutional care system are already present.

One or more of these types of specialized noninstitutional services currently exist in most communities in the United States; complex combinations of services are present in many communities; and, in a few communities, a comprehensive range of services is found. There is no question that a case can be made for the feasibility and desirability of each type of service, although how much and for whom are very much in doubt. In the typical instance, each discrete service has developed its own justification, staffing estimates, training procedures, and clientele. Certification and state surveillance of community-based services are minimal. In the typical community, moreover, adequate provision is made neither for coordinating the discrete programs administratively and financially nor for articulating them with the dominant health care delivery system. The principal issues to demonstrate regarding community and home services are, therefore, not their feasibility and desirability, but rather their efficiency, effectiveness, financial viability, and our capacity to manage a comprehensive care system (Pendleton et al. 1989).

The Cost-Effectiveness and Efficiency of Alternatives

Public discussions of alternative care programs have concentrated increasingly on the key issues of cost-effectiveness and the effective integration of non-institutional services into the existing care system. Inferences regarding costs have continued to be inconclusive, not only because the definitive evidence is lacking but also because the questions being asked are usually the wrong questions. The question typically asked is, "Are community and home care alternatives cheaper than institutionalization?" The intuitive answer would certainly be in the affirmative. This answer is misleading, however, because it avoids the issue of the cost implications of particular services for the total system of care and ignores issues of access and of quality of care. It is intuitively obvious, for example, that individuals with moderate functional impairments requiring limited support services could be maintained in a community or home setting more cheaply than in an institutional setting. This is true, to a considerable degree, because noninstitutional care costs are shifted from the public sector to the private sector, specifically to family and friends (Comptroller General of the United States 1977b; Sager 1977; Spellman and Kemper 1992). It is also intuitively obvious that a minimally impaired person who is for some reason in an institution that provides more than the required care could be managed more economically as well as more appropriately elsewhere. Enthoven (1978), Luft (1978), Ingelfinger (1978) and Aaron (1991) all note the operation of "the technologic imperative" in health care institutions; the specialized health care professionals in high-technology settings have professional, ethical, and legal reasons for trying one or more tests or procedures. These observers are convinced that in high-technology settings, the marginal utility of medical treatment—in both a medical and an economic sense of benefits in relation to investment—is frequently reached and often exceeded. Insofar as community and home care remove an individual from the technology typically found in institutional settings, reduction in the cost of care should follow. HMOs apparently reduce the total cost of care through rationing access to hospitals (Luft 1978), and proponents of the hospice movement are explicit in emphasizing care of dying patients that minimizes use of costly medical technology and maximizes use of relatively more economical psychosocial supportive therapy (Berdes 1978). Fair comparisons of the costs of hospice care and hospital care are not yet available. The results of small studies comparing hospice cost with conventional hospital cost do suggest that hospice care is cheaper; however, findings from comparisons of hospice care in inpatient settings with traditional inpatient care do not indicate savings (Mor 1987; Mor and Kidder 1985). Nonetheless, the appropriateness and defensibility of such a removal is clearly a debatable quality-of-care issue that would require far more evidence than is currently available (Breslow 1978; Donabedian 1978; Eisdorfer et al. 1989; Frazier and Hiat 1978; Tancredi and Barondess 1978). Recent evidence from a review of the cost-effectiveness of hospice care after such care became covered under Medicare has not been reassuring (Mor and Kidder 1985; Paradis and Cummings 1986).

The more severe the functional impairment of the individual, the less intuitively obvious the cost-effectiveness of community and home care becomes. A critical issue in assessing the cost-effectiveness of alternative forms of health and social services is, therefore, a determination of the degree of functional impairment and the minimal number and quality of services that would meet acceptable standards of care for persons with a known degree and kind of impairment in ability to perform normal social roles. In exploring such an issue, one can imagine an experimental or quasi-experimental design in which at least four categories of older persons emerge: 1) those whose impairments are so severe that by professional and public consensus, they would need to be in an institutional setting; 2) those whose impairments are moderate and for whom the consensus of professionals is that they might be appropriately managed in either an institutional or a noninstitutional setting; 3) those whose impairments require supportive services, but clearly in noninstitutional settings; and 4) those whose degree of well-being requires no special services. The second category is the critical one for testing hypotheses about comparative costs of alternative types of care (Smyer 1977). The first and third categories raise different questions. For example, if a person in the first category were found in the community or a person in the third category were found in a long-stay institution, we would be interested primarily in explaining an inappropriate placement. The issue of the difference in cost of maintaining third-category persons in the community or in an institution is uninteresting because it has a predetermined answer; such persons are almost certainly misplaced in institutions. A person in the first category living in the community or a person in the fourth category residing in an institution is certainly misplaced. With degree of functional impairment specified and reasonable consensus achieved regarding the type and amount of required services, one can imagine relatively definitive comparative research that might address the issue of cost-effectiveness of alternative care programs for impaired older persons. A few research studies have reflected both an understanding of and a response to these necessary conditions for drawing conclusions regarding the relative costs of alternative systems of care. These are discussed below.

The U.S. General Accounting Office in Cleveland, Ohio, designed a study to assess the impact of defined services on the well-being of a random sample of persons 65 years of age and older in that city (Comptroller General of the United States 1977a, 1977b). The design incorporated a methodology developed at the Duke University Center for the Study of Aging and Human Development (Maddox 1972, 1985; Maddox and Dellinger 1978). The Duke methodology had three elements: 1) a reliable, valid multidimensional assessment of functional status; 2) a procedure for identifying the number, quantity, and cost of basic components of commonly used services; and 3) a matrix relating the services actually received by persons of known functional status initially to their functional status at some subsequent time.

The investigators in Cleveland found that 60% of the older individuals surveyed had minimal impairments that required no special intervention or required, at most, services such as transportation; assistance with housing, social, and recreational opportunities; and, occasionally, home help. At the other extreme, 10% of the sample were severely impaired and required—and were receiving—an extensive range of supportive services. Of the 60% who were relatively unimpaired, the average individual received the equivalent of $349 (in 1975 dollars) in services each month, with 60% of this amount being provided by family and friends. Of

the 10% who were extremely impaired, the average cost per month for services received was estimated to be $845, of which 80% was provided by family and friends. This $845 is considerably above the $597 that was the average monthly cost of nursing home care in Ohio at that time. These data suggest several conclusions:

1. A large number of extremely impaired older persons are maintained in the community.
2. The extremely impaired are maintained in the community at a cost well above the cost of nursing home care.
3. The high cost of noninstitutional care is borne primarily by kin and friends rather than by public agencies.

For the extremely impaired older persons in the Cleveland study who were living in the community, the total cost of care in a noninstitutional setting was not less than that of institutional care, but the care was less costly to the public treasury, which was responsible for only 20% of the bill. What about the estimated cost of care for the 30% of older persons lying between the classifications "unimpaired" and "extremely impaired"? Such persons in Cleveland were receiving services valued at an average of $323 per month, 70% of which was provided by kin and friends. The total cost of services for this category was about half that for nursing home care, even if it had been paid entirely from public resources. Because some persons living in nursing homes—possibly 12%–14% (Health Policy Analysis Program 1978; Laurie 1978)—have an intermediate degree of functional impairment, this category is clearly critical in assessing the potential cost savings that would come from ensuring that needed care is provided outside institutions.

The estimate of 12%–14% of older persons in nursing homes whose functional impairments might be managed in noninstitutional settings is a debatable but plausible and conservative estimate based on admittedly limited data. Estimation of persons inappropriately institutionalized or receiving more than required care in institutions has varied considerably from study to study, depending on the procedures used to assess impairment and determine appropriateness of care in relation to the degree of impairment assessed. Some estimates of inappropriate care in institutions have ranged as high as 40% (Health Policy Analysis Program 1978). Current evidence does not permit a resolution of the reported variance in estimates. The consensus is only that the rate of unnecessary institutionalization and the inappropriately high levels of care are significant. Further evidence is clearly needed. With the advent of prospective reimbursement for hospitals and increasing levels of impairment among nursing home residents, the number of inappropriately placed residents in nursing homes likely has been reduced (Hawes et al. 1988). However, there is evidence that nursing homes are currently caring for a group of residents who have few or no impairments in physical functioning and no cognitive impairments. Several existing studies do, however, provide relevant illustrations of the problems of producing definitive information and present some suggestive findings.

Hurtado and colleagues (1971) at the Kaiser facility in Portland, Oregon, reported on the economic effects of introducing an extended-care facility and a home care service into a comprehensive prepayment health plan with a history of low hospitalization use among subscribers. The effect on Medicare subscribers was of particular interest. The authors demonstrated that with these new services administratively and spatially an integral part of the comprehensive care organization, hospital use in Medicare patients was reduced by 27%. Most of the observed reduction was attributable to the use of the extended care facility rather than the home care service. Moreover, the total cost of the services to Medicare patients outside the hospital service was greater than the savings from the reduced hospitalization—that is, although hospital days were reduced, the less expensive extended care and home services were used for longer periods of time, thus tending to equalize the cost of illness episodes managed primarily inside or outside the hospital service.

Similarly, Weiler and Rathbone-McCuan (1978), who are advocates of community-based care for older persons, summarized research on the cost of 10 day care facilities that variously emphasized rehabilitation or social support services. The observed range of average daily costs was from $11 to $61, and the average for the 10 facilities was about $25. This average cost for adult day care was above the national average cost of about $10 per day for nursing home care at the time of the comparison. It is important to note that the day care program reported by

Weiler and Rathbone-McCuan did not include an estimate of the out-of-pocket cost-of-living expenses of program participants.

Alan Sager (1977) provided an imaginative pilot study of the cost of alternative forms of care for impaired older persons that illustrates the problems of cost estimation. Working with a sample of individuals at the point of discharge from a hospital, he had nine professionals experienced in discharge planning estimate whether home or nursing care would be the more appropriate assignment. Home care was estimated to be more appropriate for 12% of the subjects. The assessors then proposed detailed care plans. Reasonable consensus was achieved among planners for each individual, and the estimated cost of implementing the recommended care plans was determined. The average daily cost of the estimated home care plans, with maintenance cost of board and lodging factored in, was about $52. Assessors were also asked to prescribe an alternative care plan for each individual if the person were institutionalized. The estimated cost of the services proposed for delivery in a nursing home proved to be almost exactly the same as for home care. By happenstance, nine subjects for whom home care and nursing home care plans had been developed were in fact institutionalized; the actual average cost per day was about $60. Sager's work leaves unanswered the relative importance of provider and consumer judgments about the appropriateness of care planning.

The conceptualization of Sager's study warrants special comment. First, careful attention was given to establishing professional consensus on appropriate service requirements regardless of the service site chosen. Second, total cost of services, whether public or private, was estimated. Third, experienced professional service planners proposed alternative care plans in both nursing home and home settings that proved to have the same total cost, although the actual cost of nursing home care proved to be above the estimated cost. And, fourth, at the point of discharge from the hospital, a large majority (almost 90%) of older patients considered for inclusion in the study were judged to be inappropriate for home care.

Medicus Systems Corporation (1977), under a federal contract, attempted to implement an ambitious controlled trial of the outcome of assigning appropriately selected individuals being discharged from hospitals to day care or home care programs, to a combination of both, or to a "no special care" control condition. The cost of additional services for the experimental subjects assigned to day care or home service was provided by special federal financial arrangements. For various reasons, the research study did not meet the stringent conditions of a controlled clinical trial because true random alternative assignment of subjects proved to be difficult, services received by control subjects could not be monitored carefully, and cost determination was inadequate. However, within these constraints, considerable variation in cost of services between presumably similar programs was observed. The general conclusion was that extended benefits available to participants in noninstitutional programs did appear to lower the use of traditional health services appreciably. There was some indication that total cost of care increased on the average. These conclusions are similar to those reached by Hurtado et al. (1971) in their Portland, Oregon, study.

More recent evidence on the cost-effectiveness of community-based care comes from the National Long-Term Care Demonstration (known informally as the Channeling Project), which was initiated in September 1980 by three divisions of the U.S. Department of Health and Human Services. Its objective was to assess the effects of comprehensive case management of community care on cost containment in long-term care without sacrificing quality of care for needy, impaired elderly (U.S. Department of Health and Human Services 1986). The demonstration was designed to finance some direct services and to arrange for waiver of some financial restrictions on some types of community care; but the demonstration did not include direct control over medical and nursing home care. Case management in the basic demonstration of how an existing service system might be effectively coordinated consisted in the Channeling Project of seven features: 1) outreach, 2) standard eligibility screening, 3) comprehensive assessment, 4) initial care planning, 5) service arrangement, 6) monitoring, and 7) periodic assessment. An alternative financial control model made it possible for health care managers in some demonstration sites to expand the range of services offered, to offer services on the basis of need rather than eligibility, to pool resources for strategic allocation to particular services, and to require partial copayment by recipients in some cases. The five

sites selected to test each model were operational in 1982 and continued to be fully operational through June 1984.

Over the life of the demonstration, 11,769 applicants were screened and 9,890 identified as eligible. Of these, 6,341 were randomly assigned to demonstration or control categories. Several data sources were used in the evaluation of the program's effects. In addition to telephone screening interviews, an extensive in-person survey was administered to both treatment and control groups at baseline and repeated at 6, 12, and (for half the sample) 18 months. Contact was subsequently made by telephone with a subset of informal caregivers at 6 and 12 months. Service use and cost data were collected from Medicare, Medicaid, and channeling records, and from providers directly.

Principal findings from the Channeling Project demonstration include the following:

1. Channeling's selection criteria did identify an extremely vulnerable group of older adults: 22% were unable to perform any of five activities of daily living; more than 90% were IADL-impaired (that is, unable to adequately perform instrumental activities of daily living); 53% were incontinent; a significant minority showed evidence of cognitive impairment; one-third lived alone; and more than half reported incomes of below $500 a month.

2. The demonstration, whose design was implemented essentially as planned, provided an evaluation of the effects of coordinating basic and slightly enriched services for older adults; these effects included the following:

   a) Channeling increased formal community service use.

   b) Neither type of demonstration (basic or financial model) reduced or had any major effects on the informal care being provided to participants.

   c) In spite of identifying a group of elderly persons living in the community who were at high risk for institutionalization, the demonstration did not identify the subpopulation at highest risk or reduce nursing home use.

   d) The channeling interventions did not reduce the relatively heavy use of physicians and medical services among these high-risk older adults.

e) The costs of expanded case management and community services were not offset by reductions in nursing home and other costs.

f) In general, the demonstration increased client and informal caregiver confidence and satisfaction with life.

g) The demonstration did not significantly affect client functioning or risk of mortality.

The Channeling Project was an expensive demonstration and reconfirmation of several general observations that have been made repeatedly about the organization of health care in the United States over many years. Manipulations of the system of formal care services do not appear ordinarily to reduce the availability of informal support. In the case of the Channeling Project, both the persons receiving care and their caregivers responded positively to efforts to improve care for the elderly persons for whom they were responsible. The presumption that a large number of persons in nursing homes do not need to be there has persisted for a long time without the benefit of definitive evidence. The estimates based on data generated by the Duke Older Americans Resources and Services Program and the U.S. General Accounting Office (Maddox 1985) are worth noting again because they suggest that the number of nursing home residents who might, on medical grounds, be treated more appropriately elsewhere may be 10%. On the other hand, in our estimation, possibly an equal percentage of community-dwelling elderly persons may be so disabled as to benefit from nursing home placement. In demonstrations like the Channeling Project, which emphasized comprehensive screening, it would be reasonable to assume, therefore, that some screening of community residents would lead to a recommendation for rather than against institutionalization. In any case, the demonstrated failure of the well-conceived Channeling Project to reduce institutionalization and medical care usage illustrates how such projects may add to rather than reduce or moderate total system cost for the care of older populations. Research suggests that the most likely way in which total system cost can be reduced is through a capped organizational budget that covers inpatient, outpatient, and community care services (Enthoven 1980; Evans 1985; Harrington et al. 1985; Maddox 1977). In such cases, the issue becomes one of suballocation of a specified total budget to these various services and

decentralization of health planning and delivery. Budget capping has technical merit as a cost-control strategy but it is politically quite controversial, as illustrated by an assessment of the merits of using HMOs to provide Medicare-financed care for older adults (Iglehart 1987).

The most adequate information on the cost of community and home programs designed as alternatives to institutionalization, while clearly not definitive, does not confirm the hopes of the advocates of alternative forms of care. The assertion that community and home care lowers average daily cost or total system cost is not confirmed when there is some control for the level of functional impairment of the older individual involved and for the cost-accounting procedures used. It is also evident that community and home care appears most favorable in comparison with institutional care only when public cost is considered and basic maintenance cost and other nonpublic contributions are not factored in. Further, and this is a critical issue, such evidence as there is does not indicate that total system cost is reduced by community-based care programs. On the contrary, total cost appears to be the same or perhaps slightly higher (see, for example, Hurtado et al. 1971; U.S. Department of Health and Human Services 1986).

Kemper and colleagues (1987) reviewed 16 community-care demonstration projects that sought to substitute home and community services for nursing home care and to improve patients' quality of life. All projects included case management and an expanded package of community services, including nonmedical services. As with Weissert's review of the Channeling Project, reductions in nursing home use of treatment group members, compared with control group members, were very small. In contrast to Weissert's conclusions, when reviewing only programs with a case management component, Kemper and co-workers reported that hospital use was lower among demonstration project participants than among control group members. However, the overall system costs were not reduced by the projects, and the small reduction in nursing home use was more than offset by increases in costs associated with care provided in the home and community, with the exception of the South Carolina Long Term Care Project. In this project, participation was targeted by using nursing home preadmission screening, thus producing greater reduction in nursing home use. Community care costs were kept low, case management costs were less than in other projects, and overall system costs "broke even."

Weissert and colleagues (1988) examined more than 700 citations for a meta-analysis of home and community care research to reach overall conclusions on costs and effects of home and community care for older adults by reviewing previous research findings. Twenty-seven studies were identified that tested the effects of alternatives to long-term care services that were already in place, including projects developed as alternatives to nursing homes or other home- and community-based care services. Each of the studies analyzed involved service primarily to the elderly, included at least 50 individuals, employed an experimental design with treatment and control groups, and used the individual as the primary unit of analysis. Analyses examined service recipients' risks of using a nursing home, actual nursing home and hospital use by home and community care recipients, gains or losses attributable to changes in the use of existing or new services, and the effect of home and community care services on selected domains of health status.

With few exceptions, most notably the South Carolina Long Term Care Project, which identified home and community care demonstration project recipients through that state's nursing home preadmission screening process, the targeting used in the projects reviewed was not successful in reducing cost. Nursing home admission rates among control groups were low, which suggests that targeting criteria were not discriminating those most at risk of nursing home placement. Weissert noted that targeting appears to have improved with more recent studies and the use of multivariate targeting criteria.

With regard to reductions in the use of institutional and outpatient care, Weissert reported that although most studies showed some reduction in the use of nursing homes, the use rates for hospital services were actually higher in several studies. This is an effect previously noted by others and attributed to increased surveillance and identification of unmet needs and referral for appropriate services.

The combined increased use of hospital services and additional expense for home- and community-care services rendered, coupled with the generally insignificant reduction in nursing home stays, resulted in few studies showing lower overall system costs for long-term care due to the introduction of home- and community-care services. The health status effects that were consistently reported across studies included improvements in life satisfaction for both persons receiving home- or community-care services and their caregivers, and reduction of unmet needs.

Weissert concluded that adequate evidence for developing long-term care policies will require, in addition to improved targeting, better definition of catchment areas and assurance that programs operate at full capacity; clearer delineation of subgroups served and expected outcomes relevant to each subgroup; improved utilization control and consideration of shorter treatment periods; attention to outliers (that is, very heavy users) and associated costs; and effective efforts to avoid ineffective hospital use. Weissert suggested that interventions, including housing with home and community care, merit additional study, along with prospective care financing or capitation.

In their review of evidence regarding home and community care, Hawes and colleagues (1988) complemented Weissert's finding in identifying the strength of consumer support for home and community care and the positive impact demonstrated on the well-being and psychosocial outcomes measured. Hawes also noted concerns similar to those reported by Weissert with regard to the need for improvements in targeting services to those at greatest risk of institutional care, and the need to look more carefully at congregate or sheltered housing for effects on nursing home utilization patterns. Hawes further suggested that comparison of nursing home and community care costs assumes that both service-delivery mechanisms are in adequate supply, operate equally efficiently, are priced at acceptable levels, and offer equivalent care quality. These are assumptions that both Hawes and Weissert question.

In sum, current evidence on cost-effectiveness of community care does not provide a decisive argument against such care. Economic cost is not necessarily the only or the most important consideration. It is quite possible, for instance, that costs being equal, community and home care provide good value for the money invested because the care provided is more appropriate than institutional care, is of better quality, or is more effective in maintaining functioning in the long run. Or the long-run implications may be more favorable for noninstitutional care than short-term studies have indicated.

Or public policy might favor noninstitutional care, not because its total cost is less than that of institutional care but rather because noninstitutional care transfers a significant part of the cost to the private sector. Or, by removing impaired individuals from high-technology environments, public policy that emphasizes noninstitutional care may reduce long-run system cost through reducing the use of high-cost interventions of questionable value. Each and all of these explanations are plausible, and future research must sort out the facts. Concentration on cost may, however, divert attention from what many observers believe to be the more salient problem—the inefficient and ineffective organization of care.

The Organizational Context of Health Care

We have argued above that although community and home care for impaired older persons is needed and feasible, such care is not demonstrably more economical than institutional forms of care when degree of functional impairment is controlled and total cost is determined. However, it is probable that noninstitutional care is cost-effective, we have contended, for perhaps 30% of older persons who are moderately but not severely impaired. Essential evidence does not exist that cost-effective noninstitutional care of appropriate quality can be provided for this significant category of impaired elderly within the care system as presently organized. This is so primarily for two reasons. First, currently the care system and its financing have a decidedly medical and institutional emphasis. That is, the care system is most easily accessed by individuals with a medically certifiable impairment, and access to some community services has often been contingent on the individual's having been institutionalized. Community and home services, although recognized in Medicare legislation, continue to be a small fraction (about 3%–4%) of the services financed. The concepts of preventive care and social support services have been essentially foreign to Medicare, and mental health services—and payment for these services—are limited (Berger 1978; Blazer and Maddox 1977; Glasscote 1976; Glasscote et al. 1977), although President Clinton's Health Security Plan (White House Domestic Policy Council 1993) promised to change this.

Contemporary discussions of health usually stress the desirability of taking a broad view of health in terms of functional capacity and the total well-being of individuals. That is, a philosophic interest in the social components of health and well-being is frequently expressed, and strong cases have been made for preferring social models of care to medical models (Breslow 1978; Kane and Kane 1978; Maddox 1992; Saward and Sorensen 1978). Philosophical preferences aside, the dominant care system available to older persons continues to have a decidedly medical focus. In addition, the dominant care system is highly specialized, fragmented, uncoordinated, and without a single point of entry to provide systematic, comprehensive assessment of impairment and assignment to appropriate services. One result is that each segment of the care system competes for public resources that are known to be limited. Hence, each additional service program tends to add to total system cost rather than to substitute for the cost of some other service. A striking characteristic of the care system of the United States is that its implied total annual budget is in essence unlimited and is determined retrospectively by the cumulative cost of all care programs, and total cost is known only after the costs have been incurred. This is in contrast to nationalized systems and, in fact, the prepaid comprehensive programs in this country, which assume a fixed annual budget that must be allocated among the alternative components of the system (Hollingsworth et al. 1990).

In 1971, the U.S. Department of Health, Education and Welfare (now the Department of Health and Human Services) distributed an analysis of what was described as "the crisis of health care." This document asked whether the perceived crisis was produced by 1) inferior health care as reflected in the assessed well-being of citizens; 2) the absence of essential resources; or 3) both of these. The answer in each case was negative. Although indications of health, such as mortality and morbidity statistics and life expectancy rates, in this country are not the best in the world, they are tolerable by most standards and are most distinctively different from what are found in other countries in regard to variations in health indicators by race, socioeconomic status, and locale of residence. Health indicators of white, middle-class urban populations in this country generally compare quite favorably with those of European populations; nor does this country lack resources. Our health personnel/population ratios are favorable, our hospital bed/population ratios are favorable, and our committed percentage of GNP to health (more than 10%) is among the highest in the world. Again, the most evident problem is maldistribution of resources, particularly primary care resources, rather than absence of resources. For example, 82 active physicians per 100,000 population might be found in Mississippi, whereas 228 active physicians per 100,000 population might be found in New York. Large metropolitan areas average two times more physicians per unit population than do rural areas. In recent decades, the proportion of primary care physicians has declined to the point that at the beginning of the 1990s, more than 6 in 10 active physicians were in specialty practice. The report concluded that the crisis is best described as organizational. The nation suffers, according to this analysis, from excessive fragmentation and poor coordination of existing resources. Significantly, the report did not comment directly on what Wildavsky called the Great Equation (medical care equals health), although this idea was implicit. For instance, the report did stress the importance of environmental factors that affect health, preventive care, and health education. The central illustration of a possible solution to the organizational problem identified was HMOs. This preference was justified in the report by evidence then available that HMOs are cost-effective, a conclusion supported also by current evidence (U.S. Department of Health, Education and Welfare 1977b).

Following the report by the U.S. Department of Health, Education and Welfare, legislation intended to foster HMOs emerged. The concept has been politically controversial, has had limited public acceptance, and has generated a considerable amount of rhetoric for and against (Lewis et al. 1976). Articles by Enthoven (1978) and Luft (1978) that summarized the issues and the evidence nearly two decades ago remain surprisingly current (see, for example, Eisdorfer et al. 1989). Enthoven correctly noted the absence of controlled trials in comparing alternative care systems and the consequent inability to draw definitive conclusions regarding the cost-effectiveness and quality of care provided by competing alternatives. He reviewed the incentive structures of alternative care systems and concluded that fragmented, uncoordinated systems lack any obvious incentive for control of cost. Further, if a fragmented,

uncoordinated collection of health care programs is dominated by high-technology institutions, the probability is high that a "technological imperative" will operate—that is, the availability of technology encourages high rates of use even in the face of evidence that such use has low marginal utility. This conclusion led Enthoven to argue that within a total system of care, there should be alternative care sites, some of which remove individuals from the high-technology care centers. Such removal reduces the opportunity, and the inclination, to introduce types of care that have demonstrably low return in terms of increased functioning. By implication, then, Enthoven argued that community and home care might achieve economies precisely because individuals in such settings are not, and presumably are appropriately not, at risk for high-technology therapeutic intervention. Enthoven did, however, add the caution that his general argument for alternative forms of care was not an endorsement of any specific form of care in the absence of controlled trials that take into consideration quality as well as cost.

It is worth noting in this context that some proponents of the hospice movement appear to have reached a similar conclusion (Berdes 1978). In high-technology settings, there are a variety of incentives—professional, ethical, and legal—to make extraordinary efforts to extend life by any available means and at any cost. Proponents of hospices commonly argue that such efforts are not only patently artificial but also, in the final analysis, inhumane. This conclusion leads to the deliberate exclusion of advanced technology from the hospice to a specific emphasis on the social, behavioral, and medical components of palliative, versus curative, care. Medical technology is emphasized in the hospice movement, if at all, in connection with the reduction of pain rather than with the extension of life. Evidence indicates that the promises of hospices have not automatically been fulfilled (Mor and Kidder 1985; Paradis and Cummings 1986). The cost of hospices as an alternative to hospitalization for terminal care also is not automatically cheaper. The degree of cost savings appears to be dependent on the type of hospice organization, although fair comparisons do not exist (Mor 1987). Some concern has been expressed that, over time, hospice care would become more like the institutional care it was designed to replace (Paradis and Cummings 1986). However, until recently, adequate longitudinal data that could serve as evidence in an analysis of the evolution of hospice care and expenditures were not available. Data from the state of North Carolina spanning all 14 years of state hospice history appear to provide one of the more promising sources in the resolution of the debate over changes in hospice care and its costs. A study from the Moffitt Cancer Center and Research Institute will also provide understanding of the current state of hospice expenditures by presenting the results of data that directly compare hospice and traditional institutional care for terminally ill patients.

We believe that attention to hospices as a form of community care is warranted, for both service and policy reasons. First, hospices have traditionally served a patient population whose average age is 65 years. With the population aging, observers estimate significant increase in demand for palliative care from terminally ill older adults. Second, hospices have been a form of care chosen by some of the increasing numbers of persons with advanced acquired immunodeficiency syndrome (AIDS). Third, hospices are important as a site for analyzing the organization and financing of health care. Its pioneering non–fee-for-service reimbursement package was a financing strategy designed to maintain a humane focus of care. As such, hospices may provide a model for long-term care, generally, in which the need for medical care is balanced by the need for psychosocial aspects of care (Hayslip and Leon 1992). Finally, hospices are an example of a private-sector organization using, in part, public-sector dollars and accountability to provide care; they represent the kind of mixed-sector health care provision that is occurring in many Western welfare states.

In an article by Luft (1978; see also Eisdorfer et al. 1989), a review was provided of the rhetoric and the evidence regarding the reputed savings attributed to HMOs; Luft concluded that the claimed economies are probably real and substantial. These reported savings in the total cost of care apparently were then, and are now, attributable primarily to the lower rates of hospitalization in HMOs and not to differences in the use of ambulatory care services or lengths of stay in hospitals. The studies Luft reviewed are relatively compelling because they are methodologically adequate, taking into consideration standardized age and gender rates and case mixes. Luft was not altogether certain why the apparent cost-effectiveness was consistently observed. Possibly, he argued, the HMO client is less sick or

differently disposed to use available care, although most evidence suggests that this is not the case; on the contrary, some evidence suggests that prepaid plans tend to attract a disproportionate number of chronically ill persons. Or perhaps HMOs undertreat their patients, although evidence that this is so is lacking. It should be recalled here that the research of Hurtado et al. (1971) did not show cost savings in an experiment with alternative forms of service within a particular comprehensive prepaid medical plan. One experience in the prepayment of HMOs for care of older adults under Medicare suggested that the established organizational strengths of HMOs in the cost-effective delivery of health care cannot compensate for poor fiscal management of a particular HMO (Iglehart 1987).

Constructing the Future

As noted earlier, in the discussion of Perrow's analysis of the three factors that affect service-delivery organizations, cultural and ideologic factors dominate when the technology for achieving preferred social goals is unavailable and when the existing organizational structure adversely affects the application of such technology. Many people, including many expert observers, believe that community and home care are forms of noninstitutional service delivery that are both desirable and feasible. This belief is bolstered by a number of factors, including evidence from this country and abroad that 1) programs of care for older persons outside institutional settings can be efficient and effective; 2) care in institutional settings not only is very expensive but also provides too much service for some older people and not enough for others who could benefit from minimal supportive care; and 3) appropriate technology and model organizational forms of community-based care exist that provide the basis for future development of an adequately comprehensive care system.

Beliefs, Technology, and Organization

In spite of the attractiveness of these beliefs, community and home care services have been developed slowly and with considerable cautiousness in the United States. The explanation of this apparently contradictory trend is suggested by Perrow's analysis. At the cultural level, the attractiveness of low-technology community and home care is matched by the appeal of high-technology medical care. In the abstract, both health care providers and consumers would surely respond favorably to the prospect of more noninstitutional forms of care of high quality and at low cost. In the concrete, it is not at all clear that either would respond affirmatively to more noninstitutional care if this meant fewer hospital beds, rationed access to hospitals and physicians, or reduction in the specialized tests and therapeutic procedures that are at the heart of contemporary diagnosis (Fox 1977). That is, if given the choice of a fixed amount of money to be allocated to health and welfare with more community care resulting in less institutional care, it remains to be seen where public preferences would lie.

The critical question is not whether reallocation of resources to alternative forms of care is possible. Most countries in Western Europe provide illustration of successful community care programs as integral components of their systems of care. The question is also not whether the health of populations suffers intolerably from extensive use of noninstitutional services. It does not. Every country in Western Europe has gross indicators of mortality and morbidity that compare favorably with our own (Rabin and Stockton 1987; Raffel 1985; U.S. Department of Health, Education and Welfare 1971).

The question is whether health care providers in the United States and the people they serve can live with the implications of a changed health care system in which access to specialized medical and hospital care would be rationed and the autonomy, perceived or real, of both professionals and their patients/clients would be reduced (Chapman 1978; Enthoven 1980). The evidence and the speculation are variable and suggest that American values and attitudes regarding health care are essentially contradictory. Some social survey evidence suggests that a majority of adult Americans perceive a crisis in health care delivery and identify the inaccessibility of primary care and the cost of health care as their primary concerns (Lewis et al. 1976; Maddox 1992). Fox (1977) argued that although Ivan Illich's radical critique of "medicalization" of society and his plea for "demedicalization" have some merit, health remains a central preoccupation of this society. Saward and Sorensen (1978) documented the continuing societal preoccupation with curative rather than preventive medicine.

Many individuals continue to resist modifying behavior and lifestyles that increase the risk of morbidity and mortality—cigarette smoking, overeating, physical inactivity, and nonuse of auto seat belts, for example. Of special interest are indications that social controls intended to modify risky behavior or noxious environmental factors are widely interpreted as infringements on personal freedom. It is as though, these authors conclude, freedom from regulations is more dear than life itself. Wildavsky's caustic, pessimistic essay "Doing Better and Feeling Worse" (1977) is preoccupied with the contradictory, the ironic—indeed, what he believes to be the pathologic—aspects of health care in this country. In addition to persistent belief in the wrong-headed Great Equation, he notes the "paradox of time: past success leads to future failure" (p. 106). For example, increased longevity is a human triumph that precipitates the crisis of an aging society. To save our shaky belief that investment in medicine ensures health, we displace our goals; interest in curing is displaced by interest in caring, and caring becomes equated with demonstrating that we have access to ineffective specialized technological services. Every move to increase equality in one dimension of health care increases inequality in another dimension. No society is willing and no care system is able, Wildavsky argues, to provide as much care as a population is willing to consume. We are driven by a technological imperative; there is always one more procedure to try. The cost of health care inevitably rises to a total that is provided by private insurance and federal subsidy. One is hardly surprised by the bottom line of Wildavsky's diagnosis: the politics of health care in the United States can only be described as conflicted, ambivalent, and pathological. The prognosis is not encouraging. No definitive treatment is available for our ambivalent feelings and contradictory preferences.

Perrow's analysis suggests that the persistent ideological quality of the contemporary discussion about health care constitutes evidence of the inadequacy of available technology and organizational arrangements for ensuring either curing or caring at a tolerable social cost. Our love affair with medical technology apparently is not over, but it is being pursued with less enthusiasm than before (Aaron 1991). The evidence of decreasing marginal utility of costly applications of medical technology is simply too great to be ignored (Enthoven 1980; Frazier and Hiat

1978; Ingelfinger 1978; Saward and Sorensen 1978; Tancredi and Barondess 1978). Yet there are few signs that continued discussion of "the crisis of health care" portends a radical reorganization and reallocation of health resources. After all, there is not yet even consensus about legislation on one or another form of national health insurance (Hurtado et al. 1971) or the objectives to be pursued in a national policy for long-term care of older adults (Meltzer et al. 1981). The jury has rejected President Clinton's proposed reforms (1994).

Perrow's analysis is also helpful in sensitizing the observer to an additional consequence of a plurality of ideological views about the organization and financing of health care. The policy-making arena clearly contains multiple key players, and some of the players hold a disproportionate share of the kind of organizational power to affect the direction of policy flow. So although consumers of health care services may hold a clear preference for noninstitutional forms of care, their interests may compete with the interests of health planners, politicians, health care administrators, and physicians. Robert Alford's analysis of the politics of health care planning in the United States documented how health care resources may be underallocated to groups whose interests are subordinate to those of dominant groups (Alford 1975). His analysis of the relative underdevelopment of occupational health demonstrated that the preferences and needs of workers may have been eclipsed by a dominant medical model that determined the kinds of health care provided during most of this century. What is of particular interest here, however, is that the balance of power is clearly changing in the health-policy arena today. A new actor, the health care administrator, has entered the field and has claimed an unprecedented share of the decision-making power, particularly since the implementation of Medicare. The health care administrator, whose language is that of economics and not of medical science, has altered the rules and format of the game. Stated more formally, the predominant shift in health policy in the last decade has been a move from professional control to the predominance of administrative control. Partly the result of key legislation, and partly the result of naturally occurring economic forces that have produced an unacceptable level of inflation of health care costs, it is clear that the bottom line in health planning in the 1990s will continue to focus on cost. The implications of this modulation or transfer of organizational power for the future of community-based care is, as we have argued, not entirely clear. What is clear is that the decision-making processes and the decision makers are changing.

For the foreseeable future, for better or worse, the United States seems destined to tinker incrementally with its fragmented, uncoordinated nonsystem of care. Incrementalism, a euphemism for only minor modifications of existing programs, which the British call "muddling through," has some merit in stable, democratically controlled societies (Maddox 1971). Several incremental changes at selected points in the current system of care affecting older persons do warrant at least some basis for guarded optimism about the future.

Adaptive Responses

Policymaking is not the only sphere in which the control of health care by physicians has been challenged. Public acceptance of unconditional professional autonomy and a medical monopoly of health care resources has been increasingly challenged. The origins of this challenge lie in the distant past, as Chapman (1978) has documented. The legal basis of laws regarding professional malpractice can be traced to the 14th century. In the intervening centuries, public challenge of uncontrolled professional autonomy and monopoly has been expressed through laws dealing with due process, licensure, restraint of trade, and quality control. The willingness of legislatures to limit the autonomy of medical professionals has been clearly demonstrated. Physicians, hospitals, and long-term care institutions will continue to play a vital role in the continuum of care that older persons require and in decisions about the allocation of resources to various components of the care system. The issue, therefore, is not the involvement of physicians and medical institutions in designing health care for the future, but rather the increasing involvement of nonmedical professions and nonmedical, community-based facilities in designing that future. Legislators have been reluctant to control access to high-technology medicine and to limit the proliferation and geographic concentration of highly specialized health personnel. They have also been slow to develop a plan for national health insurance and to involve government as a prudent buyer—and not just an insurer—of desired health and social services, with emphasis on preventive and primary care. Research and demonstrations assessing alternative comprehensive, prepayment care systems that integrate health and social services have not produced definitive conclusions. Orientation of consumers to realistic assessment of the relative merits of hospital- and community-based health care has been minimal. Although belief in the desirability and feasibility of more community-based services is increasing, nothing approximating a national consensus regarding the reorganization and financing of a comprehensive health care system designed to serve older persons is evident. The rejection of President Clinton's proposals for reform provides important evidence regarding the diminished prospects for change in the near future.

Organizational Development

Pragmatic, incremental experience with the organization of care in the United States has produced an outcome that, while not altogether satisfactory, is probably satisfactory enough to mitigate any inclination toward radical reorganization of care delivery in the immediate future. This same pragmatic, incremental orientation does, however, permit experimentation and model building that can provide public standards for assessing effectiveness and efficiency. In this country, elaboration of the HMO concept appears to have particular merit for responding to needs of older persons for comprehensive care.

The cost-effectiveness of HMOs has been reasonably established, and this effectiveness is usually attributed not to restriction of access to care generally but to reduction of institutionalization (Eisdorfer et al. 1989; Luft 1978). The HMO concept also emphasizes comprehensiveness of care within a fixed budget. Consider, for example, Figure 24–1 (Garfield 1970). In this figure, health is defined broadly as well-being, and attention is given to social as well as medical aspects of care and to preventive maintenance as well as "sick care." An integral and important aspect of this care system is the availability of initial screening for purposes of triage, although there is provision for bypass of screening when alternative assignment to health care, preventive maintenance, or sick care is clearly indicated. Another striking feature of this conceptualization of a care system is that although traditional medical

services are considered basic, social and psychological dimensions of care are equally basic and integral to the system. Given the origins of HMOs within the dominant medical model of care, one is hardly surprised that reference is made to paramedical staff and services with medical supervision. No violence is done to the concept by the substitution of such concepts as paraprofessional staff with professional supervision in order to transform this conventional medical model into a professional model that can include experts in social and psychological dimensions of care. Special attention is given in HMOs to programs of health education, exercise, and psychological counseling in the health care component; to provision of extended care, which could include community and home care for the impaired elderly, in the sick care component; and to geriatric clinics in the preventive maintenance component.

The HMO model of a comprehensive health maintenance organization is similar to the system of geriatric care that has operated in Glasgow, Scotland, for several decades (Kane and Kane 1978;

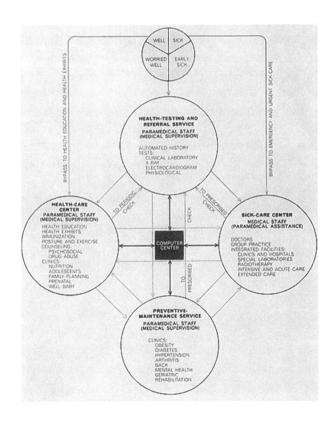

Figure 24–1. Initial concept of integrated care in a health maintenance organization.
Source. Reprinted from Garfield SR: "The Delivery of Medical Care." *Sci Am* 222:22, 1970. Used with permission.

McLachlan 1971). The Scottish model has as its focal point a primary care health center staffed by general practitioners, visiting nurses, and social workers who have been trained to work as a team. The health center personnel in this setting have access to an impressive continuum of alternative care settings, including in-home services, day care, day hospitals, sheltered housing, and inpatient hospital services with both general and specialized hospital wards, including geriatric psychiatry. Moreover, in Glasgow, community programs supplement the health services by providing special health education and a health examination coincident with retirement, as well as a variety of community support programs. The Scottish Home and Health Service, as a part of the British National Health Service, has a long tradition of integrating medical and social services and is, by definition, a comprehensive, prepaid care system. In Glasgow, professionals appear to use alternative placement of older persons judiciously and to place the impaired elderly at sites where the most appropriate care is available. Although detailed information about the cost of a comprehensive service such as that in Glasgow is not available, in general the British investment in the delivery of care runs about 5% of GNP less than in the United States.

A systematic investment of governmental resources in the development of model HMOs—and, more recently, SHMOs—to include assessment, health care, sick care, and preventive maintenance care for older persons appears to be indicated and is to be recommended. Such a decision would not preclude alternative investments in other forms of care. Yet the existence of a comprehensive system of care could provide a specific context for comparing the efficiency and effectiveness of alternative programs. In fact, the Health Care Financing Administration funded in the early 1980s a comparative study of the cost-effectiveness of SHMOs in six sites in the United States (Greenberg et al. 1988). The final report of findings has not been released. However, the apparent applicability and desirability of such a plan, as Perrow suggested, may or may not be sufficient to overcome existing organizational commitments and ideological preferences. In health planning, the best idea often turns out to be the politically feasible idea and the one that pleases those who have the authority to decide and to allocate resources.

In planning more effective integration of services and housing for older adults in community set-

tings, care planners are increasingly exploring new types of assisted-living housing (Maddox 1992).

Technological Development

Our national fascination with technology and its implementation could appropriately be directed increasingly toward problems of special relevance to caring for older persons. In the interest of serving older persons more effectively, primary attention might be given to the implementation and specific applications of two existing types of technology. Badly needed are 1) a reliable, valid, economical procedure for identifying the existence and pattern of functional impairment among older persons (Institute of Medicine 1977); and 2) the development of information systems that will facilitate the monitoring and evaluation of the efficiency and effectiveness of alternative systems of care (Breslow 1978; Donabedian 1978; Frazier and Hiat 1978; Maddox 1978, 1985; Maddox and Dellinger 1978). Assessment of the effectiveness and efficiency of care in alternative settings is contingent on the appropriateness of matching level and type of functional impairment with resources intended to maintain or restore function. Adequate procedures for systematic, comprehensive assessment of functioning exist, but these procedures are not widely available or consistently applied. As one might expect in the fragmented, uncoordinated array of services that characterizes the situation in the United States, there is no tradition of single points of entry into the care system that could provide assessment, triage, and monitoring of the outcomes of services. Experiments that include assessment of alternative systematic assessment, triage, and monitoring of older adult populations are clearly feasible and warranted in spite of the discouraging findings of the Channeling Project described earlier. Case coordination is not the sole strategy for producing cost-effective geriatric care.

Although explicit experiments in new forms of comprehensive care delivery for older persons are feasible and warranted, the opportunity to benefit from existing care programs should not be underestimated. Legislated governmental programs of care constitute social experiments from which important information can be derived (Maddox 1985; Maddox and Dellinger 1978; Schoolman and Bernstein 1978; Tancredi and Barondess 1978) if several conditions can be met. The efficiency and effectiveness of any service program can be assessed if 1) the functional status of participants can be measured at several points in time, and 2) the components of service to which participants are exposed can be specified. There is no longer any question that these conditions can be met in reasonably economic ways and in ways that are based on the types of information care programs routinely gather or could gather.

The implications of legislation in 1983 that instituted a diagnosis-related group (DRG) strategy for estimating prospectively the cost of hospitalization for Medicare recipients will be followed with interest. Consciously designed as a cost-containment measure, the DRG strategy has, in fact, since 1983 helped to reduce the average stay in hospitals for older patients by almost 1 day. Shortened hospital stays should increase interest in the greater need for and use of community-based care and in whether total Medicare costs are reduced. The evidence to date is not definitive, but in 1987, use of nonhospital services increased slightly but without evidence that this increase reduced the total Medicare bill.

As a sense of crisis about the cost and effectiveness of care for older persons escalates in the years ahead, experimentation with alternative systems of care will increase. The nation has the resources and the technology to develop an effective and efficient system of care for older persons at a bearable cost. Our capacity to develop an adequate system will hinge on our ability to reorganize the resources already at our disposal. Eisdorfer and colleagues (1989) have provided excellent suggestions for the needed comprehensive reform of health care in the United States with appropriate emphasis on home and community care.

References

Aaron HJ: Serious and Unstable Condition: Financing America's Health Care. Washington, DC, The Brookings Institution, 1991

Alford R: Health Care Politics: Ideological and Interest Group Barriers to Reform. Chicago, IL, University of Chicago Press, 1975

Ball RM: National health insurance: comments on selected issues. Science 200:864–870, 1978

Berdes C: Social Services for the Aged Dying and Bereaved in International Perspective. Washington, DC, International Federation on Aging, 1978

Berger PA: Medical treatment of mental illness. Science 200:974–981, 1978

Blazer D, Maddox G: Developing Geriatric Services in a Community Mental Health Center: A Case History of a University-Based Affiliate Clinic. Durham, NC, Duke University Center for the Study of Aging and Human Development, 1977

Blendon R, Taylor H: Views on health care: public opinion in three countries. Health Aff (Millwood) 8:149–157, 1989

Branch LG, Jette AM: Elders' use of informal long-term care assistance. Gerontologist 23:51–56, 1983

Breslow L: Risk factor intervention for health maintenance. Science 200:908–912, 1978

Chapman CB: Doctors and their autonomy. Science 200:851–855, 1978

Comptroller General of the United States: The Well-Being of Older People in Cleveland, Ohio: A Report to the Congress, April 19, 1977. Washington, DC, U.S. General Accounting Office, 1977a

Comptroller General of the United States: Home Health—The Need for a National Policy to Better Provide for the Elderly. A Report to Congress, December 30, 1977. Washington, DC, U.S. General Accounting Office, 1977b

Culliton BJ: Health care economics: the high cost of getting well. Science 200:883–885, 1978

Davies B: Care Management, Equity and Efficiency: The International Experience. Canterbury, UK, Personal Social Services Research Unit, University of Kent, 1992

Donabedian A: The quality of medical care. Science 200:856–863, 1978

Eisdorfer C, Kessler D, Spector A: Caring for the Elderly: Reshaping Health Policy. Baltimore, MD, Johns Hopkins University Press, 1989

Enthoven AC: Cutting cost without cutting the quality of care. N Engl J Med 298:1229–1238, 1978

Enthoven AC: Health Plan. Reading, MA, Addison-Wesley, 1980

Evans R: Strained Mercy: The Economics of Canadian Health Care. Toronto, Canada, Butterworths, 1985

Fox C: The medicalization and demedicalization of American society, in Doing Better and Feeling Worse: Health in the United States. Edited by Knowles JH. New York, WW Norton, 1977, pp 9–22

Frazier HS, Hiat HH: Evaluation of medical practices. Science 200:875–879, 1978

Garfield SR: The delivery of medical care. Sci Am 222:15–23, 1970

George L, Gwyther L: Caregiver well-being: a multidimensional examination of family caregivers of demented adults. Gerontologist 26:253–259, 1986

Glasscote R: Old Folks at Home: A Field Study of Nursing and Board and Care Homes. Washington, DC, Joint Information Service of the American Psychiatric Association and the National Association of Mental Health, 1976

Glasscote R, Gudeman JE, Miles D: Creative Mental Health Services for the Elderly. Washington, DC, Joint Information Service of the American Psychiatric Association and the Mental Health Association, 1977

Goldman H, Adams N, Taube C: Deinstitutionalization: the data demythologized. Hosp Community Psychiatry 34:129–134, 1983

Greenberg J, Lentz W, Greenlick M, et al: The social HMO demonstration: early experience. Health Aff (Millwood) 7:66–89, 1988

Gronfein W: Incentives and intentions in mental health policy: a comparison of Medicaid and community mental health programs. J Health Soc Behav 26:126–206, 1985

Hahn B, Lefkowitz D: Annual expenses and sources of payment for health care services (AHCPR Publ No 93-0007). National Medical Expenditure Survey Research Findings 14, Agency for Health Care Policy Research. Rockville, MD, Public Health Service, November 1992

Harrington C, Newcomer R, Estes C, et al: Long-Term Care of the Elderly: Policy Issues. Beverly Hills, CA, Sage, 1985

Hawes C, Kane RA, Powers LL, et al: The Case for a Continuum of Long-Term Care Services: Lessons From the Community-Based Care Demonstrations. Washington, DC, AARP Public Policy Institute, November 1988

Hayslip B, Leon J: Hospice Care. Newbury Park, CA, Sage, 1992

Health Policy Analysis Program: Long Term Care for the Elderly in Washington. Seattle, WA, University of Washington, Department of Health Services, 1978

High DM: Advance directives and the elderly: a study of intervention strategies to increase use. Gerontologist 33:342–349, 1993

Hollingsworth R, Hage J, Hanneman R: State Intervention in Medical Care: Consequences for Brit-ain, France, Sweden and the United States, 1890–1970. Ithaca, NY, Cornell University Press, 1990

Hurtado A, Greenlick A, Saward E: Home and Extended Care in a Comprehensive Prepayment Plan. Chicago, IL, Hospital and Research Educational Trust, 1971

Iglehart JK: Second thoughts about HMOs for Medicare patients. N Engl J Med 316:1487–1492, 1987

Ingelfinger FJ: Medicine: meritorious or meretricious? Science 200:942–945, 1978

Institute of Medicine: The Elderly and Functional Dependency. Washington, DC, National Academy of Science, 1977

Institute of Medicine: Disability in America: A National Agenda for Prevention. Washington, DC, National Academy Press, 1991

Kane RL, Kane RA: Care of the aged: old problems in need of new solutions. Science 200:913–918, 1978

Kane RL, Kane RA: A Will and a Way. New York, Columbia University Press, 1985

Kavesh W: Home care, in Annual Review of Gerontology and Geriatrics, Vol 6. Edited by Eisdorfer C. New York, Springer, 1986, pp 135–196

Kemper P, Applebaum R, Harrigan M: Community care demonstrations: what have we learned? Health Care Financing Review 8:87–100, 1987

Knowles JH (ed): Doing Better and Feeling Worse: Health in the United States. New York, WW Norton, 1977

Koren MJ: Home care: who cares? N Engl J Med 314:917–920, 1986

Lamb R: What did we really expect from deinstitutionalization? Hosp Community Psychiatry 32:105–109, 1981

Laurie WF: Employing the Duke OARS methodology in cost comparisons: home services and institutionalization. Duke University Center Reports in Advances in Research 2:2, 1978

Leader S: Home Care Benefits Under Medicare. Washington, DC, Public Policy Institute, American Association of Retired Persons, 1986

Lewis CE, Fein R, Mechanic D: A Right to Health: The Problem of Access to Primary Medical Care. New York, Wiley, 1976

Luft HS: How do health maintenance organizations achieve their "savings"? N Engl J Med 298:1336–1343, 1978

Maddox GL: Muddling through: planning for health care in England. Med Care 9:439–448, 1971

Maddox GL: Interventions and outcomes: notes on designing and implementing an experiment in health care. Int J Epidemiol 1:339–345, 1972

Maddox GL: Families as context and resource in chronic illness, in Long-Term Care: A Handbook for Researchers, Planners, and Providers. Edited by Sherwood S. New York, Spectrum, 1975, pp 317–347

Maddox GL: Community and home care: the unrealized potential of an old idea, in Care of the Elderly: Meeting the Challenge of Dependency. Edited by Exton-Smith AN, Evans JG. New York, Grune & Stratton, 1977, pp 147–160

Maddox GL: Aging, social change and social policy, in Major Social Issues: A Multidisciplinary View. Edited by Yinger M, Mausch H, Cutler S. New York, Free Press, 1978, pp 323–337

Maddox GL: An information system for planning and evaluating geriatric care: the Duke Older Americans Resources and Services Program, in Collecting Evaluation Data: Problems and Solutions. Edited by Bernstein L, Freeman H, Rossi P. Beverly Hills, CA, Sage, 1985, pp 247–262

Maddox GL: Long-term care policies in comparative perspective. Aging and Society 12:355–368, 1992

Maddox GL: Sociology of aging, in Principles of Geriatric Medicine and Gerontology. Edited by Hazzard W, Bierman E, Blass J, et al. New York, McGraw-Hill, 1994, pp 125–134

Maddox GL, Dellinger DC: Assessment of functional status in a program evaluation and resources allocation model. Annals of the American Academy of Political and Social Sciences 438:59–70, 1978

Maddox GL, Karasik R: Planning Services for Older People. Durham, NC, Duke University Center for the Study of Aging and Human Development, 1975

Maddox GL, Lawton MP: Kinship, Aging and Social Change. New York, Springer, 1993

Maddox GL, Wiley J: The scope, concepts, and methods in the study of aging, in Handbook of Aging and the Social Sciences. Edited by Binstock R, Shanas E. New York, Van Nostrand Reinhold, 1977, pp 3–34

McLachlan G: Problems and Progress in Medical Care. Oxford, UK, Oxford University Press, 1971

Medicus Systems Corporation: Evaluation of Day Care and Homemaker Demonstrations: Executive Summary: Report No 36. Chicago, IL, Medicus Systems Corporation, 1977

Meltzer J, Farrow F, Richman H: Policy Options in Long-Term Care. Chicago, IL, University of Chicago Press, 1981

Mor V: Hospice Care Systems: Structure, Process, Cost and Outcome. New York, Springer, 1987

Mor V, Kidder D: Cost savings in hospice: final results of the national hospice study. Health Serv Res 20:407–422, 1985

National Center for Health Statistics: Physical and home management activities. Advancedata 93, 1983

National Center for Health Statistics: Aging in the 1980s: use of community services. Advancedata 124, 1986

National Center for Health Statistics: Nursing and related care homes as reported from the 1986 inventory of long term care places. Advancedata 147, 1988

Palmore E: Total chance of institutionalization. Gerontologist 16:504–507, 1976

Paradis L, Cummings S: The evaluation of hospice in America toward homogeneity. J Health Soc Behav 27:370–386, 1986

Pendleton S, Capitman J, Leutz W, Omata RK. State infrastructure for long term care: a national study of state systems, 1989. Working Paper #4, Waltham, MA, Florence Heller Graduate School, Brandeis University, 1989

Perrow C: Hospitals: technology, structure, goals, in Handbook of Organizations. Edited by March JG. Chicago, Rand-McNally, 1965

Rabin D, Stockton P: Long-Term Care for the Elderly: A Factbook. New York, Oxford University Press, 1987

Raffel M: Comparative Health Systems. University Park, PA, Pennsylvania State University Press, 1985

Rodwin V: The Health Care Planning Predicament. Berkeley, CA, University of California Press, 1984

Rowland D, Lyons B (eds): Financing Home Care. Baltimore, MD, Johns Hopkins University Press, 1991

Ruchlin HS, Morris JN, Gutkin CE, et al: Expenditures for long-term care services by community elders. Health Care Financing Review 10:55–65, 1989

Sager A: Estimating the Cost of Diverting Patients from Nursing Homes to Home Care. Waltham, MA, Levinson Policy Institute, Brandeis University, 1977

Saward E, Sorensen A: The current emphasis on preventive care. Science 200:889–894, 1978

Schoolman HM, Bernstein LM: Computer use in diagnosis, prognosis, and therapy. Science 200: 926–930, 1978

Shanas E, Maddox GL: Aging, health and the organization of health resources, in Handbook of Aging and the Social Sciences. Edited by Binstock R, Shanas E. New York, Van Nostrand Reinhold, 1977, pp 592–618

Smyer MA: Differential usage and differential effects of services for impaired elderly. Duke University Center Reports on Advances in Research 1:4, 1977

Spellman BC, Kemper P: Long term care arrangements for elderly persons with disabilities: private and public roles. Home Health Care Services Quarterly 12(1/2):5–34, 1992

Tancredi LR, Barondess JA: The problem of defensive medicine. Science 200:879–883, 1978

U.S. Department of Health and Human Services: The Evaluation of the National Long-Term Care Demonstration: Final Report. Washington, DC, U.S. Department of Health and Human Services, 1986

U.S. Department of Health, Education and Welfare: Towards a Comprehensive Health Policy for the 1970s. Washington, DC, U.S. Department of Health, Education and Welfare, 1971

U.S. Department of Health, Education and Welfare: Current estimates from the health information survey, United States, 1975. Vital Health Stat 10:115, 1977a

U.S. Department of Health, Education and Welfare: Medicare: utilization of home services, 1974. Health Insurance Statistics, November 2, 1977b

U.S. General Accounting Office: Long-Term Care for the Elderly: Issues of Need, Access, and Cost. Washington, DC, U.S. General Accounting Office, 1988

U.S. Senate Special Committee on Aging: Older Americans: The Alternatives Issue, I and II. Washington, DC, U.S. Government Printing Office, 1977

U.S. Senate Special Committee on Aging: Aging America: Trends and Projections, 1985–86 Edition. Washington, DC, U.S. Department of Health and Human Services, 1985

Vogel RJ, Palmer HC (eds): Long-Term Care: Perspectives from Research and Demonstrations. Washington, DC, Health Care Financing Administration, U.S. Department of Health and Human Services, 1983

Walsh J: Federal health care spending passes the $50-billion mark. Science 200:886–888, 1978

Weiler PG, Rathbone-McCuan E: Adult Day Care: Community Work With the Elderly. New York, Springer, 1978

Weissert WG, Cready CM, Pawelak JE: The past and future of home- and community-based long-term care. Milbank Memorial Fund Quarterly 66:309–388, 1988

White House Domestic Policy Council: The President's Health Security Plan. New York, Times Books, 1993

Wildavsky A: Doing better and feeling worse: the political pathology of health policy, in Doing Better and Feeling Worse: Health in the United States. Edited by Knowles JH. New York, WW Norton, 1977, pp 105–124

CHAPTER 25

The Past and Future of Geriatric Psychiatry

Ewald W. Busse, M.D
Dan G. Blazer, M.D., Ph.D.

The Path That Geriatric Psychiatry Took in the United States

The relatively recent emergence of geriatric psychiatry in the United States is based on two centuries of interest and work by both Americans and non-Americans. Europeans, during the 18th and 19th centuries, greatly influenced American medical and lay leaders. In this review we identify and touch on the contributions of a few such public leaders, as well as behavioral scientists and physicians, whose work has been basic to the development of geriatric psychiatry. Some of these individuals have escaped the notice of modern geriatric psychiatrists, whose attention is understandably more focused on the rapidly expanding science and practice related to aging and the care of the elderly.

Among his many interests and talents, Benjamin Franklin (1706–1790) maintained a strong belief that science would eventually discover the aging process, control it, and be able to rejuvenate people. He ap-

parently was convinced that if the patriarchs of the antediluvian era could achieve extended life spans, so could the human of the future. Franklin's invention of the lightning rod derived from an interest in the power of thunder and lightning, which he thought might influence the resurrection of deceased animals and people. Two other of his inventions have contributed to the well-being of the elderly: the Franklin stove and bifocal eyeglasses (Gruman 1966).

Benjamin Rush (1745–1830), a famous American physician, patron of the American Psychiatric Association, and signer of the Declaration of Independence, wrote extensively and lucidly on a variety of subjects, including old age. In 1805, he published "An Account of the State of the Body and Mind in Old Age: With Observations on Its Diseases and Remedies" (Butterfield 1976).

G. Stanley Hall (1846–1924) was a psychologist who founded one of the first psychology departments in a university in the United States, at Johns Hopkins and, while serving as president of Clark University, was responsible for organizing a conference for which Sigmund Freud was invited to the

United States. Hall is also credited for coining the word *adolescence.* In 1922, he published a book entitled *Senescence: The Last Half of Life.* Hall organized the scattered studies and theoretical speculations concerned with the aging adult and problems of the aged. One of Hall's innovations was the study, by means of a questionnaire, of older people's religious beliefs and fears of death. Hall found that people did not necessarily show an increase in religious interest as they grew older. He also discovered that elderly persons did not become more fearful of death.

Sir William Osler (1849–1919), a distinguished physician of McGill University, the University of Pennsylvania, Johns Hopkins University, and later the University of Oxford, was a contemporary of Hall's. Osler believed that aging was closely related to the state of blood vessels in the body, and maintained that if the brain did change with aging, it was a result of hardening of the arteries.

In the 1930s, increased interest focused on age research. Walter R. Miles and his associates developed the Stanford Greater Maturity Project with the objective of investigating systematically the psychological aspects of aging. Medical research was enhanced by the publication of Edmund B. Cowdry's *Problems of Aging* (1938), which brought together discussions of physical and health-related problems in one volume. Cowdry played a major role in organizing the American Geriatric Society, the Gerontological Society of America, and the International Association of Gerontology. Also in the late 1930s, two important sociologists, Leo Simmons and Ernest W. Burgess, independently published studies on social aspects of aging. In 1945, Simmons published a pioneer study of aging in 70 preliterate societies (Simmons 1945). Ernest Burgess and his associates at the University of Chicago developed instruments to measure personality adjustment in old age. In 1946, the American Psychological Association created the division of later maturity in old age. In the same year, the first issue of the *Journal of Gerontology* was published by the Gerontological Society of America. The first national conference of that society was held in 1950, and was followed by several White House conferences, the last occurring in 1981. Also in 1950, the International Association of Gerontology was organized in Liege, Belgium. This conference has met worldwide, including in San Francisco (1960), Copenhagen (1963), Jerusalem (1975), Tokyo

(1978), New York (1985), Mexico City (1989), and Budapest (1993).

I. L. Nascher, who is frequently considered the father of geriatrics and who is thought to have coined the word *geriatric* with the publication of his text *Geriatrics: The Diseases of Old Age and Their Treatment* (1914), published an article on the aging mind the month before his death in 1944. In this paper, Nascher tabulated the characteristics of chronic brain syndrome and suggested that the condition was a primary change of senescence and that it must have a familial determinant, because he had observed the disease occurring in a mother and a daughter at approximately the same age. He believed that accelerated primary aging was a feature of heredity. Edward J. Stieglitz (1943) edited a publication entitled *Geriatric Medicine: Diagnosis and Management of Disease in the Aging and the Aged.*

In 1969, one of the first American books on aging and psychiatry was published, *Behavior and Adaptation in Late Life,* edited by Ewald W. Busse and Eric Pfeiffer. This book derived in large part from ongoing studies at Duke University of the longitudinal aspects of normal aging. Another longitudinal study of normal aging, the Baltimore Longitudinal Study on Aging, was sponsored by the National Institutes of Health. Before the appearance of the Busse and Pfeiffer book, among the best-known witnesses in the English language about geriatric psychiatry were Felix Post's *The Clinical Psychiatry of Late Life* (1965) and Zinberg and Kaufman's *Normal Psychology of the Aging Process* (1963). Many textbooks have been published on geriatric psychiatry during the last 25 years, and the present edition of Busse and Blazer's *Geriatric Psychiatry* is the third version of a text originally published in 1980 by Van Nostrand Reinhold, *Handbook of Geriatric Psychiatry.* In addition, many specialty texts have appeared on specific aspects of geriatric psychiatry, including Blazer's *Depression in Late Life* (1982a, 1993), Salzman and Lebowitz's *Anxiety in the Elderly* (1991), and a plethora of textbooks on Alzheimer's disease.

The Emergence of Geriatric Psychiatry in Professional Organizations

Authorized by the constitution of the American Psychiatric Association (APA), the APA Council on Aging was established in 1979 to address six areas of activity, including evaluation and diagnosis, training, interface problems between psychiatry and other geriatric care disciplines, design of services and third-party payment for psychiatric disorders in the elderly, decisions made by government that influence the mental health of the aged, and identifying and implementing research into the problems of geriatric psychiatry. The Council on Aging is composed of nine psychiatrists and is responsible for developing and maintaining liaison with the appropriate non-APA organizations involved in the mental health care of aging Americans, with federal agencies similarly involved, and with other APA components so involved. During the past 25 years, three psychiatrists who have a specific career emphasis on geriatric psychiatry have served as president of the APA; they are Ewald W. Busse, M.D., Jack Weinberg, M.D., and George Pollock, M.D., Ph.D.

Psychiatrists have played leading roles in the activities of two major United States societies concerned with aging—the Gerontological Society of America (GSA) and the American Geriatric Society (AGS). The GSA, founded in 1945, is a multidisciplinary organization with four distinct sections: biological sciences, medical sciences, social sciences, and psychological sciences. Three psychiatrists have served as presidents of this organization during the past generation. The AGS, established in 1942, is composed largely of physicians and members of the health care professions. Psychiatrists also have led this medical society, which gives a specific award, the Edward B. Allen Award, for Contributions to Geriatric Psychiatry. The American Association for Geriatric Psychiatry (AAGP) was founded in 1978. Its membership now exceeds 1,500. This association has taken a significant role in the effort to obtain recognition for geriatric psychiatry as a subspecialty and in establishing the certifying exam for this subspecialty.

The Administration on Aging (AOA) has had a significant impact on gerontology in the United States. It was created in 1965 to develop and coordinate research and service programs for the elderly. The AOA was originally a component of the U. S. Department of Health, Education, and Welfare. Its mission was and is in many respects quite different from that of other federal government organizations, such as the National Institutes of Health, for it primarily focuses on service and demonstration

projects. Nevertheless, the AOA has funded important projects relevant to the well-being of older adults and has usually included psychosocial interventions in these demonstration projects. The Older American Resources and Services (OARS) methodology for comprehensive geriatric assessment was developed with AOA funding and has been used in many evaluation clinics that are interdisciplinary and that employ geriatric psychiatrists (OARS 1978).

The Center for the Study of Mental Health of the Aging was established at the National Institute of Mental Health in 1975. In 1977 it received funds to support and coordinate research, research training and clinical training projects. Its original efforts focused primarily on research and clinical training, with long-term support of fellowship stipends for approved geriatric psychiatry training programs. Research training has focused on developing the Geriatric Mental Health Academic Award, which facilitated the establishment of many young geriatric psychiatrists in academic medicine who have now emerged as leaders in geriatric psychiatry. Research programs funded by the Center have included individual-initiated research grants (RO1s), research training grants (career development awards and FIRST awards), and clinical research center support. Centers at Duke University, the University of Rochester, Cornell University, Stanford University, the University of California at San Diego, and the University of Pennsylvania focus on a spectrum of psychiatric disorders afflicting older persons, including Alzheimer's disease, late-life depression, late-life schizophrenic disorders, and general neuropsychiatric disorders.

The National Institute on Aging (NIA) was established in May 1974 as part of the National Institutes of Health. The first director of the NIA was a psychiatrist, Robert N. Butler, M.D. The establishment of the NIA represents the culmination of 20 years of effort to gain government recognition and support for research on aging. Enabling legislation was passed designating the NIA as the chief federal agency responsible for promoting, coordinating, and supporting basic research and training relevant to the aging process and to the diseases and problems of the elderly. A unique aspect of the NIA's mandate was that it was to be the first component of the National Institutes of Health to be formally charged by Congress with conducting research in the biological, biomedical, behavioral, and social sciences. This broad mandate has resulted in activities that are different from those of other national research institutes. Since 1974, NIA basic research funding has increased tenfold, and many psychiatric investigators have been funded through this agency.

For many years, medical and health care education related to geriatrics received little attention. The first training program in geriatric psychiatry supported by the National Institute of Mental Health (NIMH) was established at Duke University Medical Center in 1965; this was the only such program for almost a decade. There are now a rapidly increasing number of geriatric psychiatry fellowship programs, though few of these currently receive NIMH support. These programs have been funded primarily through the Veterans Administration, state support, and support from individual medical centers. The establishment of these training programs and lobbying by groups (including the AAGP) convinced the American Board of Psychiatry and Neurology to establish an examination for added qualifications in geriatric psychiatry. The first examination was given in 1991; more than 800 persons sat for the exam and more than 500 passed it.

Geriatric Psychiatry: Present and Future

For the past several decades, psychiatry has experienced what has been called by many an "identity crisis." It is a crisis in identity that centers on the questions of what sphere of professional activity is the proper task of psychiatrists and of whether this activity provides a source of self-esteem for psychiatrists as well as unique and quality care for persons with psychiatric disorders (Busse 1972; Detre 1987). The geriatric psychiatrist, in relationship to the general psychiatrist, to the generalist physician, and to the geriatrician, has made a significant and unique contribution to resolving this so-called identity crisis. Paradoxically, the current emphasis on primary care has challenged the viability of all medical specialties during the past few years. Nevertheless, geriatric psychiatry has established itself solidly on a foundation of knowledge and skill in caring for older persons with psychiatric disorders, using the most advanced technologies and clinically proven

therapies. In most settings, the geriatric psychiatrist has established a unique and meaningful role on interdisciplinary teams caring for older adults.

The geriatric psychiatrist assumes in many ways the role of a primary care physician. He or she not only must maintain a proficiency in general medicine but also must apply the special knowledge of epidemiology as well as behavioral and social factors to patient care. For example, geriatric psychiatrists have no alternative but to recognize that many of the disorders that they treat cannot be cured or prevented, but the resultant suffering can be relieved and the disability reduced. Recognizing this fact may not in itself be inherently rewarding; however, such recognition does encourage the clinician to make observations that can contribute to a better understanding of the course of chronic illness and can also motivate investigations that may, in the future, lead to improved convalescence or even eradication of such disorders when they are recognized earlier in their course. Recent advances in the understanding of the molecular basis of Alzheimer's disease is a primary example of where such breakthroughs may occur.

To achieve the goal of effective care of the chronically ill older adult with psychiatric problems, geriatric psychiatrists must broaden their skills to include proficiency in geriatric medicine, neurology, and the neurosciences as well as focus their skills on advances in geriatric psychiatry. The proficient geriatrician and geriatric psychiatrist must be aware of aging changes that affect the human organism's capacity to respond to stress, disease, and trauma, and that eventually may result in death (Busse and Blazer 1980). Specific procedures, such as the treatment of urinary tract infection, moderate hypertension, and peripheral edema, should not require the geriatric psychiatrist to consult an internist or geriatrician for appropriate management. Although the role of the geriatric psychiatrist may be such that specialty consultation is frequent and combined management of the patient is effected by a geriatrician and geriatric psychiatrist (such as in a tertiary-care center), the skill of the geriatric psychiatrist should be of a proficiency such that, in the absence of the geriatrician, he or she can administer adequate medical care. As care moves increasingly from inpatient to ambulatory settings, the independent skills of the geriatric psychiatrist will be required even more.

At the same time, significant advances in the epidemiology, pathophysiology, diagnosis, and treatment of the most frequently encountered psychiatric disorders in late life will emerge. These disorders span at least the range described in this volume, although even a "short list" must include the dementias, the mood disorders, the anxiety disorders, the schizophrenic/light disorders, the sleep disorders, and the psychological and social factors affecting physical conditions. Advances in the neuroscience and clinical management of dementia of the Alzheimer's type alone illustrate the substantial knowledge base on which geriatric psychiatry is practiced. Previous trends have been such that when a biological etiology has been identified for a behavioral disorder, that disorder is passed from psychiatry to another specialty, usually neurology. Surely this cannot be tolerated in the future by geriatric psychiatrists. For example, geriatric psychiatrists must maintain a central role in the clinical management of the patient with dementia, especially because such a patient's primary problems are usually behavioral. To do so, however, the skills of the psychiatrist must be such that they are not overshadowed by those of the neurologist and the geriatrician.

Geriatric psychiatry may face special problems in the future regarding referrals. Managed care systems discourage referrals, and geriatric psychiatry must help identify for the primary care physician those cases in which the unique skills of the geriatric psychiatrist can contribute to cost-effective care of the older adult. Although geriatric psychiatry is a broad-based specialty, in practice it is rarely the recipient of primary referrals. Patients do not usually consider the psychiatrist as the coordinator or the provider of general medical care. The geriatric psychiatrist has special skills in the management of behavioral disorders resulting from dementing illness, the management of acute schizophrenia-like disorders, the more severe mood disorders, severe anxiety and panic disorders, complex personality and behavioral disturbances that interfere with appropriate medical management, and severe problems with sleep. Appropriate referral by the primary care physician to the geriatric psychiatrist, especially if initial therapy by the primary care physician proves ineffective, can be both cost-effective and a means of providing relief of considerable suffering in the psychiatrically impaired older adult.

Therefore, geriatric psychiatrists in the 1990s find themselves in a paradoxical situation. On the one hand, geriatric psychiatrists are better trained, and their training rests on a firmer knowledge base, than at any time in the past. Of more importance, advances in our understanding of the diagnosis and treatment of psychiatric disorders in late life have led to significantly improved and cost-effective therapies for psychiatrically disturbed older adults. On the other hand, specialty care, in particular psychiatric care, could well be a big "loser" in the battle for scarce resources for health care. Administrators of fellowship programs in geriatric medicine as well as psychiatry are finding that recruitment to these programs has been more difficult in recent years. Although training has never been better, and the original hesitation by many young physicians to treat older persons because of preconceived prejudices about aging has been largely overcome, the uncertain future of medical specialties and difficulties in reimbursing care for older persons render geriatric medicine and geriatric psychiatry less desirable financially than procedure-driven medical specialties and primary care.

Financing Psychiatric Care for Older Adults

The future of health care financing, much less the financing of psychiatric care, is uncertain at the writing of this chapter. Since the submission of President Clinton's Health Security Act in 1993, many competing proposals—ranging from single payor to basically "keep things as they are"—have emerged from Congress. The future of financing psychiatric care for older adults, however, is more predictable.

The federal government has shaped the financing of psychiatric care for older adults since the mid-1960s, with the transfer of financial responsibility from state and private insurance to Medicare and Medicaid. Medicare has tended to lead (rather than follow) health care financing reform in this country since that time. For example, the capitation of payments for certain illnesses via diagnosis-related groups (DRGs) was instituted in 1983 (although DRGs have yet to be applied to inpatient psychiatric disorders). The Omnibus Budget Reconciliation Act (OBRA) of 1987 increased coverage for outpatient psychiatric services from a total annual reimbursement of $500, with a 62.5% reimbursement of charges, to $2,200 annually for 1989. A 50% copayment remains, however. Services for the medical management of psychiatric disorders were exempted from this $2,200 limit. The OBRA Act of 1989 further improved outpatient psychiatric benefits. Effective July 1, 1990, annual dollar limits for outpatient mental health services were eliminated. Nevertheless, a 50% co-payment remains.

Inpatient services have not been capitated in terms of reimbursement for individual hospitalizations, yet a 190-day lifetime psychiatric hospitalization limit remains in effect. This limit applies to free-standing psychiatric hospitals, not to psychiatric units in general hospitals. The maximum number of days covered for a single hospitalization is 150 (though an older adult can be discharged and readmitted for the same spell).

Although Medicare benefits for psychiatric illness are far from ideal and physician payments are much lower than payments for persons currently under private insurance, private insurance reimbursement for inpatient hospitalization and outpatient care are more likely to approach current Medicare reimbursements than vice versa. Given that the Medicare system is in place, most health care economists believe that Medicare will remain relatively untouched under whatever form of health care reform emerges. Under the Clinton proposal, Medicare was to remain intact except for cost reductions.

Two additional providers of care directly impact the delivery of health services to psychiatrically impaired older adults. First, the Veterans Administration (VA) provides care for many older adults, primarily (but not exclusively) for men. The VA currently supports the most comprehensive system of care for mentally impaired older adults, including acute inpatient hospitalization, outpatient clinics, long-term care facilities, and domiciliary care. Most experts believe that the VA—because of its strong political influence in Washington—will remain relatively intact under health care reform. Blurring of the boundaries between the VA and Medicare reimbursement for mental health services may occur, however, as length of stay decreases and outpatient care replaces inpatient care. Given that the VA has an extensive network of hospitals, these hospitals could be used for a broader constituency, with reimbursements from other health plans.

A second important sector of the health delivery system to psychiatrically impaired elders is long-term care. Support for long-term care in existing health plans is limited. Therefore, many older adults must use their life savings to support long-term care until the savings are dissipated, at which time the older person becomes eligible for Medicaid support. Medicare supports long-term care only for rehabilitation and only for 120 days.

The Medicaid system reimburses about 42% of all nursing home care for older adults. The development of humane and effective treatment facilities for persons with chronic psychiatric disorders, especially persons with Alzheimer's disease and chronic schizophrenia, will depend in large part on the availability of funds to support long-term care. Although some older persons are purchasing long-term care insurance, the ability to actuate the needs of long-term care over the lifetimes of a cohort of older adults, coupled with the relatively short life of these insurance programs to date, does not ensure that long-term care will be adequately financed in the future.

Geriatric Psychiatrists and Public Health

There is an ever-increasing number of older persons in North America, and resources are limited for the psychiatric care of these elders. Therefore, geriatric psychiatrists of the future must understand the prevalence and distribution of psychiatric disorders in the population and the delivery of psychiatric services to these older adults in order to advocate for humane and cost-effective mental health care for older adults. Most older adults with psychiatric disorders do not receive any care for these conditions. Of those who do receive care, most of it is provided by primary care physicians (German et al. 1985).

In planning for more effective and efficient delivery of psychiatric services to older adults, the geriatric psychiatrist must consider interventions at one of three points in the natural course of a disorder. These points correspond to the three classic types of prevention described by public health specialists—that is, primary, secondary, and tertiary prevention (Last 1980). Primary prevention is preventing the occurrence of disease or injury. Secondary prevention is early detection and intervention.

Tertiary prevention minimizes the effects of disease and disability.

The geriatric psychiatrist can effect primary prevention by identifying potential stressful events and elements in the environment of the older adult, both social and physical, that contribute to the onset of a psychiatric disorder. For example, forced isolation and the absence of effective communication with other persons contribute to the onset of major depression and paranoid psychoses. Intervention would encourage social interaction. The appropriate use of psychotropic medications may prevent the occurrence of acute organic brain syndromes in an older adult who is bereaved. This intervention would focus on education. Early supportive intervention has been demonstrated to prevent the onset of major depression in the bereaved.

Secondary prevention requires the geriatric psychiatrist to intervene early enough in the course of an illness to facilitate the prescription of effective treatment to prevent a complicated convalescence. It is at this level that the geriatric psychiatrist may achieve the greatest success, given the limited resources available. For example, early diagnosis of major depression permits the psychiatrist to attempt a rational course of outpatient antidepressant therapy, before the complication of excess medication or neglect of physical health that may ensue during the course of a depressive illness.

Tertiary prevention is directed toward preventing the disability that may result from mental illness. Rehabilitation techniques are important in long-term care facilities, especially in the management of the patient with dementia. These techniques include reality orientation, adequate hygiene efforts, and maintenance of mobility. Although the activities themselves may not be the direct responsibility of the geriatric psychiatrist, development of a comprehensive treatment and rehabilitation plan must involve the geriatric psychiatrist.

Geriatric Psychiatry and Successful Aging

Physicians have traditionally focused on illness, and the success of the practice of medicine, including psychiatry, has been determined by the removal of illness or disability. An interest in successful aging, however, has assumed center stage in gerontological circles during the past 10–15 years (although the idea has implicitly undergirded gerontological research since its inception). The construct arose primarily as a response to a perceived need to view aging as something other than loss, decline of functioning, and approaching death. In addition, physicians working with older adults have been faulted for not looking beyond the absence of disease as a marker for health (Baltes and Baltes 1990). Criteria that have been suggested as markers of successful aging include length of life, biological health, life satisfaction and morale, cognitive efficacy, social competence and productivity, personal control, and resiliency and adaptivity (Baltes and Baltes 1990; Nowlin 1977, 1985; Palmore 1979; Rowe and Kahn 1987). Rowe and Kahn (1987) emphasized the need to explore the extent to which extrinsic factors can play positive as well as negative roles in the aging process. For example, they note studies of social support that demonstrate that the availability of perceived connectedness and membership in a network of family and friends decreases the likelihood of illness and mortality (Berkman and Syme 1979; Blazer 1982b). Rodin (1986) emphasized the positive effects on health and well-being of older adults who were involved in and asserted more control over their environments compared with persons who assumed a passive role.

Another theme that has traversed studies of successful aging is that of resiliency and adaptation. For example, Busse (1985b) equated successful aging in part to the capacity to respond with resilience to challenges arising from changes within one's body, mind, and the environment. A central task for older adults is to adopt effective strategies for dealing with losses and to be able to change goals and aspirations given either physical or psychosocial changes.

Baltes (1993) emphasized the importance of wisdom in successful aging, something that cannot be measured quantitatively. For example, he suggests that wisdom includes factual knowledge (requiring the data necessary to respond to a situation); procedural knowledge (strategies of acquiring data, making decisions, and providing advice); life-span contextualization (recognizing the inner relations, tensions, and priorities of different life domains within the context of the life span); value relativism (ability to separate one's own values from those of others); and acceptance of uncertainty (recognizing that there is no perfect solution and optimizing the resolution of a situation as well as possible). Wisdom falls generally within in the domain of *cognitive pragmatics,* which is primarily culture based and therefore potentially stable over time in persons who reach old age without specific brain pathology. In contrast, *cognitive mechanics* is roughly comparable to fluid intelligence and is primarily determined by neurophysiological function of the brain.

Not all commentators have accepted the construct of successful aging. Cole (1991) noted that this change in perspective regarding late life may be secondary to the dramatic increase in the proportion of the adult population over age 65. Specifically, as more people have aged, it is less acceptable to view aging as a time of frailty, poor health, and death. He points out that questions regarding the quality of life of the oldest old (persons age 85+) remain at the center of the health care debate regarding ordinary versus extraordinary life-extending therapies and even health care monitoring. He suggests that our society does not apply the construct of "success" to other stages of the life cycle, and that the natural consequence of the construct of successful aging is the assumption that growing old presents a problem that must be solved "successfully." Aging continues to present many problems, not the least of which are the finitude of life, preservation of personal integrity, and quality of life. Yet Cole believes our culture has distanced itself from these troubling issues, in part through its emphasis on successful aging.

It is far from clear, however, that conflict is inevitable between the themes of successful aging and the care of the frail elderly. For example, emphasis on successful aging has decreased fatalism regarding health and health habits in late life. Through diet, exercise, and strengthening (especially of the lower extremities), older persons can improve their balance, decrease their risk of falling, and improve their quality of life. On the other hand, when illness does occur that is chronic and about which outcomes are better known, there is no reason that health care professionals cannot realistically and seriously address the proper and realistic, not to mention the humane, care of these persons.

Ethical and Legal Issues

In recent years, medical ethics and legal issues associated with medical science and practice have received increased attention from media commen-

tators, religious and human rights organizations, the legal profession, and the government. The medical profession not only has responded to such pressure but has also attempted to foresee the emergence of new ethical problems and to develop applicable guidelines.

The reasons for this increased activity cannot be attributed to the existence of major defects within the generally accepted code of medical ethics, but rather are the result of rapid changes in social values and major advances in science and technology, including the extension of the length of life and the recognition that resources are limited. History clearly demonstrates that professional ethics are constantly evolving. How and why such changes or shifts occur should be understood by geriatric psychiatrists, their patients, and the public (Conold 1977; King 1982).

Accepted principles of ethical conduct or good behavior are not homogeneous throughout the world. There are a limited number of universal norms, such as the incest taboo; instead, heterogeneity of ethical principles is the rule. Ethical issues that commonly occur in the practice of geriatric psychiatry are not necessarily confined to this age group. However, elderly mentally ill patients are likely to be different from younger adult patients, and the application of ethical principles may therefore vary. A 75-year-old person is likely to have three to six chronic diseases and physical disabilities that impair, to varying degrees, work and other activities. In addition, the social and economic situation for the elderly may not be as favorable as that for younger persons. The adverse circumstances of late life make certain ethical issues more complex.

Some ethical issues in geriatric psychiatry and child psychiatry are similar but reversed. Dependency on another individual for protection, support, and survival is a shared condition of children and the frail elderly. But there is a substantial difference. The child is moving toward greater independence, whereas the frail elderly person will become increasingly dependent on others. Decisions regarding long-term care are influenced by this difference.

Ethical and legal issues that are particularly relevant to geriatric psychiatry include informed consent and the patient's "right to know"; competency and the appointment of a guardian or some alternative; and advance directives, such as the living will and its association with withdrawal of life-support systems. Physician-assisted suicide falls under the latter category.

Informed Consent and the Right to Know

The concept of informed consent implies a highly rational process (Busse 1985a). It requires that the source and the content of the communication be clear and complete and that the patient be an intelligent, rather stable individual capable of questioning any point requiring clarification. Unfortunately, the geriatric psychiatrist recognizes that an elderly individual who is beginning to show signs of brain deterioration may actually fluctuate in his or her ability to understand and communicate. Consequently, the geropsychiatrist must double-check questionable patients. Another alternative is to have present an advocate for the patient. Informed consent and the concept of the patient's right to know are almost synonymous. The right to know is inherent in consent. Furthermore, mental competence is a required condition for informed consent. Decisions that are made by a so-called normal person as well as decisions made by a "sick" person are influenced by a number of interacting determinants. These include intelligence, both inherent and acquired (education); response to situation stress; biologic defects, particularly of the central nervous system or perhaps perceptual changes; current emotional status; personal and social values; loyalties and religious convictions; legal constraints and consequences; and socioeconomic and environmental factors (Busse 1985a).

Intelligent elderly patients with impaired perception can make faulty interpretations of information provided to them because of their failure to hear or see properly. Some elderly persons do not admit to defects; consequently, such patients should have provided to them not only verbal information, but also written statements and illustrated material. When perceptual difficulties are evident, a valuable person is a family member who, through experience, knows when to assist the patient.

There are individuals who are limited in capacity to deal with informed consent but who are legally competent. The autonomy of the individual, which is central to informed consent, is a status that is not always welcomed by the patient. There are patients who prefer that the physician maintain a paternalistic attitude—that is, they believe the physician will make the correct decision. Similarly, there are professionals and lay persons who believe that a patient who has detailed, accurate knowledge of his or her disease may experience considerable stress and suffering because of this knowledge. Therefore, they believe that providing such extensive, accurate knowledge is not actually in the best interest of the patient.

There are times when a patient is not able to fully participate in the process of informed consent because he or she lacks the necessary ability to understand complex medical problems. The question then arises as to the obligation of the physician either to take the time to educate the person to a level of complete understanding or to present the complex situation in a simplified manner that expedites the patient's decision. The first approach can be time-consuming, whereas the second contains a strong element of paternalism. The term *fiduciary* describes an important relationship between the patient and the physician, the lawyer and the client, or the clergy member and the parishioner. A fiduciary relationship is based on confidence and trust. A fiduciary is a person who stands in a special relationship of trust, confidence, or responsibility in her or his obligation to another person or persons, and this relationship is the essence of informed consent (Dyer 1982).

Informed consent, which was originally an ethical concept, is becoming an important and changing legal issue. Gutheil (1987) reported that in a 10-year study performed at the Risk Management Foundation, out of 1,200 cases, only 159 had an informed-consent component. However, this component will become an increasingly important forensic problem. For example, *hindsight allegation* can result from the patient's actually experiencing the harm and bad outcome and then claiming in retrospect that he or she was not adequately informed.

The failure to provide informed consent has been recognized by the courts as a complex information process focusing on the medical matters under question. The courts have recognized that there are difficulties in communication of scientific information by the trained physician to the untrained patient and almost limitless risk in any proposed treatments. Consequently, the legal position has been that what the patient has a right to know must be harmonized with the patient's recognition that an undue burden should not be placed on the physician. However, the physician owes to the patient the duty to disclose any reasonable matter or significant medical information that the physician possesses or reasonably should possess that is material to an intelligent decision by the patient of whether to undergo a proposed procedure. Furthermore, the legal stance has been that an informed physician should possess that knowledge which is held by the average qualified physician or, in the case of specialty care, by the average qualified physician specialist. The court standard, therefore, has been a peer-group comparison and not a patient-centered standard.

Furthermore, the courts now have decided that the physician must provide medical information that is "material to the intelligent decision by the patient" (Gutheil 1987, p. 5). The physician is expected to know, or "should know," of the patient's position in regard to the disclosed risk or risks that are associated with the decision to submit or not to submit to surgery or treatment. This new court interpretation emphasizes the importance of a physician's empathic judgments.

Although not yet explicitly recognized by the courts, it is evident that the ability of a "reasonable" person to make a complicated decision is influenced by numerous personal attitudes, values, and experiences. Many such influences may be essentially unknown (that is, they may reside in the unconscious of the patient) and may not be apparent to the physician. These new legal developments emphasize the importance for the geriatric psychiatrist to include in his or her clinical records an adequate summary of the process of informed consent, reviewing the medical information that has been given to the patient and the patient's reaction to this information, and documenting particularly pertinent questions and responses.

Competency

The terms *incompetent* and *competent,* as legally used in the United States, do not necessarily represent extreme or opposing points along a continuum. A competent individual has the quality or condition that makes him or her capable of participating in certain legally recognized activities. In addition, a competent person is responsible for his or her own acts. A person is considered competent until declared incompetent. Incompetence is a term used to denote the lack of capacity to legally consent or to make a contract.

In addition there are specific areas in which a person can be declared incompetent. A person may be unable to give informed consent, to have testamentary capacity (that is, to execute a last will and testament), or to be held responsible for certain illegal acts. If an individual is considered incompetent in one area, it does not necessarily make that person incompetent in other areas. Competence is not an all-or-nothing mental condition and may be limited and/or intermittent. Competence is usually an accepted condition in which it appears that an individual has the capacity to cope with common events of everyday life. Unfortunately, the degree of competence is subject to variation when the individual is faced with a new, acute situation that requires a solution. Alzheimer's disease, for example, is held to be a condition characterized by a steady deterioration, devoid of periods of plateau or actual periods of restoration. Nevertheless, longitudinal studies suggest that in many individuals there are episodes of organic mental impairment—that is, an exacerbation and remission. Consequently, there are fluctuations in the mental competence of such patients. Observers at different times may justifiably reach opposing conclusions.

Geriatric psychiatrists should be thoroughly acquainted with the laws of the state in which they practice. In many states an incompetent adult or child is one who lacks mental capacity to manage himself or herself and his or her own affairs, or who lacks sufficient capacity to make or communicate important decisions concerning persons, family, or property. De facto competence is based on a person's understanding of what is being proposed—medical treatment, hospitalization, and so on. Psychiatrists are asked to give their opinions about patients' de facto competence as a prelude to formal legal review. De facto competence differs distinctly from de jure competence, which is competence due to a status under the law—that is, the person has not been declared legally incompetent and therefore is presumed to be competent for a variety of purposes, unless the person has been found to be legally incompetent for a specific purpose. By definition of the law, de jure competence is not given to children or adolescents because they are considered incompetent up to specified ages. Consequently, because of age alone, under certain circumstances, they are unable to perform certain activities, such as purchase alcoholic beverages.

It is sometimes necessary for the geriatric psychiatrist to become involved in legal procedures to determine the status of competency; in such procedures, if the person is declared incompetent, the court appoints a guardian. Guardians may be divided into several classes: a guardian of the estate, a guardian of the person, or a guardian of both the estate and the person. Guardianship ad litem permits a person appointed by the court to represent another person who lacks capacity in a particular procedure or for a particular purpose. All states have laws that allow a guardian to be appointed if a person is no longer able to manage his or her own affairs. This usually becomes obvious when he or she is unable to handle property or financial affairs. The laws in most states require that a concerned individual file for a procedure to be carried out that establishes guardianship. This procedure usually involves a hearing of some sort. Some states require that a patient be examined by professionals before the court hearing. These professionals are often assigned by the court. Unfortunately, hearings can be embarrassing, particularly if the mentally impaired individual does not want to have a guardian. Although the procedure varies from state to state, often the judge or presiding legal authority will recognize that the hearing can be a traumatic procedure and will structure the hearing to reduce the trauma to the individual and to the family or interested parties.

A person who has been declared incompetent can be assigned to a hospital or a facility as a voluntary patient with written approval from the person's guardian. Nevertheless, as described above, determination of guardianship is frequently a complicated matter. A preferred solution is a power of attorney. Power of attorney must be given freely, and the person giving it must be competent at the time. A power of attorney limits the authority that it sets forth in the document. In most states, power of attorney given by a competent person immediately becomes nonfunctional when the person becomes incompetent. All types of power of attorney are revocable. If an older person is at risk for becoming mentally incapacitated in the future, it is desirable to set up what is referred to as a *durable power of attorney.*

At times, protective services are required for older adults because a guardian has not been iden-

tified. In such cases, a *conservatorship* denotes the condition in which the court provides control over a person's property or person in place of a guardian.

Advance Directives, Living Wills, and Life Support

A penultimate, or "living," will has been declared a legal instrument or procedure in many states. A living will is a written document prepared and signed by a person while mentally competent. A living will specifies the circumstances under which a person will permit the cessation of extraordinary treatment to prolong life and allow death to occur in accordance with the natural progression of a person's disease. A penultimate will can include instructions that, in the event that the individual becomes mentally incompetent, he or she is willing to participate in research activity that has little or no likelihood of personal therapeutic benefit but would add to the understanding of the disease process and may benefit the lives of others. A written living will is an important component of the medical record, particularly for those who are terminally ill. It must be properly signed and in conformity with state laws. The existence of such a document not only is of great comfort to the patient, but it permits the physician to behave in accordance with the desires of the patient and considerably reduces the burden and emotional conflict for the nursing and supporting staff of a facility and for the patient's loved ones.

A variant of the living will, and a required procedure on admission to the hospital, is the *advance medical directive.* In the wake of the U.S. Supreme Court's decision in *Cruzan v. the State of Missouri Department of Health,* the U.S. Congress, in 1991, decided to reinforce the right of an individual to refuse any and all medical interventions, including life-sustaining measures. It was decreed in the Patient Self-Determination Act (1991) that all hospitals, nursing facilities, hospital programs, and health maintenance organizations that serve Medicare and Medicaid patients must provide each of their adult patients with written information of their right to make decisions about their medical care. This information must be consistent with state laws, and patients should be aware that they have a right to execute a living will or a durable power of attorney.

These advance directives, however, were accompanied by numerous complications. Often, a living will is not sufficiently specific for a physician or health care surrogate to make a firm decision. Changes that followed the initial act included the development of the health care durable (persisting when incompetent or incapacitated) power of attorney and the addendum called the *medical directive.* The medical directive is composed of a list of specific procedures and what should or should not be implemented should the situation arise. Examples are cardiopulmonary resuscitation (CPR), mechanical breathing, artificial nutrition, artificial hydration, and so forth. The importance of having these specific topics is reflected in the number of publications that have emerged since that time. For patients to make an informed decision, education is required; specifically, patients must understand their chances of survival after certain interventions. If they do survive an intervention, what is the length of life expectation and the quality of life under those circumstances? Even so, the use of advance directives by older persons remains relatively low. Education does not appear to increase significantly the use of these directives. The most common reasons for nonuse are more complicated than the lack of information or the lack of encouragement from health professionals. There is a significant difference between people *saying* that they are interested in and support, or even in their saying that they want, advance directives to be implemented and their *willingness to sign a legal document* specifying which procedures will be implemented in their own care. They do not go through the relatively easy steps of carrying it out. It appears that elderly people often defer action because they believe that their present status does not urgently call for advance directives. In addition, some assume that if their status changes abruptly, decisions can be made by family members. Among some older persons, there is concern that the living will or advance directive could be misused and that a commitment made today could be altered by medical advances tomorrow.

There have been numerous discussions regarding the motivation on the part of the individual to make advance directives. There is the recurring question, Is the individual interested in avoiding pain and prolonged discomfort? Is the directive altruistic, in a sense that it helps other individuals and reduces the cost of caring for a person who is terminally ill or in a vegetative state? The altruistic factor is critical, because it indicates the patient's willingness to sacrifice in order to reduce stress and financial cost to others.

Studies have been carried out to determine how the do-not-resuscitate (DNR) order is used and how such orders affect the cost of caring for patients who die during a hospital stay. In one such study, Baksoud et al. (1993) found that all patients who had died with DNR orders had a mean total charge of $57,334. However, those patients who had the order written during hospitalization had a much higher mean charge ($70,193) than did those who were admitted with a DNR order ($10,631). Unfortunately, this study does not specify the preexisting conditions, and it does not clarify whether those with preadmission DNR orders were patients with previous admissions and greater knowledge of their poor prognosis. It is noted that those patients who died without ever having issued a DNR order had lower hospitalization costs than those who died after a DNR order was written.

It may be an illusion that wider use of advance directives will substantially reduce costs. In a recent study, Emmanuel and Emmanuel (1994) observed that focusing on Medicare expenditures distorts the costs of dying. Further, they observed that if all Americans refused aggressive inpatient intervention or chose hospice care, the total savings on all health care spending would be 3.3%, whereas the savings would be 6.1% of Medicare expenditures. The situation is further complicated by the lack of predictability in the dying process, changing medical practices (particularly when many dying patients do not have resuscitation orders), and the lack of "empirical evidence indicating that the patients are receiving more treatment than desired" (p. 540). Nevertheless, the practicing physician is still confronted with the decision of when to withhold life-sustaining efforts.

A 1992 report suggested that the cost of treating patients with life-threatening diseases who have advance directives as compared with a control group of patients without advance directives shows no significant positive or negative effect of such directives. Included in this evaluation of possible differences were medical treatments, charges, and other variables such as cognitive functioning, patient satisfaction, and quality of life (Schneiderman et al. 1992).

A decision regarding the withholding of life-sustaining efforts should follow certain guidelines:

1) the patient should not have a temporary but treatable psychiatric disorder that is influencing the decision; 2) the decision should be carefully considered and should not be impulsive—a reasonable amount of time for consideration should be insisted on before a decision; 3) there should be no undue influence by faculty or heirs, particularly those who would financially benefit from the patient's death; 4) the patient must understand the risks and benefits that relate to withholding continuing care and treatment; 5) in certain unusual situations, a patient should be kept alive to allow for a full assessment and a resolution of certain problems, especially legal ones. Some degree of irrationality is normal.

It should be kept in mind that the surrogate who is chosen by the patient may have considerable difficulty in making a decision, given that the surrogate must try to integrate the values of the patient into his or her own value system. Further, on occasion, the surrogate may be incompetent. Unfortunately, there is no clear procedure for coping with incompetent surrogates, and legal consultation is certainly justified. However, under these circumstances, it appears preferable to keep the patient alive pending a judicial determination.

Euthanasia and Assisted Suicide

According to *Merriam-Webster's Collegiate Dictionary* (1994), euthanasia is

> the act or practice of killing or permitting the death of hopelessly sick or injured individuals . . . in a relatively painless way for reasons of mercy. (p. 347)

In *Stedman's Medical Dictionary* (1990), it is defined as

> a quiet, painless death; the intentional putting to death of a person with an incurable or painful disease. (p. 544)

These two definitions do not clarify the involvement of the patient in the decision process. Twenty years ago, an intense discussion developed in the Netherlands because of a case in which a doctor administered, at the patient's request, a lethal dose of medication to a woman suffering from a terminal disease. Subsequently it was found that euthanasia is widely practiced in cases of terminal illnesses in

the Netherlands. In many instances, it appears that the practice was better referred to as *assisted suicide* rather than as "euthanasia request by medically ill patients" (Huyse and van Tilburg 1993, p. 733). After a long discussion in January 1990, the minister of justice of the Netherlands established a committee to assess the extent of euthanasia practice in the Netherlands and the circumstances surrounding such practice. The definition of euthanasia was "the intentional termination of life by someone other than the person concerned at that person's request by means of prescription, supply, or administration of drugs" (Huyse and van Tilburg 1993, p. 733). Reliable data at that time were lacking. In late 1990, it was estimated that euthanasia accounted for 1.8% of all deaths in the Netherlands. Of the 2,300 cases of euthanasia, 1,500 were carried out by general practitioners outside of hospitals. Physician-assisted suicide was reported in another 400 cases. Patients with cancer accounted for the majority of those involved in euthanasia, and age was the second most common associated factor. In 1990, guidelines were formulated to guide doctors who perform euthanasia at the request of physically ill patients. A report must be submitted that includes four parts: three parts involved with questions concerning the patient and the fourth part addressing how the euthanasia was performed. Attitudes and the recordings of euthanasia are obviously influenced by legal proceedings and by cultural and individual values. This is another important consideration when one is comparing definitions and implementations in one nation with those in another.

In recent years in the United States, the role of Dr. Jack Kevorkian in assisted suicide has resulted in considerable debate and differences of opinion among members of the public, and within the government, the judicial system, and the medical profession. At present, the Ethics Committee of the American Psychiatric Association concurs with the position of the American Medical Association: that it is inappropriate for physicians to participate in execution or any other procedures that would purposely cause the death of a patient. Further, "physician-assisted suicide, like euthanasia, is contrary to the traditional prohibition against using the tools of medicine to cause a patient's death" (American Medical Association 1991, p. 60).

The complexity of the debate is evident. Geriatric psychiatrists are and will be involved. The issues must be clarified and attention must be given to the moral dilemma of "how best to permit parties to honor their own values without coercing unwilling others" (Haavi Morreim 1994, p. 34).

References

American Medical Association: Code of Medical Ethics. Chicago, IL, American Medical Association, 1991

Baksoud A, Jahnigen D, Skibinski C: Do-not-resuscitate orders and the cost of death. Arch Intern Med 153:1249–1253, 1993

Baltes PB: The aging mind: potential and limits. Gerontologist 33:580–594, 1993

Baltes PB, Baltes MM: Successful Aging: Perspectives From the Behavioral Sciences. New York, Cambridge University Press, 1990

Berkman LF, Syme LS: Social network, host resistance, and mortality: a 9-year follow-up study of Alameda County residents. Am J Epidemiol 109:186–204, 1979

Blazer DG: Depression in Late Life. St. Louis, MO, CV Mosby, 1982a

Blazer DG: Social support and mortality in an elderly community population. Am J Epidemiol 115:684–694, 1982b

Blazer DG: Depression in Late Life, 2nd Edition. St. Louis, MO, CV Mosby, 1993

Busse EW: The presidential address: there are decisions to be made. Am J Psychiatry 129:33–41, 1972

Busse EW: Ethical issues in geriatric psychiatry, in Psychiatry. Edited by Pichot P, Berner P, Wolf R, et al. New York, Plenum, 1985a, pp 149–153

Busse EW: Mental health and mental illness, in Normal Aging III. Edited by Palmer E, Busse EW, Maddox AW, et al. Durham, NC, Duke University Press, 1985b, pp 81–91

Busse EW, Blazer DG (eds): Handbook of Geriatric Psychiatry. New York, Van Nostrand Reinhold, 1980

Busse EW, Pfeiffer E (eds): Behavior and Adaptation in Late Life. Boston, MA, Little, Brown, 1969

Butterfield LH: Benjamin Rush, the American Revolution and the American Millenium. Harvard Medical Alumni Bulletin 50:16–22, 1976

Cole TR: The Journey of Life: A Cultural History of Aging in America. New York, Cambridge University Press, 1991

Conold DE: Codes of medical ethics, in Encyclopedia of Medical Ethics, Vol 1. New York, Free Press, 1977, pp 162–171

Cowdry EV: Problems of Aging: Biological and Medical Aspects. Baltimore, MD, Williams & Wilkins, 1938

Detre T: The future of geriatric psychiatry. Am J Psychiatry 144:621–625, 1987

Dyer AR: Assessment of competence to give informed consent, in Proceedings: Conference on Senile Dementia and Related Diseases—Ethical and Legal Issues. Washington, DC, National Institute on Aging, 1982, pp 227–237

Emmanuel E, Emmanuel L: The economics of dying: the illusion of cost saving at the end of life. N Engl J Med 331:540–544, 1994

German PS, Shapiro S, Skinner EA: Mental health of the elderly: use of health and mental health services. J Am Geriatr Soc 33:246–252, 1985

Gruman GJ: A history of ideas about the prolongation of life: the evolution of prolongevity hypotheses to 1800, in Transaction Services, Vol 56, part 9. Philadelphia, PA, American Philosophical Society, 1966

Gutheil TC: Forensic psychiatry—survey of informed consent—Risk Management Foundation. American Association of Geriatric Psychiatry Newsletter 9:84–85, 1987

Haavi Morreim E: Profoundly diminished life: the casualties of coercion. Hastings Cent Rep (January–February):33–41, 1994

Hall GS: Senescence: The Last Half of Life. New York, Appleton, 1922

High DM: Advance directives and the elderly: a study of intervention strategies to increase use. Gerontologist 33:342–349, 1993

Huyse FJ, van Tilburg W: Euthanasia policy in the Netherlands: the role of consultation-liaison psychiatrists. Hosp Community Psychiatry 44:733–738, 1993

King IW: The old code of medical ethics and some problems it had to face. JAMA 248:2329–2333, 1982

Last JM (ed): Public Health and Preventive Medicine, 11th Edition. New York, Appleton-Century-Crofts, 1980

Merriam Webster's Collegiate Dictionary, 10th Edition. Springfield, MA, Merriam-Webster, 1994

Nascher IL: Geriatrics: the diseases of old age and their treatment. Philadelphia, PA, P. Blokiston's Sons, 1914

Nascher IL: The aging mind. Medical Record 157: 669, 1944

Nowlin JB: Successful aging. Black Aging 2:4–6, 1977

Nowlin JB: Successful aging, in Normal Aging III. Edited by Palmer E, Busse EW, Maddox AW, et al. Durham, NC, Duke University Press, 1985, pp 34–46

OARS: Multidimensional Functional Assessment: The OARS Methodology, 2nd Edition. Durham, NC, Center for the Study of Aging at Duke University, 1978

Palmore E: Predictors of successful aging. Gerontologist 19:427–431, 1979

The Patient Self-Determination Act, December 12, 1991 (See APA *Updates,* December 1992)

Post F: The Clinical Psychiatry of Late Life. Oxford, UK, Pergamon, 1965

Rodin J: Control and well-being in the elderly. Science 233:1231–1274, 1986

Rowe JW, Kahn RL: Human aging: usual and successful. Science 237:143–149, 1987

Salzman C, Lebowitz BD (eds): Anxiety in the Elderly: Treatment and Research. New York, Springer, 1991

Schneiderman L, Kronick R, Kaplan R, et al: Effects of offering advance directives on medical treatments and costs. Ann Intern Med 117:599–606, 1992

Simmons LW: The Role of the Aged in Primitive Societies. New Haven, CT, Yale University Press, 1945

Stedman's Medical Dictionary, 25th Edition. Baltimore, MD, Williams & Wilkins, 1990

Stieglitz EJ: Geriatric Medicine: Diagnosis and Management of Disease in the Aging and the Aged. Philadelphia, PA, WB Saunders, 1943

Zinberg NE, Kaufman I: Normal Psychology of the Aging Process. New York, International Universities Press, 1963

Index

*Page numbers printed in **boldface** type refer to tables or figures.*

A Question of Madness, 8
AAGP. *See* American Association for Geriatric Psychiatry
Abdomen, focus on, 243
Abkhazians, 8
Abnormal Involuntary Movement Scale (AIMS), 185
Absorption, gastric, 40
Acetophenazine, 362
Acetyl-CoA. *See* Acetylcoenzyme A
Acetylcholine (ACh), 63, 74, 75–78, 86
Acetylcholinesterase (AChE), 75–76
Acetylcoenzyme A (acetyl-CoA), 75
Acetylsalicylic acid, 302
ACh. *See* Acetylcholine
AChE. *See* Acetylcholinesterase
Acidosis, respiratory, 195
Acquired immunodeficiency syndrome (AIDS), 14
dementia complex, 226–227
ACTH. *See* Adrenocorticotropic hormone
Active listening, 253
Activities of daily living (ADL)
impairment, relationship to psychiatric disorders, 136–138
scales, 43
Activity groups, 404, 405
Activity theory of aging, 19
Acuity, age-related changes in, 49–51
Acupuncture, 301
Acute brain syndrome, 271
Acute stress disorder, 281
Addiction, to alcohol, 346
Adenosine triphosphate (ATP), 73
Adenosine, 75

Adjustment disorder with anxious mood, differential diagnosis of, 250
Adjustment disorder with depressed mood, differential diagnosis of, 245
Adjustment disorders in late life, 323–325
acute *vs.* chronic, 323
prevalence of, 323–324
psychosocial stressors and, 323–325
ADL. *See* Activities of daily living
Adrenal dysfunction, psychotic symptoms and, 269
Adrenocorticotropic hormone (ACTH), 88
Advance directives, 469–471
Advanced sleep phase syndrome, depression and, 249
Adverse drug effects, in nursing home populations, 415
Aerobic conditioning, in elderly persons, 389
Aerobic fitness, sleep disturbances and, 337
Afebrile infection, 41–42
Affect
as a factor in mental status examination, 180
defined, 180
Affective disorders, 134
positron-emission tomography and evaluation of, 199
Aflatoxin, 98
Age
and epidemiologic distribution of psychiatric disorders, 159
help-seeking behavior and, 145

and recovery from psychiatric disorders, 142
relationship to psychiatric disorder, 131, 140
Age changes and social/economic factors, 129–130
Age stratification theory of aging, 19
Aging
advantages of, 11
astrology and, 10
attitudes toward, 8–10
crystallized intelligence and, 18
definition of, 11–16
fluid intelligence and, 18
functional change and, 42–43
how it feels to grow old, 10–11
impaired homeostasis and increased vulnerability to disease with, 28
interaction between physiology and pathology, 27–29
mitochondrial DNA role in, 97–98
neuropsychological perspective on, 111–112
normal
vs. pathological changes, 25
subtypes of, 26–27
physiology of
age-related changes in major organ systems, 29–42
overview of, 25–26
variability in changes among individuals, 26
premature, models of, 20–22.
See also Hutchinson-Gilford syndrome; Progeria(s); Werner's syndrome

Aging *(continued)*
  primary, 11–12
  psychological theories of,
    18–19
      stage theory of
        adult cognitive
          development, 18–19
  psychology of, 105–118
  redundant theory of, 8
  secondary, 12
  selected biological theories of
      "aging clock" theory, 13
      cellular theories, 13
      cross-linkage theory, 15
      deliberate biological
        programming, 14
      error theories, 13
      eversion theory, 15
      exhaustion theory, 13
      fault-hit approach, 14
      free radical theory, 14
      genetics and, 15–16
      glycosylation, 15
      immune system and,
        14–15
      integrative approaches, 13
      meta-aging, 13
      organ-based, 13
      population-based, 13
      program theories, 13
      somatic mutation theory,
        13
      stochastic theories, 13–14
      watch-spring theory, 13
  social theories of
      activity theory, 19
      age stratification, 19
      continuity approach, 19
      disengagement theory, 19
      homogeneity and
        heterogeneity
        theories, 20
      life events and stress
        theory, 20
      minority-group theory, 20
      modernization theory, 20
  successful
      geriatric psychiatry and,
        465–466
      vs. unsuccessful, 116–118
      vs. usual, 26–27
  telomeres and, 97
  wisdom and, 18
"Aging clock" theory of aging, 13

Agitated behaviors, in dementia
    of the Alzheimer's type,
    treatment of, 222
Agitated dementia, 184
  buspirone and, 284
Agitated depression, in nursing
    home populations, 414–415
Agitation
  as a factor in mental status
    examination, 180
  as a manifestation of
    cardiovascular disease, 194
      hypoparathyroidism
        and, 195
      in nursing home
        populations, 415
Agoraphobia, 186, 280
  antidepressants in, 284
AGS. *See* American Geriatric
    Society
AIDS. *See* Acquired immuno-
    deficiency syndrome
AIMS. *See* Abnormal Involuntary
    Movement Scale
Akathisia, 362
  in nursing home populations,
    415
  interference with medication
    compliance, 274
Alchemy, 6
Alcohol
  as an anxiolytic, 283
  dementia and, 214. *See also*
      Alcohol abuse/dependence
  effects on cholesterol, 384
  interactions with drugs, 346
  pharmacological properties of,
    343–344
Alcohol abuse/dependence, 134,
    136, 138, 186, 239
  abuse *vs.* dependence, 348
  addiction, 346
  diagnostic workup for, 347–348
  differential diagnosis of, 250
  genetic predisposition to, 347
  major patterns of, 144
  mortality and, 345–346
  physical consequences of,
    344–346
  prevalence in elderly persons,
    342
  recovery from, social factors
    that affect, 144–145
  risk factors for, 342–343

scope of problem in elderly
    persons, 341–342
  sleep characteristics in, 346
  tolerance, 346
  treatment for
      detoxification centers, 349
      disulfiram prophylaxis,
        349–350
      inpatient *vs.* outpatient,
        349
      long-term goals of,
        349–350
      self-help groups in, 350
      withdrawal as a first step
        in, 349
  withdrawal, 283, 346–347
      interference with
        dexamethasone
        suppression test
        accuracy, 196
      psychotic symptoms
        and, 269
Alcohol use
  cognitive function and,
    165–166
  gender differences in, 17
  history of, 341
  hypothermia and, 41
  sleep disturbances and, 332
Alcohol-induced dementia,
    psychotic symptoms and,
    269
Alcohol-induced persisting
    amnestic disorder, 228
Alcoholic amnestic dementia, 345
  vs. dementia of the
    Alzheimer's type, 345
Alcoholics Anonymous (AA), 350
Alcoholism. *See* Alcohol
    abuse/dependence
Aldosterone, 30
Alkalosis, 195
Alpha-adrenergic receptor
    agonists, effects on
    growth hormone, 241
Alpha-methyldopa, 178
Alprazolam, 284, 370, 373
Aluminum intoxication, possible
    role in pathogenesis of
    dementia of the
    Alzheimer's type
    pathogenesis, 67.
    See also Dementia of
    the Alzheimer's type

Aluminum toxicity, dementia of the Alzheimer's type and, 197

Alzheimer's Disease Assessment Scale (ADAS), 221

Alzheimer's Disease Diagnostic and Treatment Centers, State of California, 224

Alzheimer, Alois, 64

American Association for Geriatric Psychiatry (AAGP), 461

American Geriatric Society (AGS), 460, 461

American Psychiatric Association Council on Aging, 460–461

Amino acids, as components of neurotransmitter molecules, 78

Aminoglycosides, effects of renal function on dosage, 38

Aminoketones, use in elderly patients, 369

Amitriptyline, 364, 365
  sleep disturbances and, 336

Amnesia, electroconvulsive therapy and, 256

Amnestic disorders, 213, 228–229
  alcoholism as a cause of, 228–229
  etiology of, 228
  head trauma as a cause of, 228
  memory impairment in, 228

Amoxapine, 365

Amphetamine, 368

Amyotrophic lateral sclerosis, 62

Analgesics, 302
  interactions with alcohol, 346

Androgen clearance, 33

Androgens, 30

Androstenedione, 33

Angel dust. See Phencyclidine

Angina pectoris
  anxiety disorders and, 282
  hypothyroidism and, 32

Anomia, 215

Anoxia, dementia and, 214

Antediluvian theme, 4–5

Antianxiety drugs, 178

Anticoagulants, coumarin-type, interactions with alcohol, 346

Anticonvulsants, interactions with alcohol, 346

Antidepressants, 178, 238–239, 283
  anxiety disorders and, 284–285
  in dementia of the Alzheimer's type, 221–222
  hypothermia and, 41
  misuse of, in nursing homes, 417–418
  treatment of nocturnal delirium with, 333
  use in elderly patients, 364–371

Antihistamines, 283, 285, 374
  sleep disturbances and, 336

Antihypertensives, sleep disturbances and, 331

Antioxidant vitamins, 387

Antipsychotic drugs
  cardiotoxicity of, 195
  in dementia of the Alzheimer's type, 222
  misuse of, in nursing homes, 417–418
  side effects of, 362
  treatment of nocturnal delirium with, 333
  use in elderly patients, 361–363

Antisocial personality disorder, 186

Anxiety
  hypoglycemia and, 195

Anxiety disorders, 134, 136, 138, 186, 239
  acute stress disorder, 281
  agoraphobia without history of panic disorder, 280
  diagnostic workup and differential diagnosis, 282–283
  DSM-IV diagnostic classification, 279–281, **280**
  differential diagnosis of, 250
  due to a general medical condition, 282
  epidemiology of, 282
  generalized anxiety disorder, 280–281
  laboratory tests to evaluate, 283
  not otherwise specified, 282
  obsessive-compulsive disorder, 281–282
  panic disorder, 280
  pharmacological management, 283–285, 373–374
  posttraumatic stress disorder, 281

psychological treatments, 285–286
  psychometric assessment for, 283
  social phobia, 280
  specific phobia, 280
  substance-induced, 282
  symptoms of, 279

Anxiety in the Elderly, 460

Anxiety rating scales, 283

Anxiety-depression syndromes, mixed, buspirone and, 284

Anxiolytic drugs, 283. See also Anxiety disorders, pharmacological management
  effects on norepinephrine, 83

Anxious depression, 184

Aortic sclerosis, 34

Apathy
  in dementia of the Alzheimer's type, 218
  in nursing home populations, 415

Aphasia, 165, 215
  in dementia of the Alzheimer's type, 218

Apolipoprotein E$_4$ (apo-E), dementia of the Alzheimer's type and, 68, 101

Apoptosis, 63

Apraxia, 165, 215
  in dementia of the Alzheimer's type, 218

Arrhythmias, cardiac
  hypothermia and, 41
  tricyclic antidepressants and, 194

Arteriosclerosis, vs. atherosclerosis, 29

Arthritis, behavioral factors and, 116

Aslan, Professor Anna, 7

Aspartate, 75

Aspirin, 302, 376
  nutritional effects of, 383

Assessment, functional, 43–44

Assisted suicide, 471–472

Ataxia
  in acquired immunodeficiency syndrome (AIDS) dementia complex, 227
  thiamine deficiency and, 229

Ataxia telangiectasia, association with aging process, 16
Atenolol, 37, 285
Atherosclerosis
  vs. arteriosclerosis, 29
  dietary modification and, 384
  increased risk after menopause, 29
ATP. See Adenosine triphosphate
Atrial fibrillation, hypothyroidism and, 32
Atrophic gastritis, 383
  alcohol abuse and, 345
  vs. gastric atrophy, 40
Attachment theory
  bereavement and, 314
  vs. disengagement, 19
Attention, 108, 108
  impairment in, 226, 332
Attitudinal biases, in self-reports of symptoms, 176
Atypical depression. See Depression not otherwise specified (NOS)
Audition, age–related changes in, 54–55
Auditory threshold, age-related changes in, 54
Aurora, 3
Auto-anti-idiotypic antibody production, 27
Autoimmune disease, reduced incidence among elderly persons, 27
Avian pancreatic polypeptide, 86
Azapirones, 283

Backward masking, test of image retention, 52
Bacon, Roger, 5, 6
Baltimore Longitudinal Study on Aging, 460
Barbiturates, 283
  interference with dexamethasone suppression test accuracy, 196
  nutritional effects of, 383
  sleep disturbances and, 334–335
Barton, Walter E., 10–11
BDI. See Beck Depression Inventory
Beck Anxiety Inventory, 283

Beck Depression Inventory (BDI), 183, 206
Behavior and Adaptation in Late Life, 460
Behavioral disturbances, in nursing home populations, 414
Behavioral factors
  arthritis and, 116
  chronic pain and, 116
  cigarette smoking and, 116
  coping, 116
  coronary heart disease and, 116
  dementia and, 116
  diabetes and, 116
  hypertension and, 116
  stroke and, 116
Behavioral medicine, applications in geriatric populations, 115–116
Behavioral therapy, 401
Benzodiazepines, 283, 284, 361, 373–374
  abuse of, 353
  in dementia of the Alzheimer's type, 222
  depression and, 245
  effects on norepinephrine, 83
  interference with dexamethasone suppression test accuracy, 196
  sleep disturbances and, 334, 335
  toxicity symptoms, 353
  treatment of nocturnal delirium with, 333
  withdrawal symptoms, 353
Bereavement, 138
  complicated, 245, 316–317
    treatment of, 321–322
  differential diagnosis of, 242, 244–245
  epidemiology of, 313–314
  longitudinal studies of, 317–318
  multiple losses and, 315
  normal symptoms of, 244, 316–317
  pathological grief, 245, 316–317
  pharmacotherapy for, 321
  phases of adaptation to, 314–315
  psychotherapy for, 321–323

risk factors for negative outcome of grief, 318–321
self-help groups for, 322–323
sleep disorders and, 332
theories about adjustment to permanent loss, 314–315
treatments for, 321–323
uncomplicated vs. complicated, 245, 316–317
  treatment of, 322–323
Bereavement overload, 315
Beta-adrenergic stimulation, response of elderly persons to, 35
Beta-amyloid, role in pathogenesis of dementia of the Alzheimer's type, 67–68, 223
Beta-blockers, 178, 283, 374
  depression and, 245
  somatic anxiety and, 285
  treatment of nocturnal delirium with, 333
Beta-carotene, 14, 387
Beta-endorphin, 88
Bible, longevity reported in, 4–5
Biliary tract, 40–41
Binswanger's disease, 69
Biogenic amines, 74
Biomedical tests. See Diagnostic workup of geriatric patient, laboratory testing in
Biophosphonates, 34
Biosenescence. See Aging
Bipolar disorder
  differential diagnosis of, 242
  in late life, 240
  in nursing home patients, 237
  linkage studies in, 101
  recovery from 142–144
  heritability of, 240–241
Bizarre delusions, in late-onset schizophrenia, 268
Blessed Dementia Index, 183
Blindness, from cataracts, 29
Blood pressure, systolic, 29, 35. See also Hypertension
Blood urea nitrogen (BUN), in evaluation of dementia, 216
Body mass, hypothermia and, 41
Bone loss, postmenopausal, 33. See also Osteoporosis

BPRS. *See* Brief Psychiatric Rating Scale
Braceland, Francis, 11
Bradykinesia, in acquired immunodeficiency syndrome (AIDS) dementia complex, 227
Bradykinin, 86
Brain infection, cerebrospinal fluid testing and, 197
Brain proteins, abnormalities in dementia of the Alzheimer's type, 219
Brain tumors
    dementia and, 225
    psychotic symptoms and, 269
Brief dynamic therapy, 399–400
    group, 405
Brief Psychiatric Rating Scale (BPRS), 184
Brief psychotic disorder, 270
Brinkley, John Romulus, 4
Bromocriptine, 363
Bromosulfophthalein retention test, 40
Brown-Séquard, Dr. Charles Edouard, 4
Bupropion, 254, 284, 369
Buspirone, 284, 369, 370, 374
    in dementia of the Alzheimer's type, 222
Busse, Ewald W., 460
Butyrophenones, 362

Caffeine, sleep disturbances and, 332
CAGE questions, to screen for alcohol problems, 347
Calcitonin, 34
Calcium, 385, 386, 386
Caloric intake profile, lifetime, 382
Caloric intake, recommendations in elderly persons, 386
cAMP. *See* Urinary cyclic adenosine monophosphate
Cancer
    anxiety disorder and, 250
    breast, in postmenopausal *vs.* premenopausal women, 27
    depression and, 246
    dietary modification and, 384
    effect on nutritional needs, 382

gender differences in mortality from, 17
interference with dexamethasone suppression test accuracy, 196
and interference with fever development, 41
vitamin E and, 387
Werner's syndrome and, 21–22
Cancer screening, recommendations for elderly persons, 44
Carbamazepine, 361, 370, 371
    in dementia of the Alzheimer's type, 222
    interference with dexamethasone suppression test accuracy, 196
    seasonal affective disorder and, 243
Carbidopa, sleep disturbances and, 334
Carbohydrate intolerance of aging, 31
Carbohydrate metabolism, age-related changes in, 30–31
Carbohydrates, dietary recommendations in elderly persons, 386
Carcinogens, dietary, 384
Cardiac arrhythmias
    anxiety disorders and, 282
    neuroleptic drugs and, 195
    tricyclic antidepressants and, 194, 195
Cardiac function studies, in elderly persons, 34
Cardiac hypertrophy, 35
Cardiac output, 34, 35
Cardiotoxicity
    of antipsychotic drugs, 195
    of tricyclic antidepressants, 194
Cardiovascular disease
    behavioral factors and, 116
    depression and, 245, 246
    dietary modification and, 384
    psychiatric manifestations of, in geriatric patients, 194
CARE. *See* Comprehensive Assessment and Referral Evaluation

Caregivers
    family role of, 179
    support groups for, 406–407
Caregiving
    relationship to psychiatric disorder, 137
    stress of, 116
Carrel, Alexis, 6–7
Carroll Rating Scale for Depression, 184, 206
CAT scan. *See* Computed tomography
CAT. *See* Choline acetyltransferase
Cataracts, 29, 49
    Werner's syndrome and, 21, 97
Catechol-*O*-methyl transferase (COMT), 79
Catecholamines, 30, 74, 79
    hypothermia and, 41
Cell immortality, myth of, 6–7
Cellular theories of aging, 13
Centenarians, 4, 8
    studies involving, 117
Center for Epidemiologic Studies Depression Scale (CES-D), 100–101, 158, 183, 193, 235
Center for the Study of Mental Health of Aging, 461
Cerebral atrophy, evaluation with computed tomography, 197
Cerebrospinal fluid (CSF)
    biochemical tests of, 196–197
    recommended uses of, 197
Cerebrovascular accident. *See* Stroke
Cerebrovascular disease, 64
Cervical lipodysplasia, association with aging process, 16
CES-D. *See* Center for Epidemiologic Studies Depression Scale
CHD. *See* Coronary heart disease
Childbearing, relationship to psychiatric disorder, 135
Childhood traumas, relationship to psychiatric disorder, 131, 135, 140
Chlorazepate, 284
Chlordiazepoxide, 284, 373
Chloride, abnormal blood levels, psychiatric symptoms and, 195

Chlorpromazine, 361, 368
Chlorprothixene, 362
Chlorthalidone, 37
Cholecystokinin, 80
Cholesterol control, dietary
    modification and, 384
Cholesterol, high-density
    lipoprotein, 31
Cholestyramine, nutritional
    effects of, 383
Choline, 376
Choline acetyltransferase (CAT),
    75, 77
Cholinergic systems, **76**
Cholinergic-deficiency
    hypothesis, in dementia of
    the Alzheimer's type,
    219–220
    treatment implications, 220–221
Chromium, dietary, 387
Chronic anxiety symptoms,
    buspirone and, 284
Chronic decubitus ulcers, 387
Chronic early-onset
    schizophrenia, 267,
    268–269
Chronic fatigue syndrome,
    depression and, 245
Chronic illness, 141
    and recovery from psychiatric
        disorders, 143
    relationship to psychiatric
        disorders, 136
Chronic obstructive pulmonary
    disease, anxiety disorders
    and, 283
Chronic pain
    behavioral factors and, 116
    depression and, 245, 247–248
    treatment of, 301–302
Chronic stress, 136, 141
    recovery from psychiatric
        disorders, 142
    relationship to psychiatric
        disorder, 131
Chronobiological disturbances.
    See Sleep, circadian
    physiology of
Church attendance, psychiatric
    disorders and, 136
Cicero, Marcus Tullius, 8–9
CIDI. *See* Composite
    International Diagnostic
    Interview

Cigarette smoking, 39
    and death from ischemic heart
        disease, 18
    behavioral factors and, 116
    gender differences in, 17
Circadian physiology, sleep and,
    330–331
Circadian rhythm
    desynchronization of, 241
    unstable, interference with
        dexamethasone suppression
        test accuracy, 196
Cirrhosis, alcohol abuse and, 344
Claudication, dietary
    modification and, 384
Climacteric, male, 32–33
Clinical chemistry screen, 191,
    195, 251
Clinical Psychiatry of Late Life, 460
Clomipramine, 284, 365
Clonazepam, sleep disturbances
    and, 334
Clonidine, 178
    depression and, 245
    effects on growth hormone,
        241
Clorazepate, 373
Clozapine, 362
Cobalamin. *See* Vitamin B$_{12}$
Cobalt, dietary, 387
Cockayne's syndrome,
    association with aging
    process, 16
Cognition, impaired, and
    depressive disorder, 240
Cognitive changes,
    hypothyroidism and, 246
Cognitive disorders, 213–229. *See
    also* Dementia of the
    Alzheimer's type
    amnestic disorders, 213,
        228–229
    dementia, 213, 214–227
        elements in evaluation
            of, **215**
Cognitive functioning, 108–109
    alcohol abuse and, 345
    health and, 109
    rating scales for, 182–183, 202
Cognitive impairment, 43, 186.
    See also Cognitive
    disorders; Dementia
    behavioral therapy in patients
        with, 401

environmental toxins and, 165
impact of nutrition on, 165
neurosyphilis and, 165
prevalence of, 159–162, **160**
relationship to psychiatric
    disorders, 136
sleep disorders and, 334
Cognitive therapy, 321–322
Cognitive-behavior therapy,
    321–322, 400–401, 407
    in anxiety disorders, 285
    group, 404–405
    for mood disorders, 253
Cohort, definition of, 130
Cohort differences in psychiatric
    disorders
    age changes and, 139–141
    social/economic factors in, 130
Colchicine, nutritional effects of,
    383
Cold intolerance, 246
Collagen structure, changes in,
    with aging, 15
Colon, 41
Color perception, age-related
    changes in, 53
Communication, factors relating
    to, 186–187
Community-based care
    advantages of, 438–439
    community services and,
        440–442
    constructing the future of,
        450–455
    current focus on, 439–440
Compassionate Friends, 323
Competency, legal definitions of,
    468–469
Compliance, with
    pharmacotherapy, 376
Composite International
    Diagnostic Interview
    (CIDI), 186
Comprehensive Assessment and
    Referral Evaluation
    (CARE), 185
Compulsions, defined, 281
Computed axial tomography. *See*
    Computed tomography
Computed tomography (CT),
    197–198
    in evaluation of dementia, 216
COMT. *See* Catechol-*O*-methyl
    transferase

Concentration, impairment in, 181, 226, 332
Confusion, 270
    electroconvulsive therapy and, 256
    as a manifestation of cardiovascular disease, 194
    thiamine deficiency and, 229
Congestive heart failure
    dietary modification and, 385
    effect on nutritional needs, 382
    hypothermia and, 41
    hypothyroidism and, 32
Congruence theories, and help-seeking behaviors, 146
Constipation, 41, 246
    hypothyroidism and, 32
    in nursing home populations, 415
Continuity approach to aging, 19
Contrast sensitivity, age-related changes in, 51
Coping
    and stress, personality influence on, 114
    risk of disease and, 116
Coping behavior
    age-related stressors and, 324–325
    influence on prognosis of late-life depression, 239–240
Coping strategies, relationship to psychiatric disorder, 131
Copper, dietary, 387
Cor pulmonale, 332
Cornaro, Luigi, 10
Coronary artery disease, alcohol abuse and, 344
Coronary heart disease (CHD)
    behavioral factors and, 116
    postmenopausal, 33
    trace minerals and, 387
Corticosteroids, 302
    sleep disturbances and, 332
    synthetic, interference with dexamethasone suppression test accuracy, 196
Corticotropin-releasing factor (CRF), 87–89
Cortisol, depressive disorders and, 241
Cowdry, Edmund B., 460

Creatinine clearance, 38
Creutzfeldt-Jakob's disease, dementia and, 16, 64, 224, 225–226, 227
CRF. See Corticotropin-releasing factor
Cross-linkage theory of aging, 15
Cruzan v. the State of Missouri Department of Health, 469
Crystallized intelligence, 18
    vs. fluid intelligence, 112
CT. See Computed tomography
Cushing's disease, interference with dexamethasone suppression test accuracy, 196
Cyavana, legend of, 5
Cyclandelate, 375
Cyclic antidepressants, sleep disturbances and, 335

DA. See Dopamine
DAG. See Diacylglycerol
Dale, Sir Henry, 74
Dance groups, 404, 405
Dantrolene, 363
DAT. See Dementia of the Alzheimer's type
Dehydration
    convulsions and, 195
    delirium and, 195
    dietary modification and, 384
    lethargy and, 195
Dehydroepiandrosterone, 30
Deinstitutionalization, 436–437
Delayed sleep phase syndrome, depression and, 249
Deliberate biological programming theory of aging, 14
Delirium, 213
    abnormal chloride blood levels and, 195
    abnormal sodium blood levels and, 195
    alcohol withdrawal and, 349
    vs. dementia, 214
    diagnosis of, 227–228
    drug toxicity as a cause of, 227
    DSM-IV diagnostic criteria for, **227**
    environmental stressors as a cause of, 228
    etiology of, 227–228, **228**

    in late-onset paranoid and schizophrenic disorders, 270–271
    metabolic disorders as a cause of, 227
    in nursing home populations, 414–415
    overhydration and, 195
    somatostatin and, 89
    systemic illness as a cause of, 227
    treatment of, 228
Delusional depression, 181
Delusional disorder, late-life, 269–270
Delusions of persecution, acute brain syndrome and, 271
Dementia, 64–69, 180, 213. See also Dementia of the Alzheimer's type
    agitated, 184
        buspirone and, 284
    anoxia as a cause of, 214
    behavioral factors and, 116
    alcohol abuse and, 214, 345
    beta-blockers in, 285
    brain tumor as a cause of, 225
    clinical features of, 214
    Creutzfeldt-Jakob's disease as a cause of, 224, 227
    vs. delirium, 214
    vs. depression, 214–217
    dexamethasone suppression test in diagnosis of, 196
    differential diagnosis of, 214–217
    drug toxicity as a cause of, 217
    electroencephalograph findings in, 200–201
    etiological studies of, 164–166
    evaluation of
        with computed tomography, 197
        history, 216
        laboratory tests, 216
        medical inventory, 216
        mental status examination, 215–216
        physical examination, 216
        screening neurological examination, 216
        urinalysis, 216
    head trauma as a cause of, 214, 224

Dementia *(continued)*
  human immunodeficiency
    virus (HIV) disease as a
    cause of, 224, 226–227
  Huntington's disease as a
    cause of, 224
  hypothyroidism as a cause of,
    216, 224, 226
  intracranial radiation and, 225
  laboratory tests in patients
    with, 195
  Lewy body diseases as a cause
    of, 225
  misdiagnosis of, 195
  multi-infarct. *See* Vascular
    dementia
  neurosyphilis as a cause of,
    227
  normal-pressure
    hydrocephalus as a cause
    of, 224, 226
  in nursing home populations,
    414–415
  Parkinson's disease as a cause
    of, 224, 225
  pharmacotherapy for, 375–376
  Pick's disease as a cause of,
    224, 225–226
  positron-emission
    tomography and
    evaluation of, 199
  prevalence of, 159–162, **160**
  psychotic symptoms and, 269
  rating scales for, 183
  retarded, 184
  reversible causes of, 195,
    216–217
  rheumatoid cerebrovasculitis
    as a cause of, 217
  senile, genetic determinants
    of, 16. *See also* Dementia of
    the Alzheimer's type
  sleep disturbances and, 333
  subdural hematoma as a cause
    of, 216, 217
  and transitional paranoid
    reactions, 267
  treating anxiety and agitation
    with trazodone, 285
  vascular. *See* Vascular dementia
  vitamin B$_{12}$ deficiency and, 225
Dementia of the Alzheimer's
    type, 16, 64, 68–69, 74, 213,
    217–223, 252

  accuracy of antemortem
    diagnosis, 218–219
  agitated disruptive behaviors,
    treatment of, 222
  vs. alcoholic amnestic
    dementia, 345
  aluminum toxicity and, 197
  apolipoprotein E and, 101
  behavioral therapy in, 401
  caregivers, support groups for,
    406–407
  chemical neurotransmitters
    and, 76–77, 78
  clinical course, 218
  clinical features of, 214
  corticotropin-releasing factor
    and, 88
  vs. Creutzfeldt-Jakob's
    disease, 65
  depression and, 200, 249
  vs. depression, 215
  DSM-IV diagnostic criteria for,
    217
  Down's syndrome and, 101,
    165
  early-onset familial, 223
  early-onset *vs.* late-onset, 100,
    223
  electroencephalograph
    findings in, 201
  ergoloid mesylates in, 376
  etiological studies of,
    164–166
  hallucinations and, 269
  heritability of, 99–100
  hypotheses for pathogenesis
    of, 67–68
  inheritance pattern, 99
  magnetic resonance imaging
    and, 198, 216
  Mattis Dementia Rating Scale
    in evaluation of, 216
  molecular genetics and, 95,
    222–223
  morphological changes in,
    65–69
  neuronal changes in, 62–63
  neuropathological findings in,
    217–218
  neuropeptides and, 63
  norepinephrine-containing
    neurons in, 83
  in nursing home populations,
    414

  pathophysiology of, 219–222
    brain neurotransmitter
      abnormalities, 219–221
        cholinergic-deficiency
          hypothesis,
          219–220
        implications for
          pharmacological
          treatment, 220–221
  personality change in, 114
  vs. Pick's disease, 65
  positron-emission
    tomography and
    evaluation of, 199
  prevalence of, 159–162, **160**
  psychotic symptoms and, 269
  role of beta-amyloid in
    pathogenesis, 223
  sleep disturbances and, 218, 333
  somatostatin and, 89
  special care units in nursing
    homes for, 419–420
  tacrine hydrochloride therapy
    for, 76 219, 220–221
  treatment of, 221–222
  vasodilators in, 375
Dementing disorders, treatable
    components of, in nursing
    home populations, 414
Demographic variables, and risk
    of psychiatric disorders,
    134, 140
Deoxyribonucleic acid (DNA)
  discovery of, 96
  mitochondrial, 97–98
  nuclear (nDNA), defined, 97
  recombinant, 96
Deprenyl, 367
Depression. *See also* Depressive
    disorders; Mood disorders
  anxious, 184
  atypical. *See* Depression not
    otherwise specified
  bereavement and. *See*
    Bereavement, pathological
    grief
  chronic, misdiagnosis of, 195
  effect on nutritional needs, 382
  hypochondriasis and, 293
  mixed, electroencephalograph
    findings in, 200–201
  not otherwise specified
    (NOS), differential
    diagnosis of, 244

positron-emission
tomography findings in, 199
psychotic
differential diagnosis of,
243
electroconvulsive
therapy and, 243
electroencephalograph
sleep findings in, 200
nihilistic delusions in, 243
tricyclic antidepressants
and, 200, 243
rapid-cycling, and
hypothyroidism, 193
rating scales for, 183–184
reactive, 243
symptoms of
secondary to
hypothyroidism, 195
withdrawn, 184
Depression in Late Life, 460
Depressive disorders
in nursing home populations,
415–416
treatment of, 415–416
sleep disturbances and,
332–333
social factors and, 241–242
Depressive neurosis. *See*
Dysthymic disorder
Depressive pseudodementia,
214–215
Depressive symptoms
in nursing home populations,
414
sleep disorders and, 334
Depth perception, age-related
changes in, 51
Desipramine, 254, 284, 336, 365
Detoxification centers, 349
Dexamethasone suppression test
(DST), 191–192, 193,
196215, 239, 241, 251
Dextroamphetamine, 370
Diabetes mellitus
behavioral factors and, 116
depression and, 245
dietary modification and, 385
hypothermia and, 41
and stroke risk, 31
and vision loss, 53
presentation in elderly *vs.*
persons, 28
Werner's syndrome and, 21, 97

Diacylglycerol (DAG), 73
Diagnostic and Statistical Manual
of Mental Disorders (DSM),
186, 235, 282
DSM-III, 166, 137, 192, 205,
265, 269, 348, 414
Epidemiological
Catchment Area
studies, criteria used
in, 265
paranoid disorder in,
269
personality disorder
criteria used in
structured interviews,
205
DSM-III-R, 132, 155, 158, 161,
186, 192, 235, 236, 242, 266,
348, 414, 415, 416
bereavement
(complicated/
uncomplicated) in,
245, 316
delusional disorder in,
269
depression not
otherwise specified
(NOS) in, 244
dysthymic disorder in,
239
hypochondriasis
(hypochondriacal
neurosis) in, 291, 293
interview schedules,
criteria used as basis
for, 159
late-onset schizophrenia
in, 266, 268
multi-infarct dementia
in, 223
organic mental disorder
in, 213
personality disorder
criteria used in
structured interviews,
205
primary degenerative
dementia of the
Alzheimer's type in,
217
psychotic depression in,
200
seasonal affective
disorder in, 243

sexual disorders
category in, 302
somatoform pain
disorder in, 296,
298–299, **299**
DSM-IV, 158, 162, 175, 182, 186,
192, 214, 218, 235, 268, 270,
360
alcohol-induced
persisting amnestic
disorder in, 228
anxiety disorders in,
279–281, **280**
bereavement
(uncomplicated) in,
245
cognitive disorders
category in, 213
delirium due to a general
medical condition
criteria in, **227**
delusional disorder in,
270
dementia due to other
disorders, coding in,
224
dementia of the
Alzheimer's type
criteria in, **217**
Global Assessment Scale
as Axis V in, 184
hypochondriasis criteria
in, 291, **292**
pain disorder criteria in,
298–299, **299**
sexual dysfunction due
to a general medical
condition in, 302
vascular dementia
criteria in, **223**
Diagnostic Interview Schedule
(DIS), 159, 186
Diagnostic workup of the geriatric
patient, laboratory testing
in, 191–206
cerebrospinal fluid tests,
196–197
clinical chemistry screen, 195
value of, 191
computed tomography,
197–198
dexamethasone suppression
test, 191–192, 196
electrocardiogram, 194–195

Diagnostic workup of the geriatric patient, laboratory testing in (continued)
  electroencephalography, 192, 200–201
  magnetic resonance imaging, 191, 197, 198–199
  methodological criteria for, 192
  plain radiographs, 197
  polysomnography, 192, 193–194
  positron-emission tomography, 197, 198, 199
  psychodiagnostics laboratory, 201–206
  sensitivity, 192–193
  single photon emission computed tomography, 200
  specificity, 192–193
  structured interviews and, 205
  thyrotropin-releasing hormone stimulation test, 195–196
  tricyclic antidepressant plasma levels, 191
  validity, 192–193
  psychiatric interview, 185–187
Diastolic filling, 35
Diastolic function, 35
Diazepam, 284, 373, 376
  alcohol withdrawal and, 347
Dibenzoxapines, 362
Diet history, 381
Diet
  barriers to adequate, 383–384
  disease control and, 385–386
  as preventive therapy, 384
  recommendations in elderly persons, 386–387
  as therapeutic intervention, 384–385
Digoxin, 376
  effects of renal function on dosage, 38
Dihydroindolones, 362
Dihydrotestosterone, 32–33
Dihydroxyphenylacetic acid, 79
1,25-Dihydroxy-vitamin D_3, 31, 40
Dilantin, nutritional effects of, 383
Diphenhydramine, 285
  sleep disturbances and, 336
DIS. See Diagnostic Interview Schedule

Disease prevention in elderly persons, 44–45
Diseases
  atypical or altered presentation in elderly persons, 42
  coexistence of multiple, 42
Disengagement theory of aging, 19
Disordered perception, 270
Disordered thinking, 270–271
Disulfiram, 349-350
Diuretics, sleep disturbances and, 331
Diverticulosis, dietary modification and, 384
Divided attention, 108
DNA. See Deoxyribonucleic acid
Do-not-resuscitate order, 470
Dominance, genetic, defined, 95
DOPAC. See Dihydroxy-phenylacetic acid
Dopamine (DA), 74, 78, 79–81, 86
Dopamine neurons, pathways in human brain, **80**
Dorsal column stimulation, and pain control, 301
Down's syndrome
  association with aging process, 16, 67, 68, 98, 165
  and dementia of the Alzheimer's type, 222
  positron-emission tomography and evaluation of, 199
Doxepin, 336, 364, 365, 366
  mood disorders and, 254
Dramatic activity groups, 404, 405
Drug abuse/dependence
  behavioral and social factors in, 352–353
  diagnostic workup for, 353–354
  etiology of, 350–351
  iatrogenic contributors to, 353
  scope of the problem, 351–352
  treatment of, 354
Drug disposition, in elderly persons, 360
Drug toxicity
  and delirium, 227
  dementia and, 217
Drug-taking behavior, in elderly patients, 376

DSM. See Diagnostic and Statistical Manual of Mental Disorders
DST. See Dexamethasone suppression test
Duke Longitudinal Studies of Aging, 292, 295
Duodenum, 40
Dwarfism, Hutchinson-Gilford syndrome and, 20, 98
Dying-back phenomenon, 62
Dynamic psychotherapy, in anxiety disorders, 285
Dynorphin, 86
Dysphoria, 180
Dyspnea, 35
Dysthymic disorder, 186, 239
  differential diagnosis of, 243–244

Early-onset schizophrenia, chronic, 267, 268–269
ECA. See Epidemiologic Catchment Area
ECG. See Electrocardiogram
Edema, alcohol abuse and, 345
Education, 140
  relationship to psychiatric disorder, 131, 134–135
EEG. See Electroencephalogram
Ejection fraction, left ventricular, 35
Electrocardiogram (ECG)
  in evaluation of geriatric patient, 194–195
  in evaluation of sleep disorders, 194
  precaution before pharmacotherapy, 254
Electroconvulsive therapy (ECT), 238–239
  direct electroencephalograph monitoring during, 255
  electrocardiogram findings as contraindication for, 194
  medical workup before, 255
  Parkinson's disease and, 247
  psychotic depression and, 243
  risks and side effects in elderly patients, 256
  seizure duration, 256
  unilateral vs. bilateral electrode placement, 255
  withdrawal of medication before, 255

Electroencephalogram (EEG), 192
  findings in dementia, 200–201
  findings in mixed depression, 200–201
Electroencephalogram, sleep. See Polysomnography
Electroencephalographic sleep in psychotic depression, 200
Electrolyte abnormalities, 195
  psychotic symptoms and, 269
Electromyogram, submental. See Polysomnography
Electrooculogram, 194. See also Polysomnography
Eledioisin, 86
Elixir of life, 6
Emptying, gastric, 40
Enabling factors, in help-seeking behaviors, 145
Encephalitis, psychotic symptoms and, 269
Encephalopathy
  alcoholism and, 228
  psychotic symptoms and, 269
End diastolic volume, left ventricular, 35
Endocrine changes
  aging and, 13
  with aging, 13
Endocrine disorders, anxiety disorders and, 282
Endocrine disturbances, depression and, 245
Endocrine factors, interference with dexamethasone suppression test accuracy, 196
Endocrine secretion patterns, role in depressive disorders, 241
Endocrine systems, age-related changes in, 29–30
Endorphins, 63, 86
Enkephalins, 86
Environmental stressors, delirium and, 228
Environmental toxins, cognitive impairment and, 165
Eos, 3
EPI. See Epinephrine
Epidemiologic Catchment Area (ECA) studies, 127, 159, 186, 265, 330, 342, 414

Epilepsy
  glutamic acid and, 84
  positron-emission tomography and evaluation of, 199
  temporal lobe, anxiety disorders and, 283
Epinephrine (EPI), 74, 79
Episodic/semantic memory model, 107
EPS. See Extrapyramidal side effects
Erectile dysfunction, 305
Ergoloid mesylates, 375–376
Error theories of aging, 13
Erythromycin, 372
Escapee, family role of, 179
Esophagus, 40
Estradiol, 33
Estrogen, 385
  postmenopausal deficiency in, 33
Estrone, 33
Ethnicity. See Race/ethnicity
Eukaryotic cells, defined, 97
Euthanasia, 471–472
Eversion theory of aging, 15
Executive function, deficits in, in dementia of the Alzheimer's type, 218
Exercise
  effects on sleep, 331
  in elderly persons
    activity initiation, 390–391
    benefits of, 391
    correlation of age and activity, 388
    etiology of inactivity, 388–389
    fitness assessment, 390
    hazards of, 391
    injury risk assessment, 390
    types of activity, 389
  psychological impact of, 116
Exercise tolerance, decreased, 246
Exhaustion theory of aging, 13
Existential psychotherapy, 403
Explicit/implicit memory model, 107
Expressive psychotherapy groups, 405

Extrapyramidal side effects (EPS)
  psychoactive drugs and, 362, 368–369
  antiparkinsonian medication for, 375
Facilitator, family role of, 178
Failure to thrive, in nursing home populations, 416
Family roles, in psychiatric evaluation of geriatric patient, 178–179
Family support, assessment of, 179–180
Family therapy, 407
Far vision, age-related changes in, 50
Fat, dietary recommendations in elderly persons, 386
Fat stores, body, assessment of, 382
Fatigue, exercise and, 391
Fault/hit theory of aging, 14
Fearfulness, 279
Fertility, relationship to psychiatric disorder, 131
Fiber, dietary
  dietary modification and, 384
  recommendations in elderly persons, 386
Fibroblasts, features of, Werner's syndrome and, 21
Fibromyalgia, depression and, 245
Flaccid paralysis, 195
Flexibility, physical, importance of in elderly persons, 389
Flicker fusion threshold, age-related changes in, 52
Fluid intelligence, 18
  vs. crystallized intelligence, 112
Fluoxetine, 254, 284, 367, 369
  interaction with warfarin, 178
Fluphenazine, 285, 362
Flurazepam, 284, 373
Folate deficiency, 43, 251, 375
  psychotic symptoms and, 269
Folic acid, 40, 383, 387
  alcohol abuse and, 345
  cognitive function and, 165
Follicle-stimulating hormone (FSH), in aging men, 33
Fountain of Youth legends, 5, 7
Franklin, Benjamin, 459

Free radicals, oxygen, 97, 387
  theory of aging, 14
Free thyroxine (T_4) index, 195
Freud, Sigmund, 314, 396
FSH. *See* Follicle-stimulating
  hormone
Functional disability, assessment
  targets
    activities of daily living, 43
    cognitive impairment, 43
    falls and impaired mobility, 43
    losses, 43
    nutritional deficiency, 43
    sensory impairment, 43
    social and economic status, 43
    urinary incontinence, 43
    psychiatric disorders and, 136

G proteins, 77
GABA. *See* Gamma-aminobutyric
  acid
GAD. *See* Glutamic acid
  decarboxylase
GAL. *See* Galanin
Galanin (GAL), 76
Galton, Sir Francis, 95
Gamma-aminobutyric acid
  (GABA), 74, 78–79, 86, 376
Gastric atrophy, *vs.* atrophic
  gastritis, 40
Gastrointestinal system,
  age-related changes in,
  40–41
    alcohol abuse and, 344–345
    biliary tract, 40–41
    colon, 41
    esophagus, 40
    liver, 40–41
    pancreas, 40–41
    small intestine, 40–41
    stomach and duodenum, 40
Gate-control theory of pain, 301
GDS. *See* Geriatric Depression
  Scale
Gender
  and epidemiologic
    distribution of psychiatric
    disorders, 159
  and recovery from psychiatric
    disorders, 142
  late paraphrenia and, 271
  relationship to psychiatric
    disorder, 131, 134, 140
  sleep patterns and, 331

Gender differences
  in alcohol consumption, 17
  in cigarette smoking, 17
  in immune system capacities, 17
  in ischemic heart disease, 17
  in life expectancy, 16–18
  in mortality, 17
  in Type A behavior, 17
  risk-taking behavior and, 17, 18
Gene mapping, 96
General assessment scales,
  184–185
Generalized anxiety disorder, 280
  benzodiazepines in, 284
  differential diagnosis of, 250
Genetic testing and counseling,
    cautions concerning, 102
Genetics
  aging and, 15–16, 95–102
  alcohol abuse/dependence
    and, 347
  history of, 95–96
  molecular, 101
  population, 98–101
  quantitative, defined, 99
Genogram, in evaluating
    psychiatric disorders in
    geriatric patients, 177
Genome, human, 96
Georgia Centenarian Study, 117
Georgia, Republic of,
    centenarians in, 8
Geriatric Depression Scale
    (GDS), 183–184, 235
Geriatric Institute of Bucharest, 7
*Geriatric Medicine: Diagnosis and
    Management of Disease in
    the Aging and the Aged,* 460
Geriatric Mental State Schedule,
    185–186
Geriatric neuropsychology,
    111–112
Geriatric psychiatrists, and
    public health, 464–465
Geriatric psychiatry
  board certification in, 462
  current and future issues,
    462–463
  ethical and legal issues in,
    466–472
  professional organizations
    and, 460–462
  successful aging and, 465–466
  in the United States, 459–460

*Geriatrics: The Diseases of Old
    Age and Their Treatment,*
    460
Gerocomy, 4, 6
Gerontocomia, 9
Gerontological Society of
    America (GSA), 460, 461
Gerovital H_3, 7, 376
Gerstmann-Sträussler syndrome,
    16
Gey, George O., 7
GFR. *See* Glomerular filtration
  rate
Ghandi, Mahatma, 4
Gilgamesh, myth of, 5–6
Glaucoma, 49, 53
Global Assessment Scale (GAS),
    184
Global Deterioration Scale,
    202
Glomerular filtration rate, 31
GLU. *See* Glutamic acid
Glucose regulation, dietary
    modification and, 385
Glutamate. *See* Glutamic acid
Glutamic acid (GLU), 75, 78,
    84–85, 86
Glutamic acid decarboxylase
    (GAD), 78
Glycine, 75, 78
Glycosylation and aging, 15
Gonadotropin-releasing
    hormone, 33
Grief
  pathological, 245, 316–317
    vs. bereavement, 245
  risk factors for negative
    outcome in, 318–321
Grief counseling, 322. *See also*
    Bereavement, treatments
    for
Grief therapy, 322. *See also*
    Bereavement, treatments
    for
Group therapy, for elderly
    patients, 404–407. *See also*
    Activity groups
Growth hormone, 241
GSA. *See* Gerontological Society
    of America
GTP. *See* Guanosine triphosphate
Guanosine, 73
Guanosine triphosphate (GTP),
    73

Guided autobiographical groups, 405

Gustation, age-related changes in, 55

HACU. *See* High-affinity choline uptake (transporter)

Hall, G. Stanley, 459–460

Hallucinations, 180, 265
alcohol withdrawal and, 349
and dementia of the Alzheimer's type, 269
in late-onset schizophrenia, 268
and schizophrenia-like symptoms in late life, 272
sensory impairment and, 272

Haloperidol, 273–274, 285, 362, 374
in dementia of the Alzheimer's type, 222

Halstead Category Test, 203

Halstead Finger Tapping Test, 203

Halstead-Reitan Neuropsychological Test Battery, 202, 203

Hamilton Anxiety Scale (HAS), 283

Hamilton Rating Scale for Depression, 184, 206

HAS. *See* Hamilton Anxiety Scale

Head trauma
amnestic disorders and, 228
dementia and, 214, 224

Headache, electroconvulsive therapy and, 256

Health belief models, and help-seeking behaviors, 146

Health care, for older persons, 436–438
organizational context of, 448–450

Health maintenance organizations (HMOs), psychiatric treatment and, 147

Health promotion in elderly persons, 44–45

Health services, factors that affect use of, 145–146, 166–168

Health, impact on behavior, 115

Hearing. *See* Audition

Heart, age-related changes in, 34–37

Heart disease, trace minerals and, 387

Heart failure
dietary modification and, 385
effect on nutritional needs, 382

Heart rate, 34, maximal, 35

Heat stroke. *See* Hyperthermia

Height/weight tables, application to elderly persons, 381

HeLa cells, 7

Help seeking for psychiatric disorders, 145–147

Hematocrit, aging and changes in, 27

Hera, 5

Heritability
defined, 99
of dementia of the Alzheimer's type, 99–100
of mood disorders, 100

Herodotus, 5

Heterogeneity theory of aging, 20

Hiatus hernia, 40

High-affinity choline uptake (HACU) transporter, in Dementia of the Alzheimer's type, 76–77

High-density lipoprotein, 31

Hip fractures, 385

Histamine, 78, 85–86
forms of receptors, 85–86

HIV. *See* Human immuno-deficiency virus disease

Homogeneity theory of aging, 20

Homosexuality, aging and, 307

Homovanillic acid (HVA), 79

Hormones, posterior pituitary, 86. *See also* Oxytocin; Neuropeptides; Vasopressin

Hot flashes, menopausal, 33

5-HT. *See* Serotonin (5-hydroxytryptamine)

Human development, in elders, 396–397

Human Genome Project, 96

Human immunodeficiency virus (HIV) disease, dementia and, 224, 226–227

Human pancreatic polypeptide, 86

Huntington's chorea, 74
dementia and, 224
positron-emission tomography and, 199
somatostatin and, 89

Hunza, centenarians in, 8

Hutchinson-Gilford syndrome, 20–22
characteristic features of, 20
genetic transmission of, 98

HVA. *See* Homovanillic acid

Hydergine, 375–376

Hydrazine-type monoamine oxidase inhibitors, 367

Hydrocephalus
normal-pressure, dementia and, 224, 226
psychotic symptoms and, 269

Hydrochlorothiazide, 376

5-Hydroxyindoleacetic acid, 241, 247

5-Hydroxytryptamine (5-HT). *See* Serotonin

Hydroxyzine, 285

Hyperbaric oxygen therapy, 376

Hypercalcemia, hyperpara-thyroidism and, 195

Hyperglycemia, 195

Hyperinsulinemia, postprandial, 31

Hyperinsulinism, psychiatric manifestations of, 195

Hyperkinesis, 279

Hyperparathyroidism, 31
hypercalcemia and, 195
normocalcemic, 32
psychiatric manifestations of, 195

Hypersomnolence, 332

Hypertension, 35–37
behavioral factors and, 116
benefits of treating, 36–37
dietary modification and, 385
in elderly persons, 36–37
isolated systolic, 35
benefits of treating, 37
risk of, 36
systolic-diastolic, 35
trace minerals and, 387
transient systolic, electroconvulsive therapy and, 256

Hyperthermia, 41

Hyperthyroidism, 193, 251
    anxiety disorders and, 282
    depression and, 245, 246
Hyperventilation, 195, 279
Hypnosis, as a test for
        registration, 182
Hypnotic medications. *See*
        Sedative-hypnotic drugs
Hypobetalipoproteinemia, life
        expectancy and, 16
Hypocalcemia, psychiatric
        manifestations of, 195
Hypochondriasis
    brief psychotherapy for,
        295–296
    comorbidity in, 293
    course of illness, 295
    depression in, 293
    description of, 291–292
    DSM-IV diagnostic criteria for,
        292, **292**
    differential diagnosis of, 250
    epidemiology of, 293–294
    etiology of, 292
    genesis of, 294
    high bodily concern and, 292
    psychodynamics of, 294–295
    remission, 295
    risk factors for, 295
    therapeutic techniques for,
        292–293296–298
Hypoglycemia
    anxiety disorders and, 282
    psychiatric manifestations of,
        195
Hypoglycemic agents, oral,
        interactions with alcohol,
        346
Hypoparathyroidism
    hypocalcemia and, 195
    psychiatric manifestations of,
        195
Hypoproteinemia, alcohol abuse
        and, 345
Hyporborean theme, 4
Hypothalamic-pituitary-adrenal
        axis, dysregulation of, 241
Hypothalamus, 13
    changes in, with aging, 13
Hypothermia
    accidental, 41
    in frail elderly persons, 28–29
    neurotensin and, 86
    paradoxical, with sepsis, 41

Hypothyroidism, 32, 224, 226, 251
    dementia and, 216
    depression and, 245, 246
    hypothermia and, 41
    and interference with fever
        development, 41
    and rapid-cycling depression,
        193
    subclinical, 195

Ibn-Snia, 6
Ibuprofen, 302
ICD. *See* International
        Classification of Diseases
Identified patient, family role of,
        179
Illness
    behavior, 42
    acute, effect on nutritional
        needs, 382
    chronic, 141
        and recovery from
            psychiatric disorders,
            143
        relationship to
            psychiatric disorder,
            136
    systemic
        delirium and, 227
        dietary modification
            and, 386
Imipramine, 284, 365, 366
    binding, 252
    in dementia of the
        Alzheimer's type, 221
Immaturity, physical,
        Hutchinson-Gilford
        syndrome and, 20, 98
Immune system
    assessment of function, 382
    effects of aging on, 27
    gender differences in
        capacities of, 17
    theories of aging and,
        14–15
Impotence, sexual, 305
Inactivity
    etiology of, 388–389
    in nursing home populations,
        415
Income, 140
    relationship to psychiatric
        disorder, 131, 135
Incontinence, urinary, 43

Indolamines, 74
Infection
    brain, cerebrospinal fluid
        testing and, 197
    chronic, effect on nutritional
        needs, 382
    interference with
        dexamethasone
        suppression test accuracy,
        196
    and reversible dementia, 195
Influenza virus vaccination, 44
Information-processing
        impairment, alcohol abuse
        and, 345
Informed consent and the right
        to know, 467–468
Inosine 3'-triphosphate (IP3), 73
Insomnia, 334. *See also* Sleep,
        disorders of
    pharmacotherapy for,
        374–375
    rationale for early
        intervention, 330
    risks of benzodiazepine
        treatment in, 336
Institutionalization, alternatives
        to, 434–435
    cost-effectiveness of,
        442–448
Insulin, 30
Intellect
    impact of cerebral atrophy on,
        197
    impairment of, 181
Intellectual functioning, 108
    aging and, 108
    assessment instruments for,
        202–203
Intelligence
    assessment of, 182
    crystallized, 18
    fluid *vs.* crystallized, 112
    fluid, 18
Intelligence testing
    contributions of, 202
    elements of, 202–203
Intensity recruitment
        phenomenon, 57
Intercourse. *See* Sexual activity
Interleukin-1, reduced
        production of, 42
International Association of
        Gerontology, 460

International Classification of Diseases (ICD), 186
ICD-10
hypochondriasis disorder in, 291, 292
persistent somatoform pain disorder in, 299
Interpersonal psychotherapy, 401–403
Intestinal transit time, 383
Intimacy in late life, 307–308
Intracranial blood vessel hemorrhage, cerebro-spinal fluid testing and, 197
Intracranial radiation, dementia and, 225
Iodine, dietary, 387
IP3. See Inosine 3'-triphosphate
Iron, dietary, 383
deficiency
alcohol abuse and, 345
dietary modification and, 385
Irritability, in dementia of the Alzheimer's type, 218
Ischemic heart disease
age differences in incidence of, 18
gender differences in, 17
mortality attributable to cigarette smoking, 18
Ischemic stroke, dementia and, 214
Isocarboxazid, 368, 369
Isoxsuprine, 375

Journal of Gerontology, 460

Kassinin, 86
Ketoacidosis, hyperglycemia and, 195
Kevorkian, Dr. Jack, 471
Kidney. See Renal system
King Aeson, 3–4
King David, 4
Klinefelter's syndrome, association with aging process, 16
Korsakoff's psychosis, 228
Kynurenine, 82
Kyphosis, 385

L-dopa, sleep disturbances and, 331–332, 334

Lactase deficiency, dietary modification and, 385
Lacunae, in vascular dementia, 69
Late paraphrenia, gender and, 271
Late-onset panic disorder, 280
Late-onset schizophrenia, 267, 268
Lateral Dominance Examination, 203
Lateral gaze palsy, thiamine deficiency and, 229
Lawrence-Seip syndrome, association with aging process, 16
Lazarus Ways of Coping Scales, 116–118
Learning capacities, aging and, 112–113
Learning disorders, glutamic acid and, 84
Lecithin, 376
Lens opacification. See Cataracts
Lepeshinskaya, O. B., 8
Lethargy
dehydration and, 195
hyperglycemia and, 195
overhydration and, 195
Level-of-processing memory model, 107
Lewy body diseases, dementia and, 225
LH. See Luteinizing hormone
Life, length of. See Longevity
Life, prolongation of, 3–8
Life events and stress theory of aging, 20
Life expectancy
demographics and, 16–17
hypobetalipoproteinemia and, 16
sex (gender) differences in, 16–18
Life review therapy, 403, 404, 405–406
group, 405–406
Life span, human, 8
Life support, legal and ethical implications of, 469
Ligands, described, 73
Light therapy
seasonal affective disorder and, 243
sleep disturbances and, 335, 337

Light-headedness, respiratory alkalosis and, 195
Lipofuscin, 13, 67
Lithium carbonate, 361, 367, 371
drug abuse diagnostic workup and, 353–354
seasonal affective disorder and, 243
Liver, 40–41
cancer, aflatoxin implicated in, 98
function, alcohol abuse and, 344
Living wills, 469–471
Lobar sclerosis. See Pick's disease
Loewi, Otto, 74
Long-term care, 436
financing of, 464
Long-term memory, 106
Longevity
environmental factors in, 96
gender differences in, 16, 96
genetic factors in, 96–97
mitochondrial DNA and, 97–98
reported in Bible, 4–5
successful vs. unsuccessful aging, 116–118
Lorazepam, 284, 373
Loss(es). See also Bereavement
adjustment disorders and, 324
multiple (bereavement overload), 315
phases of adaptation to, 314.
coping mechanisms for, 272–273
Loudness recruitment phenomenon, 54
Loxapine, 362
in dementia of the Alzheimer's type, 222
LSD. See Lysergic acid diethylamide
Lung. See Pulmonary system
Luria–Nebraska Neuropsychological Battery, 203
Luteinizing hormone, in aging men, 33
Lysergic acid diethylamide (LSD), 81

Macular degeneration, 49, 53
Magnesium, dietary, 387

Magnetic resonance imaging
(MRI), 191, 197, 198–199
in evaluation of dementia, 216
vascular dementia and, 193
Major depression. *See* Depressive
disorders
Malignancy(ies). *See* Cancer
Malnutrition
consequences of, 382–383
hypothermia and, 41
interference with dexa-
methasone suppression test
accuracy, 196
Manager, family role of 178–179
Manganese, dietary, 387
Mania
episodes in later life, 237, 240
pharmacotherapy for, 361
positron-emission
tomography findings in, 199
psychotic symptoms and, 269
Manic delirium, 237
Manic-depressive illness. *See*
Bipolar disorder
MAO. *See* Monoamine oxidase
MAOIs. *See* Monoamine oxidase
inhibitors
Maprotiline, 364, 365, 366
Marital separation, relationship
to psychiatric disorder, 139
Marital status, 140
depression and, 166
and recovery from psychiatric
disorders, 143
relationship to psychiatric
disorder, 131, 135
Marital therapy, 407
Marriage trends in late life, 305
Mattis Dementia Rating Scale, 202
in evaluation of dementia, 216
Maximianus, 9
MCMI-I. *See* Millon Clinical
Multiaxial Inventory–I
MCMI-II. *See* Millon Clinical
Multiaxial Inventory–II
MDS. *See* Minimum Data Set
Measure of My Days, The, 396
Medea, 3–4
Medicaid, 148, 436, 437, 463, 464
Medical illness, depression and,
245
Medicare, 148, 436, 463, 464
Prospective Payment System
(PPS), 420

Medication cost, 377
Medication history, importance
of, in geriatric patients, 178
Medications
psychotic symptoms and, 269
symptoms of anxiety and, 283
Medvedev, Roy, 8
Medvedev, Zhores, 7–8
Melancholic depression, in later
life, 242
Memory
assessment of, instruments for,
203
disorders, glutamic acid and,
84
dysfunction, as a factor in
mental status examination,
181
functioning, 106–107
aging and, 106–107
theoretical models of,
106–107
impairment, 270
alcohol abuse and, 345
amnestic disorders and,
228
in dementia of the
Alzheimer's type, 218
electroconvulsive
therapy and, 256
information-processing model
of, 106–107
long-term, defined, 106
loss, hypothyroidism and, 32
primary, defined, 106
secondary, defined, 106
sensory, defined, 106
short-term, defined, 106
tertiary, defined, 106
testing of, 181–182
vitamin C and, 165
and written information,
109–110
Mendel, Gregor, 95
Meningioma, Werner's
syndrome and, 22
Menopause, 29, 33
estrogen replacement therapy
and, 34
influence on life expectancy, 17
Mental disorders, organic,
pathology of, 64–69
Mental health outcomes,
indicators of, 131–132

Mental health services, factors
that affect use of, 145–146,
166–168
Mental status examination, in
psychiatric evaluation of
geriatric patient, 180–182
Mental Status Questionnaire,
182
Mescaline, 81
Mesoridazine, 361
Messenger RNA, dopamine and,
81
Met-enkephalin, 80
Meta-aging, theory of, 13
Metabolic disorders, delirium
and, 227
Metchnikoff, Elie, 4
3-Methoxy-4-
hydroxyphenylglycol
(MHPG), 220
Methyldopa, depression and, 245
Methylphenidate, 254, 370–371
Metoprolol, 285
MHPB. *See* 3-Methoxy-4-
hydroxyphenylglycol
Midarm circumference
measurement, 382
Midtown Manhattan Study, 237
Millon Clinical Multiaxial
Inventory–I (MCMI-I), 204
Millon Clinical Multiaxial
Inventory–II (MCMI-II),
204
Minerals, dietary
recommendations in
elderly persons, 386
Mini-Mental State Exam
(MMSE), 43, 158, 160, 165,
182, 202
in evaluation of dementia, 216
Minimum Data Set (MDS), 418
Minnesota Multiphasic
Personality Inventory
(MMPI), 114, 192, 203, 204
Minnesota Multiphasic
Personality Inventory—2
(MMPI-2), 204
Minority-group theory of aging,
20
Mitochondrial DNA, role in
aging, 97–98
MMPI-2. *See* Minnesota
Multiphasic Personality
Inventory—2

MMPI. *See* Minnesota Multiphasic Personality Inventory
MMSE. *See* Mini-Mental State Exam
Modernization theory of aging, 20
Molindone, 362
Monoamine oxidase (MAO), 79, 241
Monoamine oxidase activity, platelet, 252
Monoamine oxidase inhibitors (MAOIs), 254
    use in elderly patients, 367–369
Montgomery-Åsberg Rating Scale for Depression, 184, 206
Mood
    as a factor in mental status examination, 180
    defined, 180
Mood disorder due to a medical condition. *See* Organic mood syndrome
Mood disorders, 134, 136, 138, 139, 180, 186, 235–257. *See also* Affective disorders
    blunted adrenocorticotropic hormone response and, 88
    conceptualization of late-life depression, 235–236
    corticotropin-releasing factor and, 88
    dexamethasone suppression test in diagnosis of, 196
    diagnostic workup of depressed older adult, 250–253
    differential diagnosis of
        adjustment disorder with depressed mood, 245
        alcohol use/abuse, 250
        anxiety, 250
        bereavement, 242, 244–245
        bipolar disorder, 242
        depression and medical illness, 245–248
        depression not otherwise specified, 244
        dysthymic disorder, 243–244

hypochondriasis, 250
        major depressive disorder, 242–243
        normal aging and, 248
        organic mental disorders, 248–249
        organic mood syndrome, 245
        primary sleep disorder, 249
        psychotic depression, 243
        schizophrenia, 249
        seasonal affective disorder, 243
    epidemiology of late-life mortality, 237. *See also* Suicide
        prevalence, 236–237
        prognosis, 238–240
        risk factors for, 240–242
    gender differences in, 240–241
    heritability of, 100, 240–241
    hypothyroidism and, 32
    marital status and, 166
    molecular genetics and, 95
    recovery from, 142–144
    risk factors for, 136–138
    sleep disturbances and, 332–333
    somatostatin and, 89
    thyrotropin-releasing hormone and, 86
    treatment
        active listening, 253
        electroconvulsive therapy, 254–256
        family therapy, 256–257
        pastoral counseling, 253
        pharmacotherapy, 254
        psychotherapy, 253
        unipolar depression, recovery from, 142–144
Mood-stabilizing drugs
    treatment of nocturnal delirium with, 333
    use in elderly patients, 371–373
Morbidity, due to acute illness or trauma, 28
Mortality
    alcohol abuse and, 345–346
    gender differences in causes of, 17
    obstructive sleep apnea and risk of, 332

Motility, gastric, 40
Motor coordination, deficits in, in dementia of the Alzheimer's type, 218
Motor hyperactivity, in dementia of the Alzheimer's type, 218
"Mourning and Melancholia," 314
Movement disorders, anxiety disorders and, 283
MRI. Magnetic resonance imaging
mRNA. *See* Messenger RNA
Multi-infarct dementia. *See* Vascular dementia
Multiple sclerosis
    psychotic symptoms and, 269
    somatostatin and, 89
Muscarinic receptors, 77, 78
Muscle wasting, alcohol abuse and, 345
Muscular twitching
    overhydration and, 195
    potassium disorders and, 195
Musculoskeletal injuries, exercise and, 391
Music groups, 404, 405
Mutism, in acquired immunodeficiency syndrome (AIDS) dementia complex, 226
Myocardial infarction, 384. *See also* Cardiovascular disease
    prevention of, 37
Myocardium, response to adrenergic stimulation, 35
Myoclonus, sleep disturbances and, 332
Myotonic dystrophy, association with aging process, 16
Myxedema, 246

NAMCS. *See* National Ambulatory Medical Care Surveys
Napping, sleep disturbances and, 332
Narcoanalysis, as a test for registration, 182
Nascher, I. L. 460
National Ambulatory Medical Care Surveys (NAMCS), 147

National Institute on Aging, 8, 13, 461–462

Nature *vs.* nurture debate, twin studies and, 95

Near vision, age-related changes in, 50

Negative predictive value, of laboratory tests, 192

Nei Ching, 301

Neighborhood stability, psychiatric disorders and, 136

Neihans, Paul, 4

Neomycin, nutritional effects of, 383

Neuroactive peptides. *See* Neuropeptides

Neuroanatomy, 61–64

Neurobehavioral Cognitive Status Examination, 202

Neurobehavioral Rating Scale, 202

Neuroleptic drugs, 273, 283, 361, 369
    cardiac arrhythmias and, 194, 195
    misuse of, in nursing homes, 417–418
    in nursing home populations, 415

Neuroleptic malignant syndrome, 362–363
    bromocriptine in, 363
    dantrolene in, 363

Neurological disorders, psychotic symptoms and, 269

Neurological examination, in diagnostic workup of depressed older adult, 251

Neuromedin N, 86

Neurons
    age-related changes in, 62–63
    plasticity process and, 64
    programmed death of (apoptosis), 63
    synaptic communication between, 73. *See also* Neurotransmitters

Neuropeptide Y, 77, 78, 86

Neuropeptides, 63, 75, 86–89
    cholecystokinin, 80
    corticotropin-releasing factor, 87–89

families of, 86
galanin, 76
met-enkephalin, 80
neuromedin N, 86
neuropeptide Y, 77, 78, 86
neurotensin, 80, 86–87
somatostatin, 63, 77, 78, 89
substance P, 78, 86
thyrotropin-releasing hormone, 87

Neuropsychological testing batteries, 203
    contributions of, 202
    elements of, 202–203

Neuropsychology, geriatric, 111–112

Neurosyphilis
    cognitive impairment and, 165
    dementia and, 227
    psychotic symptoms and, 269

Neurotensin, 80, 86–87

Neurotransmitters, 196. *See also* Neuropeptides
    abnormalities in dementia of the Alzheimer's type, 219–220
    acetylcholine, 63, 74, 75–78, 86
    adenosine triphosphate, 73
    adenosine, 75
    aspartate, 75
    biogenic amines, 74
    catecholamines, 74, 79
    criteria for, 75
    dopamine, 74, 78, 79–81, 86
    epinephrine, 74, 79
    gamma-aminobutyric acid, 74, 78–79, 86
    glutamic acid, 75, 78, 84–85, 86
    glycine, 75, 78
    guanosine triphosphate, 73
    guanosine, 75
    histamine, 78, 85–86
    norepinephrine, 35, 74, 77, 79, 82–84, 86
    role in depressive disorders, 241
    serine, 75
    serotonin, 74, 77, 78, 81–82, 86
    synaptic transmission process, **74**
    vasoactive intestinal peptide, 78

Niacin deficiency, psychotic symptoms and, 269

Nicotinic acid, 375

Nicotinic receptors, 77, 78

Nifedipine, 373

Nihilistic delusions, in psychotic depression, 243

Nitric oxide, neurotransmitter status of, 75

NMR. *See* Magnetic resonance imaging

Nocturnal delirium (sundowning)
    behavioral techniques in treating, 333
    etiology of, 333
    sleep disturbances and, 333

Nocturnal myoclonus, sleep disturbances and, 332

Nocturnal neurosis, 280

Noradrenergic system, deficits in, in dementia of the Alzheimer's type, 220

Norepinephrine, 35, 74, 77, 79, 82–84, 86, 220, 241
    effects of anxiolytic drugs on, 83

Norepinephrine uptake inhibitor drugs, 83

Normal Psychology of the Aging Process, 460

Normal-pressure hydrocephalus, dementia and, 224, 226

Nortriptyline, 254, 284, 336, 365, 366

NPH. *See* Normal-pressure hydrocephalus

Nuclear magnetic resonance imaging. *See* Magnetic resonance imaging

Nursing Home Reform Amendments, 418

Nursing homes. *See also* Long-term care; Nursing home populations
    federal regulations and psychiatric care in, 418–419
    mental health care in, service delivery model, 420–423, 427
    populations in
        clinical features of psychiatric disorders in, 414–418
        epidemiological perspectives on, 413

problems related to lack of
mental health service in,
416–418
special care units in, 419–420
studies of psychosocial
interventions, **423–427**
Nutrition
cognitive function and, 165
in elderly persons, 381–383
Nutritional deficiency, 43
Nutritional needs, variation with
age and health, 382–383
Nutritional status, documenting,
381–382
Nylidrin, 375
Nystagmus, thiamine deficiency
and, 229

OARS. *See* Older American
Resources and Services
Obesity, 382
dietary modification and, 385
obstructive sleep apnea and,
332
OBRA. *See* Omnibus Budget
Reconciliation Act
Obsessions, defined, 281
Obsessive-compulsive disorder,
186, 239, 281–282
antidepressants in, 284
benzodiazepines in, 284
selective serotonin reuptake
inhibitors in, 285
Obstructive sleep apnea, 332
Occupation
and epidemiologic
distribution of psychiatric
disorders, 159
relationship to psychiatric
disorder, 131, 135, 140
Octreotide, 89
Older American Resources and
Services, methodology for
geriatric assessment, 461
Older Americans Resources and
Services (OARS)
Multidimensional
Functional Assessment
Questionnaire, 185
Olfaction, age-related changes
in, 55–56
Omnibus Budget Reconciliation
Act (OBRA), 167, 418,
463–464

Opiate antagonists, 376
Opiates, interactions with
alcohol, 346
Opioids, endogenous, 86. *See also*
Dynorphin; Endorphins;
Enkephalins;
Neuropeptides
Oral contraceptives, 372
Oral-history groups, 404, 405
Organic brain syndrome. *See*
Cognitive disorders
Organic mental disorders. *See
also* Cognitive disorders
differential diagnosis of,
248–249
Organic mood syndrome,
differential diagnosis of,
245
Orthostatic hypotension, and
tricyclic antidepressants,
194
Osler, Sir William, 10, 460
Osteomalacia, alcohol abuse and,
344
Osteoporosis, 34
dietary modification and, 385
exercise and, 391
increased risk after
menopause, 29
Werner's syndrome and, 97
Ovarian function, menopause
and, 33
Overhydration
and delirium, 195
muscular twitching and, 195
Oxazepam, 284, 373
Oxprenolol, 285
Oxygen free radicals, 97, 387
Oxytocin, 86

Pain
age-related changes in
perception of, 56–57
disorder
clinical implications of
pain, 300
depression and, 200–301
DSM-IV diagnostic
criteria for, 298–299,
299
pain clinics and, 302
somatoform, DSM-III-R
diagnostic criteria for,
299

techniques for relief of
pain, 301
treatment of chronic
pain, 301–302
chronic
behavioral factors and,
116
depression and, 245
in nursing home populations,
415
relief, techniques for, 301
Palpitations, 279
Pancreas, 40–41
Pancreatic dysfunction,
psychotic symptoms and,
269
Pancreatic polypeptide–related
peptides, 86
Panic attacks, 279, 280
Panic disorder, 186, 280
antidepressants in, 284
benzodiazepines in, 284
selective serotonin reuptake
inhibitors in, 284, 285
Papaverine, 375
Parallel distributed memory
model, 107
Paralysis, flaccid, 195
Paranoid
delusions, 265
disorders, late-onset, factors
associated with,
270–273
ideation, acute brain
syndrome and, 271
psychosis, 184
symptoms, treatment of,
273–275
Paraphilias. *See* Sexual behavior
and disorders
Paraphrenia, late, 266, late, 267,
268
Parathyroid
age-related changes in
function, 31–32
dysfunction, psychotic
symptoms and, 269
Paresthesias
potassium disorders and, 195
respiratory alkalosis and, 195
Parkinson's disease, 74, 80
dementia and, 224, 225
depression and, 245, 247
hypothermia and, 41

Parkinson's disease *(continued)*
  positron-emission
    tomography and
    evaluation of, 199
  as treatment analog for
    dementia of the
    Alzheimer's type, 219
  with dementia, somatostatin
    and, 89
Paroxetine, 254, 284, 369
PASARR. *See* Preadmission
    Screening and Annual
    Resident Review
Pastoral counseling, 253
Pathological grief, *vs.*
    bereavement, 245
Patient Self-Determination Act, 469
Patient-controlled analgesia
    (PCA), 302
Pausanias, 5
PCA. *See* Patient-controlled
    analgesia
PCP. *See* Phencyclidine
Pepsinogen, secretion of, 40
Peptide histidine leucine, 86
Peptide histidine methionine, 86
Peptide YY, 86
Peptides, glucagon-regulated, 86.
    See also Neuropeptides;
    Peptide histidine leucine;
    Peptide histidine
    methionine; Vasoactive
    intestinal peptide
Perception
  as a factor in mental status
    examination, 180
  defined, 180
Perikaryon, structural
    degeneration in, 62
Peripheral neuropathy, alcohol
    abuse and, 345
Peripheral resistance,
    cardiovascular, 34
Peripheral vision, age-related
    changes in, 51–52
Peroneal palsy, in depressed
    older adult, 251
Perphenazine, 362
Persecutory ideation, 265
Personality
  assessment, instruments for,
    203–206
  changes, in dementia of the
    Alzheimer's type, 218

coping and, 114
coronary-prone, 116. *See also*
    Type A behavior
  effects on social interactions
    and attributions, 114–115
  development, patterns of,
    113–114
  pathology, and depressive
    disorder, 240
Personality Disorders
    Examination, 205
PET. *See* Positron-emission
    tomography
Pfeiffer, Eric, 460
Pharmacodynamics, defined, 335
Pharmacokinetics, defined, 335
Pharmacotherapy, in elderly
    populations
  compliance issues, 376
  general considerations,
    359–360
  special considerations, 376–377
Phencyclidine (PCP), 84
Phenelzine, 284, 367, 368, 369
Phenothiazines, 195, 273, 361
Phentolamine, 368
Phenylephrine, 368
Phenylpropanolamine, 368
Phenytoin, 373
  interference with dexa-
    methasone suppression test
    accuracy, 196
Phobias, 279
  social, 280
  specific, 280
Phototherapy, 334, 337
  seasonal affective disorder
    and, 243
Physical activity, reduced,
    hypothermia and, 41
Physical fitness, effects on
    cardiac function in elderly
    persons, 34
Physical illness, occult, in
    nursing home
    populations, 415
Physical restraints, in nursing
    homes, 416, 417
Physostigmine, 376
  use in dementia of the
    Alzheimer's type, 220
Pick's bodies, 68, 226
Pick's disease, 64, 68–69
  dementia and, 224, 225–226

Piperidine, 361
Piracetam, 376
Pituitary gland, 13
  changes in, with aging, 13
Platelet-binding density of
    tritiated imipramine,
    depression and, 252
Pliny, 4, 5
Pneumococcal vaccination, 44
Polypeptide-related peptides,
    pancreatic, 86. *See also*
    Avian pancreatic
    polypeptide; Human
    pancreatic polypeptide;
    Neuropeptides;
    Neuropeptide Y;
    Peptide YY
Polypeptides, neuroactive. *See*
    Neuropeptides
Polysomnography, 192, 193–194,
    252, 334
Pool of Youth, 5
Pope Innocent VIII, 4
Population genetics, 98–101
Positive predictive value, of
    laboratory tests, 192
Positron-emission tomography
    (PET), 197, 198, 199
  and affective disorders,
    evaluation of, 199
  and dementia of the
    Alzheimer's type,
    evaluation of, 199
  and dementia, evaluation of,
    199
  and depression, findings in,
    199
  and Down's syndrome,
    evaluation of, 199
  and epilepsy, evaluation of, 199
  Huntington's disease, findings
    in, 199
  and mania, findings in, 199
  and Parkinson's disease,
    evaluation of, 199
  and schizophrenia, evaluation
    of, 199
Potassium disorders, 195
Postprandial hyperinsulinemia, 31
Posttraumatic stress disorder
    (PTSD), 281
Poverty, 136
PPS. *See* Prospective Payment
    System

Prazepam, 373
Preadmission Screening and Annual Resident Review (PASARR), 418
Pregnancy, interference with dexamethasone suppression test accuracy, 196
Premature aging, Down's syndrome and, 98. *See also* Hutchinson-Gilford syndrome; Progeria(s); Werner's syndrome
Premature ventricular contractions, electro-convulsive therapy and, 256
Presbycusis, aging and, 110
Prescription drugs, abuse of, 351
Presenile dementia. *See* Dementia of the Alzheimer's type
Present State Examination (PSE), 159, 185–186
Primary degenerative dementia of the Alzheimer's type. *See* Dementia of the Alzheimer's type
Primary sleep disorder depression and, 249 differential diagnosis of, 249
Proband, defined, 98
Problem solving, aging and, 110
Problems of Aging, 460
Procaine hydrochloride, 7
Prochlorperazine, 362
Progeria(s), 16, 20–22, 97. *See also* Hutchinson-Gilford syndrome; Werner's syndrome
Program theories of aging, 13
Prohormones, 86
Projective assessment techniques, 205–206
Promazine, 361
Propoxyphene, 372
Propranolol, 178, 285, 376
Prospective Payment System (PPS), 420
Prostacyclins, role in pain generation, 302
Prostaglandins, role in pain generation, 302
Protective factors and psychiatric disorders, 137–138

Protein
    dietary recommendations in elderly persons, 386
    malnutrition, alcohol abuse and, 345
    stores, body, assessment of, 382
Protriptyline, 366
PSE. *See* Present State Examination
Pseudodementia, 248
    depressive, 214–215
    sleep disorders and, 334
Pseudoephedrine, 368
Pseudoephedrine hydrochloride, 283
Pseudoexophthalmos, Werner's syndrome and, 21
Pseudosenility, Hutchinson-Gilford syndrome and, 20, 98
Psilocin, 81
Psychiatric care for older adults, financing, 463–464
Psychiatric disorders
    age changes *vs.* cohort differences, 129–130
    diagnostic measures of, 132
    diagnostic measures *vs.* symptom scales in, 133
    epidemiological distribution of, 159–162
    epidemiology of, 155–168
        approach to case identification, 157–159
        use of symptom scales in, 157–159
        etiological studies in, 164–166
        historical studies in, 162–164
    help seeking for
        mental health service use, 145–146
        sector choice for treatment, 146–147
    protective factors and, 136–138, 141
        church attendance, 136
        coping efforts, 131, 138, 138
        religious activities, 136
    public policies and programs concerning, 147–148
    recovery from, social factors that affect, 141–145

social risk factors for
        cohort differences in, 139–141
        demographic variables in, 131, 134
        marital separation, 139
        methodological issues, 132–134
        provoking agents, 131, 138, 141
        stress-buffering hypothesis, 138, 144
        studies concerning, 133–134
        theoretical model of, 130–132
            evidence bearing on, 134–138
        urban *vs.* rural residence, 136
        vulnerability, 131–132, 136–138, 141
    social/economic factors related to, 129–149
    symptoms scales for, 133
Psychiatric interview of geriatric patient
    communication factors, 186–187
    elements of, **176**
    family assessment, 178–180
        identifying family roles, 178–179
    history, 175–178
    mental status examination, 180–182
    rating scales in, 182–185
    structured interviews and, 185–186
Psychiatric Status Schedule, 185
Psychoanalysis, as a test for registration, 182
Psychodiagnostics laboratory, use of services of, 201–206
Psychodynamic therapy, 399
    time-limited, 407
Psychometric tests. *See* Psychiatric interview of geriatric patient, rating scales in
Psychomotor
    agitation, 270
    retardation, 180, 246, 270
        in depressed older adult, 251

Psychosis
    hypoparathyroidism and, 195
    induced by organic causes,
        267, 269
    paranoid, 184
    pharmacotherapy of patients
        with, 360–361
Psychosocial stressors
    adjustment disorders and,
        323–325
    age-related, 324–325
Psychotherapy
    bereavement and, 321–323
    grief and, 321–323
    group, 321
        common themes and
            issues in, 408-409
        practical considerations
            in, 409
    in later life
        historical perspectives
            against, 396
        individual
            psychotherapies for
            elders, 399–403
        inherent challenges in,
            397–398
        overview, 395–396
        treatment goals, 403–404
Psychotic depression
    differential diagnosis of,
        243
    electroconvulsive
        therapy and, 243
    electroencephalographic
        sleep in, 200
    nihilistic delusions in, 243
    psychotic symptoms
        and, 269
    tricyclic antidepressants
        and, 200, 243
Psychotic disorder, brief, 270
Psychotic symptoms, in nursing
    home populations, 414
Psychotropic drugs
    misuse of, in nursing homes,
        417–418
    use among older persons, 166,
        167
PTSD. See Posttraumatic stress
    disorder
Pulmonary
    embolism, anxiety disorders
        and, 283

failure, effect on nutritional
    needs, 382
function and, 28
    aging and, 28
hypertension, 332
system, age-related changes
    in, 38–40
        control of respiration, 39
        gas exchange, 39
        pulmonary defense
            mechanisms, 39–40
        pulmonary mechanics, 39
Pulmonary venous congestion, 35

Race/ethnicity
    and epidemiologic
        distribution of psychiatric
        disorders, 159
    help-seeking behavior and, 145
    relationship to psychiatric
        disorder, 131, 134, 140
Radiation, intracranial, dementia
    and, 225
Radioactive iodine uptake, 251
Radiographs, plain, 197
Rapid eye movement (REM)
    density, depression and, 252
    latency, 192, 200
        depression and, 248, 252
    sleep, 200
Rating scales, 182–185, 202
    for anxiety, 283
RDC. See Research Diagnostic
    Criteria
Reactive depression, 243
Reality orientation groups, 404,
    405 406
Recall, as a memory process, 181,
    182
Recessive characteristic, genetic,
    defined, 95
Recombinant DNA, 96
Redundant theory of aging, 8
Registration, as a memory
    process, 181–182
Reitan–Indiana Aphasia
    Examination, 203
Reitan–Klove Sensory–
    Perceptual Examination, 203
Rejuvenists, 4
Religious activities
    influence on depression, 239–240
    psychiatric disorders and, 136
REM. See Rapid eye movement

Reminiscence therapy
    group, 405–406
    individual, 403, 404
Remotivation/resocialization
    groups, 404, 405
Renal failure
    and interference with fever
        development, 41
    dietary modification and, 384
    dietary modification and,
        385–386
Renal mass
    decreases in, 31
    loss of, with aging, 37
Renal system, age-related
    changes in, 37–38
    glomerular filtration rate, 38
    renal blood flow, 38
    serum creatinine, 38
Renin, 30
Reproductive system,
        age-related changes in
    female, 33
    male, 32–33
Republic of Georgia,
    centenarians in, 8
Research Diagnostic Criteria
    (RDC), 132, 162, 181, 200,
        243
Reserpine, 37, 369
    depression and, 245
Resident Assessment Protocols
    (RAPs), 418–419
Restless legs, sleep disturbances
    and, 332
Restriction fragment length
        polymorphisms (RFLPs),
        100
Retarded dementia, 184
Retention, as a memory process,
    181, 182
Retirement groups, 404, 405
RFLPs. See Restriction fragment
    length polymorphisms
Rheumatoid arthritis, behavioral
    factors and, 116
Rheumatoid cerebrovasculitis,
    dementia and, 217
Rise and Fall of T. D. Lysenko, 8
Risk-taking behavior, gender
    differences in, 17
River of Immortality, 5
Rorschach test, 205
Rush, Benjamin, 459

SADS-L. *See* Schedule for Affective Disorders and Schizophrenia, Lifetime Version

Saliva, age-related changes in, 55

Sandoz Clinical Assessment—Geriatric Scale (SCAG), 184

Sarcoma, Werner's syndrome and, 22

SCAG. *See* Sandoz Clinical Assessment—Geriatric Scale

Schedule for Affective Disorders and Schizophrenia (SADS), 246

Schedule for Affective Disorders and Schizophrenia, Lifetime Version (SADS-L), 159, 206

Schedule of Recent Events, 166

Schizoaffective disorder, 270

Schizophrenia, 134, 138, 186, 252, 265
  controversy surrounding diagnosis in the elderly, 266
  depression and, 249
  differential diagnosis of, 249
  effects of dopamine blockade in, 80
  historical perspectives, 266–267
  vs. late paraphrenia, 360
  pharmacotherapy for, 360–361
  positron-emission tomography and evaluation of, 199
  somatostatin and, 89

Schizophrenia-like psychotic symptoms, 360

Schizophrenia-like symptoms in late life
  coping with loss and, 272–273
  diagnostic evaluation of, 270
  differential diagnosis of
    affective disorders with psychotic features, 269
    chronic early-onset schizophrenia, 267, 268–269
    late paraphrenia, 267, 268
    late-life delusional disorder, 269–270
    late-onset schizophrenia, 267, 268

psychosis induced by organic causes, 267, 269
    suspiciousness, 267
    transitional paranoid reaction, 267–268
  family psychiatric history and, 272
  marital status and, 272
  poor social and occupational adjustment and, 271
  sensory impairment and, 271
  social isolation and, 271
  treatment of, 273–275

Schizophrenic disorders, late-onset
  factors associated with, 270–273
  molecular genetics and, 95

Schizophreniform disorder, 186, 265, 270
  evaluation of, 180

SCID. *See* Structured Clinical Interview for DSM-III-R

SCL-90-R. *See* Symptom Checklist 90—Revised

Seashore Rhythm Test, 203

Seasonal affective disorder
  carbamazepine and, 243
  diagnostic criteria for, 243
  differential diagnosis of, 243
  light therapy and, 243
  lithium carbonate and, 243

Second-messenger species, described, 73

Secondary memory, 106

Sedative-hypnotic drugs
  hypothermia and, 41
  interactions with alcohol, 346
  sleep disturbances and, 335
  withdrawal from, 283

Seizure disorders, psychotic symptoms and, 269

Seizures, alcohol withdrawal and, 349

Selective attention, 108

Selective serotonin reuptake inhibitors (SSRIs), 254
  use in elderly patients, 369

Selectivity theory, 114–115

Selenium, dietary, 387

Self-esteem, loss of, in dysthymic disorder, 243–244

Self-help groups, 406
  alcohol abuse/dependence treatment and, 350
  bereavement and, 322–323

Senescence. *See* Aging

Senescence: The Last Half of Life, 460

Senile dementia. *See* Dementia of the Alzheimer's type

Sensitivity, of laboratory tests for psychiatric disorders, 192–193

Sensory changes, as barriers to an adequate diet, 383

Sensory deprivation, in nursing home populations, 414–415

Sensory impairment, 43. *See also specific sensory systems*
  schizophrenia-like symptoms in late life and, 272

Sensory overload, in nursing home populations, 414–415

Serine, 75

Serotonergic abnormalities, in dementia of the Alzheimer's type, implications for treatment, 221–222

Serotonergic systems, **82**

Serotonin (5-hydroxy-tryptamine), 74, 77, 78, 81–82, 86, 241, 247
  central nervous system receptors for, 81

Serotonin systems, deficits in, in dementia of the Alzheimer's type, 220

Sertraline, 254, 284, 369

Serum electrolytes, in evaluation of dementia, 216

Sexual activity in late life, 243, 302–303
  attitudes toward, 304–305
  intimacy, 307–308
  among aging men, 33

Sexual behavior and disorders, 302–308

Sexual dysfunction due to a general medical condition, 302

Sexual dysfunction in late life, 305–306

Sexuality
    and institutionalized elderly
        persons, 308
    illness and disability affecting,
        306–307
    psychological changes that
        affect, 303–304
Shivering, hypothermia and, 41
Short Portable Mental Status
    Questionnaire (SPMSQ),
    158, 182
Short-term memory, 106
SIDP. *See* Structured Interview
    for DSM-III Personality
    Disorders
SIDP-R. *See* Structured Interview
    for DSM-III Personality
    Disorders–Revised
Silicone, dietary, 387
Sine-wave grating, in contrast
    sensitivity testing, 51
Single photon emission computed
    tomography (SPECT), 200
Sinus bradycardia, hypothermia
    and, 41
Sleep
    age-related changes in, 329–331
    circadian physiology and,
        330–331
    deprivation, 331
    disorders of
        approach to in elderly
            persons, 329–330
        bereavement and, 332
        cognitive impairment
            and, 334
        dementia and, 332–333
        depressive symptoms
            and, 334
        diagnosis of, 193–194
        evaluation of sleep/wake
            complaints in elderly
            persons, 334
        medications that may
            precipitate, 331–332
        mood disorders and,
            332–333
        nocturnal myoclonus
            and, 332
        Parkinson's disease and,
            334
        restless legs and, 332
        sleep-disordered
            breathing, 332

    treatment
        nonpharmacological,
            334–335, 337
        pharmacological, 335–336
    disturbances, from
        menopausal hot flashes, 29
    electroencephalograph
        activity in, 330
    exercise and, 331
    gender effects on, 331
    need *vs.* ability, 331
Sleep apnea syndrome,
    depression and, 249
Sleep cycle disruption, role in
    depressive disorders, 241
Sleep deprivation, studies of, 331
Sleep hygiene, 334
Sleep medications,
    over-the-counter, 336
Sleep restriction, 337
Sleep/wake cycle
    changes in elderly persons,
        330–331
    disruptions, in dementia of
        the Alzheimer's type, 218
Small intestine, 40–41
"Smart genes," 96
Smell, sense of. *See* Olfaction
Smoking. *See* Cigarette smoking
Social class, and epidemiologic
    distribution of psychiatric
    disorders, 159
Social integration, relationship to
    psychiatric disorder,
    140–141
Social interactions, effects of
    personality on, 114–115
Social isolation, schizophrenia-
    like symptoms in late life
    and, 271
Social phobia, 280
Social support
    depressive disorders and,
        241–242
    help-seeking behavior and, 145
    impact of, 115, 137–138
    major dimensions of, 137
    psychiatric disorders and, 166
    and recovery from psychiatric
        disorders, 143
    relationship to psychiatric
        disorders, 131
Social withdrawal, in nursing
    home populations, 415

Socioeconomic status
    and recovery from psychiatric
        disorders, 142
    relationship to psychiatric
        disorder, 134, 135
Sodium
    abnormal blood levels,
        psychiatric symptoms and,
        195
    dietary, 385–386
Soluble beta-amyloid precursor
    protein (sβPP), in
    diagnosis of dementia of
    the Alzheimer's type, 218
Somatic disorders, 134
Somatic mutation theory of
    aging, 13
Somatization disorder, 186
Somatoform disorders, 291–302
Somatoform pain disorder. *See*
    Pain disorder
Somatomedins, 30
Somatostatin, 63, 77, 78, 89
Somatotropin release–inhibiting
    factor (SRIF). *See*
    Somatostatin
Somesthesis, age-related changes
    in, 56–57
Soviet Institute of Gerontology, 8
Soviet Union, rejuvenation in,
    7–8
Specificity, of laboratory tests for
    psychiatric disorders,
    192–193
SPECT. *See* Single photon
    emission computed
    tomography
Speech
    comprehension, aging and, 110
    perception, age-related
        changes in, 54–55
Speech Sounds Perception Test,
    203
Spinal cord stimulation, and
    pain control, 301
SPMSQ. *See* Short Portable
    Mental Status
    Questionnaire
SSRIs. *See* Selective serotonin
    reuptake inhibitors
Stage theory of adult cognitive
    development, 18–19
Stanford Greater Maturity
    Project, 460

Stanford-Binet Intelligence Scale, 202
State-Trait Anxiety Inventory, 283
Status epilepticus, electroconvulsive therapy and, 256
Steroid hormones, 30
Steroids, 283, 372
Stieglitz, Edward J., 460
Stimulant drugs, 370–371
Stochastic theories of aging, 13–14
Stomach, 40
Strength of Grip Test, 203
Stress
    and recovery from psychiatric disorders, 142
    chronic, 136, 141
Stress and coping, personality influence on, 114
Stress disorder
    acute, 281
    posttraumatic, 281
Stress theory of aging, 20
Stress-buffering hypothesis, 138, 144
Stressors
    adjustment disorder and, 245
    psychosocial
        adjustment disorders and, 323–325
        age-related, 324–325
Stroke
    behavioral factors and, 116
    depression and, 245, 246–247
    dietary modification and, 384
    glutamic acid and, 84
    hypothermia and, 41
    prevention of, 37
Stroke volume, 35
Stroke work, 35
Structured Clinical Interview for DSM-III-R (SCID), 186, 205
Structured Interview for DSM-III Personality Disorders (SIDP), 205
Structured Interview for DSM-III-R Personality Disorders–Revised (SIDP-R), 205
Structured interviews, 185–186, 205
Subdural hematoma, dementia and, 216

Substance abuse/dependence, 134. See also Alcohol abuse/dependence; Drug abuse/dependence
    and reversible dementia, 195
Substance P, 78, 86
Substance withdrawal, psychotic symptoms and, 269
Substance-induced anxiety disorders, 282
Substance-induced mood disorder. See Organic mood syndrome
Substitution hypothesis, and help-seeking behaviors, 146
Successful aging, 26–27
    geriatric psychiatry and, 465–466
Succinic semialdehyde, 78
Sudden death, exercise and, 391
Suicidal ideation, as a factor in mental status examination, 181
Suicide
    assisted, 471–472
    with concurrent hypochondriasis and depression, 250
    epidemiology of, 237
    gender differences in, 17
    rates, among older persons, 163–164
    risk, assessment for, 250
Sundowning. See Nocturnal delirium
Superoxide, 14, 97
Superoxide dismutase, 14, 97
Supplementation hypothesis, and help-seeking behaviors, 146
Support groups, 406
    bereavement and, 322–323
Supportive psychotherapy, 399
Suspiciousness, 265, 267
Sweating response, delayed, and hyperthermia, 41
Sympathomimetic amines, 283
Symptom Checklist 90—Revised (SCL-90-R), 283
Symptom scales, 158–159
Systemic hypertension, 332
Systemic lupus erythematosus, psychotic symptoms and, 269

Systolic ejection murmurs, nonradiating, 34
Systolic hypertension. See Hypertension
Szilard, Leo, 14

Tachykinins, 86. See also Bradykinin; Eledoisin; Kassinin; Neuropeptides; Substance P
Tacrine hydrochloride, 76, 376
    and dementia of the Alzheimer's type, 219, 220–221
Tactile Form Recognition Test, 203
Tactual Performance Test, 203
Tardive dyskinesia, 80, 273, 362
Taste perception. See Gustation
TAT. See Thematic Apperception Test
Telomeres, role in aging, 97
Temazepam, 284, 373
Temperature sensitivity, impaired, and hyperthermia, 41
Temporal arteritis, psychotic symptoms and, 269
Temporal lobe epilepsy, anxiety disorders and, 283
Tertiary memory, 106
Testosterone, 30, 32–33
Tetanus-diphtheria toxoid vaccination, 44
Tetracyclic antidepressants, use in elderly patients, 364–367
Tetrahydroaminoacridine (THA). See Tacrine hydrochloride
THA (Tetrahydroaminoacridine), See Tacrine hydrochloride
Thematic Apperception Test (TAT), 205–206
Theophylline, 372
    sleep disturbances and, 331
Thermoregulation
    age-related changes in, 41–42
    psychoactive medications affecting, 41
Thiamine (vitamin B_1)
    alcohol abuse and, 345
    deficiency
        alcoholism and, 228
        clinical manifestations of, 229
        psychotic symptoms and, 269

Thioridazine, 195, 273, 361
    in dementia of the
        Alzheimer's type, 222
Thiothixene, 362, 374
Thioxanthenes, 362
Thought-content disturbances,
    as a factor in mental status
    examination, 180-181
Thromboxane, role in pain
    generation, 302
Thyroid axis, dysregulation of,
    241
Thyroid dysfunction
    and reversible dementia, 195
    psychotic symptoms and, 269
Thyroid function
    age-related changes in, 32
    importance of tests for, 195
Thyroid hormone, 30
Thyroid replacement therapies,
    283
Thyroid-stimulating hormone
    (TSH), 32, 195, 251. See also
    Thyrotropin-releasing
    hormone (TRH)
    stimulation test
Thyrotropin-releasing hormone
    (TRH), 32, 87
    stimulation test, 195–196, 216,
        241, 252
Thyroxine (T$_4$), 32
    radioimmunoassay, 195, 251
TIPS. See Tridimensional
    Interview of Personality
    Style
Tithonus, 3
Tolerance, to alcohol, 346
Touch, sense of. See Somesthesis
Toxicology screen, 195
Trail Making Test, 203
Tranquilizers
    hyperthermia and, 41
    hypothermia and, 41
    interactions with alcohol, 346
Transcutaneous electronic nerve
    stimulation (TENS), and
    pain control, 301
Transient cognitive disturbances,
    270
Transitional paranoid reaction,
    267–268
Transportation, access to, impact
    on psychiatric disorders,
    136

Tranylcypromine, 367
Trauma
    cerebrospinal fluid testing
        and, 197
    increased morbidity among
        elderly persons, 28
    childhood, 140
        relationship to psychiatric
            disorder, 131
Trazodone, 254, 284, 285, 336,
    369–370
    in dementia of the
        Alzheimer's type, 222
TRH. See Thyrotropin-releasing
    hormone
Triamterene, 376
Triazolam, 335–336, 373
Triceps skinfold thickness
    measurement, 382
Tricyclic antidepressants (TCAs),
    178
    cardiac arrhythmias and, 194,
        195
    cardiotoxicity of, 194
    drug abuse diagnostic workup
        and, 353
    mood disorders and, 254
    orthostatic hypotension and,
        194
    plasma levels of, 191
    precipitation of depressive
        symptoms, 245
    response of patients with
        psychotic depression, 200
    seasonal affective disorder
        and, 243
    sleep disturbances and, 334,
        336
    use in elderly patients, 364–367
Tridimensional Interview of
    Personality Style (TIPS),
    205
Tridimensional Personality
    Questionnaire, 205
Trifluoperazine, 273, 362
Triglycerides, 31
3,5,3'-Triiodothyronine. See
    Triiodothyronine (T$_3$) resin
    uptake test
Triiodothyronine (T$_3$), 365, 367
    resin uptake test, 32, 251
    uptake, 195
Trimethoprim, nutritional effects
    of, 383

Trimipramine, 364
Tritiated imipramine,
    platelet-binding density
    of, 252
TSH. See Thyroid-stimulating
    hormone
Turner's syndrome, association
    with aging process, 16
Twins
    dizygotic, defined, 95
    monozygotic, defined, 95
    registries of, 98
Type A behavior, gender
    differences in, 17
Tyramine, 368

Undernourishment, alcohol
    abuse and, 344
Underreporting of illness, 42
Unemployment, psychiatric
    disorders and, 136
Unipolar depression. See
    Depressive disorders
Urban vs. rural residence,
    psychiatric disorders and,
    136
Urethra, postmenopausal
    atrophic changes in, 33
Urinalysis, in evaluation of
    dementia, 216
Urinary cyclic adenosine
    monophosphate (cAMP),
    31
Urinary incontinence, 43
Urinary retention, in nursing
    home populations, 415
Usual aging, 26–27

Vaccinations, recommendations
    for elderly persons, 44
Vagina, postmenopausal atrophic
    changes in, 33
Validation therapy, 406
Validity, of laboratory tests for
    psychiatric disorders,
    192–193
Valproate, 369, 372–373
    in dementia of the
        Alzheimer's type, 222
Valproic acid. See Valproate
Vascular dementia, 69, 178, 180,
    214. See also Dementia
    computed tomography and,
    223–224

defined, 223
diagnosis of, 223–224
    Alzheimer's Disease
        Diagnostic and
        Treatment Centers
        proposed criteria for,
        224
DSM-IV diagnostic criteria for,
    223
in nursing home populations,
    414
interference with
    dexamethasone
    suppression test accuracy,
    196
magnetic resonance imaging
    and, 193, 216, 223–224
psychotic symptoms and, 269
rating scales for, 183
vs. dementia of the
    Alzheimer's type, 224
Vasoactive intestinal peptide, 86
Vasodilation, delayed, and
    hyperthermia, 41
Vasodilators, 375
Vasopressin, 63, 86
Venlafaxine, in dementia of the
    Alzheimer's type,
    221–222
Ventricle, age-related changes in,
    35
Ventricular arrhythmias,
    electroconvulsive therapy
    and, 256
Ventricular dilatation,
    significance in geriatric
    patients, 197–198
Verapamil, 372, 373
Vertebral compression fractures,
    electroconvulsive therapy
    and, 256
Veterans Administration,
    provision of psychiatric
    care, 464
Victim, family role of, 178
Viejos, 8
Vilcabamba, centenarians in, 8
Vision
    age-related changes in, 49–53
    pathology affecting, 53
Visual acuity, dynamic, 52–53
Visual-spatial skills, deficits in, in
    dementia of the
    Alzheimer's type, 218

Vita Sobria, 10
Vitamin A, 387
    absorption of, 40
Vitamin B$_2$ deficiency, depression
    and, 247
Vitamin B$_6$ deficiency, depression
    and, 247
Vitamin B$_{12}$ (cobalamin), 387
    alcohol abuse and, 345
    deficiency, 40, 251
        dementia and, 225, 226
        depression and, 247
        psychotic symptoms
            and, 269
        and reversible dementia,
            195
    serum level, in evaluation of
        dementia, 216
Vitamin B group, 247, 387. *See
    also* Folate deficiency;
    Folic acid; Thiamine
    (vitamin B$_1$); *individual
    B vitamins*
Vitamin C, 14, 383, 387
    cognitive function and, 165
Vitamin D$_3$, 383, 385, 387
    alcohol abuse and, 344
Vitamin E, 14, 387
Vitamin K, 383
Vitamins. *See also individual
    vitamins*
    alcohol abuse and, 345
    deficiencies
        cognitive function and,
            165
        psychotic symptoms
            and, 269
    multiple, 376
        1,25-dihydroxy-vitamin
            D$_3$, 31, 40
Vitamin supplementation, 34, 40,
    349, 375, 383, 387
Voluntary organizations,
    psychiatric disorders and,
    136
Vomiting, interference with
    dexamethasone
    suppression test accuracy,
    196
Voronoff, Serge, 4

WAIS-R. *See* Wechsler Adult
    Intelligence Scale—
    Revised

Wandering, in dementia of the
    Alzheimer's type, 218
Warfarin, 372
    interaction with fluoxetine,
        178
Watch-spring theory of aging, 13
Water, intake of,
    recommendations in
    elderly persons, 386
Weakness
    acidosis and, 195
    hypoglycemia and, 195
    hypothyroidism and, 32
    overhydration and, 195
Wechsler Adult Intelligence Scale
    (WAIS), 111
Wechsler Adult Intelligence
    Scale—Revised (WAIS-R),
    110, 111, 202–203
Wechsler Memory
    Scale—Revised (WMS-R),
    203
Weight loss
    in depressed older adult,
        251
    rapid, interference with
        dexamethasone
        suppression test accuracy,
        196
Werner's syndrome
    association with aging
        process, 16
    characteristic features of, 21,
        97
    genetic transmission of, 97
Wernicke-Korsakoff syndrome/
    disease, 228, 345
Widowhood groups, 404, 405
Wisdom, and aging, 18
Withdrawal
    from abused drugs, 354
    from alcohol, 346–347, 349
    social, in nursing home
        populations, 415
Withdrawn depression, 184
WMS-R. *See* Wechsler Memory
    Scale—Revised
World Health Organization
    International
    Classification of Diseases.
    See International
    Classification of Diseases
Worry, 279
Writing groups, 404, 405

X rays, plain, 197

Youth, fountain of, 5
Youth, prolongation of, 3–8

Zerbi, Gabriele, 9
Zeus, 3, 5
Zinc supplementation,
    386–387

Zolpidem, 374–375
    sleep disturbances and, 336
Zung Self-Rating Depression
    Scale, 183, 235